Autism and Child Psychopathology Series

Series Editor:

Johnny L. Matson
Department of Psychology
Louisiana State University
Baton Rouge, LA, USA

More information about this series at http://www.springer.com/series/8665

Robert D. Friedberg
Jennifer K. Paternostro
Editors

Handbook of Cognitive Behavioral Therapy for Pediatric Medical Conditions

Springer

Editors
Robert D. Friedberg
Child Emphasis Area
Palo Alto University
Palo Alto, CA, USA

Jennifer K. Paternostro
Division of Developmental and
Behavioral Pediatrics, Stead Family
Department of Pediatrics
University of Iowa Stead Family
Children's Hospital
Iowa City, IA, USA

ISSN 2192-922X ISSN 2192-9238 (electronic)
Autism and Child Psychopathology Series
ISBN 978-3-030-21685-6   ISBN 978-3-030-21683-2 (eBook)
https://doi.org/10.1007/978-3-030-21683-2

© Springer Nature Switzerland AG 2019
This work is subject to copyright. All rights are reserved by the Publisher, whether the whole or part of the material is concerned, specifically the rights of translation, reprinting, reuse of illustrations, recitation, broadcasting, reproduction on microfilms or in any other physical way, and transmission or information storage and retrieval, electronic adaptation, computer software, or by similar or dissimilar methodology now known or hereafter developed.
The use of general descriptive names, registered names, trademarks, service marks, etc. in this publication does not imply, even in the absence of a specific statement, that such names are exempt from the relevant protective laws and regulations and therefore free for general use.
The publisher, the authors, and the editors are safe to assume that the advice and information in this book are believed to be true and accurate at the date of publication. Neither the publisher nor the authors or the editors give a warranty, express or implied, with respect to the material contained herein or for any errors or omissions that may have been made. The publisher remains neutral with regard to jurisdictional claims in published maps and institutional affiliations.

This Springer imprint is published by the registered company Springer Nature Switzerland AG
The registered company address is: Gewerbestrasse 11, 6330 Cham, Switzerland

To my mother, Rachelle Friedberg; my grandparents, Rose and Frank Derewitz; my love of my life, Barbara Friedberg; and my daughter, Rebecca, who always makes me proud, look I made a hat where there never was a hat!!

RDF

I would like to dedicate this project to my parents, Karen and Tony Paternostro; to my brother, Kevin Paternostro; and to my incredible partner, Alex Wiese. I cannot thank them enough for their unconditional love and support.

JKP

Acknowledgments

First and foremost, I thank my loving partner, Barbara A. Friedberg, for the ongoing daily sacrifices she makes so I can thrive as a person and professional. Second, I am grateful for my friend, colleague, and coauthor, Dr. Jennifer Paternostro, who epitomizes excellence in pediatric psychology and *seizes the day* routinely! Next, I want to express my gratitude to the many outstanding contributors to this handbook—your work humbles me! Additionally, I could not have accomplished much in my career without the help of my mentors and longtime friends Drs. Julian Meltzoff, Constance Dalenberg, Christine Padesky, Aaron Beck, Judith Beck, Raymond Fidaleo, James Shenk, Jessica McClure, Kathleen Mooney, James Dobbins, Brenda Mobley, Victor McCarley, Janeece Warfield, Stuart Kaplan, Fauzia Mahr, Amanda Pearl, and Allen Miller. Of course, I want to recognize the many patients who entrusted their care to me over the years.

As an early career psychologist, there are countless numbers of individuals who have cultivated dedication and passion for the field of pediatric psychology. First, words cannot express how grateful I am to have had the opportunity to train under Dr. Robert Friedberg. You have been a life-changing mentor and, now, colleague. I cannot thank you enough for all that you have done for me. Next, I want to acknowledge Dr. Friedberg's exceptional contributions that made this handbook possible. I am truly inspired by your work. Furthermore, to the village that stood beside me as I navigated graduate school and beyond—Andrea Alioto, Micaela Birt, Lauren Fussner, Xiaolong Li, Christie Mead, Amie Haas, Michael Harris, Kayla Albrecht McMenamin, and Karen and Tony Paternostro—*Thank You*! Finally, a special shout out to my fiancé, Alex Wiese, for your unparalleled dedication to an equal and loving partnership.

Contents

1   **Introduction: Knowledge, Actionable Practices, and Urgency**.................................. 1
Jennifer K. Paternostro and Robert D. Friedberg

Part I   Broad Conceptual Issues

2   **The Value of Integrated Pediatric Behavioral Health Care** 11
Robert D. Friedberg and Jennifer K. Paternostro

3   **Diversity Issues in Pediatric Behavioral Health Care** 21
Jessica M. Valenzuela, Kristina Tatum, and Joyce H. L. Lui

4   **Ethical Issues Applying CBT in Pediatric Medical Settings**.... 41
Gerald P. Koocher and Jeanne S. Hoffman

5   **Emotional Regulation and Pediatric Behavior Health Problems** 49
Carisa Parrish, Hannah Fajer, and Alison Papadakis

6   **Motivational Interviewing** 69
Kathryn Jeter, Stephen Gillaspy, and Thad R. Leffingwell

7   **Cognitive Behavioral Therapy with Youth: Essential Foundations and Elementary Practices** 87
Robert D. Friedberg and Jennifer K. Paternostro

8   **Necessary Adaptations to CBT with Pediatric Patients** 103
Corinne Catarozoli, Lara Brodzinsky, Christina G. Salley, Samantha P. Miller, Becky H. Lois, and Johanna L. Carpenter

9   **DBT for Multi-Problem Adolescents**...................... 119
Alec L. Miller and Casey T. O'Brien

10   **DBT Adaptations with Pediatric Patients**................... 137
Becky H. Lois, Vincent P. Corcoran, and Alec L. Miller

11   **Pharmacological Interventions** 151
Rahil R. Jummani and Jess P. Shatkin

Part II Working with Specific Populations

12 Cognitive Behavioral Therapy in Primary Care 173
Carisa Parrish and Kathryn Van Eck

13 Cognitive Behavioral Therapy in Pediatric Patients with Chronic Widespread Musculoskeletal Pain 185
Lauren M. Fussner and Anne M. Lynch-Jordan

14 Cognitive Behavioral Therapy for Functional Abdominal Pain Disorders 201
Kari Baber and Kelly A. O' Neil Rodriguez

15 Cognitive Behavioral Therapy for Enuresis 219
Edward R. Christophersen and Christina M. Low Kapalu

16 Cognitive Behavioral Therapy for Encopresis 239
Christina M. Low Kapalu and Edward R. Christophersen

17 Cognitive-Behavioral Therapy for Chronic Headache Disorders in Children and Adolescents 261
Karen Kaczynski

18 Cognitive Behavioral Treatment for Pediatric Sleep Difficulties 279
Karla K. Fehr, Danielle Chambers, and Jennifer Ramasami

19 Cognitive Behavioral Therapy for Pediatric Epilepsy and Psychogenic Non-epileptic Seizures 295
Karla K. Fehr, Julia Doss, Abby Hughes-Scalise, and Meghan M. D. Littles

20 Cognitive Behavioral Therapy in Pediatric Oncology: Flexible Application of Core Principles 315
Christina G. Salley and Corinne Catarozoli

21 Cognitive Behavioral Therapy for Children and Adolescents with Diabetes 329
Johanna L. Carpenter and Christina Cammarata

22 Cognitive Behavioral Therapy for Youth with Asthma: Anxiety as an Example 345
Ashley H. Clawson, Nicole Ruppe, Cara Nwankwo, Alexandra Blair, Marissa Baudino, and Nighat Mehdi

23 Cognitive-Behavioral Therapy for Pediatric Obesity 369
Carolina M. Bejarano, Arwen M. Marker, and Christopher C. Cushing

24 Working with Transgender and Gender Expansive Youth 385
Andrea Carolina Tabuenca and Krista Hayward Basile

25 Noncompliance and Nonadherence 407
Kathleen L. Lemanek and Heather Yardley

Part III Special Topics

26 Training Issues in Pediatric Psychology 419
Ryan R. Landoll, Corinn A. Elmore, Andrea F. Weiss,
and Julia A. Garza

27 Financial Issues 433
Allen R. Miller

**28 Conclusion: What Have We Learned
and Where Do We Go from Here?** 445
Jennifer K. Paternostro and Robert D. Friedberg

Index 453

Contributors

Kari Baber, Ph.D. Department of Child and Adolescent Psychiatry and Behavioral Sciences, The Children's Hospital of Philadelphia, Philadelphia, PA, USA

Department of Pediatrics/Division of Gastroenterology, Hepatology and Nutrition, The Children's Hospital of Philadelphia, Philadelphia, PA, USA

Krista Hayward Basile, M.H.S. Palo Alto University, Palo Alto, CA, USA

Marissa Baudino, M.S. Department of Psychology, Oklahoma State University, Center for Pediatric Psychology, Stillwater, OK, USA

Carolina M. Bejarano, M.A. Clinical Child Psychology Program and Life Span Institute, University of Kansas, Lawrence, KS, USA

Alexandra Blair Department of Psychology, Oklahoma State University, Center for Pediatric Psychology, Stillwater, OK, USA

Lara Brodzinsky, Psy.D. Department of Child and Adolescent Psychiatry, Child Study Center, Hassenfeld Children's Hospital at NYU Langone, New York, NY, USA

Christina Cammarata, Ph.D., A.B.P.P. Division of Behavioral Health, Department of Pediatrics, Nemours/Alfred I. duPont Hospital for Children and Sidney Kimmel Medical College, Thomas Jefferson University, Wilmington, DE, USA

Johanna L. Carpenter, Ph.D. Division of Behavioral Health, Department of Pediatrics, Nemours/Alfred I. duPont Hospital for Children and Sidney Kimmel Medical College, Thomas Jefferson University, Wilmington, DE, USA

Corinne Catarozoli, Ph.D. Weill Cornell Medicine, New York, NY, USA

Danielle Chambers, M.A. Department of Psychology, Southern Illinois University, Carbondale, IL, USA

Edward R. Christophersen, Ph.D., A.B.P.P., F.A.A.P. (Hon.) Children's Mercy Hospital—Kansas, Overland Park, KS, USA

Children's Mercy Hospital—Kansas City, Kansas City, MO, USA

Ashley H. Clawson, Ph.D. Department of Psychology, Oklahoma State University, Center for Pediatric Psychology, Stillwater, OK, USA

Vincent P. Corcoran, M.A. Clinical Psychology Doctoral Program, Graduate School for Arts and Sciences, Fordham University, Bronx, NY, USA

Christopher C. Cushing, Ph.D. Clinical Child Psychology Program and Life Span Institute, University of Kansas, Lawrence, KS, USA

Julia Doss, Psy.D. Minnesota Epilepsy Group and Children's Hospitals and Clinics, St. Paul, MN, USA

Corinn A. Elmore, Ph.D. Pediatric and Adolescent Primary Care Medical Homes, Walter Reed National Military Medical Center, Bethesda, MD, USA

Hannah B. Fajer Department of Psychological and Brain Sciences, Johns Hopkins University, Baltimore, MD, USA

Karla K. Fehr, Ph.D. Department of Psychology, Southern Illinois University, Carbondale, IL, USA

Robert D. Friedberg, Ph.D., A.B.P.P. Child Emphasis Area, Palo Alto University, Palo Alto, CA, USA

Lauren M. Fussner, Ph.D. Yale Medicine Child Study Center, New Haven, CT, USA

Julia A. Garza, B.A. Uniformed Services University of the Health Sciences, Bethesda, MD, USA

Stephen Gillaspy, Ph.D. Section of General and Community Pediatrics, University of Oklahoma Health Sciences Center, Oklahoma City, OK, USA

Jeanne S. Hoffman, Ph.D., A.B.P.P. Tripler Army Medical Center, Honolulu, HI, USA

Abby Hughes-Scalise, Ph.D. United Family Medicine Residency, St. Paul, Eagan, MN, USA

Kathryn Jeter, Ph.D. Section of General and Community Pediatrics, University of Oklahoma Health Sciences Center, Oklahoma City, OK, USA

Rahil R. Jummani, M.D. Department of Child and Adolescent Psychiatry, Hassenfeld Children's Hospital at NYU Langone, Child Study Center, New York, NY, USA

Karen Kaczynski, Ph.D. Pediatric Headache Program, Division of Pain Medicine, Department of Anesthesia, Perioperative, and Pain Medicine, Boston Children's Hospital and Harvard Medical School, Waltham, MA, USA

Gerald P. Koocher, Ph.D., A.B.P.P. Quincy College, Quincy, MA, USA

Ryan R. Landoll, Ph.D., A.B.P.P., Maj., U.S.A.F. Uniformed Services University of the Health Sciences, Bethesda, MD, USA

Thad R. Leffingwell, Ph.D. Department of Psychology, Oklahoma State University, Stillwater, OK, USA

Kathleen L. Lemanek, Ph.D. The Ohio State University, Nationwide Children's Hospital, Columbus, OH, USA

Meghan M. D. Littles, B.S. Department of Psychology, Southern Illinois University, Carbondale, IL, USA

Becky H. Lois, Ph.D. Department of Child and Adolescent Psychiatry, Child Study Center, Hassenfeld Children's Hospital at NYU Langone, New York, NY, USA

Christina M. Low Kapalu, Ph.D. Children's Mercy Hospital—Kansas City, Kansas City, MO, USA

University of Missouri Kansas City School of Medicine, Kansas City, MO, USA

Joyce H. L. Lui, Ph.D. University of California at Los Angeles, Los Angeles, CA, USA

Anne M. Lynch-Jordan, Ph.D. University of Cincinnati College of Medicine, Cincinnati Children's Hospital Medical Center, Cincinnati, OH, USA

Arwen M. Marker, M.A. Clinical Child Psychology Program and Life Span Institute, University of Kansas, Lawrence, KS, USA

Nighat Mehdi, M.D. Department of Pediatrics, Pulmonary and Cystic Fibrosis Center, OU Children's Physician, Oklahoma City, OK, USA

Alec L. Miller, Psy.D. Cognitive and Behavioral Consultants, LLP (Westchester and Manhattan), White Plains, NY, USA

Allen R. Miller, Ph.D., M.B.A. Beck Institute for Cognitive Behavior Therapy, Bala Cynwyd, PA, USA

Samantha P. Miller, Ph.D. Dell Children's Medical Center Chronic Disease Program, Dell Medical Group, University of Texas at Austin, Austin, TX, USA

Cara Nwankwo, B.A. Department of Psychology, Oklahoma State University, Center for Pediatric Psychology, Stillwater, OK, USA

Casey T. O'Brien, Psy.D. Cognitive and Behavioral Consultants, LLP (Westchester and Manhattan), White Plains, NY, USA

Alison A. Papadakis, Ph.D. Department of Psychological and Brain Sciences, Johns Hopkins University, Baltimore, MD, USA

Carisa Parrish, Ph.D. Division of Child and Adolescent Psychiatry, Department of Psychiatry and Behavioral Sciences, Johns Hopkins University School of Medicine, Baltimore, MD, USA

Jennifer K. Paternostro, Ph.D. Division of Developmental and Behavioral Pediatrics, Stead Family Department of Pediatrics, University of Iowa Stead Family Children's Hospital, Iowa City, IA, USA

Jennifer Ramasami, M.A. Department of Psychology, Southern Illinois University, Carbondale, IL, USA

Kelly A. O' Neil Rodriguez, Ph.D. Department of Child and Adolescent Psychiatry and Behavioral Sciences, The Children's Hospital of Philadelphia, Philadelphia, PA, USA

Department of Pediatrics/Division of Gastroenterology, Hepatology and Nutrition, The Children's Hospital of Philadelphia, Philadelphia, PA, USA

Nicole Ruppe, B.S. Department of Psychology, Oklahoma State University, Center for Pediatric Psychology, Stillwater, OK, USA

Christina G. Salley, Ph.D. Department of Child and Adolescent Psychiatry, NYU School of Medicine and Hassenfeld Children's Hospital at NYU Langone, New York, NY, USA

Jess P. Shatkin, M.D., M.P.H. Department of Child and Adolescent Psychiatry, Child and Adolescent Mental Health Studies (CAMS), NYU College of Arts and Science and Hassenfeld Children's Hospital at NYU Langone, Child Study Center, New York, NY, USA

Andrea Carolina Tabuenca, Ph.D. Stanford University, Stanford, CA, USA

Kristina Tatum, M.S. College of Psychology, Nova Southeastern University, Fort Lauderdale, FL, USA

Jessica M. Valenzuela, Ph.D. College of Psychology, Nova Southeastern University, Fort Lauderdale, FL, USA

Kathryn Van Eck, Ph.D. Division of Child and Adolescent Psychiatry, Department of Psychiatry and Behavioral Sciences, Johns Hopkins University School of Medicine, Baltimore, MD, USA

Andrea F. Weiss, Malcolm Grow Medical Clinics and Surgery Center, Joint Base Andrews, MD, USA

Heather Yardley, Ph.D. Department of Pediatric Psychology and Neuropsychology, The Ohio State University and Nationwide Children's Hospital, Columbus, OH, USA

About the Editors

Robert D. Friedberg, Ph.D., A.B.P.P. obtained his doctorate in clinical psychology from the California School of Professional Psychology, San Diego, and completed his postdoctoral fellowship at the Center for Cognitive Therapy, Newport Beach. Currently, he is a Tenured Full Professor, Head of the Child and Family Emphasis Area, and Director of the Center for the Study and Treatment of Anxious Youth at Palo Alto University. He is a Board Certified Diplomate in Cognitive Behavioral Therapy, a Former Extramural Scholar at the Beck Institute for Cognitive Behavioral Therapy, a Founding Fellow of the Academy of Cognitive Therapy, a Fellow of APA Division 53 (Society of Clinical Child and Adolescent Psychology), and a Fellow of the Association for Behavioral and Cognitive Therapy. He is the Author of eight books, including Clinical Practice of Cognitive Therapy with Children and Adolescents (2015, Guilford Press, with Jessica M. McClure) as well as many journal articles, book chapters, and national and international presentations.

Jennifer K. Paternostro, Ph.D. was awarded her doctorate in clinical psychology from Palo Alto University in July 2017. She completed her postdoctoral fellowship in Pediatric Psychology at Oregon Health & Science University in Portland, OR. She specializes in integrated behavioral health for children with chronic health conditions. Currently, she is a Clinical Assistant Professor in the Division of Developmental and Behavioral Pediatrics at the University of Iowa Stead Family Department of Pediatrics, where she is developing integrated health psychology programs in pediatric pulmonology and endocrinology.

Introduction: Knowledge, Actionable Practices, and Urgency

Jennifer K. Paternostro and Robert D. Friedberg

I have been impressed with the urgency of doing. Knowing is not enough, we must apply. Being willing is not enough, we must do.
Leonardo Da Vinci

Delivering Cognitive Behavioral Therapy to young patients challenged by various medical conditions represents an evolving frontier in behavioral health care. In order to traverse this fertile ground, practitioners require state-of-the-science findings and effective clinical practices. The chapters in this handbook provide precisely this type of material. This book reflects the work of 55 contributors from 25 different institutions. The diverse topics are addressed in ways that ideally facilitate the easy transfer from page to practice. In this introductory chapter, we summarize each individual chapter underscoring the salient issues.

Part I of the handbook focuses on broad conceptual issues. The book kicks off by highlighting the value of integrated behavioral health care in pediatric medical settings. Friedberg and Paternostro first describe the current state of affairs as it relates to integrated care practices, as well as efforts to pursue the Triple Aim of Health Care—enhanced patient care experience, decreased per capita health expenditures, and improved population health outcomes. Various integrated care models are presented including collaborative and coordinated care options, co-located services, and fully integrated systems. The chapter then delves into common psychological problems and issues that often present in pediatric primary and specialty care clinics. Friedberg and Paternostro argue that pediatric psychologists and behavioral health providers are uniquely skilled in addressing general parenting concerns (e.g., toilet training, discipline, feeding), and developmental, emotional, and behavioral issues that arise in pediatric medical offices. The chapter concludes with a discussion on the value of integrated service delivery models to the patient population served, health care providers, and stakeholders.

By the year 2020, racial/ethnic minority children in the United States will make up the majority of the population. Although this indicates an exciting time of growth in our country, health disparities (e.g., overall health outcomes, oral health, mental

J. K. Paternostro (✉)
Division of Developmental and Behavioral Pediatrics, Stead Family Department of Pediatrics, University of Iowa Stead Family Children's Hospital,
Iowa City, IA, USA
e-mail: jennifer-paternostro@uiowa.edu

R. D. Friedberg
Child Emphasis Area, Palo Alto University,
Palo Alto, CA, USA
e-mail: rfriedberg@paloaltou.edu

health, increased risk of chronic illness) are far too prevalent among minority youth. Moreover, health disparities are not exclusive to racial and ethnic minorities. Sexual minority youth also experience poorer health outcomes and have higher rates of mental health issues. Valenzuela, Tatum, and Lui provide an insightful overview of evidence-based treatments for diverse pediatric patients and their families. In addition, the authors examine challenges of providing culturally competent care, while emphasizing the importance of adapting to the individual's cultural experience. Specific recommendations for cultural adaptations of evidence-based treatments are provided. Next, the authors identify distinct considerations in working with African-American populations, immigrant youth and their families, and sexual minorities. Historical and systemic barriers to quality care conclude the chapter.

Providing competent, quality, and evidence-based care in pediatric medical settings is associated with unique ethical considerations and challenges. Koocher and Hoffman offer specific knowledge and skills required to deliver ethical care including optimizing treatment manuals while maintaining fidelity, and collaborating with physician colleagues. Moreover, the authors contend that developing a basic understanding of common medical conditions and associated treatment regimens is a basic ethical obligation. Further, attention is explicitly directed to informed consent and assent processes. Since integrated care often requires ongoing collaboration between medical providers and behavioral health clinicians, nuances of confidentiality are reviewed. Potential ethical dilemmas and infractions in pediatric medical settings are explored. Specific examples are provided to further illustrate these concerns.

Parrish, Fajer, and Papadakis' chapter explains the critical role emotion regulation plays in pediatric psychology. When youth are diagnosed with a medical condition, whether acute or chronic, undoubtedly, resources for regulating distress are triggered. The chapter begins with two compelling case vignettes that demonstrate the emotional impact children and families often face when presented with a medical condition or unexpected medical events. Moreover, adjustment to diagnosis and subsequent adherence to complex medical regimens may provoke significant familial stress and conflict. Emotion regulation is a critical component of psychosocial functioning and adjustment and thus requires tailored intervention. The authors illustrate the relevance of emotional regulation to understanding and treating pediatric patients and their families. Next, Parrish and colleagues provide a comprehensive review of emotion regulation focused interventions and resources for clinicians that aid in the treatment of youth with medical conditions.

Motivational Interviewing (MI) is a patient-centered approach to addressing behavioral change. MI is well equipped to assist patients in successfully managing chronic medical conditions and adherence to complex treatment regimens. Jeter, Gillaspy, and Leffingwell detail essential components of MI as well as necessary modifications for working with pediatric patients diagnosed with medical conditions. Furthermore, the authors review empirical evidence of MI for various referral questions such as adherence and pediatric health behaviors (e.g., asthma, obesity, diabetes). The chapter concludes with an overview of training requirements and resources for MI interventions.

In Chap. 7, Friedberg and Paternostro introduce the foundational elements of traditional Cognitive Behavioral Therapy with youth. The chapter begins with a brief overview of the theoretical underpinnings of learning theory, which prioritizes classical conditioning, operant conditioning, and social learning theory in understanding human behavior. An updated review of the literature is provided with specific attention to the empirical status of CBT for disruptive behavior disorders, depressive disorders, and anxiety spectrum disorders. Next, the authors describe core components of modular CBT, which are well suited to adapt to pediatric settings. The chapter ends with a pertinent case example of a 9-year-old patient with anxiety and functional gastrointestinal and neurological distress, who begins a course of modular CBT.

Treatment for patients diagnosed with pediatric medical conditions commonly requires modifications to traditional practice. Accordingly, Catarozoli and colleagues present necessary adaptations to the CBT framework to fit pediatric populations. Pediatric medical settings are replete with comorbid mental health challenges. Budding research supports the use of CBT for pediatric medical conditions, with noted improvement in both mental and physical health outcomes. The nuances of providing CBT for pediatric populations in medical settings are explored. Inclusion of alternative CBT spectrum approaches such as Dialectical Behavior Therapy, Acceptance and Commitment Therapy, and Parent–Child Interaction Therapy to meet the unique needs of this population is emphasized. Additionally, consistent with the patient-centered care model, the authors suggest ongoing collaboration and consultation with other medical providers may be indicated. Next, the chapter provides a comprehensive directory of ways to adjust cognitive and behavioral interventions for pediatric patients presenting with medical complexity.

Dialectical Behavior Therapy (DBT) revolutionized the field of clinical psychology. Originally developed by Marsha Linehan in 1993, DBT has become the first-line treatment for suicidal behavior and Borderline Personality Disorder. Miller and O'Brien provide an overview of the theories, modes, functions, and interventions of DBT as well as its application to adolescents with high-risk behaviors. Next, clinical practices in medical and school-based settings are presented. Empirical evidence of DBT-A for treating multi-problem youth is well supported in the literature for a variety of presenting concerns. The chapter concludes with a clinical vignette of a 17-year-old who presents for a comprehensive DBT-A program with a past mental health history of Major Depressive Disorder, Generalized Anxiety Disorder, Social Anxiety Disorder, and Alcohol Use Disorder.

Building off of the previous chapter, Lois, Corcoran, and Miller explain how to adapt DBT techniques for youth with chronic medical illness (CMI). Living with a CMI can be a difficult and daunting task that requires substantial self-management skills including adhering to complex treatment regimens, attending follow up and routine medical appointments, and following dietary restrictions. This chapter highlights the specific challenges associated with living with a CMI and the impact chronic illness has on one's mental health. Using a DBT framework, the authors explore various systems-level issues that compound an already complicated situation for patients and their families. Although DBT-CMI research is in its infancy, the authors provide a brief look into the current empirical literature. Throughout the chapter, Lois and colleagues seamlessly interweave "how to" examples into their description of the DBT-CMI protocol and case examples.

The diagnosis and management of an acute or chronic medical condition can be extremely taxing on pediatric patients and their families. Chronic medical conditions are commonly associated with extensive medical intervention, prolonged hospitalizations, changes in daily routines, and complex self-management tasks. Therefore, it is understandable that patients are at higher risks for notable anxiety, post-traumatic stress disorder, depression, and/or disruptive behavior. Jummani and Shatkin provide a comprehensive overview of pharmacological interventions for youth with medical conditions who may be experiencing moderate to severe psychopathology. Along with a basic explanation of specific medications used in pediatric populations, the chapter reviews the empirical evidence supporting the use of psychopharmacological intervention across mental health diagnoses. Moreover, the chapter serves as an excellent resource for clinicians looking for a quick reference on pharmacological interventions in integrated care settings.

Part II addresses clinical work with specific populations. Parrish and Van Eyck begin with a review of CBT interventions in pediatric primary care. Pediatric primary care settings are frequently visited by children and their families. Children are generally seen by their pediatrician at least once per year and often report a trusting and collaborative relationship. Thus, the primary care office is a convenient place to receive behavioral health support and connect with a mental health provider. Parrish and Van Eck argue that integrated primary care settings provide a multitude of benefits for both the patient and medical providers, who are often treating mental health problems alone and without necessary adjunctive support. The authors then examine the literature on distinct models of integrated care practices and highlight the all too common discrepancy between research and clinical application. The chapter concludes with two case vignettes that demonstrate CBT implementation in a pediatric primary care setting.

The remainder of this section focuses on behavioral health management of acute and chronic medical conditions. Fussner and Lynch-Jordan introduce CBT strategies for patients with widespread musculoskeletal pain. Chronic pain is often associated with substantial declines in daily functioning and can become debilitating if left untreated. Furthermore, chronic pain increases risk for mental health conditions. The chapter nicely illustrates the biopsychosocial model of widespread musculoskeletal by synthesizing the extant literature and clinical case examples. The importance of taking a multidisciplinary team-based approach to treatment is delineated. Next, the authors provide a framework for working with pediatric patients with chronic pain, using CBT components to increase functioning. A sample treatment course is broken down session by session. Additionally, resources for ongoing assessment are recommended. Given the significant impact chronic pain has on the entire family, the authors suggest specific intervention guidelines for caregivers.

Functional gastrointestinal disorders (FGID) and functional abdominal pain include an activation of symptoms within the gastrointestinal tract. FGIDs are very common in pediatric patients. The physical symptoms can be embarrassing to young patients and impact their quality of life. Furthermore, functional disorders are associated with higher rates of anxiety and depressive symptoms. Physical symptoms of FGIDs are akin to the physical manifestations of anxiety and depression. Thus, Baber and Rodriquez present CBT interventions for FGIDs with specific emphasis on functional abdominal pain. Using a clinical case example, the authors highlight the biopsychosocial model as it relates to functional abdominal pain. Evidence for the "brain–gut axis" and the interaction between physiological and psychological factors is outlined and discussed. Psychoeducation on the brain–gut axis is a foundational element in the treatment of functional disorders. To address worry associated with gastrointestinal symptoms, graded engagement and exposures are key features of treatment with this population. Throughout the chapter, the authors equip readers with tangible scripts and intervention strategies pertinent to addressing functional GI distress.

The next two chapters focus of behavioral interventions for enuresis and encopresis in pediatric patients. First, Christophersen and Kapalu present the assessment and treatment of enuresis. Enuresis is defined as repeated voiding of urine (either voluntary or intentional) in a place other than the toilet. For a diagnosis of enuresis to be warranted, urinary accidents must occur twice per week for at least 3 months or cause clinically significant distress or impairment. The authors provide an overview of the prevalence of enuresis, cultural considerations, and the course and prognosis of the disorder. The chapter is divided into nocturnal enuresis (nighttime wetting) and diurnal enuresis (daytime wetting) sections. For both conditions, a thorough medical and psychosocial assessment of the maintaining factors impacting the youth's enuresis is discussed, and behavioral interventions for treating this population is explored. The bell-and-pad or urine-alarm training is the first-line treatment intervention for nocturnal enuresis. The urine alarm utilizes both classical and operant conditioning paradigms, which lay the foundation of behavioral interventions. Additional behavioral interventions for enuresis include dry-bed training, cleanliness training, positive practice, nighttime awakening, retention-control training, positive reinforcement, and over-learning. Each of these interventions is illustrated using clinical case examples to highlight the individual treatment components.

Encopresis is the second of the two main elimination disorders that commonly occur in childhood. Also known as fecal incontinence, encopresis is defined as repeatedly passing stool in inappropriate locations such as onto the floor or in underwear/pull-ups. Similar to enuresis, encopresis is considered a biobehavioral or biopsychobehavioral disorder that is treated and managed with both medical and psychosocial intervention. Kapalu and Christophersen begin the chapter by documenting the prevalence and etiology of encopresis. The role of constipation in the development and maintenance of encopresis is provided. In order to develop pertinent treatment targets, a thorough psychosocial assessment is suggested. Kapalu and Christophersen explain common behavioral interventions including adherence to bowel regimen, reinforcement schedules for appropriate toileting behaviors, toilet training routines, access to preferred activities while completing scheduled toilet sits, and effective parental responses. The chapter concludes with a case example to highlight key components of assessment and treatment of encopresis.

Kaczynski describes the debilitating impact headache disorders have on individuals' daily functioning. With approximately 60% of youth experiencing headaches of varying degrees of intensity and duration, headaches are considered a widespread condition. This chapter dives into the different types of headaches that regularly affect pediatric patients as well as the impact headaches have on a children's functioning and quality of life. Mood disruption, sleep problems, school difficulties, participation in extracurricular activities, family dynamics, and peer relationships can all be affected by chronic headache. Kaczynski then presents the biopsychosocial framework for treating pediatric chronic headache. The emphasis on multidisciplinary treatment is described along with alternative approaches to care. Furthermore, the utility of psychological intervention including relaxation training, CBT, and biofeedback is explored using clinical case examples that highlight treatment targets and techniques.

Pediatric sleep disturbances impact approximately 20–40% of children. Without proper sleep hygiene and adequate sleep per night, children's as well as their families' daily functioning is ruptured. Fehr, Chambers, and Ramasami begin the chapter with a review of the literature on healthy and disrupted sleep. The authors then present the biopsychosocial conceptualization of sleep disturbance using a clinical case example of a 4-year-old with bedtime resistance and sleep avoidance. Additional sleep disorders are reviewed, including delayed sleep-wake phase disorder, parasomnias, obstructive sleep apnea, and narcolepsy. Next, the authors describe the treatment components recommended for sleep difficulties. More specifically, parental education, sleep hygiene training to increase sleep promoting behaviors, establishing regular bedtime routines, contingency procedures such as reinforcement and extinction, bedtime fading, chronotherapy, scheduled awakenings, and traditional CBT are illustrated. The chapter ends with a case example that embodies individual treatment components to sleep disruption.

Chapter 19 is focused on pediatric epilepsy and is separated into two sections: epilepsy and psychogenic non-epileptic seizures. Consequently, the chapter illustrates the nuances of CBT for each condition. Seizure disorders increase risk for developing mood and behavioral problems in youth and can become a major source of ongoing stress. Therefore, addressing these components is critical for continuous adjustment and improving quality of life. For each section, Fehr, Doss, Hughes-Scalise, and Littles describe treatment components including adjustment to diagnosis, adherence to complex treatment regimens, and psychosocial comorbidities. The goal of treatment for patients with epilepsy is an emphasis on maximizing quality of life and psychosocial functioning. Psychogenic non-epileptic seizures (PNES) is a conversion disorder, as described by the DSM-5. Accordingly, PNES is believed to develop as a response to psychological stress, and biopsychosocial model suggests that unresolved distress produces adverse physiological and emotional responses. A case example is used to illustrate the course of CBT treatment with this population.

It is no surprise that children diagnosed with cancer are at greater risk for developing emotional, behavioral, and social problems than their healthy peers. Invasive treatments, painful surgeries, repeated hospitalizations, and office visits often lead to significant emotional burden and distress. Salley and Catarozoli's chapter focuses on the biopsychosocial assessment and treatment of childhood cancer. Considering important factors unique to those who are battling cancer, the authors describe flexible adaptations of CBT interventions. Notably, there are distinct modifications for cognitive restructuring. Salley and Catarozoli also provide helpful guidelines for parental involvement, behavior management, emotional regulation, and coping with somatic complaints. A case example of a 12-year-old boy with acute lymphocytic leukemia concludes the chapter.

The impact of psychosocial factors on disease management in pediatric patients with diabetes is well established. In this next chapter, Carpenter and Cammarata augment the biopsychosocial model of diabetes management with special considerations unique to patients with diabetes. Their contribution begins with a brief introduction of insulin-dependent diabetes mellitus as well as biological and psychosocial variables that impact adherence to diabetes self-management. Further, the authors discuss the importance of assessing for executive functioning deficits/delays and diabetes distress. To help illustrate the concept of diabetes distress, a case example of a 14-year-old boy with type 1 diabetes is provided. Evidence-based treatment approaches commonly utilized in the psychosocial treatment of diabetes including behavioral family systems therapy for diabetes (BFST-D), behavioral rewards systems, problem-solving skills training, and traditional components of CBT are explored. In addition, strategies to address diabetes distress, diabetes-related fear or resistance to injections, and fear of hypoglycemia are noted.

Asthma is the most common medical condition among youth. Asthma is characterized by recurrent and intermittent respiratory symptoms and airway obstruction that often include symptoms of wheezing, shortness of breath, coughing, chest tightness, and airway limitation. In Chap. 22, Clawson and colleagues explain the biopsychosocial conceptualization and treatment of anxiety in youth with asthma and describe learning processes that may contribute to increased anxiety in this population. CBT interventions that integrate asthma-related concepts and education are promising and may significantly benefit youth with comorbid asthma and anxiety. Case material augments these salient points.

Pediatric obesity has become an epidemic in the United States. Obesity plagues 18.5% of children and adolescents, and these numbers are growing. Children who are obese are at greater risk of developing cardiovascular disease, type 2 diabetes, chronic sleep problems, respiratory distress, poor academic achievement, and mental health issues. Empirically supported interventions for treating pediatric obesity have been found effective in maintaining weight loss up to 1 year post intervention as well as demonstrated improvement in health-related quality of life. Bejarno, Marker, and Cushing explain the biopsychosocial conceptualization of pediatric obesity. Next, initial assessment of obesity is described and includes screening of body mass index (BMI) along with more traditional mental health screening measures. The chapter then delves into specific treatment components to addressing pediatric obesity using rich clinical material.

Historically, transgender and gender expansive youth have been misunderstood and mistreated in both the medical/mental health field and society. In their chapter, Tabuenca and Basile present information aiming to increase clinicians' understanding and treatment of this vulnerable population. They discuss common misconceptions and the lack of social awareness affecting these young people. Further, the authors describe the changes in how clinicians treat transgender and gender expansive youth by providing gender-affirmative care. Empirically supported interventions include a family-based intervention to increase familial support of the patient and trans-affirmative CBT. A detailed case example is provided emphasize treatment components.

Part 2 of the book ends with a chapter that focuses on noncompliance and nonadherence with patients suffering from chronic medical conditions. Medical nonadherence is an ongoing challenge for providers working with pediatric patients and their families. The chapter begins with a clinical case example of an 18-year-old with type 1 diabetes and poor adherence to his medical regimen. Lemanek and Yardley provide the definition and prevalence of nonadherence among pediatric patients. The authors go on to discuss theoretical models of adherence such as the health belief model, theory of planned behavior, and transtheoretical model. Measures of adherence are provided as a resource for clinicians. Finally, cognitive behavioral intervention components for medical nonadherence conclude the chapter.

The third section of the book focuses on special topics related to delivering cognitive behavioral therapy to pediatric patients diagnosed with medical conditions. In Chap. 26, Landoll, Elmore, Weiss, and Garza explicate the crucial factors central to training issues in pediatric psychology. The authors illustrate the current competency guidelines for working in pediatric primary care and present a brief overview of well-established training programs that emphasize integrated primary care. According to Landoll and colleagues, the Children's Hospital of Philadelphia, Montefiore Medical Center/Albert Einstein School of Medicine, and MetroHealth are leading the way with innovative training initiatives for pediatric psychologists. A helpful review of continuing education and brief training opportunities that utilize modalities such as seminars, workshops, and conferences are also presented.

In Chap. 27, Miller astutely describes the many business and financial considerations associated with working in a pediatric medical setting. Financial issues are paramount in building sustainable clinical practice yet these pivotal concerns are often neglected. The current financial structure of reimbursement for behavioral health services is presented. Obtaining adequate and fair reimbursement is an essential task for the field. One option for demonstrating service necessity in integrated setting is employing outcome measures as well as patient and provider feedback that support value-added benefits. Outcome measures are critical for quantifying the quality of services and creating an argument for behavioral health integration. Miller also explains the financial models that shape the delivery of CBT and various barriers to integration.

Paternostro and Friedberg conclude the text with a brief commentary on common themes and future challenges. These 28 chapters collectively present knowledge guided by contemporary theories and empirical findings. Further, the book offers readers actionable practices that are portable to various settings and populations. If the information rests passively on pages, knowledge is inert. We urge readers to apply the content contained in this text to the vulnerable patients they serve. Carrying around a medical condition accompanied by psychological distress is a weighty burden. These patients deserve the urgent action that impressed Da Vinci. We are proud to introduce this text to readers.

Part I

Broad Conceptual Issues

The Value of Integrated Pediatric Behavioral Health Care

Robert D. Friedberg and Jennifer K. Paternostro

Introduction

The health-care system in the United States is in desperate need of a complete overhaul. Despite spending nearly three times as much on healthcare expenditures than comparable countries, the United States has one of the lowest life expectancies, highest maternal and infant mortality rates, and highest prevalence of preventable diseases (OECD 2017). The discrepancy between healthcare spending and population health outcomes demands critical attention to the development of alternative care models.

Integrated behavioral health care is a forward leaning initiative. Janicke et al. (2015) predicted that integrated services will become a practice exemplar in the coming decade. The confluence of several factors fuel the call for integrated behavioral health-care services (Foy 2015; Hunter et al. 2018; Reiter et al. 2018). The Patient Protection and Affordable Care Act (ACA; Public Law No.111–148111th Congress: Patient Protection and Affordable Care Act 2010) and the Triple Aim of Health Care are major determinants. The Triple Aim advocates for improved patient experience, cost-containment, and a population health focus (Berwick et al. 2008). Behavioral health concerns represent many of the top concerns for consulting a pediatrician (Kazak et al. 2017; Yogman et al. 2018; also see Chap. 12 of this volume). The majority of children with developmental, behavioral, and emotional needs are often first identified and treated in the primary care setting (Committee on Psychosocial Aspects of Child and Family Health and Task Force on Mental Health 2009). Further, pediatric primary care offices are desirable places to market psychosocial treatments (Becker et al. 2018).

Integrated pediatric behavioral health care (IPBHC) seeks to attenuate the isolated nature of stand-alone behavioral health-care clinics and/or mental health-care carve-out services (Freeman et al. 2018). A focus on accountability, accessibility, prevention, and fiscal responsibility drives integration efforts. Asarnow et al. (2015) argued that "effective behavioral health care is particularly critical for pediatric populations, with potentially large benefits over a life-time (p. 930)." Ladd et al. (2017) commented that external referrals for behavioral health problems are challenging due to the lack of trained professionals in most communities. Therefore, treating these patients within the pediatric medical setting is crucial.

R. D. Friedberg (✉)
Child Emphasis Area, Palo Alto University,
Palo Alto, CA, USA
e-mail: rfriedberg@paloaltou.edu

J. K. Paternostro
Division of Developmental and Behavioral Pediatrics,
Stead Family Department of Pediatrics,
University of Iowa Stead Family Children's Hospital,
Iowa City, IA, USA
e-mail: jennifer-paternostro@uiowa.edu

Behavioral health is being integrated in both primary care and pediatric subspecialties. Freeman et al. (2018) claimed "primary care is the front door to the health care system (p. 197)." More specifically, primary care offices are seen as the default mental health clinic (Bray 2010). Tynan and Woods (2013) mentioned that OB-GYN, family medicine, and other specialty clinics (e.g., oncology, endocrine, GI, etc.) are likely to welcome behavioral health specialists. There is a call for behavioral health specialists to be fully integrated throughout the physical health-care system from emergency rooms to primary care to specialty clinics (Bray 2010).

The biopsychosocial model of health and wellness is endemic to IPBHC (Giese and Waugh 2017). When describing the biopsychosocial model, Engel (1977) stated that psychological factors influence the initiation, maintenance, and exacerbation of physical disorders. Physiological, socio-cultural, psychological, and behavioral factors are all causally interactive in a holistic perspective or illness (Williams and Zahka 2017). Yogman et al. (2018) remarked "Integration of care also reframes the behavioral health/physical health dichotomy as a unified concept of whole person health and emphasizes coordination of care between providers so that patients' receive comprehensive and non-redundant services (p. 461)."

This chapter defines integrated care and speaks to its value. Common psychological complaints that present to primary care and specialty clinics are briefly reviewed. Finally, value-added benefits offered by IPBHC are delineated.

Definition of Integrated Care

Integrated pediatric behavioral health care is traditionally classified into three domains: coordinated, co-located, and fully integrated (Ader et al. 2015; Asarnow et al. 2017). Coordinated care is characterized by physicians and behavioral health-care providers working in separate facilities but communicating about shared patients through various platforms. In co-located practices, physicians and behavioral health clinicians practice in the same location and collaborate on patient care. Fully integrated services are marked by both behavioral health-care specialists being part of the same treatment team necessitating a variety of systemic changes. Ader et al. (2015) explained, "seamless integration demands a system redesign including the blending of separate practice cultures, introduction of new workflows, an integrated team-based approach to treatment, and consideration of available reimbursement options (p. 910)."

Integrated care models are characterized by several features (Blount 2003; Richardson et al. 2017). Giese and Waugh (2017) stated that integrated care paradigms emphasize patient-centered care, team-based delivery systems, population health, and stepped care models. A common treatment plan incorporating both behavioral health and medical interventions is typical. Sandoval et al. (2018) claimed integrated care creates routine clinical pathways for patients with behavioral health concerns. Multiple providers pool their individual interventions to patients, and outcomes are systematically measured. Further, they asserted that flexibility, tolerance for change, and professional commitment are common values. Finally, a focus on reducing mental health stigma and accountability through measurement-based care defines integrated systems. In sum, Yogman et al. (2018) maintained, "Integration of care also reframes the behavioral health/physical health dichotomy as a unified concept of whole-person health, and emphasizes coordination of care between providers so that patients receive comprehensive and nonredundant services (p. 461)."

One of the most widely established integrated care models is Primary Care Behavioral Health (PCBH; Robinson and Reiter 2016). Reiter et al. (2018) described PCBH as a team-based primary care approach that addresses pediatric health conditions using a biopsychosocial framework. PCBH models incorporate behavioral health consultants (BHC) into the everyday workflow of pediatric primary care clinics. Primary responsibilities include assisting patients with managing their health conditions, providing same-day consultation, sharing clinic space and resources with the primary care team, engaging with the majority of patients who present to clinic, improving the teams' use of biopsychosocial assessment and intervention, and retaining a routine presence in the biopsychosocial care of patients. Furthermore, BHC are allotted 15- to 30-min consultation and follow-up visits to assist in meeting the behavioral health needs of patients and their families. BHC may also act as a stepped-care triage service for those who need more intensive services.

Since the inception of integrated models of care, innovative behavioral health programs, such as PCBH, have greatly expanded. However, the literature on the effectiveness of these programs remains limited among pediatric populations. In an effort to improve availability and access to quality behavioral health services, the Deepwater Horizon Medical Benefits Class Action Settlement developed the Mental and Behavioral Health Capacity Project (MBHCP) to assess the effectiveness of a variety of integrated care models for underserved populations (Hansel et al. 2017). Results of two different MBHCP programs located in Florida and Louisiana demonstrated statistically significant decreases in child behavior and parenting stress, as well as 87% reporting satisfaction in services provided (Hansel et al. 2017). Albeit limited, an increased number of integrated behavioral health-care programs are being developed and assessed for effectiveness and feasibility in both primary and specialty care settings.

In response to the obstacles facing the sustainability and feasibility of behavioral health integration, several health-care organizations are piloting innovative programs intended to improve integration efforts proposed by the Triple Aim. The Novel Interventions in Children's Healthcare (NICH; Harris et al. 2013) was developed to address the complex psychosocial needs of pediatric patients and their families who are at-risk for avoidable medical complications (Harris et al. 2018). NICH utilizes alternative payment models to promote quality improvement and effective allocation of health-care resources that accentuate intensive behavioral health integration. Additionally, NICH strives to simultaneously address the Triple Aim of enriching patients' care experiences, boosting population health status, and decreasing health-care costs.

The integration of behavioral health services within the context of pediatric primary and specialty care settings is increasingly becoming the gold standard of integrated care. Despite decades of research illustrating the importance of providing holistic care to pediatric patients and their families, a sustainable service delivery model has yet to be identified. However, in order to deliver integrated behavioral health services, payment reform and the development of innovative programming that increase access and quality of care are crucial.

Psychological Problems in Pediatric Primary and Specialty Care

The number of behavioral health concerns that arise in pediatric medical settings has soared over the past several decades (Slomski 2012). Mental health conditions account for the top five disabilities among children in the United States, which are ranked above physical illness and disabilities (Halfon et al. 2012; Yogman et al. 2018). Approximately one in five children are diagnosed with a developmental or behavioral health disorder that greatly impacts the individual patient, family, and community (Halfon et al. 2012; Perou et al. 2013). Common psychological problems that surface in pediatric primary and specialty care settings include general parenting issues, developmental concerns, mental health problems, adjustment to chronic illness, and adherence to treatment regimens (also see Chap. 12 of this volume).

General Parenting Issues and Developmental Concerns

Pediatric primary care settings are designed to provide children and their families with ongoing and routine health care at all stages of development. Frequent contact with pediatricians affords families the opportunity to discuss any physical, emotional, or environmental concerns that may develop throughout childhood. In addition, the American Academy of Pediatrics created the Bright Future guidelines to bolster health promotion, disease prevention, and optimal growth for all families who present to primary care (Hagan et al. 2017). On average, pediatricians are allotted approximately 18 min of face-to-face time for each well-child visit (Halfon et al. 2011). Thus, the opportunity to fully explore and address behavioral health concerns, physical examinations, and Bright Future guidelines is extremely limited.

Alternatively, behavioral health providers could be tasked with providing developmental, behavioral, or psychosocial screening, and parental guidance on typical development (e.g., toilet training, sleep practices, or discipline). In a recent study examining the scope of behavioral health consultation, Talmi et al. (2016) found approximately 20% of behavioral health consultations addressed developmental concerns and anticipatory guidance. Developmental and anticipatory guidance consultations generally attend to common parenting questions such as toilet training, discipline and time out implementation, limit setting, tantrums, noncompliance, aggression, disruptive behavior, obesity, picky eating, homework compliance, school behavior, and sleep problems/bedtime resistance. With expertise in child development and behavior, behavioral health providers are well equipped to further support efforts to provide holistic care in pediatric primary care settings.

Attention Deficit/Hyperactivity Disorder

As the most common neurodevelopmental disorder diagnosed in childhood, attention deficit/hyperactivity disorder (ADHD) is usually first identified in the pediatric primary care office (Perou et al. 2013; Visser et al. 2015; also see Chap. 12 of this volume). In 2016, approximately 5.4 million children in the United States had a current diagnosis of ADHD, and almost two-thirds (62%) were prescribed medication (Danielson et al. 2018). Furthermore, the prevalence rates of ADHD and prescribing practices have increased substantially from 2007 to approximately present day (Visser et al. 2014). The growing number of children and adolescents diagnosed with ADHD in primary care settings highlights the critical need for improved access to evidence-based intervention.

The literature identified the combination of medication management and behavioral therapy as a well-established treatment for youth with ADHD (Hinshaw and Arnold 2015). However, in pediatric primary care offices that do not provide integrated behavioral health services, medication management becomes the first-line approach to ADHD treatment. With the increasing rates of ADHD in pediatric populations, integrated care is crucial for adequately supporting these patients and their families. In a recent study comparing a fully integrated primary care office to a co-located model of behavioral health care, the results suggested significantly higher rates of standardized assessment guideline adherence, greater collaboration and contact with the patient's school, and improved behavioral observation in the integrated practice setting (Moore et al. 2018). Furthermore, families received more parent/caregiver education on ADHD, behavior management training, and school advocacy, and families attended a greater number of clinical visits and medication management follow-up in the integrated model (Moore et al. 2018). Thus, it is not enough to improve access solely through co-located service models, and greater collaboration and integration among pediatric providers is indicated.

Anxiety/Depression

The average age of onset is approximately 6 years for anxiety disorders and early adolescence, or 13 years, for mood disorders (Merikangas et al. 2010). Bor et al. (2014) postulate that the prevalence of internalizing disorders in adolescent females is rising (also see Chap. 12 of this volume). Although mental health diagnoses can lead to significant problems if left untreated, more than half of individuals do not receive adequate treatment (Merikangas et al. 2010; Stancin and Perrin 2014). Integrated behavioral health in the treatment of targeted mental health problems demonstrates significant benefit in symptom reduction compared to usual care models (Asarnow et al. 2015). Therefore, there is considerable opportunity for early identification and intervention in integrated pediatric primary care, as youth frequently present to these settings.

Adjustment and Adherence in Specialty Care

When faced with a chronic medical condition, mental health problems can become exacerbated. Youth with chronic medical conditions are often seen more regularly by their specialty care doctor. Thus, integrated behavioral health in specialty care is also recommended. The pediatric diabetes literature (also see Chap. 21 of this volume) is furthest along in capturing the benefit of integrated service delivery models. According to a recent systematic review and meta-analysis, the rates of anxiety and mood disorders in youth with type 1 diabetes are approximately 32% and 30%, respectively (Buchberger et al. 2016). There is a dramatic increase in the prevalence of mental health disorders in the T1D population than in normative samples. However, developing research suggests that addressing diabetes distress and associated burden of living with a chronic medical condition may play a critical role in better understanding and supporting pediatric patients with diabetes.

Diabetes distress is a relatively new concept and describes the negative emotional reactions that emerge as a response to the burden of living with diabetes (Hagger et al. 2016). Diabetes distress is correlated with suboptimal glycemic control, poor adherence to treatment regimen, lower self-efficacy, and reduced self-care (Hagger et al. 2016). Other chronic health conditions are beginning to explore disease distress as a key player in disease management. Pediatric psychologists and/or other behavioral health providers are well suited to provide holistic care for pediatric patients with chronic health conditions. Psychologists can provide short-term intervention aimed at addressing disease distress and burnout of chronic disease management through intervention strategies including cognitive restructuring, problem-solving barriers to adherence, and goal setting (Hagger et al. 2016; also see Chap. 25 of this volume). Furthermore, early psychological screening and routine monitoring of distress and burnout in specialty care clinics add an additional layer of support and resources to patients and their families.

Value of Integrated Care

IPBHC delivers numerous value-added benefits to patients, providers, and payers. One-stop shopping, decreased stigma, greater access to care, improved clinical efficiency, better outcomes, enhanced patient experience, decreased physician burden, increased focus on prevention/population health, and cost-savings can be realized through integrated care. In the following section, each of these advantages are explained and discussed.

One-stop shopping (Asarnow et al. 2017; Ader et al. 2015; Kelly and Coons 2012; Yogman et al. 2018) is a consumer-friendly and patient-centered way to provide care. Addressing behavioral health issues in a trusted and familiar place where physical ailments are treated is convenient and destigmatizing. IPBHC decreases stigma regarding receiving mental health care (Campo et al. 2015; Hansel et al. 2017; Stancin and Perrin 2014; Tynan 2016; Berkout and Gross 2013). Campo et al. (2015) explained, "Integration challenges stigma by communicating that health is a unitary construct that cannot be parsed into physical health and mental health, and it has the potential to change patient, family, and health care professionals' attitudes and beliefs as well as address structural barriers to care (p. E1–E2)." A continuum of care where services are simplified and administrative obstacles are avoided facilitates better access (Campo et al. 2015). Since pediatricians are a trusted resource, patients are more likely to follow through with these referrals, which are also located in the same setting (Berkout and Gross 2013; Polaha et al. 2011).

McMillan et al. (2016) noted, "The American Academy of Child and Adolescent Psychiatry (AACAP) is well aware that the 8700 child and adolescent psychiatrists in the United States, many of whom do not engage in full-time practice, are not able to meet all the mental health needs of America's children (p. 5)." Orwat et al. (2018) concluded that due to shortages of child psychiatrists and other mental health professionals, a high number of uninsured youths, and poor reimbursement policies, led to approximately 64% of young people experiencing depressive symptoms not receiving care. There is wide agreement that IPBHC increases access and promotes greater service utilization (Ader et al. 2015; Davis et al. 2015; Hansel et al. 2017; Tynan and Woods 2013). Simply, greater access is realized when more patients are served in an efficient and effective manner (Campo et al. 2015; Hansel et al. 2017; Ward-Zimmerman and Cannata 2012). Further, racially and ethnically diverse youth may be well served by integrated pediatric behavioral health-care clinics (Arora et al. 2017). Improved access will attenuate health disparities. In their review, Arora et al. (2017) noted that marginalized populations may prefer integrated services due to decreased stigma and financial barriers.

IPBHC facilitates workflow by curbside/hallway consultations and warm handoffs (Davis et al. 2015; Freeman et al. 2018). Warm handoffs refer to in-person referrals that occur in the presence of patients. In general, the physician typically introduces patients to the behavioral health specialist, explains the reason for referral, communicates the clinician's competence, and declares how they can be helpful (Ader et al. 2015). Warm handoffs propel increased access (Davis et al. 2015; Reiter et al. 2018). Reiter et al. (2018) claimed that warm handoffs facilitate same-day appointments, eliminate frequency of no-show appointments, and reinforce team-based care. Moreover, stigma is reduced by warm handoffs (Ader et al. 2015).

The focus on value-based payment models calls for an increased attention on tractionable outcomes (Freeman et al. 2018). Examples of compelling outcome metrics include cost-savings, lowered medication dosages, decreased lengths of hospital stays, reduced emergency room visits, fewer missed school days, and less unnecessary utilization of specialty medical services (Janicke et al. 2015). Better patient care outcomes are realized by IPBHC (Herbst et al. 2018; Bucholz et al. 2018; Cohen et al. 2015; Davis et al. 2015; Gomez et al. 2014; Kazak et al. 2017). In their meta-analysis, Asarnow et al. (2015) found that young patients receiving integrated care had a 66% greater probability of obtaining a more favorable outcome than youth in treatment-as-usual settings. Patient satisfaction and experience with care also increased in IPBHC settings (Yogman et al. 2018). Integrated care settings were associated with greater clinical efficiency (Aupont et al. 2012; Ward-Zimmerman and Cannata 2012). Finally, both patients and physicians appear to favor IBHC services over other more siloed delivery systems (Asarnow et al. 2005; Kolko et al. 2014; Polaha et al. 2011; Rozenman and Piacentini 2016). Sixty-three percent of parents sought help from pediatricians for behavioral health problems compared to only 24% who consulted mental health specialists (Polaha et al. 2011).

IPBHC decreases the workload burden for pediatricians. McMillan et al. (2018) lamented that pediatricians are ill-equipped to care for patients with behavioral health concerns. Treating behavioral health problems imposes significant time demands on pediatricians (Meadows et al. 2011). Meadows et al. (2011) found that when patients present with behavioral health-care concerns, appointments last 2.5 times longer than appointments addressing medical complaints. Furthermore, pediatric residents are more comfortable assessing behavioral health problems than treating them (Ladd et al. 2017). Increased collaboration between pediatricians and behavioral health clinicians in integrated settings can decrease physician burden (McMillan et al. 2018; Tynan 2016; Yogman et al. 2018). IPBHC settings facilitate closer collaboration between providers. Additionally, co-locating pediatric and behavioral health training programs expand skill sets in all the trainees (McMillan et al. 2018). Further, they also discovered that reimbursement for pediatricians' treatment of behavioral complaints was offered at a far lower rate (e.g., approximately 119 dollars for a medical visit compared to approximately 79 dollars for a behavioral health visit). Kelly and Coons (2012) learned that 92% of pediatric staff reported less burden due to IPBHC. Cummings et al. (2011) called these benefits "physician leveraging," which is defined as "releasing them to perform procedures more in keeping with their medical training (p. 44)."

Preventative care is intimately tied to a population health focus. Giese and Waugh (2017) maintained that an emphasis on population health "shifts the health care system from a diagnose-and-treat-disease model to a whole health continuum (p. 7)." Janicke et al. (2015) rightly lauded the previous clinical child and pediatric psychology efforts at preventing substance abuse, conduct disorders, bullying, and depression in youth. Hunter et al. (2017) listed anxiety chronic pain, diabetes, insomnia, and tobacco use as additional targets for early intervention and prevention projects.

Although the research is in its infancy, IPBHC can yield cost-savings (Cohen et al. 2015; Tynan 2016; Yogman et al. 2018). For example, integrated care practices reduced spending for patients by over 50% (Yogman et al. 2018). Additionally, Yogman et al. (2018) noted there was a decrease in emergency room spending for patients receiving integrated care. Despite potential cost benefits, funding issues for integrated behavioral health care are cumbersome and complicated.

New business models are necessary to implement and sustain IPBHC practices (Robinson et al. 2018; also see Chap. 27 of this volume). Tynan (2016) argued that public and private financing options should be developed to support IPBHC. They identified restrictions on same-day billing for mental health and physical health care as well as lack of reimbursement for health collaborative care, nonphysician delivered services, prevention and treatment for mental health diagnoses. Tynan (2016) offered several recommendations for mitigating problems including unbundling service, finding Common Procedural Terminology Codes (CPT) that are reimbursable for psychologists and negotiating with Medicaid to ensure parity with Medicare. Hansel et al. (2017) advocated for training integrated clinic staff in the ICD-10. They explained, "Direct billing and contracts would not be possible without training practitioners in the ICD-10 system, as reimbursement is often contingent on a diagnosable condition that falls under the category of an F code (p. s22)." The use of Health and Behavior Assessment and Intervention Codes for payment is essential (Freeman et al. 2018).

Miller et al. (2017) proposed the adoption of a global or capitated payment system to fund IPBHC services. Perrin (2017) explained that capitation is "payment based on the number of patients attributed to the provider(s) potentially adjusted for risk (p. S86)." Capitation rates are derived from actuarial claims data and are paid out on a per member per month (PMPM) basis (Freeman et al. 2018). Global payment structures allow a health-care organization to determine the appropriate integrated care team, and subsequent services, for each individual patient using a fixed prepayment arrangement. Freeman et al. (2018) noted that information technology, population risk adjustments, and patient engagement/management processes must be in place for capitation to be successful.

Conclusion

The next decade will likely see a rise in integrated pediatric behavioral health-care services (IPBHC). Continued theory-building, empirical research, innovative practices, and robust training programs are necessary to sustain growth. In order to make good on promises, IPBHC will need to be subject to both more randomized clinical trials and cost-effectiveness studies. Additionally, the emerging workforce must receive more specialized training. Doctoral, predoctoral, and postdoctoral programs will need to modify their pedagogical practices to develop new competencies in trainees (also see Chap. 26 of this volume). As Jonas Salk noted, "the reward for work done well is the opportunity to do more." Ideally, the future will yield greater opportunities for work in integrated care settings due to the hard work completed by academicians and clinicians.

References

Ader, J., Stille, C. J., Keller, D., Miller, B. F., Barrs, M. S., & Perrin, J. M. (2015). The medical home and integrated behavioral health: Advancing the policy agenda. *Pediatrics, 135*, 909–917.

Arora, P. G., Godoy, L., & Hodgkinson, S. (2017). Serving the underserved: Cultural considerations in behavioral health integration in pediatric primary care. *Professional Psychology: Research and Practice, 48*, 139–148.

Asarnow, J. R., Jaycox, L. H., Duan, N., LaBorde, A. P., Rea, M. M., Murray, P., et al. (2005). Effectiveness of a quality improvement intervention for adolescent depression in primary care clinics: A randomized controlled trial. *Journal of the American Medical Association, 193*, 311–319.

Asarnow, J. R., Rozenman, M., Wiblin, J., & Zeltzer, L. (2015). Integrated medical-behavioral care compared with usual primary care for child and adolescent behavioral health: A meta-analysis. *JAMA Pediatrics, 169*, 929–937.

Asarnow, J. R., Kolko, D. J., Miranda, J., & Kazak, A. E. (2017). The pediatric patient-centered medical home: Innovative models for improving behavioral health. *American Psychologist, 72*, 13–27.

Aupont, O., Doerfler, L., Connor, D. F., Tisminetzky, M., & McLaughlin, T. J. (2012). A collaborative care model to improve access to pediatric mental health services. *Administration and Policy in Mental Health Services and Research, 40*, 264–273.

Becker, S. J., Helseth, S. A., Frank, H. E., Escobar, K. I., & Weeks, B. J. (2018). Parent preferences and experiences with psychological treatment: Results from a direct-to-consumer survey using the marketing mix framework. *Professional Psychology: Research and Practice, 49*, 167–176.

Berkout, O. V., & Gross, A. M. (2013). Externalizing behavior challenges within primary care settings. *Aggression and Violent Behavior, 18*, 491–495.

Berwick, D. W., Nolan, T. W., & Whittington, J. (2008). The triple aim: Care, health, and cost. *Health Affairs, 27*, 759–769.

Blount, A. (2003). Integrated primary care: Organizing the evidence. *Families, Systems, and Health, 21*, 121–133.

Bor, W., Dean, A. J., Najman, J., & Hayatbakhsh, R. (2014). Are child and adolescent mental health problems increasing in the 21st century? *Australian & New Zealand Journal of Psychiatry, 48*(7), 606–616.

Bray, J. H. (2010). The future of psychology practice and science. *American Psychologist, 65*, 355–369.

Buchberger, B., Huppertz, H., Krabbe, L., Lux, B., Mattivi, J. T., & Siafarikas, A. (2016). Symptoms of depression and anxiety in youth with type 1 diabetes: A systematic review and meta-analysis. *Psychoneuroendocrinology, 70*, 70–84.

Bucholz, M., Burnett, B., Margolis, K., Millar, A., & Talmi, A. (2018). Early childhood behavioral health integration and activities and healthy steps: Sustaining practice averting costs. *Clinical Practice in Pediatric Psychology, 6*, 140–151.

Campo, J. V., Bridge, J. A., & Fontanella, C. A. (2015). Access to mental health services: Implementing an integrated solution. *JAMA Pediatrics, 164*(4), 299–300.

Cohen, D. J., Balasubramanian, B. A., Davis, M., Hall, J., Gunn, R., Strange, C., et al. (2015). Understanding care integration from the ground up: Five organizing constructs that shape integrated practices. *Journal of the American Board of Family Medicine, 28*(S1), S7–S20.

Committee on Psychosocial Aspects of Child and Family Health and Task Force on Mental Health. (2009). Policy statement—the future of pediatrics: Mental health competencies for pediatric primary care. *Pediatrics, 124*, 410–421.

Cummings, N. A., O'Donohue, W. T., & Cummings, J. L. (2011). The financial dimensions of integrated behavioral primary care. In N. A. Cummings & W. T. O'Donohue (Eds.), *Understanding the behavioral health care crisis* (pp. 33–57). New York: Routledge.

Danielson, M. L., Bitsko, R. H., Ghandour, R. M., Holbrook, J. R., Kogan, M. D., & Blumberg, S. J. (2018). Prevalence of parent-reported ADHD diagnosis and associated treatment among U.S. children and adolescents, 2016. *Journal of Child & Adolescent Psychology, 47*(2), 199–212.

Davis, M. M., Balasubramanian, B. A., Cifuentes, M., Hall, J., Gunn, R., Fernald, D., et al. (2015). Clinician staffing, scheduling, and engagement strategies among primary care practices delivering integrated care. *Journal of the American Board of Family Medicine, 28*, S32–S40.

Engel, G. (1977). The need for a new medical model: A challenge for biomedicine. *Science, 196*, 129–136.

Foy, J. M. (2015). The medical home and integrated behavioral health. *Pediatrics, 135*(5), 930–931.

Freeman, D. S., Manson, L., Howard, J., & Hornberger, J. (2018). Financing the primary care behavioral health model. *Journal of Clinical Psychology in Medical Settings, 25*, 197–209.

Giese, A. A., & Waugh, M. (2017). Conceptual framework for integrated care: Multiple perspectives to achieve integrated care. In R. E. Feinstein, J. V. Connelly, & M. S. Feinstein (Eds.), *Integrating behavioral health and primary care* (pp. 3–16). New York: Oxford.

Gomez, D., Bridges, A. J., Andrews, A. R., III, Cavell, T. A., Pastrana, F. A., Gregus, S. J., et al. (2014). Delivering parent management in an integrated primary care setting: Description and preliminary outcome data. *Cognitive and Behavioral Practice, 21*, 296–309.

Hagan, J. F., Shaw, J. S., & Duncan, P. M. (Eds.). (2017). *Bright futures: Guidelines for health supervision of infants, children, and adolescents* (4th ed.). Elk Grove Village, IL: American Academy of Pediatrics.

Hagger, V., Hendrieckx, C., Sturt, J., Skinner, T. C., & Speight, J. (2016). Diabetes distress among adolescents with type 1 diabetes: A systematic review. *Current Diabetes Reports, 16*(1), 1–14.

Halfon, N., Stevens, G. D., Larson, K., & Olson, L. M. (2011). Duration of a well-child visit: Association with content, family-centeredness, and satisfaction. *Pediatrics, 128*, 657–664.

Halfon, N., Houtrow, A., Larson, K., & Newacheck, P. W. (2012). The changing landscape of disability in childhood. *The Future of Children, 22*, 13–42.

Hansel, T., Rohrer, G., Osofsky, J., Osofsky, H., Arthur, E., & Barker, C. (2017). Integration of mental and behavioral health in pediatric health care clinics. *Journal of Public Health Management & Practice, 23*, S19–S24.

Harris, M. A., Spiro, K., Heywood, M., Wagner, D., Hoehn, D., Hatten, A., et al. (2013). Novel interventions in children's health care (NICH): Innovative treatment for youth with complex medical conditions. *Clinical Practice in Pediatric Psychology, 1*(2), 137–145.

Harris, M. A., Teplitsky, L., Nagra, H., Spiro, K., & Wagner, D. V. (2018). Single (aim)-minded strategies for demonstrating value to payers for youth with medical complexity. *Clinical Practice in Pediatric Psychology, 6*(2), 152–163.

Herbst, R. B. J., Margolis, K. L., McClelland, B. B., Herndon, J. L., Millar, A. M., & Talmi, A. (2018). Sustaining integrated behavioral health practice without sacrificing the continuum. *Clinical Practice in Pediatric Psychology, 6*, 117–128.

Hinshaw, S. P., & Arnold, L. E. (2015). Attention-deficit/hyperactivity disorder, multimodal treatment, and longitudinal outcome: Evidence, paradox, and challenge. *WIREs Cognitive Science, 6*, 39–52.

Hunter, C. L., Goodie, J. L., Oordt, M. S., & Dobmeyer, A. C. (2017). *Integrated behavioral health in primary care: A step x step guidance for assessment and intervention*. Washington, DC: American Psychological Association.

Hunter, C. L., Dobmeyer, A. C., & Reiter, J. T. (2018). Integrating behavioral health services into primary care: Spotlight on the primary care behavioral health model of service delivery. *Journal of Clinical Psychology in Medical Settings, 25*, 105–108.

Janicke, D. M., Fritz, A. M., & Rozensky, R. H. (2015). Healthcare reform and preparing the future clinical child and adolescent workforce. *Journal of Clinical Child and Adolescent Psychology, 44*, 1030–1039.

Kazak, A. E., Nash, J. M., Hiroto, K., & Kaslow, N. J. (2017). Psychologists in patient-centered medical homes (PCMHs): Roles, evidence, opportunities, and challenges. *American Psychologist, 72*, 1–12.

Kelly, J. F., & Coons, H. L. (2012). Integrated healthcare and professional psychology: Is the setting right for you? *Professional Psychology: Research and Practice, 43*, 586–595.

Kolko, D. J., Camp, J., Kilbourne, A. M., Hart, J., Sakolsky, D., & Wisniewski, S. (2014). Collaborative care outcomes for pediatric behavioral health problems: A cluster randomized trial. *Pediatrics, 133*(4), e981–e992.

Ladd, I., Kettlewell, P., Shahidullah, J., Dehart, K., Bogaczyck, T., & Larson, S. (2017). Treating behavioral health conditions: What worries pediatric residents? *Journal of Patient-Centered Research and Reviews, 4*(3), 191.

McMillan, J. A., Land, M., & Leslie, L. K. (2016). Pediatric residency education and the behavioral and mental health crisis: A call to action. *Pediatrics, 139*(1), 1–7.

McMillan, J. A., Land, M. L., Jr., Rodday, A. M., Wills, K., Green, C. M., & Leslie, L. K. (2018). Report of a joint association of pediatric program directors—American Board of Pediatrics workshop: Preparing future pediatricians for the mental health crisis. *Journal of Pediatrics, 201*, 285–291.

Meadows, T., Valleley, R., Haack, M. K., Thorson, R., & Evans, J. (2011). Physician "costs" in providing behavioral health in primary care. *Clinical Pediatrics, 50*, 447–455.

Merikangas, K. R., He, J., Burstein, M., Swanson, S. A., Avenevoli, S., Cui, L., et al. (2010). Lifetime prevalence of mental disorders in U.S. adolescents: Results from the national comorbidity survey replication adolescent supplement (NCS-A). *Journal of the American Academy of Child & Adolescent Psychiatry, 49*(10), 980–989.

Miller, B. F., Ross, K. M., Davis, M. M., Melek, S. P., Kathol, R., & Gordon, P. (2017). Payment reform in the patient-centered medical home: Enabling and sustaining integrated behavioral health care. *American Psychologist, 72*(1), 55–68.

Moore, J. A., Karch, K., Sherina, V., Guiffre, A., Jee, S., & Garfunkel, L. C. (2018). Practice procedures in models of primary care collaboration for children with ADHD. *Families, Systems, and Health, 36*(1), 73–86.

OECD. (2017). *Health at a Glance 2017: OECD Indicators*. Paris: OECD. https://doi.org/10.1787/health_glance-2017-en.

Orwat, J., Kumaria, S., & Dentato, M. P. (2018). Financing and delivery of behavioral health in the United States. In C. D. Moniz & S. H. Gorin (Eds.), *Behavioral and mental health care policy and practice* (pp. 78–102). New York: Routledge.

Perou, R., Bitsko, R. H., Blumberg, S. J., Pastor, P., Ghandour, R. M., Gfroerer, J. C., et al. (2013). Mental health surveillance among children—United States, 2005-2011. *Morbidity and Mortality Weekly Report, 62*, 1–35.

Perrin, J. M. (2017). Innovative health care financing strategies for children and youth with special needs. *Pediatrics, 139*, S85–S88.

Polaha, J., Dalton, W. T., & Allen, S. (2011). The prevalence of emotional and behavioral problems in pediatric primary clinics serving rural children. *Journal of Pediatric Psychology, 36*, 352–360.

Public Law No. 111–148, 111th Congress: Patient Protection & Affordable Care Act. (2010). 124 STAT.119. Retrieved from http://www.gpo.gov/fdsys/pkg/PLAW/111publ148/pdf/PLAW-111publ48.pdf.

Reiter, J. T., Dobmeyer, A. C., & Hunter, C. (2018). The primary care behavioral health (PCBH) model: An overview and operational definition. *Journal of Clinical Psychology in Settings, 25*, 109–126.

Richardson, L. P., McCarty, C. A., Radovic, A., & Suleiman, A. B. (2017). Research in the integration of behavioral health for adolescents and young adults in primary care settings: A systematic review. *Journal of Adolescent Health, 60*, 261–269.

Robinson, P. J., & Reiter, J. T. (2016). *Behavioral consultation and primary care: A guide to integrating services* (2nd ed.). Geneva: Springer.

Robinson, P., Oymaja, J., Beachy, B., Goodie, J., Sprague, L., Bell, J., et al. (2018). Creating a primary care workforce: Strategies for leaders, clinicians, and nurses. *Journal of Clinical Psychology in Medical Settings, 25*, 169–186.

Rozenman, M., & Piacentini, J. (2016). Pediatric primary care as a stepped care setting for youth anxiety: Commentary on "What steps to take? How to approach concerning anxiety in youth". *Clinical Psychology: Science and Practice, 23*, 230–233.

Sandoval, B. E., Bell, J., Khatri, P., & Robinson, P. J. (2018). Toward a unified integration approach: Uniting diverse primary care strategies under primary care behavioral health model (PCMH). *Journal of Clinical Psychology in Medical Settings, 25*, 187–196.

Slomski, A. (2012). Chronic mental health issues in children now loom larger than physical problems. *Journal of the American Medical Association, 308*, 223–225.

Stancin, T., & Perrin, E. C. (2014). Psychologists and pediatricians: Opportunities for collaboration in primary care. *American Psychologist, 69*(4), 332–343.

Talmi, A., Muther, E. F., Margolis, K., Buchholz, M., Asherin, R., & Bunik, M. (2016). The scope of behavioral health integration in a pediatric primary care setting. *Journal of Pediatric Psychology, 41*(10), 1120–1132.

Tynan, W. D. (2016). Commentary: Integrated primary care psychology evolving with the affordable care act. *Journal of Pediatric Psychology, 41*(10), 1165–1167.

Tynan, W. D., & Woods, K. E. (2013). Emerging issues: Psychology's place in the primary care pediatric medical home. *Clinical Practice in Pediatric Psychology, 1*(4), 380–385.

Visser, S. N., Danielson, M. L., Bitsko, R. H., Holbrook, J. R., Kogan, M. D., Ghandour, R. M., et al. (2014). Trends in the parent-report of health care provider-diagnosed and medicated attention-deficit/hyperactivity disorder: United States, 2003-2011. *Journal of the American Academy of Child & Adolescent Psychiatry, 53*(1), 34–46.

Visser, S. N., Zablotsky, B., Holbrook, J. R., Danielson, M. L., & Bitsko, R. H. (2015). Diagnostic experiences of children with attention-deficit/hyperactivity disorder. *National Health Statistics Report, 81*, 1–7.

Ward-Zimmerman, B., & Cannata, E. (2012). Partnering with pediatric primary care: Lessons learned through collaborative co-location. *Professional Psychology: Research and Practice, 43*, 596–605.

Williams, S. E., & Zahka, N. E. (2017). *Treating somatic symptoms in children and adolescents*. New York: Guilford.

Yogman, M. W., Betjemann, S., Sagaser, A., & Brecher, L. (2018). Integrated behavioral health care in pediatric primary care: A quality improvement project. *Clinical Pediatrics, 57*(4), 461–470.

Diversity Issues in Pediatric Behavioral Health Care

Jessica M. Valenzuela, Kristina Tatum, and Joyce H. L. Lui

Impact of Minority Status in Pediatric Health

Existing US population trends and a significant relationship between minority status (both racial/ethnic and sexual) and health outcome suggest the importance of competence in working with diverse pediatric populations. In the USA, racial/ethnic minority children will be a "minority majority" by 2020. The US Census projects that by 2020, less than one-half of children will be non-Hispanic, White, with the racial/ethnic composition of children changing more quickly than that of older cohorts (Vespa et al. 2018). Immigration is likely to become the primary driver of population growth in the USA. In fact, the proportion of the US population that is foreign born is projected to be higher by 2030 than at any time in the last century (2018). This is likely to be costly for our health systems given that, in just a 3-year period (between 2003 and 2006), the Joint Center for Economic and Political Studies estimates that existing health inequalities for racial/ethnic minorities cost more than one trillion dollars (LaVeist et al. 2009).

Decades of data across disciplines point to significant differences in racial/ethnic minority youths' overall health, health behavior, oral health, mental health, and risk for chronic illness (e.g., diabetes and cardiovascular disease). Some examples of disparities in key national indicators of well-being include increased risk of low birth weight and infant mortality experienced by African-American mothers, increased risk of obesity in African-American and Mexican-American youth, and increased risk of asthma in African-American and Puerto Rican youth, especially those living in poverty (Federal Interagency Forum on Child & Family Studies 2017). In addition, the 2017 Youth Risk Behavior Surveillance (YRBS; Kann et al. 2018) demonstrates higher rates of depressed mood in Hispanic youth and higher rates of suicide attempts in Black females. Disparities are also alarming among sexual minority youth who identify as lesbian, gay, or bisexual. In fact, there is consistent evidence indicating that sexual minority youth experience poor health outcomes including increased odds of asthma, sexually transmitted infections, and multiple behavioral and mental health concerns including attempted suicide, depression, substance use, and eating disorders (Coker et al. 2010; Marshal et al. 2011; Strutz et al. 2015).

J. M. Valenzuela (✉) · K. Tatum
College of Psychology, Nova Southeastern University, Fort Lauderdale, FL, USA
e-mail: jv637@nova.edu

J. H. L. Lui
University of California at Los Angeles, Los Angeles, CA, USA

In addition to increased risk in the general population, health disparities exist in the outcomes of minority youth who receive care for chronic conditions. African-American children with asthma have lower quality of life and higher rates of emergency room visits, hospitalizations, and mortality, and many of these disparities remain after adjusting for disease severity (Harper et al. 2015; Haselkorn et al. 2008). Similarly, racial/ethnic minority youth with type 1 diabetes have higher rates of poor glycemic control across a variety of ethnic groups (Naranjo et al. 2015). In particular, African-American youth with diabetes experience more frequent life-threatening complications like diabetic ketoacidosis and severe hypoglycemia and have a twofold increased risk for diabetes death compared to non-Hispanic, White youth (Saydah et al. 2017).

Pediatric psychologists provide evidence-based clinical care in health settings as part of multidisciplinary teams. They play an important role in "address(ing) the psychological aspects of illness, injury, and the promotion of health behaviors in children, adolescents, and families" (Aylward et al. 2009, p. 3). As such, psychologists in pediatric primary and specialty care have a role in addressing health disparities affecting youth and families, a critical public health concern. The literature reviewed below suggests that both evidence-based clinical practice at the individual and family level, as well as participation in systems-level changes within health settings and communities (discussed briefly at the end of the chapter) may meaningfully improve the outcomes of youth from diverse, minority backgrounds.

Evidence-Based Treatment for Diverse Pediatric Patients and Families

Evidence-based treatments (EBTs) provided by psychologists in pediatric health settings frequently target improving a patient and family's adjustment to injury or chronic condition, treatment adherence, lifestyle behavior change, and/or comorbid behavioral health issues. A wealth of research on common behavioral concerns such as depression, anxiety, and disruptive behavior problems has pointed to a higher risk of these diagnoses among youth with chronic health conditions (Pinquart and Shen 2011). EBTs for these presenting concerns have been largely designed and tested in non-Hispanic, White youth and families. However, there is growing evidence that available EBTs also hold promise for diverse, minority youth. EBTs have been shown to have meaningful benefit for racial/ethnic minority youth, and a growing literature suggests potential benefit for sexual minority youth as well (Huey et al. 2014; Safren et al. 2001).

Huey and Polo (2017) systematically reviewed the literature and found that current EBTs targeting a variety of concerns ranging from depression and suicidal behavior to ADHD benefited racial/ethnic minority youth (note that existing research primarily included African-American and Latino youth). The authors reported on 45 interventions, examining them based on revised criteria for "well-established" treatment that included a requirement for the treatment to be tested in a largely racial/ethnic minority sample (at least 75%) and for the effectiveness of the treatment in minority youth to be specifically examined. Among the interventions reviewed, only motivational interviewing was classified as "well established." However, 22 additional treatments were categorized as "probably efficacious" for racial/ethnic minority youth. The authors note that "cognitive-behavioral psychotherapies predominated, accounting for more than 53%" of the EBTs that were effective in racial/ethnic minority populations (Huey and Polo 2017, p. 362). The authors further synthesized 18 meta-analyses evaluating treatment outcomes in racial/ethnic minority youth and found a majority of studies demonstrating "few ethnic differences in youth treatment outcomes." Their review provides strong evidence that existing EBTs for common behavioral concerns are largely effective in racial/ethnic minority youth.

Beyond traditional mood and behavioral concerns, there is also a need for EBTs to address disease management (e.g., medication administration) and other health behavior change (e.g., increased physical activity, safe sex behaviors) among racial/ethnic and sexual minority youth. Significant disparities in these health behaviors have been documented in the literature across a variety of chronic conditions (e.g., Diabetes—Hilliard et al. 2013; HIV—Simoni et al. 2012; Obesity—Kirkpatrick et al. 2012; Organ transplantation—Thammana et al. 2014) and can have serious consequences including neuropathy, graft loss, additional morbidity, and early death. Unfortunately, there has been limited research examining the impact of EBTs on minority youths' health behaviors. Existing studies are limited by homogeneous samples and a lack of reporting on patient minority status (including race/ethnicity, sexual orientation, and other important characteristics; Kahana et al. 2008).

Notably, at least two meta-analyses have found that motivational interviewing, aimed at improving health behaviors, had larger effect sizes in samples "comprised primarily or exclusively of people from ethnic minority groups" (Hettema et al. 2005, p. 105; Lundahl et al. 2010) and that these effect sizes are further increased by combining motivational interviewing with other EBTs. A recent meta-analysis of motivation interviewing and pediatric health behavior change found a modest effect that was not impacted by racial/ethnic minority status of youth (Gayes and Steele 2014). More broadly, meta-analyses focused on disease management and medication adherence in underrepresented, culturally diverse adults have also demonstrated modest improvements for minority individuals targeted by a variety of interventions (e.g., technology-assisted, educational, behavioral strategies; Conn et al. 2014; Manias and Williams 2010). It is important to note that these studies are often limited by dichotomous comparison groups (i.e., all racial/ethnic minority youth versus all non-Hispanic, White youth) and that this practice may lead to inaccuracies in the interpretation of findings. While there are some important limitations to the existing research examining the impact of existing interventions on health behavior change in minority individuals, there appears to be some growing consensus that minority individuals can benefit from EBT and that this might extend to youth who present in medical settings.

Adaptation of Evidence-Based Treatments (EBTs)

Cultural adaptation of EBTs is sometimes considered a controversial and ill-defined matter. A wide range of terms such as "culturally adapted," 'culturally competent," "culturally responsive," "culturally sensitive," and "culturally tailored" have been used, sometimes interchangeably, when referring to the adaptation of interventions for a specific group (Huey et al. 2014). One concise definition for "cultural adaptation" is "the systematic modification of an EBT to consider language, culture and context in such a way that is compatible with a client's cultural patterns, meanings and values" (Bernal et al. 2009; p. 361–2). Notably, the definition speaks to the importance of adapting to an *individual* patient's cultural context.

In reality, clinicians almost universally agree that a balance between a systematic empirically supported approach and the personalization of clinical practice to an individual and their context results in the best treatment response (Norcross and Wampold 2011). In fact, the American Psychological Association definition of evidence-based practice is consistent with this idea: "the integration of the best available research with clinical expertise in the context of patient characteristics, *culture* [emphasis added] and preferences" (APA Presidential Task Force on Evidence Based Practice 2006, p. 280). The rationale for cultural adaptation of EBTs includes research findings related to minority youth and families' reduced access to and retention in treatment, engagement in treatment, satisfaction with treatment and the provider–patient relationship, and other documented disparities (Barrera et al. 2017). However, evidence of the benefits of cultural adaptation to minority groups has sometimes been mixed.

According to an APA interdivisional taskforce on evidence-based psychotherapy relationships, culture was found to be one of four transdiagnostic characteristics identified as "demonstrably effective in adapting psychotherapy" based on the existing research (Norcross and Wampold 2011). Specifically, task force members found that treatment targeting a specific cultural group ($d = 0.51$) was much more effective than treatment targeting individuals more broadly ($d = 0.18$) and that treatment benefits were related to the number of culturally adapted components described in the study ($r = 0.28$; Smith et al. 2011). These findings strongly suggest that when psychological treatments are adapted by culture, they are more effective for youth and adults.

Other meta-analyses have been more equivocal regarding cultural adaptation. Huey et al. (2014) reviewed ten recent meta-analyses aimed at evaluating adaptations of existing treatments. They found that while culturally adapted interventions were effective for youth and adults, it was not clear if cultural adaptation provided any benefit above and beyond standard EBT. They note that their analysis was limited by the existence of few studies comparing culturally adapted treatments to non-adapted treatments (most had conventional control groups). Additionally, while most of these research syntheses have focused on mental health outcomes, a recent meta-analysis by Healey et al. (2017) included other health outcomes in their analysis of culturally adapted EBTs. They found mixed results with only 17 of 31 studies demonstrating improved outcomes in culturally adapted EBTs. The authors attribute the mixed findings, in part, to the fact that there are variations within cultural groups that must be considered by clinicians and over-generalization in treatment adaptation may lead to less beneficial results.

Another finding of note from the research on cultural adaptation of EBT is the ubiquity with which it occurs. One study found that, across meta-analyses, more than half of EBTs for racial/ethnic minority youth were adapted in some way (Huey et al. 2014). In addition to cultural adaptations that are developed prior to "broad scale implementation," it is well documented that clinicians implementing EBTs in local communities further adapt EBTs (sometimes called "local adaptation") for better fit with their systems and populations (Barrera et al. 2017). While there is no consensus in the literature regarding how EBTs should be adapted, there appears to be a growing movement aimed at encouraging clinicians to find "flexibility within fidelity" and to tailor EBTs meaningfully to culture and developmental considerations (Hamilton et al. 2008). There is a great potential value in making treatments more accessible and "tailoring the content to address contextual realities" through cultural adaptation (Friedberg et al. 2014).

Recommendations vary regarding when to systematically adapt an existing EBT. Castro et al. (2010) argue that cultural adaptation is particularly "justifiable" in cases where there is evidence that:

1. Patients and families from a particular group are not effectively engaged in treatment (i.e., do not participate or are not retained in treatment),
2. Unique risk and resilience factors exist for a particular group and may be different from those taken into consideration when an EBT was developed and tested (e.g., immigrants with refugee status who have experienced war-related violence might need unique components to PTSD treatment),
3. Patients from a particular group are presenting consistently with a unique presentation or symptom (e.g., Haitian families of HIV-positive youth with significant concerns that the patient's illness was supernaturally induced), and/or
4. An intervention that has been faithfully administered is less effective for a particular group (suggesting it should be adapted to be effective).

In addition, it is helpful to note that clinicians will often find that EBTs, particularly cognitive behavioral approaches, provide considerable flexibility for adaptation. However, if making a justifiable (as evidenced by the above) cultural adaptation requires a significant departure from fidelity to the original EBT, it may mean that the existing EBT is not a good fit for the given patient (Domenech Rodríguez and Bernal 2012).

There are several models for culturally adapting EBT, which have been used throughout the literature in developing treatments for racial/ethnic minority children and adolescents with various mental health concerns ranging from disruptive behavior (e.g., Domenech Rodríguez et al. 2011) to depression (e.g., Nicolas et al. 2009). These frameworks have most often been applied to cognitive behavioral and behavioral EBTs, and use a staged approach including review of existing research and community involvement in making treatment adaptation decisions. This is sometimes referred to as a combination of "top-down" and "bottom-up" approaches." Adaptation using one of these approaches ultimately leads to a research trial evaluating the outcomes of the culturally adapted EBT (Barrera et al. 2013). For general and specific guidelines for gathering data on which to base cultural adaptations, see Domenech Rodríguez and Bernal (2012). Unfortunately, these frameworks have less frequently been used in research on youth with medical conditions, and very few condition-specific frameworks have been developed to culturally adapt EBTs for health behavior change (e.g., HIV Prevention—Wingood and DiClemente 2008).

Of interest in clinical practice are the kinds of cultural adaptations that are most often made in EBTs. Resnicow et al. (2002) have traditionally made a distinction between surface (e.g., language translation, images of diverse youth included in materials) and deep adaptations (e.g., changes in the content of the intervention or processes). More recently, Healey et al. (2017) have argued that there are three domains in which EBTs may be adapted:

1. Assessing needs from the community's perspective and involving community members in intervention delivery (e.g., African-American youth with diabetes review materials for adaptation and provide peer education).
2. Changing service delivery structure or processes, which includes offering treatment in a more accessible location or telehealth, matching therapists culturally or linguistically to the patient, translating materials, and other additions or changes to the treatment.
3. Adapting the content (the most common kind of cultural adaption found in the health and mental health literature), which includes changes in the allusions, metaphors or images used during treatment, and incorporation of patient's cultural values and beliefs. These adaptations were sometimes broadly based on a racial/ethnic cultural group, but at other times, they were individually adapted (e.g., changing content based on patient's level of acculturation).

Of note, the clinicians' awareness of risk and resilience factors found in the literature for specific groups may be important but should be supplemented by patient and community input regarding the accessibility, sensitivity, and relevance of various issues and strategies in treatment.

Integrating bottom-up and top-down approaches in adapting EBTs may allow clinicians to better address the treatment needs of diverse pediatric populations. Notably, intervention science is moving towards more personalized approaches that are likely to lead to improvements for working with individuals from diverse backgrounds including racial/ethnic and sexual minority youth and families. Ng and Weisz (2016) have described the potential benefits of cultural adaptations as well as modular therapies, sequential adaptive interventions, measurement feedback systems, distillation and matching strategies, and incorporation of individualized metrics as just a few ways to personalize treatment. This is truly an exciting time for working with pediatric populations with medical conditions as we are on the precipice of a "revolution" in terms of both the diversity of the families we work with and the ways in which we can bring EBTs to bear to meet their needs (Friedberg et al. 2014).

Evidence-Based Assessment with Diverse Patient Populations

Competent evidence-based assessment will always be critical in order to successfully personalize EBT to the specific needs and strengths of patients. However, traditional assessment tools have many potential limitations in pediatric practice with diverse populations including limited information about validity in other cultures, lack of access to multiple normative samples, and lack of translation to other languages. Beyond the need to use culturally valid measures in patients' preferred language, competent evidence-based assessment means that providers conduct culturally informed interviews, consider potential sources of bias across observations, and interpret patterns from multiple sources of information with a clear understanding of the patient and family's context including multicultural influences (Valenzuela et al. 2017).

Existing research suggests that clinician bias may lead to diagnostic errors when working with minority youth. Two examples of bias include clinicians' interpretation of African-American youths' pain experiences (e.g., Hoffman et al. 2016) and clinician bias contributing to disproportionate psychotic disorder diagnoses in African-American and Latino youth (e.g., Schwartz and Blankenship 2014). Given the potential for clinician bias, any framework for assessing diverse youth and families should include "safeguards." Assessments of risk and protective factors, diagnostic impressions, and case conceptualization should be considered hypotheses that the clinician is frequently testing in their work. Furthermore, careful integration of information from multiple sources is needed, along with consideration of the patient and family's cultural context and the possible impact of cross-cultural communication and oppressive experiences within the health-care system. It may be that inclusion of community leaders and experts is important for competent practice in some cases. For example, a published case of a Middle Eastern youth with an eating disorder diagnosis found that consultation with an imam regarding Muslim prayer rituals was important in order for sensitive treatment planning with the patient and family (Hilliard et al. 2012).

Frameworks for culturally informed assessment often include suggestions for open-ended interview questions that improve provider's understanding of important contextual factors. Notably, the DSM-5 includes one of the most comprehensive efforts at "changing the way clinicians conduct a diagnostic interview so that the perspective of the patient (and caregiver) become(s) at least as important as the signs/symptoms identified by the clinician" (Lewis-Fernández et al. 2016). The Cultural Formulation Interview (CFI) includes supplementary modules for school-age children and adolescents, and its prompts can be helpful for clinicians seeking to understand how cultural concerns, such as immigration-related problems or discrimination, impact the presenting concern. Clinicians may choose to adapt their clinical interviews to include prompts from the CFI and/or other semi-structured interviews to elicit information about patients' cultural context.

Furthermore, when deciding which domains are relevant for a given patient, it is recommended that clinicians consider the domains put forth by Hays (2008) in the ADDRESSING framework. The acronym is shorthand for the importance of assessing a number of multicultural dimensions: Age and generational status, Disability, Religion and spiritual orientation, Ethnic and racial identity, Socioeconomic status, Sexual orientation, Indigenous heritage, National origin, and Gender. Notably, it is important to consider multiple areas of the individual's identity and the family's culture and how they interact (e.g., in working with a transgender adolescent diagnosed with a chronic condition, family members' responses to the patient's gender minority status and involvement in disease management may be influenced by the family's acculturation level, and cultural values and beliefs).

In addition to the frameworks identified above, some condition-specific frameworks have been developed to guide providers in culturally competent conceptualization and treatment planning. For example, Maloney et al. (2005) conceptual model of sociocultural issues in pediatric organ transplantation includes questions about the patient and family's world view and neighborhood risks based on the pediatric transplant and diversity literature. Disease-specific models are lacking in number, however, in part because of the need for more research to understand the ways in which culture and minority status impact the typical trajectories of youth with specific conditions. For example, recent research suggests that the typical trajectories of family conflict, autonomy support, transfer of care, and disease management behavior in adolescents with type 1 diabetes may differ for Hispanic versus non-Hispanic, White youth with the disease (Nicholl et al. 2019). Further research regarding specific groups may also result in an understanding of unique barriers, strengths, and mechanisms to consider in assessment with diverse populations.

Culturally relevant domains that have been shown to influence health are particularly important to be aware of and to assess. These domains may be directly related to the referring questions or goals or may be important contextual variables to consider in case of conceptualization and treatment planning. As noted above, many of these issues are best assessed through a culturally informed clinical interview (Valenzuela et al. 2017). The section below focuses on several relevant domains with examples of their considerable influence in work with youth diagnosed with medical conditions. The domains listed are not exhaustive (e.g., disability, indigenous heritage, and spirituality are not included).

Cultural Domains Relevant to Risk and Resiliency in Pediatric Health

Considerations in Working with African-American Youth and Families in the USA

As discussed, research documents health disparities for African-American youth in health outcomes and access to quality interventions (described more below). Individual and familial factors that affect health disparities must be considered within the backdrop of historic marginalization, ongoing systemic discrimination, and a resulting mistrust of the health-care system within the African-American community (Feagin and Bennefield 2014). The Tuskegee experiment is one of several well-known and salient reminders of maltreatment of African-American patients, where treatment for syphilis was intentionally withheld from African-American men participating in the study. Race-based mistrust of the health-care system and providers continues to permeate. For example, Breland-Nobel and colleagues (2011) found that African-American young adults and their parents reported not trusting providers. They recommend that clinicians be aware of the potential need to explicitly address issues of culturally embedded (mis)trust of doctors and health-care systems. In addition, clinicians may want to consider using motivational interviewing techniques (Miller and Rollnick 2013) to explore ambivalence about initiating treatment, or adapting the intervention to increase relevancy and sensitivity to African-American culture (e.g., incorporation of African-American community members in efforts to encourage youth and family involvement in treatment efforts).

Research continues to document that African-Americans experience racism and discrimination in the health-care system. A recent meta-analysis found that racism was associated with more negative patient experiences in health service, including lower trust, less satisfaction, lower perceived quality of care, compromised patient–provider communication, and delays in accessing health care (Ben et al. 2017). Similar findings of the deleterious effects of racism and discrimination on health extend to the pediatric population. Thakur et al. (2017) found that African-American children who reported experiencing discrimination had 78% greater odds of having asthma and 97% greater odds of poor asthma control relative to African-American children who did not report experiencing discrimination. It is critical for providers to assess for experiences of discrimination when working with African-American youth and consider how such experiences may or may not influence the etiology and maintenance of presenting concerns as well as whether or how experiences of discrimination may impact treatment. For example, due to concerns of racial profiling, African-American parents may be reluctant to allow their children to be outdoors to engage in physical activity due to high police presence in the neighborhood. Providers should strive to create a therapeutic norm and a safe environment for talking about race and racial issues. At the same time, clinicians should exercise care when discussing discrimination to not further marginalize youth and families. For example, when employing cognitive restructuring techniques, it is often not helpful to challenge the validity of cognitions related to discrimination and oppression. Rather, it may be more appropriate to assess the helpfulness of thoughts and beliefs related to discrimination and help youth develop more positive self-talk, identify personal strengths, and develop adaptive coping skills (Hays 2009).

Additional factors to consider when working with African-American youth and families in health-care settings include assessing for culture-specific beliefs about the causes of mental health conditions (e.g., contagion vs. medical causes vs. normative reaction) and attention to differences in the potential meaning of nonadherence to treatment regimens. For example, Ward and Brown (2015) found that African-American participants believed that depression was a normal reaction to life circumstances, thus not warranting treatment. The authors described their addition of a treatment module with culturally sensitive education about the diagnostic process and treatment options in order to enhance engagement in treatment. Assessing for beliefs in mental illness or psychological processes can help inform clinicians which strategies to use to best engage youth and their families. Providers should also be mindful of cultural differences in the meaning of disease management behaviors for racial minority youth. For example, Peek et al. (2008) found that African-American individuals with diabetes perceived nonadherence to their treatment plan as an acceptable method to express control and to indicate active participation in treatment decisions. This example highlights the importance of having open discussions with patients and families and to be mindful to not automatically assume the underlying motivations for noncompliance in treatment.

Consistent with a strength-based approach to care, providers should also be aware of protective and resiliency factors when working with African-American youth and families. Notably, research indicates that positive racial/ethnic identity through racial socialization can serve as a protective factor for African-American youth (Seaton et al. 2012). Providers can assess the ways in which parents communicate information about race and discrimination to their children and normalize communication that fosters racial pride and preparation for bias. These messages have been associated with positive outcomes in many domains including academic, psychological adjustment, and family functioning, and helped buffer the negative consequences of perceived discrimination on health outcomes (Jones and Neblett 2017; Okeke-Adeyanju et al. 2014; Reynolds and Gonzales-Backen 2017). These consistent findings suggest the importance of supporting families in maintaining their cultural traditions (e.g., supporting families with healthy ethnic food recommendations as opposed to providing recommendations for diet that are not culturally syntonic), as well as the potential value in exposing youth to same race role models (e.g., African-American athletes with well-managed diabetes). In addition, clinicians can work with families to develop positive self-statements for coping in cognitive-behavioral treatments that incorporate racial pride, and coping strategies that incorporate preparation for bias (e.g., how to interact with authority figures and how to stay safe) as needed.

Additional strengths that have been found in African-American youth and families include religiosity and strong extended family/kinship support that may be leveraged in treatment. Individuals from African-American cultures tend to rely on informal supports such as churches, family, and friends to manage psychological symptoms (Hays and Aranda 2016). Respecting and encouraging the use of religious and spiritual coping strategies (e.g., praying, using biblical stories for analogies) can enhance trust and rapport. Due to the importance of extended families and community supports, it may be important to identify and incorporate individuals beyond the nuclear family in treatment. For example, Lofton et al. (2016) reviewed culturally adapted obesity interventions for African-American youth and identified joint-youth interventions (i.e., involving family members) and building relationships between mentors and youth as important elements of treatment adaptations.

Considerations in Working with Immigrant Youth and Families in the USA

Although access to care generally improves with successive generations for immigrant families (BeLue et al. 2014), Calvo and Hawkins (2015) found that health disparities persist for immigrant youth and families even to the third-generation (native-born children of native-born parents). There are many unique psychosocial factors that may impact the health of immigrant families including language barriers, separation from and loss of extended family/support system, decrease in socioeconomic status after migration, lack of knowledge of the US health-care system, acculturation stress (stressful experiences or reactions from adjusting to a new country; Berry 2006), and traumatic experiences in the country of origin or from the migration process, all of which may compromise health. Being cognizant of these unique risk factors and systematically assessing for them can aid in treatment conceptualization and planning when working with immigrant populations.

Linguistically competent services have been found to be especially important in pediatric health care. Professional interpretation services can help overcome language barriers with a number of caveats. Clinicians should discuss the parameters of such services with families and be familiar with the considerable challenges of tetradic (parent, child, provider, and interpreter) communication (Pope et al. 2016). In addition, having knowledge of culture-bound syndromes may facilitate communication and understanding especially when conditions or symptoms do not translate well into English (e.g., "gaz" in Haitian culture, "nervios" in some Hispanic cultures). Whenever possible, it may be helpful to encourage youth and/or parents to engage in treatment components in their native language, such as completing cognitive restructuring in their primary language, as thoughts may be distorted or lost in translation (Weiss et al. 2011). Addressing beliefs about mental health and providing psychoeducation to increase understanding and familiarity of mental health disorders as well as the process of psychotherapy may be important for immigrant families, especially if psychotherapy is uncommon in the youth's native culture/country.

Attending to acculturative and traumatic stress not only in immigrant youth but also in their parents is critical (Preciado and D'Anna-Hernandez 2017; Zeiders et al. 2016). In one study, two-thirds of immigrant youth reported experiencing at least one traumatic event, and these stressors varied throughout the migration process in ways that uniquely predicted child mental health outcomes (Cleary et al. 2017). Therefore, providers should routinely screen for trauma symptoms and specifically ask about immigration history when working with immigrant youth. Acculturative stress and stress related to managing a bicultural home may also be significant in immigrant families. In one parent-training example, Parra-Cardona et al. (2012) found that attending to both parents' stress as an immigrant and the unique challenges of navigating a bicultural family were associated with high rates of engagement, retention, and satisfaction among Latino immigrants. Providers should assess for acculturation and related stress in youth and parents/other family members and explore whether varying levels of acculturation exist and how that may impact treatment (e.g., Is an acculturation gap between youth and parents creating parent–child conflict that is interfering with adherence to a medical regimen?). Parents may require referrals for individual services to help manage their own psychological distress associated with the immigration experience.

In addition to a host of culturally relevant risk factors, immigrant families have been documented to have unique resiliency, sometimes highlighted in the literature as the "immigrant paradox." The "immigrant paradox" refers to recent or less acculturated immigrants demonstrating better health outcomes relative to native-born or more acculturated counterparts from the same race or ethnicity despite more adverse socioeconomic circumstances. Research indicates that this counterintuitive finding may be due to immigrant youth and families maintaining aspects of their native cultural lifestyles and behaviors that are protective, such as a more active lifestyle and less consumption of high-fat, processed food relative to US norms (Banna et al. 2012; Delavari et al. 2013). Relatedly, immigrant families also tend to have stronger family cohesion and social support (e.g., more likely to be two-parent households; Akresh and Frank 2008; Child Trends 2014), which are protective against psychological distress. Another explanation involves a selection bias where families that successfully migrate to another country are those that already have physical and psychological strengths to enable them to make such a difficult transition (Akresh and Frank 2008). However, the immigrant paradox does not appear to be universal as scholars have found that it does not generalize across races, ethnicities, age groups, and genders (John et al. 2012; Teruya and Bazargan-Hejazi 2013). Thus, while it is important for providers to assess for strengths associated with immigrant status, particularly protective behaviors fostered by a family's native culture that may be leveraged in treatment (e.g., continuing to promote an active lifestyle), providers should also be mindful of the complexity and heterogeneity that exist among immigrant families.

Hays (2009) recommended that clinicians assess for and build upon cultural strengths to provide culturally competent care. When working with immigrant youth and families, it is important to ask about culturally accepted ways of coping and encourage the continuation of these strategies even if they are not traditionally included in CBT. Promoting culturally accepted coping can help buffer the loss of extended family support systems as a result of migration. For example, youth and families may be encouraged to engage in culturally syntonic self-care activities for behavioral activation. Cultural beliefs and values and strong cultural identity can oftentimes protect immigrant youth from psychological problems. For example, the concept of "familismo" in Latino cultures (i.e., commitment and loyalty to family) has been associated with positive adjustment, particularly serving as a protective factor against internalizing symptoms (Valdivieso-Mora et al. 2016). Thus, it may be important for providers to consult and collaborate with family members and extended family and encourage them to be a part of the treatment process. Similarly, for Chinese immigrants, Chinese principles may be used to illustrate CBT concepts to enhance understanding and motivation. For example, the use of coping skills can be framed as a way to rebalance one's Qi if in keeping with the families' beliefs and traditions.

Considerations in Working with LGBTQ Youth and Their Families

Many have suggested that literature focused on competence in working with racial and ethnic minority clients has been useful in developing frameworks for improving care with sexual and gender minority individuals (Boroughs et al. 2015). Sexual minority here refers to individuals who are not exclusively heterosexual in their sexual attraction or behavior, while gender minority refers to individuals who identify in ways that do not fit into binary definitions of gender (including transgender and gender nonconforming youth). While sexual and gender minority status have been associated with increased stress, health, and mental health risk, they are not conceptualized as mental disorders.

Homosexuality was historically defined as mental illness until 1973 and "conversion" or "reparation" therapies seeking to "eradicate homosexuality," despite being banned in several states and evidence demonstrating potential harm to patients, continue to be practiced across the USA (Drescher et al. 2016; Herek 2010). Therefore, it is important to note that the American Psychological Association "encourages mental health professionals to… utilize affirmative multiculturally competent and client-centered approaches that recognize the impact of social stigma on sexual minorities" (Anton 2010, p. 464). Also, of note, while the most recent Diagnostic and Statistical Manual of Mental Disorders includes a diagnosis of "gender dysphoria," there is a clear distinction made between gender dysphoria and gender nonconformity, which is not a mental disorder (DSM-5; APA 2013). Specifically, the American Psychological

Association has resolved that "diverse gender expressions, regardless of gender identity, and diverse gender identities, beyond a binary classification, are normal and positive variations of the human experience" (APA and NASP 2015). A few important domains of consideration for clinicians working with sexual and gender minority youth in health-care settings are discussed here.

Understanding patients' sexual orientation and gender identity is key to competent care (Levine 2013). However, there is evidence that providers are often uncomfortable discussing sexuality with youth and frequently use non-inclusive language in ways that are stressful to youth (e.g., "do you have a girlfriend/boyfriend?" Alexander et al. 2014; Fuzzell et al. 2016). Furthermore, institutional policies and practices may be problematic for sexual and gender minority parents (e.g., practices that do not allow two mothers to be present during a procedure but allow two opposite sex parents, questionnaires that ask about parent's relationship status in non-inclusive ways, etc.). Recommendations for competent care include ongoing training for providers and staff, review of existing policies/practices that may be discriminatory, and creating a safe environment for youth and families (e.g., using visible signage in clinics such as those indicating clinics are a 'Safe Zone;" Oransky et al. 2018). Resources developed by the UC Davis Health system (https://myhs.ucdmc.ucdavis.edu/web/lgbti) may be helpful to pediatric providers in health settings. These include recommended interview questions for adolescents and young adults (e.g., "Some of the teens I work with have feelings of attraction to members of the same sex. This is perfectly OK, but it worries some teens a lot. So I'm wondering, do you have ever these kinds of feelings or worries?"); trainings for health-care providers, students, and staff; as well as information about how to incorporate sexual orientation and gender identity data into the electronic health record (Callahan et al. 2015).

Beyond assessing patient orientation/identity and improving non-inclusive or heterosexist language, providers should also assess for potential stigma-related stress experienced by sexual and gender minority youth in their care. Stigma-related stress in this population includes objective stressful events including discrimination as well as a patient's expectation/vigilance surrounding these events and internalization of negative attitudes towards the self. These stressors have been consistently implicated in health disparities that exist for sexual and gender minority youth (Meyer 2003; Hatzenbuehler 2009; Hendricks and Testa 2012). It is important that clinicians ask youth about stressors commonly experienced by sexual and gender minority youth—especially those experienced in the school and home environments (Higa et al. 2014).

Hostile peer interactions, school climate, and bullying are experienced by a majority of sexual and gender minority youth and are related to health outcomes such as suicide risk and substance use (Berlan et al. 2010; Earnshaw et al. 2016; Kosciw et al. 2016; Reisner et al. 2015). Current studies suggest that youth are "coming out" at younger ages today than ever before. This may be associated with increased exposure to harassment and "intense interpersonal regulation of gender and sexuality" by peers at younger developmental stages (Russell and Fish 2016). Providers should educate families about these stressors and their rights related to bullying and harassment, advocate for changes to policies and practices that can improve outcomes for all sexual and gender minority youth (e.g., the adoption of comprehensive bullying/harassment policies), and plan treatment according to each patient's specific needs in these contexts. For example, cognitive behavioral strategies aimed at increasing pleasurable activities, reducing isolation and social anxiety, using problem-solving skills to decrease stress and find safe spaces, and addressing cognitive distortions (e.g., beliefs such as "something must be wrong with me if I am this way") have all been recommended (Perry et al. 2017; Safren et al. 2001).

A strength-based and affirmative approach has been preferred in most existing treatment guidelines and recommendations for sexual and gender minority youth (e.g., APA 2012; Austin and Craig 2015). Family and peer acceptance and support have been consistently identified as protective factors and are associated with improved outcomes for sexual and gender minority youth including greater sense of well-being and self-acceptance, reduced depressive symptoms and suicidal thoughts, and increased self-esteem (Shilo and Savaya 2011; Snapp et al. 2015). Of note, Snapp et al. (2015) found that family acceptance during adolescence predicted multiple positive adjustment outcomes in young adulthood. Further, family acceptance was the strongest predictor of positive outcomes, beyond peer and community support. Clinicians in pediatric health settings are already familiar with the importance of family support in trauma, injury rehabilitation, and chronic disease management. When working with gender and sexual minority youth in these contexts, it is particularly important to understand the potential influence of minority status on family support and relationships. Ryan's (2013) Family Acceptance Project provides evidence-based resources including family educational booklets available in several languages, faith-based materials for parents, and provider and family training videos (https://familyproject.sfsu.edu/). These resources provide a spectrum of ways in which to engage families "where they are," such as reducing harm and rejection behaviors among parents who may not accept their child's orientation/identity and promoting comfort in communication within families with greater levels of acceptance.

Systemic and Contextual Barriers to Quality Care for Diverse Youth and Families

Beyond cultural considerations, it is important for clinicians to be mindful of common roadblocks faced by marginalized groups and how these challenges can increase the difficulty of obtaining quality care (Avila and Bramlett 2013; Chando et al. 2013). Underutilization of services has often been linked to racial/ethnic and sexual minority status. Social determinants of health such as low education, poverty, lack of insurance, and stigma have been demonstrated to impede access to quality care for minority youth (Beck et al. 2018; Dreyer 2013). In addition to assessing important cultural domains, providers should systematically assess social determinants of health that may impact patients' access to care and health outcomes (e.g., access to transportation, housing, and quality food; Garg et al. 2015). Assessing for social determinants of health can lead to more effective care by ensuring that treatment recommendations are meaningful/feasible (e.g., not recommending purchasing fresh fruits and vegetables to youth and families who are homeless and lack appropriate refrigeration) and by the provision of resources necessary to address specific barriers (e.g., providing support for health insurance access, transportation voucher program information).

Disparities also exist in health literacy and health-related communication experienced by minority youth and families such that interventions to improve communication could lead to higher quality care (IOM 2011). Low health literacy among parents/caregivers has been associated with poor health-care navigation, fewer prevention-related medical encounters, and less satisfaction with the quality of collaboration with health-care providers (Yin et al. 2012), resulting in poorer health outcomes among minority youth. For example, Pulgarón and colleagues (2014) found that low health literacy such as numeracy skills among parents of youth with type 1 diabetes was positively correlated with poorer disease outcomes in diabetes management. Additionally, higher health literacy, including reading and numeracy skills, among parents/caregivers of children with asthma has been associated with better disease outcomes, such as better asthma control and parental asthma knowledge (Harrington et al. 2015). Ensuring that education is provided in multiple formats, with simple language explanations and frequent checks for youth and family understanding can be helpful. Furthermore, existing health literacy toolkits may be helpful to providers in making changes to their practice (DeWalt et al. 2010; Silberholz et al. 2017).

Beyond literacy, disparities in health communication include differences in provider communication with patients/caregivers. Studies have found differences in relationship-building talk, information exchange, and decision-making processes for racial/ethnic minority patients compared to those for non-Hispanic, White patients during medical encounters (Cox et al. 2012). These differences are associated with less patient/caregiver satisfaction with care and poorer disease management (Valenzuela and Smith 2015). Awareness of these disparities in care and efforts to incorporate developmentally appropriate provider–caregiver–patient interactions into patient encounters may be important efforts in reducing existing gaps in the quality of care received by minority youth and families.

Finally, we note the significance of limitations of the existing research for improving our practice and the outcomes of minority youth and families. Researchers should seek to specifically describe patient populations on important minority status variables including patient race, ethnicity, immigrant status/acculturation, sexual orientation, and gender identity whenever possible. In addition, racial and ethnic minority youth, lower income youth, and other marginalized groups are currently underrepresented in research (Robinson et al. 2016). Recruitment and retention of minority youth and families must be addressed in order to further our understanding of EBT for the diverse youth and families we serve. Disparities in research participation are related to historic mistrust, limited representation among research staff, limited knowledge about research, and other barriers (e.g., Raphael et al. 2017). Strategies for improving minority research participation have been described (e.g., Flores et al. 2017; Brannon et al. 2013; Ireland et al. 2015) and include optimizing cultural/linguistic competency, staff training on participant relationships and trust, electronic tracking, reinforcing study importance for children, families, and communities, and other strategies.

Conclusion

This chapter highlights the significant health disparities that exist for the racial/ethnic, sexual, and gender minority youth that we serve in medical settings. As the US population has transformed, these disparities have been costly and have changed the face of the work that clinicians do. We are optimistic given evidence that existing treatments, including cognitive behavioral therapies, can improve the outcomes of minority youth and families. The implementation of systems of care that increase marginalized youth and families' access to these treatments is one of many new frontiers that needs to be embarked upon in our field.

Existing treatments are beneficial for diverse populations based on the extent to which they can be faithfully but flexibly applied. This chapter has reviewed important culturally relevant domains for consideration including historic mistrust, stigma, acculturative stress, and discrimination that are important to understand and assess in order to address the needs of minority youth and families. In addition, we have highlighted how movements towards personalization of treatment, including cultural adaptations, modular therapy programs, and adaptive intervention techniques, will benefit minority patients with unique risk and resiliency profiles and influential cultural and contextual influences. These new approaches are also likely to be favored by clinicians, who prefer flexible and tailored treatment approaches (versus rigid manualization of care).

Clinicians should continue to be innovative in addressing youth and families' needs as the populations they care for continue to change. Beyond cultural factors, we have noted the need for clinicians to be well connected in their communities and to assess for social determinants of health that are often significant barriers to patient wellness. "The train has left the station," and pediatric providers across the USA will be working within "majority minority" health-care environments. The need to address the existing gaps in the health of minority youth is one of our most urgent priorities.

References

Akresh, I. R., & Frank, R. (2008). Health selection among new immigrants. *American Journal of Public Health, 98*(11), 2058–2064. https://doi.org/10.2105/AJPH.2006.100974.

Alexander, S. C., Fortenberry, J. D., Pollak, K. I., Bravender, T., Østbye, T., & Shields, C. G. (2014). Physicians' use of inclusive sexual orientation language during teenage annual visits. *LGBT Health, 1*(4), 283–291. https://doi.org/10.1089/lgbt.2014.0035.

American Psychiatric Association. (2013). *Diagnostic and statistical manual of mental disorders (DSM-5)* (5th ed.). Arlington, VA: American Psychiatric Publishing. https://doi.org/10.1176/appi.books.9780890425596.

American Psychological Association. (2012). Guidelines for psychological practice with lesbian, gay, and bisexual clients. *The American Psychologist, 67*(1), 10–42. https://doi.org/10.1037/a0024659.

American Psychological Association & National Association of School Psychologists. (2015). *Resolution on gender and sexual orientation diversity in children and adolescents in schools*. Retrieved from http://www.apa.org/about/policy/orientation-diversity.aspx

American Psychological Association Presidential Task Force on Evidence-Based Practice. (2006). Evidence-based practice in psychology. *American Psychologist, 61*(4), 271. https://doi.org/10.1037/0003-066X.61.4.271.

Anton, B. S. (2010). Proceedings of the American Psychological Association for the legislative year 2009: Minutes of the annual meeting of the council of representatives and minutes of the meetings of the board of directors. *American Psychologist, 65*(5), 385–475. https://doi.org/10.1037/a0019553.

Austin, A., & Craig, S. L. (2015). Transgender affirmative cognitive behavioral therapy: Clinical considerations and applications. *Professional Psychology: Research and Practice, 46*(1), 21. https://doi.org/10.1037/a0038642.

Avila, R. M., & Bramlett, M. D. (2013). Language and immigrant status effects on disparities in Hispanic children's health status and access to health care. *Maternal and Child Health Journal, 17*(3), 415–423. https://doi.org/10.1007/s10995-012-0988-9.

Aylward, B. S., Bender, J. A., Graves, M. M., & Roberts, M. C. (2009). Historical developments and trends in pediatric psychology. In M. C. Roberts & R. G. Steele (Eds.), *Handbook of pediatric psychology* (4th ed., pp. 3–18). New York, NY: Guilford Press.

Banna, J. C., Kaiser, L., Drake, C., & Townsend, M. (2012). Acculturation, physical activity and television viewing in Hispanic women: Findings from the 2005 California Women's Health Survey. *Public Health Nutrition, 15*, 198–207. https://doi.org/10.1017/S1368980011001273.

Barrera, M., Jr., Castro, F. G., Strycker, L. A., & Toobert, D. J. (2013). Cultural adaptations of behavioral health interventions: A progress report. *Journal of Consulting and Clinical Psychology, 81*(2), 196–205. https://doi.org/10.1037/a0027085.

Barrera, M., Jr., Berkel, C., & Castro, F. G. (2017). Directions for the advancement of culturally adapted preventive interventions: Local adaptations, engagement, and sustainability. *Prevention Science, 18*(6), 640–648. https://doi.org/10.1007/s11121-016-0705-9.

Beck, A. F., Cohen, A. J., Colvin, J. D., Fichtenberg, C. M., Fleegler, E. W., Garg, A., et al. (2018). Perspectives from the Society for Pediatric Research: Interventions targeting social needs in pediatric clinical care. *Pediatric Research, 83*(6), 1–12. https://doi.org/10.1038/s41390-018-0012-1.

BeLue, R., Miranda, P., Elewonibi, B., & Hillemeier, M. (2014). The association of generation status and health insurance among US children. *Pediatrics, 134*, 307–314. https://doi.org/10.1542/peds.2013-3337.

Ben, J., Cormack, D., Harris, R., & Paradies, Y. (2017). Racism and health service utilisation: A systematic review and meta-analysis. *PLoS One, 12*, e0189900. https://doi.org/10.1371/journal.pone.0189900.

Berlan, E. D., Corliss, H. L., Field, A. E., Goodman, E., & Austin, S. B. (2010). Sexual orientation and bullying among adolescents in the growing up today study. *Journal of Adolescent Health, 46*(4), 366–371. https://doi.org/10.1016/j.jadohealth.2009.10.015.

Bernal, G., Jiménez-Chafey, M. I., & Domenech Rodríguez, M. M. (2009). Cultural adaptation of treatments: A resource for considering culture in evidence-based practice. *Professional Psychology: Research and Practice, 40*(4), 361–368. https://doi.org/10.1037/a0016401.

Berry, J. W. (2006). Acculturative stress. In T. Wong & G. Wong (Eds.), *Handbook of multicultural perspectives on stress and coping* (pp. 287–295). Dallas, TX: Spring Publications.

Boroughs, M. S., Bedoya, C. A., O'Cleirigh, C., & Safren, S. A. (2015). Toward defining, measuring, and evaluating LGBT cultural competence for psychologists. *Clinical Psychology: Science and Practice, 22*(2), 151–171. https://doi.org/10.1111/cpsp.12098.

Brannon, E. E., Kuhl, E. S., Boles, R. E., Aylward, B. S., Benoit Ratcliff, M., Valenzuela, J. M., et al. (2013). Strategies for recruitment and retention of families from low-income, ethnic minority backgrounds in a longitudinal study of caregiver feeding and child weight. *Children's Health Care, 42*(3), 198–213. https://doi.org/10.1080/02739615.2013.816590.

Breland-Noble, A., Bell, C., Burriss, A., & AAKOMA Project Adult Advisory Board. (2011). "Mama just won't accept this": Adult perspectives on engaging depressed African American teens in clinical research and treatment. *Journal of Clinical Psychology in Medical Settings, 18*, 225–234. https://doi.org/10.1007/s10880-011-9235-6.

Callahan, E. J., Sitkin, N., Ton, H., Eidson-Ton, W. S., Weckstein, J., & Latimore, D. (2015). Introducing sexual orientation and gender identity into the electronic health record: One academic health center's experience. *Academic Medicine, 90*(2), 154–160. https://doi.org/10.1097/ACM.0000000000000467.

Calvo, R., & Hawkins, S. (2015). Disparities in quality of healthcare of children from immigrant families in the US. *Maternal and Child Health Journal, 19*, 2223–2232. https://doi.org/10.1007/s10995-015-1740-z.

Castro, F. G., Barrera, M., Jr., & Steiker, L. K. H. (2010). Issues and challenges in the design of culturally adapted evidence-based interventions. *Annual Review of Clinical Psychology, 6*, 213–239. https://doi.org/10.1146/annurev-clinpsy-033109-132032.

Chando, S., Tiro, J. A., Harris, T. R., Kobrin, S., & Breen, N. (2013). Effects of socioeconomic status and health care access on low levels of human papillomavirus vaccination among Spanish-speaking Hispanics in California. *American Journal of Public Health, 103*(2), 270–272. https://doi.org/10.2105/AJPH.2012.300920.

Child Trends Data Bank. (2014, October). *Immigrant children: Indicators of child and youth well-being.* Retrieved from https://www.childtrends.org/wp-content/uploads/2013/07/110_Immigrant_Children.pdf

Cleary, S. D., Snead, R., Dietz-Chavez, D., Rivera, I., & Edberg, M. (2017). Immigrant trauma and mental health outcomes among Latino youth. *Journal of Immigrant and Minority Health., 20*, 1053. https://doi.org/10.1007/s10903-017-0673-6.

Coker, T. R., Austin, S. B., & Schuster, M. A. (2010). The health and health care of lesbian, gay, and bisexual adolescents. *Annual Review of Public Health, 31*, 457–477. https://doi.org/10.1146/annurev.publhealth.012809.103636.

Conn, V. S., Enriquez, M., Ruppar, T. M., & Chan, K. C. (2014). Cultural relevance in medication adherence interventions with underrepresented adults: Systematic review and meta-analysis of outcomes. *Preventive Medicine: An International Journal Devoted to Practice and Theory, 69*, 239–247. https://doi.org/10.1016/j.ypmed.2014.10.021.

Cox, E. D., Nackers, K. A., Young, H. N., Moreno, M. A., Levy, J. F., & Mangione-Smith, R. M. (2012). Influence of race and socioeconomic status on engagement in pediatric primary care. *Patient Education and Counseling, 87*(3), 319–326. https://doi.org/10.1016/j.pec.2011.09.012.

Delavari, M., Sønderlund, A. L., Swinburn, B., Mellor, D., & Renzaho, A. (2013). Acculturation and obesity among migrant populations in high income countries–a systematic review. *BMC Public Health, 13*(1), 458. https://doi.org/10.1186/1471-2458-13-458.

DeWalt, D. A., Callahan, L. F., Hawk, V. H., Broucksou, K. A., Hink, A., Rudd, R., & Brach, C. (2010). *Health literacy universal precautions toolkit* (pp. 1–227). Rockville, MD: Agency for Healthcare Research and Quality. https://doi.org/10.1016/j.outlook.2010.12.002.

Domenech Rodríguez, M. M., & Bernal, G. (2012). Bridging the gap between research and practice in a multicultural world. In G. Bernal & M. M. D. Rodríguez (Eds.), *Cultural adaptations: Tools for evidence-based practice with diverse populations* (pp. 265–287). Washington, DC: American Psychological Association. https://doi.org/10.1037/13752-013.

Domenech Rodríguez, M. M. D., Baumann, A. A., & Schwartz, A. L. (2011). Cultural adaptation of an evidence-based intervention: From theory to practice in a Latino/a community context. *American Journal of Community Psychology, 47*(1–2), 170–186. https://doi.org/10.1007/s10464-010-9371-4.

Drescher, J., Schwartz, A., Casoy, F., McIntosh, C. A., Hurley, B., Ashley, K., et al. (2016). The growing regulation of conversion therapy. *Journal of Medical Regulation, 102*(2), 7–12. https://doi.org/10.30770/2572-1852-102.2.7.

Dreyer, B. P. (2013). To create a better world for children and families: the case for ending childhood poverty. *Academic Pediatrics, 13*(2), 83–90. https://doi.org/10.1016/j.acap.2013.01.005.

Earnshaw, V. A., Bogart, L. M., Poteat, V. P., Reisner, S. L., & Schuster, M. A. (2016). Bullying among lesbian, gay, bisexual, and transgender youth. *Pediatric Clinics, 63*(6), 999–1010. https://doi.org/10.1016/j.pcl.2016.07.004.

Feagin, J., & Bennefield, Z. (2014). Systemic racism and US health care. *Social Science & Medicine, 103*, 7–14. https://doi.org/10.1016/j.socscimed.2013.09.006.

Federal Interagency Forum on Child and Family Statistics. (2017). *America's children: Key national indicators of well-being, 2017.* Washington, DC: U.S. Government Printing Office. Retrieved from https://www.childstats.gov/americaschildren/members.asp

Flores, G., Portillo, A., Lin, H., Walker, C., Fierro, M., Henry, M., & Massey, K. (2017). A successful approach to minimizing attrition in racial/ethnic minority, low-income populations. *Contemporary Clinical Trials Communications, 5*, 168–174. https://doi.org/10.1016/j.conctc.2017.01.009.

Friedberg, R. D., Hoyman, L. C., Behar, S., Tabbarah, S., Pacholec, N. M., Keller, M., & Thordarson, M. A. (2014). We've come a long way, baby!: Evolution and revolution in CBT with youth. *Journal of Rational-Emotive & Cognitive-Behavior Therapy, 32*(1), 4–14. https://doi.org/10.1007/s10942-014-0178-3.

Fuzzell, L., Fedesco, H. N., Alexander, S. C., Fortenberry, J. D., & Shields, C. G. (2016). "I just think that doctors need to ask more questions": Sexual minority and majority adolescents' experiences talking about sexuality with healthcare providers. *Patient Education and Counseling, 99*(9), 1467–1472. https://doi.org/10.1016/j.pec.2016.06.004.

Garg, A., Toy, S., Tripodis, Y., Silverstein, M., & Freeman, E. (2015). Addressing social determinants of health at well child care visits: A cluster RCT. *Pediatrics, 135*(2), e296–e304. https://doi.org/10.1542/peds.2014-2888.

Gayes, L. A., & Steele, R. G. (2014). A meta-analysis of motivational interviewing interventions for pediatric health behavior change. *Journal of Consulting and Clinical Psychology, 82*(3), 521–535. https://doi.org/10.1037/a0035917.

Hamilton, J. D., Kendall, P. C., Gosch, E., Furr, J. M., & Sood, E. (2008). Flexibility within fidelity. *Journal of the American Academy of Child & Adolescent Psychiatry, 47*(9), 987–993. https://doi.org/10.1097/CHI.0b013e31817eed2f.

Harper, F. W. K., Eggly, S., Crider, B., Kobayashi, H., Meert, K. L., Ball, A., et al. (2015). Patient- and family-centered care as an approach to reducing disparities in asthma outcomes in urban African American children: A review of the literature. *Journal of the National Medical Association, 107*(2), 4–17. https://doi.org/10.1016/S0027-9684(15)30019-5.

Harrington, K. F., Zhang, B., Magruder, T., Bailey, W. C., & Gerald, L. B. (2015). The impact of parent's health literacy on pediatric asthma outcomes. *Pediatric Allergy, Immunology, and Pulmonology, 28*(1), 20–26. https://doi.org/10.1089/ped.2014.0379.

Haselkorn, T., Lee, J. H., Mink, D. R., Weiss, S. T., & TENOR Study Group. (2008). Racial disparities in asthma-related health outcomes in severe or difficult-to-treat asthma. *Annals of Allergy, Asthma & Immunology, 101*(3), 256–263. https://doi.org/10.1016/S1081-1206(10)60490-5.

Hatzenbuehler, M. L. (2009). How does sexual minority stigma "get under the skin"? A psychological mediation framework. *Psychological Bulletin, 135*(5), 707. https://doi.org/10.1037/a0016441.

Hays, P. A. (2008). *Addressing cultural complexities in practice: Assessment, diagnosis, and therapy*. Washington, DC: American Psychological Association. https://doi.org/10.1037/11650-000.

Hays, P. A. (2009). Integrating evidence-based practice, cognitive–behavior therapy, and multicultural therapy: Ten steps for culturally competent practice. *Professional Psychology: Research and Practice, 40*(4), 354–360.

Hays, K., & Aranda, M. P. (2016). Faith-based mental health interventions with African-Americans: A review. *Research on Social Work Practice, 26*(7), 777–789. https://doi.org/10.1177/1049731515569356.

Healey, P., Stager, M. L., Woodmass, K., Dettlaff, A. J., Vergara, A., Janke, R., & Wells, S. J. (2017). Cultural adaptations to augment health and mental health services: A systematic review. *BMC Health Services Research, 17*(1), 8. https://doi.org/10.1186/s12913-016-1953-x.

Hendricks, M. L., & Testa, R. J. (2012). A conceptual framework for clinical work with transgender and gender nonconforming clients: An adaptation of the minority stress model. *Professional Psychology: Research and Practice, 43*(5), 460–467. https://doi.org/10.1037/a0029597.

Herek, G. M. (2010). Sexual orientation differences as deficits: Science and stigma in the history of American psychology. *Perspectives on Psychological Science, 5*(6), 693–699. https://doi.org/10.1177/1745691610388770.

Hettema, J., Steele, J., & Miller, W. R. (2005). Motivational interviewing. *Annual Review of Clinical Psychology, 1*(1), 91–111. https://doi.org/10.1146/annurev.clinpsy.1.102803.143833.

Higa, D., Hoppe, M. J., Lindhorst, T., Mincer, S., Beadnell, B., Morrison, D. M., et al. (2014). Negative and positive factors associated with the well-being of lesbian, gay, bisexual, transgender, queer, and questioning (LGBTQ) youth. *Youth & Society, 46*(5), 663–687. https://doi.org/10.1177/0044118X12449630.

Hilliard, M. E., Ernst, M. M., Gray, W. N., Saeed, S. A., & Cortina, S. (2012). Adapting pediatric psychology interventions: Lessons learned in treating families from the middle east. *Journal of Pediatric Psychology, 37*(8), 882–892. https://doi.org/10.1093/jpepsy/jsr084.

Hilliard, M. E., Wu, Y. P., Rausch, J., Dolan, L. M., & Hood, K. K. (2013). Predictors of deteriorations in diabetes management and control in adolescents with type 1 diabetes. *Journal of Adolescent Health, 52*(1), 28–34. https://doi.org/10.1016/j.jadohealth.2012.05.009.

Hoffman, K. M., Trawalter, S., Axt, J. R., & Oliver, M. N. (2016). Racial bias in pain assessment and treatment recommendations, and false beliefs about biological differences between blacks and whites. *PNAS Proceedings of the National Academy of Sciences of the United States of America, 113*(16), 4296–4301. https://doi.org/10.1073/pnas.1516047113.

Huey, S. J., Jr., & Polo, A. J. (2017). Evidence-based psychotherapies with ethnic minority children and adolescents. In J. R. Weisz & A. E. Kazdin (Eds.), *Evidence-based psychotherapies for children and adolescents* (3rd ed., pp. 361–378). New York, NY: Guilford Press.

Huey, S. J., Jr., Tilley, J. L., Jones, E. O., & Smith, C. A. (2014). The contribution of cultural competence to evidence-based care for ethnically diverse populations. *Annual Review of Clinical Psychology, 10*, 305–338. https://doi.org/10.1146/annurev-clinpsy-032813-153729.

Institute of Medicine. (2011). *Innovations in health literacy research: Workshop summary*. Washington, DC: The National Academies Press. https://doi.org/10.17226/13016.

Ireland, K. A., Manders, A. J., Corkey, B. E., & Lenders, C. M. (2015). Recruitment in a pediatric clinical research trial targeting underserved populations: Efforts and challenges. *Journal of Obesity & Weight Loss Therapy, 5*(3), 262. https://doi.org/10.4172/2165-7904.1000262.

John, D. A., de Castro, A. B., Martin, D. P., Duran, B., & Takeuchi, D. T. (2012). Does an immigrant health paradox exist among Asian Americans? Associations of nativity and occupational class with self-rated health and mental disorders. *Social Science & Medicine, 75*(12), 2085–2098. https://doi.org/10.1016/j.socscimed.2012.01.035.

Jones, S. C. T., & Neblett, E. W. (2017). Future directions in research on racism-related stress and racial-ethnic protective factors for black youth. *Journal of Clinical Child and Adolescent Psychology, 46*(5), 754–766. https://doi.org/10.1080/15374416.2016.1146991.

Kahana, S., Drotar, D., & Frazier, T. (2008). Meta-analysis of psychological interventions to promote adherence to treatment in pediatric chronic health conditions. *Journal of Pediatric Psychology, 33*(6), 590–611. https://doi.org/10.1093/jpepsy/jsm128.

Kann, L., McManus, T., Harris, W. A., Shanklin, S. L., Flint, K. H., Queen, B., et al. (2018). Youth Risk Behavior Surveillance—United States, 2017. *MMWR Surveillance Summaries, 67*(8), 1–114. https://doi.org/10.15585/mmwr.ss6708a1.

Kirkpatrick, S. I., Dodd, K. W., Reedy, J., & Krebs-Smith, S. M. (2012). Income and race/ethnicity are associated with adherence to food-based dietary guidance among US adults and children. *Journal of the Academy of*

Nutrition and Dietetics, 112(5), 624–635. https://doi.org/10.1016/j.jand.2011.11.012.
Kosciw, J. G., Greytak, E. A., Giga, N. M., Villenas, C., & Danischewski, D. J. (2016). The 2015 National School Climate Survey: The experiences of lesbian, gay, bisexual, transgender, and queer youth in our Nation's schools. Gay, lesbian and straight education network. New York: GLSEN.
LaVeist, T. A., Gaskin, D. J., & Richard, P. (2009). The economic burden of health inequalities in the United States. Washington, DC: Joint Center for Political and Economic Studies.
Levine, D. A. (2013). Office-based care for lesbian, gay, bisexual, transgender, and questioning youth. Pediatrics, 132(1), e297–e313. https://doi.org/10.1542/peds.2013-1283.
Lewis-Fernández, R., Aggarwal, N. K., Hinton, L., Hinton, D. E., & Kirmayer, L. J. (2016). DSM-5 handbook on the cultural formulation interview. Arlington, VA: American Psychiatric Publishing.
Lofton, S., Julion, W. A., McNaughton, D. B., Bergren, M. D., & Keim, K. S. (2016). A systematic review of literature on culturally adapted obesity prevention interventions for African-American youth. The Journal of School Nursing, 32(1), 32–46. https://doi.org/10.1177/1059840515605508.
Lundahl, B. W., Kunz, C., Brownell, C., Tollefson, D., & Burke, B. L. (2010). A meta-analysis of motivational interviewing: Twenty-five years of empirical studies. Research on Social Work Practice, 20(2), 137–160. https://doi.org/10.1177/1049731509347850.
Maloney, R., Clay, D. L., & Robinson, J. (2005). Sociocultural issues in pediatric transplantation: A conceptual model. Journal of Pediatric Psychology, 30(3), 235–246. https://doi.org/10.1093/jpepsy/jsi034.
Manias, E., & Williams, A. (2010). Medication adherence in people of culturally and linguistically diverse backgrounds: A meta-analysis. Annals of Pharmacotherapy, 44(6), 964–982. https://doi.org/10.1345/aph.1M572.
Marshal, M. P., Dietz, L. J., Friedman, M. S., Stall, R., Smith, H. A., McGinley, J., et al. (2011). Suicidality and depression disparities between sexual minority and heterosexual youth: A meta-analytic review. Journal of Adolescent Health, 49(2), 115–123. https://doi.org/10.1016/j.jadohealth.2011.02.005.
Meyer, I. H. (2003). Prejudice, social stress, and mental health in lesbian, gay, and bisexual populations: Conceptual issues and research evidence. Psychological Bulletin, 129(5), 674–697. https://doi.org/10.1037/0033-2909.129.5.674.
Miller, W., & Rollnick, S. (2013). Motivational interviewing: Helping people change (3rd ed.). New York, NY: Guildford Press.
Naranjo, D., D Schwartz, D., & M Delamater, A. (2015). Diabetes in ethnically diverse youth: Disparate burden and intervention approaches. Current Diabetes Reviews, 11(4), 251–260. https://doi.org/10.2174/1573399811666150421115846.
Ng, M. Y., & Weisz, J. R. (2016). Annual research review: Building a science of personalized intervention for youth mental health. Journal of Child Psychology and Psychiatry, 57(3), 216–236. https://doi.org/10.1111/jcpp.12470.
Nicholl, M. C., Valenzuela, J. M., Lit, K., DeLucia, C., Shoulberg, A. M., Rohan, J. M., ... & Delamater, A. M. (2019). Featured article: comparison of diabetes management trajectories in Hispanic versus white Non-Hispanic youth with Type 1 Diabetes across early adolescence. Journal of pediatric psychology, 44(6), 631–641. https://doi.org/10.1093/jpepsy/jsz011.
Nicolas, G., Arntz, D. L., Hirsch, B., & Schmiedigen, A. (2009). Cultural adaptation of a group treatment for Haitian American adolescents. Professional Psychology: Research and Practice, 40(4), 378–384. https://doi.org/10.1037/a0016307.
Norcross, J. C., & Wampold, B. E. (2011). What works for whom: Tailoring psychotherapy to the person. Journal of Clinical Psychology, 67(2), 127–132. https://doi.org/10.1002/jclp.20764.
Okeke-Adeyanju, N., Taylor, L. C., Craig, A. B., Smith, R. E., Thomas, A., Boyle, A. E., & DeRosier, M. E. (2014). Celebrating the strengths of black youth: Increasing self-esteem and implications for prevention. The Journal of Primary Prevention, 35(5), 357–369. https://doi.org/10.1007/s10935-014-0356-1.
Oransky, M., Burke, E. Z., & Steever, J. (2018). An interdisciplinary model for meeting the mental health needs of transgender adolescents and young adults: the Mount Sinai Adolescent Health Center approach. Cognitive and Behavioral Practice. https://doi.org/10.1016/j.cbpra.2018.03.002.
Parra-Cardona, J. R., Domenech-Rodriguez, M., Forgatch, M., Sullivan, C., Bybee, D., Holtrop, K., et al. (2012). Culturally adapting an evidence-based parenting intervention for Latino immigrants: The need to integrate fidelity and cultural relevance. Family Process, 51(1), 56–72. https://doi.org/10.1111/j.1545-5300.2012.01386.x.
Peek, M. E., Quinn, M. T., Gorawara-Bhat, R., Odoms-Young, A., Wilson, S. C., & Chin, M. H. (2008). How is shared decision-making defined among African-Americans with diabetes? Patient Education and Counseling, 72(3), 450–458. https://doi.org/10.1016/j.pec.2008.05.018.
Perry, N. S., Chaplo, S. D., & Baucom, K. J. W. (2017). The impact of cumulative minority stress on cognitive behavioral treatment with gender minority individuals: Case study and clinical recommendations. Cognitive and Behavioral Practice, 24(4), 472–483. https://doi.org/10.1016/j.cbpra.2016.12.004.
Pinquart, M., & Shen, Y. (2011). Behavior problems in children and adolescents with chronic physical illness: A meta-analysis. Journal of Pediatric Psychology, 36(9), 1003–1016. https://doi.org/10.1093/jpepsy/jsr042.
Pope, C. A., Escobar-Gomez, M., Davis, B. H., Roberts, J. R., O'Brien, E. S., Hinton, E., & Darden, P. M. (2016). The challenge of tetradic relationships in medically interpreted pediatric primary care visits: A descriptive study of communication practices. Patient Education and Counseling, 99, 542–548. https://doi.org/10.1016/j.pec.2015.10.032.

Preciado, A., & D'Anna-Hernandez, K. (2017). Acculturative stress is associated with trajectory of anxiety symptoms during pregnancy in Mexican-American women. *Journal of Anxiety Disorders, 48*, 28–35. https://doi.org/10.1016/j.janxdis.2016.10.005.

Pulgarón, E. R., Sanders, L. M., Patiño-Fernandez, A. M., Wile, D., Sanchez, J., Rothman, R. L., & Delamater, A. M. (2014). Glycemic control in young children with diabetes: The role of parental health literacy. *Patient Education and Counseling, 94*(1), 67–70. https://doi.org/10.1016/j.pec.2013.09.002.

Raphael, J. L., Lion, K. C., & Bearer, C. F. (2017). Policy solutions to recruiting and retaining minority children in research. *Pediatric Research, 82*(2), 180. https://doi.org/10.1038/pr.2017.119.

Reisner, S. L., Greytak, E. A., Parsons, J. T., & Ybarra, M. L. (2015). Gender minority social stress in adolescence: Disparities in adolescent bullying and substance use by gender identity. *Journal of Sex Research, 52*(3), 243–256. https://doi.org/10.1080/00224499.2014.886321.

Resnicow, K., Jackson, A., Braithwaite, R., DiIorio, C., Blisset, D., Rahotep, S., & Periasamy, S. (2002). Healthy body/healthy Spirit: A church-based nutrition and physical activity intervention. *Health Education Research, 17*(5), 562–563. https://doi.org/10.1093/her/17.5.562.

Reynolds, J. E., & Gonzales-Backen, M. A. (2017). Ethnic-racial socialization and the mental health of African-Americans: A critical review. *Journal of Family Theory & Review, 9*(2), 182–200. https://doi.org/10.1111/jftr.12192.

Robinson, L., Adair, P., Coffey, M., Harris, R., & Burnside, G. (2016). Identifying the participant characteristics that predict recruitment and retention of participants to randomised controlled trials involving children: a systematic review. *Trials, 17*(1), 294. https://doi.org/10.1186/s13063-016-1415-0.

Russell, S. T., & Fish, J. N. (2016). Mental health in lesbian, gay, bisexual, and transgender (LGBT) youth. *Annual Review of Clinical Psychology, 12*, 465–487. https://doi.org/10.1146/annurev-clinpsy-021815-093153.

Ryan, C. (2013). Generating a revolution in prevention, wellness, and care for LGBT children and youth. *Temple Political & Civil Rights Law Review, 23*(2), 331–344.

Safren, S. A., Hollander, G., Hart, T. A., & Heimberg, R. G. (2001). Cognitive-behavioral therapy with lesbian, gay, and bisexual youth. *Cognitive and Behavioral Practice, 8*(3), 215–223. https://doi.org/10.1016/S1077-7229(01)80056-0.

Saydah, S., Imperatore, G., Cheng, Y., Geiss, L. S., & Albright, A. (2017). Disparities in diabetes deaths among children and adolescents—United States, 2000–2014. *Morbidity and Mortality Weekly Report, 66*, 502. https://doi.org/10.15585/mmwr.mm6619a4.

Schwartz, R. C., & Blankenship, D. M. (2014). Racial disparities in psychotic disorder diagnosis: A review of empirical literature. *World Journal of Psychiatry, 4*(4), 133. https://doi.org/10.5498/wjp.v4.i4.133.

Seaton, E. K., Yip, T., Morgan-Lopez, A., & Sellers, R. M. (2012). Racial discrimination and racial socialization as predictors of African-American adolescents' racial identity development using latent transition analysis. *Developmental Psychology, 48*(2), 448–458. https://doi.org/10.1037/a0025328.

Shilo, G., & Savaya, R. (2011). Effects of family and friend support on LGB youths' mental health and sexual orientation milestones. Family relations: An interdisciplinary. *Journal of Applied Family Studies, 60*(3), 318–330. https://doi.org/10.1111/j.1741-3729.2011.00648.x.

Silberholz, E. A., Brodie, N., Spector, N. D., & Pattishall, A. E. (2017). Disparities in access to care in marginalized populations. *Current Opinion in Pediatrics, 29*(6), 718–727. https://doi.org/10.1097/MOP.0000000000000549.

Simoni, J. M., Huh, D., Wilson, I. B., Shen, J., Goggin, K., Reynolds, N. R., et al. (2012). Racial/ethnic disparities in ART adherence in the United States: Findings from the MACH14 study. *Journal of Acquired Immune Deficiency Syndromes, 60*, 466–472. https://doi.org/10.1097/QAI.0b013e31825db0bd.

Smith, T., Rodriguez, M., & Bernal, G. (2011). Culture. *Journal of Clinical Psychology, 67*, 166–175. https://doi.org/10.1002/jclp.20757.

Snapp, S. D., Watson, R. J., Russell, S. T., Diaz, R. M., & Ryan, C. (2015). Social support nnetworks for LGBT young adults: Low cost strategies for positive adjustment. Family Relations: An Interdisciplinary. *Journal of Applied Family Studies, 64*(3), 420–430. https://doi.org/10.1111/fare.12124.

Strutz, K. L., Herring, A. H., & Halpern, C. T. (2015). Health disparities among young adult sexual minorities in the US. *American Journal of Preventive Medicine, 48*(1), 76–88. https://doi.org/10.1016/j.amepre.2014.07.038.

Teruya, S. A., & Bazargan-Hejazi, S. (2013). The immigrant and Hispanic paradoxes: A systematic review of their predictions and effects. *Hispanic Journal of Behavioral Sciences, 35*(4), 486–509. https://doi.org/10.1177/0739986313499004.

Thakur, N., Barcelo, N. E., Borrell, L. N., Singh, S., Eng, C., Davis, A., et al. (2017). Perceived discrimination associated with asthma and related outcomes in minority youth: The GALA II and SAGE II studies. *Chest, 151*(4), 804–812. https://doi.org/10.1016/j.chest.2016.11.027.

Thammana, R. V., Knechtle, S. J., Romero, R., Heffron, T. G., Daniels, C. T., & Patzer, R. E. (2014). Racial and socioeconomic disparities in pediatric and young adult liver transplant outcomes. *Liver Transplantation, 20*(1), 100–115. https://doi.org/10.1002/lt.23769.

Valdivieso-Mora, E., Peet, C. L., Garnier-Villarreal, M., Salazar-Villanea, M., & Johnson, D. K. (2016). A systematic review of the relationship between familism and mental health outcomes in Latino population. *Frontiers in Psychology, 7*, 13. https://doi.org/10.3389/fpsyg.

Valenzuela, J. M., & Smith, L. (2015). Topical review: Provider–patient interactions: An important consideration for racial/ethnic health disparitics in youth. *Journal of Pediatric Psychology, 41*(4), 473–480. https://doi.org/10.1093/jpepsy/jsv086.

Valenzuela, J. M., Pulgaron, E. R., Salamon, K. S., & Patiño-Fernandez, A. M. (2017). Evidence-based assessment strategies for working with ethnic minority youth. *Clinical Practice in Pediatric Psychology, 5*(1), 108–120. https://doi.org/10.1037/cpp0000183.

Vespa, J., Armstrong, D. M., & Medina, L. (2018). *Demographic turning points for the US: Population projections for 2020 to 2060 (Report No. P25-1144)*. Retrieved from https://www.census.gov/library/publications/2018/demo/p25-1144.html

Ward, E. C., & Brown, R. L. (2015). A culturally adapted depression intervention for African American adults experiencing depression: Oh happy day. *American Journal of Orthopsychiatry, 85*(1), 11–22. https://doi.org/10.1037/ort0000027.

Weiss, B. J., Singh, J. S., & Hope, D. A. (2011). Cognitive-behavioral therapy for immigrants presenting with social anxiety disorder: Two case studies. *Clinical Case Studies, 10*(4), 324. https://doi.org/10.1177/1534650111420706.

Wingood, G. M., & DiClemente, R. J. (2008). The ADAPT-ITT model: A novel method of adapting evidence-based HIV interventions. *Journal of Acquired Immune Deficiency Syndromes, 47*, S40–S46. https://doi.org/10.1097/QAI.0b013e3181605df1.

Yin, H. S., Dreyer, B. P., Vivar, K. L., MacFarland, S., van Schaick, L., & Mendelsohn, A. L. (2012). Perceived barriers to care and attitudes towards shared decision-making among low socioeconomic status parents: Role of health literacy. *Academic Pediatrics, 12*(2), 117–124. https://doi.org/10.1016/j.acap.2012.01.001.

Zeiders, K. H., Umaña-Taylor, A. J., Jahromi, L. B., Updegraff, K. A., & White, R. M. B. (2016). Discrimination and acculturation stress: A longitudinal study of children's well-being from prenatal development to 5 years of age. *Journal of Developmental and Behavioral Pediatrics, 37*(7), 557–564. https://doi.org/10.1097/DBP.0000000000000321.

Ethical Issues Applying CBT in Pediatric Medical Settings

Gerald P. Koocher and Jeanne S. Hoffman

As medicine has increasingly focused on evidence-based treatments, we have seen a growing trend toward integration of behavioral health services within medical practices and hospitals. CBT interventions fit comfortably within this model. CBT has demonstrated efficacy in treating children across a range of diagnoses including anxiety (Loades 2015; McMurtry et al. 2017), depression (Allen et al. 2018), obsessive-compulsive disorder (McGuire et al. 2018; Turner et al. 2018), and pediatric bipolar disorder (Isaia et al. 2018). Effectiveness in treating a number of physical conditions or complaints affecting children also appear in the literature, including pain (Allen et al. 2018; McMurtry et al. 2017), headache (Law et al. 2017; Ernst et al. 2015), and chronic fatigue syndrome (Loades 2015). CBTs also may prove useful in addressing behaviors that result from medical conditions and/or their treatment, for example, inflammatory bowel disease (IBD; Reigada et al. 2015), sleep problems (Caporino et al. 2017), needle phobia (Birnie et al. 2018), and pain (Allen et al. 2018).

Some definitions will help to clarify our approach. For simplicity sake, we will use the word "children" to refer to any patient treated in a pediatric setting who falls below the age of legal majority. Our definition of CBT encompasses a number of specific treatments with the unifying characteristic of having empirical support and components that involve a behavioral change focus and a reflective element related to thoughts and emotions. Implementation of CBT with child patients will require a degree of receptive and expressive language and self-reflective ability to participate fully in treatment. Therefore, we will need to consider the role of parents and guardians in treatment decision-making. In addition, for some young patients, the focus of treatment may be their parents.

Readers of this volume will doubtlessly have familiarity with the importance of conceptualizing the assessment and treatment of children and adolescents differently than adults from a clinical and developmental perspective. We recognize the need to take account of variations in intellectual, emotional, social, and personality development and incorporate such thinking when developing or modifying treatment approaches to accommodate differences between child and adult patients. CBTs pose special subsets of problems that require sensitivity to developmental considerations

---

The views expressed in this manuscript are those of the authors and do not reflect the official policy or position of the Department of the Army, Department of Defense, or the US Government.

G. P. Koocher (✉)
Quincy College, Quincy, MA, USA

J. S. Hoffman
Tripler Army Medical Center, Honolulu, HI, USA

in order to provide ethically sound assessment, treatment, and research in pediatric settings. For example, some CBT approaches may exceed the developmental competence of young children and some exposure-based therapeutic approaches may not lend themselves to sound pediatric care. The clinician must specifically assess each child patient to assess the applicability of a generic CBT or treatment manual. Using clinical case examples, we will illustrate the key concerns and possible solutions.

Clinical Competence and Optimizing Treatment Quality

Even if one assumes that the practitioner already has the education, training, and experience necessary to work effectively with children, incremental expertise in CBT approaches is essential. CBT includes a wide range of therapeutic techniques requiring specific knowledge and skills, typically presented in the form of treatment manuals or protocols. Such manuals can provide necessary but not sufficient information for the practitioner (Norcross et al. 2017). Manualized treatments clearly outline treatment steps and increase the probability of fidelity to treatment protocols but can pose risks when not supported by clinical skills and training. In medical settings, trainees are often involved in direct patient service delivery but with an assumption that treatment will occur under the supervision of clinicians experienced in these techniques. The ability to properly assess the problem, select treatment options, and tailor a treatment plan to a particular patient and clinical context is essential to ethical care.

In pediatric settings, an added challenge involves the range of medical conditions and symptoms that accompany referrals for psychotherapeutic intervention (Hoffman and Koocher 2018). The child psychotherapist will frequently need to interface with other medical team members who have highly variable degrees of psychological knowledge and mindedness. In addition to inter-professional practice competence, the clinician will need to know about the fundamentals of pediatric medical problems they will encounter. A parallel understanding of medical conditions presenting as psychological symptoms will also prove essential. This latter skill requires the clinician to recognize medical issues when referrals arrive framed as psychological in nature.

A basic understanding of medical treatments and resulting "normal pediatric reactions" will enable the clinician to readily engage with the medical team in ways that add significant patient care value. Some referrals will reach the psychologist directly from non-medical sources or without an appropriate physical assessment. Assuring that we practice with beneficence (aiming to treat patients well) and non-maleficence (doing no harm) requires that we recognize the limits of our skills and have all aspects of patient assessment conducted by those competent to do so.

For example, the child referred for treatment of chronic enuresis should be pre-screened for urinary tract problems and the child with abdominal pain should be cleared by a gastroenterologist. However, the therapist should also recognize their own expertise in child behaviors and treatment and not be intimidated by referring physicians who make what seems to be a prescriptive referral. Each child deserves a thorough assessment by the behavioral health specialist as to problem definition and determination of the most appropriate treatment. Similarly, parents' preferences must be taken into consideration in the context of acceptable treatment options. For example, some parents may express a preference for a trial of medication rather than CBT or may seek to veto the use of an exposure therapy. Rather than regarding prescriptive referrals or parental preferences as obstacles, the competent practitioner can seize the opportunity to offer thoughtful psychoeducation regarding treatment approaches. At the same time, because support of parents and other professionals in the child's life (e.g., physicians and teachers) may prove essential for success, the practitioner must have the experience and flexibility to adapt manualized treatments in order to better fit the case context.

As with any intervention around a medical problem, early termination from treatment may lead to adverse outcomes. Research on family-based psychosocial treatments has identified some characteristics likely associated with families who drop out of treatment or do not adhere to recommendations or homework follow-through. High parental stress and low baseline parental coping are associated with early termination. Worsening of the child's symptoms during treatment also predispose the family to premature termination. Conversely, improvement in children's global functioning is associated with reduced dropout across treatments (Isaia et al. 2018). Well-informed, attentive, and nimble therapists can take steps to identify hazards and provide additional family supports or prompt modifications to treatment protocols when parents report that the child's condition is not improving or worsening.

In one case, an eager novice psychology intern was assigned to treat a high school sophomore who reported anxiety and depression at the start of the school year. The patient had undergone surgical treatment for endometriosis in the early summer and had developed symptoms of urinary urgency that complicated her days at school. After the first visit, the intern arrived at supervision feeling anxious herself and told the supervisor that the patient said very little, leaving the intern at a loss for which of the manualized treatments she had studied should be applied. The supervisor gently noted that it would be important to first assess and understand the patient's context and concern. The supervisor suggested eliciting the patient's narrative of her experience by asking, "Tell me about what happened when you got sick and had the surgery. What have the symptoms been like recently and how do they affect you?" As the patient gave her account to the intern over coming sessions, she provided the young therapist with details of her experience, cognitions, emotions, and symptoms in a way that enabled building a therapeutic alliance and helping the trainee to target intervention more precisely to the patient's symptoms.

In another case, the parents of a child presenting with very active and oppositional behavior expressed a wish to have the child medicated. With careful interviewing, it became clear that both parents worked full time and did not feel able to commit participating in regular therapy sessions. They saw medication as a fast and easy solution. Explanations of why medication per se was not indicated and would not solve the root problem, paired with offers for a weekend CBT parent-training program and follow-up coaching by telephone, fit their need and proved effective.

Autonomy and the Challenge of Consent

As adults, we expect a high degree of autonomy in our medical care as evidenced through a process of well-informed consent. In that context, we expect our care providers to give us all of the information we might reasonably need to make a decision in a form that we can understand and process. We can also choose to decline treatments that are recommended or offered for ourselves. Unless we are deemed legally incompetent, we have a right to our decisions based on thoughtful, well-reasoned bases or even arbitrary preferences (e.g., "I know my physician said that I need to lose weight, but I'd rather not limit my diet and exercise more. Is there a pill I can take instead?"). On the other hand, suppose the pediatrician recommends an immunization for your child and the 5-year-old refuses (e.g., "I don't want it. It will hurt."). Most parents, who understand the benefits preventing a future serious illness, will decide that these benefits outweigh the discomfort a moment of injection pain. In such situations, a parent will authorize the injection even if doing so means restraining their child for a short time. In this context, parents grant permission for the treatment (i.e., a form of proxy consent because people can only consent for themselves).

Child patients arriving at a practitioner's office for mental health treatment typically present because some adult (i.e., parent, physician, teacher, etc.) has decided that professional intervention is warranted. In some situations, parents and caregivers may want to solicit the assent of the child, who cannot give legal consent for themselves. However, true assent means granting veto power. One would not want to allow a child, who lacks the developmental capacity to understand the future consequences of a medical treatment or procedure (including mental health care), to have veto authority over a likely beneficial or life-saving treatment. In some treatment contexts involving distress-inducing techniques, patient engagement and education with continuing discussion of goals and process may help to enhance cooperation (Gola et al. 2016; Sookman 2015). However, the circumstances change if/when there is no real benefit to the child (e.g., a medical student would like to perform a redundant practice examination, but the child is tired, anxious, or otherwise opposed.). In situations where no potential direct benefit to the child exists, the child's preferences deserve heavy weight even if they seem arbitrary.

Adolescents may have the intellectual capacity to make many important treatment decisions, but the legal system has offered mixed guidance. For example, in most states, adolescents may seek treatment for pregnancy, substance abuse, sexually transmitted diseases, and, in some states, psychotherapy without parental consent (Koocher and Keith-Spiegel 2016). In many states, adolescents also have the right to have an objection heard in court, if parents seek inpatient mental health treatment for them against their will (Koocher and Keith-Spiegel 2016). It follows that adolescents' have the right to withhold assent for some types of treatment in some situations.

Because CBT's effectiveness, as with most psychotherapy, flows in part from a collaborative process (Sookman 2015; Gola et al. 2016), developing individualized cooperation with child patients of any age is essential. Thus, the consent/assent process becomes inextricably intertwined with forging and maintaining a therapeutic alliance. The key ethical principles such as beneficence and non-maleficence come into play here. Juggling these variables requires a degree of flexibility that some treatment-manual-bound clinicians may find challenging.

For example, suppose a clinician proposes use of an exposure-type intervention for a child with phobic anxiety and the child resists. In many circumstances, alternative therapeutic approaches could be deployed and the therapist should make the range of treatment options available for discussion. In other cases, the clinician may have a potential conflict (e.g., lacking competence in alternative approaches or wanting to enroll the patient in a clinical trial requiring random assignment to different treatment groups). In all such instances, the child patient's preferences deserve prime consideration for ethical and clinical reasons of consent, as well as beneficence and non-maleficence. The therapeutic relationship forged in decision-making about treatment planning can become as important and powerful an effect as the technique applied.

As hinted at above, clinical research with CBTs can trigger a number of potential ethical concerns for consideration during the design phase and execution of a psychotherapy treatment study. Randomization to treatment groups, use of a wait-list or other control group, or enrolling children who may be entering a critical developmental period of development all raise critical -risk to benefit calculations (Haman and Hollon 2009). If a study offers treatment as usual, often referred to as TAU, compared with an alternative deemed to have a potential for better outcomes, the participation of children may have strong benefits. However, delayed treatment or no treatment control conditions demand caution. When parent or guardian permission is required, a careful explanation of risks and benefits is warranted with special attention to avoid a "therapeutic misconception" (Koocher and Keith-Spiegel 2016). Such a misconception refers to a circumstance in which the participant or permission-giver wrongly assumes that treatment will occur even when randomization to a no-treatment-control group is an option. Similarly, reimbursement for participation, methods of patient recruitment, and exclusion rules also create a need to balance scientific rigor with the patients' best interests, beneficence, non-maleficence, and respect for people's rights and dignity (Haman and Hollon 2009). In some instances, compensation offered may constitute an unreasonable temptation for participation in clinical research that poses substantial misunderstood risk (Koocher 2005).

Confidentiality

Confidentiality with respect to CBT with children does not raise unique issues. The usual reporting mandates for child abuse or neglect and policies regarding requests to access a child patient's records remain the same as that with other treatment models. When the patient is a child, parents or guardians generally have full legal entitlement to record access. Therapists should recognize the unique problems that arise when working with minors or families and should remain sensitive to each individual's right to privacy and confidentiality in such circumstances. From the outset of any such relationship, all parties should receive information about the specific nature of the confidential relationship. A discussion about what sorts of information might be shared and with whom should be raised early. This is not a difficult or burdensome process when done as a routine practice (Koocher and Keith-Spiegel 2016).

Large medical practices and health-care systems will typically maintain electronic medical records (EMRs) and increasingly move toward interoperable EMRs. The term *EMR* refers to a system of accessing patient medical data electronically, while the concept of interoperability reaches across providers and systems. Apart from observing all of the standard confidentiality caveats inherent in ethical codes and HIPAA regulations, CBT does not create incremental or unusual risks. Detailed discussions of confidentiality issues involving minors in medical settings are available elsewhere (Hoffman and Koocher 2018; Koocher and Keith-Spiegel 2016).

Non-maleficence Hazards

Exposure-based CBT has been referred to as the "Cruelest Cure" having "a public relations problem" (Olatunji et al. 2009) with reference to adult patients. However, the same authors note that the degree to which non-maleficence issues become problematic in implementing exposure-based treatments depends largely on therapists' ability to create and foster a safe and professional context. Competence and consent clearly play significant roles in this process. Gola et al. (2016) suggest using developmentally appropriate language, describing steps in the procedure carefully, and continuing to discuss any issues that arise throughout treatment. Solid clinical skills, close supervision of trainees, and the careful crafting of developmentally appropriate exposure items to maximize the tolerability of treatment is particularly important. Ideally, therapeutic exposure should be developmentally appropriate and not exceed what might occur naturally outside of the office and should unfold gradually, rather than as "flooding" or implosive paradigms (Levis and Castelda 2005).

Hoping to mitigate clinicians' concerns, McGuire and his colleagues (2018) editorialized exposure-based CBT used to treat pediatric obsessive-compulsive disorder and found that a sizable proportion of clinicians express hesitancy regarding the use of exposure treatments because of anticipated negative patient and parent reactions. They focused on three commonly reported clinician concerns related to supposed concerns (e.g., treatment attrition, harm to the therapeutic relationship, and lowered treatment satisfaction) among youth who received exposure-based CBT compared with a non-exposure-based treatment group. They noted that some exposure-based CBT does elicit discomfort and distress but found no empirical support for the belief that exposure-based CBT increased the adverse effects measured. The analysis is encouraging, and in many respects, withholding an effective treatment based on groundless concerns might qualify as unethical. Nevertheless, it will behoove clinicians who plan to deploy exposure-based CBT with children to do so with appropriate developmental perspectives.

Mélange of Misconduct

Several other types of potential ethical infractions deserve mention, not because they occur commonly, but because they deserve careful avoidance. These include some issues related to CBT as a "brand-name" psychotherapy, boundary challenges, protocol deviations, and unwarranted applications or claims.

Some forms of psychotherapy have acquired a kind of brand name salience much the same as the brand "Kleenex," owned by the Kimberly-Clark Corporation, is often used in everyday speech to describe any facial tissue regardless of brand. The field of psychotherapy has brands such as psychoanalysis, eye movement desensitization and reprocessing (EMDR), client-centered therapy, rational emotive therapy (RET), and others with varying degrees of cachet. When a layperson uses the word "psychoanalyze," they most likely do not have in mind lying on a couch and free associating. Because of a substantial body of research on cognitive and behavioral therapies, the name "CBT" has acquired a degree of brand salience to the point that many people seek it out without fully understanding that the label covers a range of approaches targeting different problems that may not generalize well across patient, symptoms, or pathology.

What does it mean when a physician prescribes CBT for a patient? Do patients understand what they are seeking when they walk into a psychologist's office asking for CBT? What authority permits clinicians to advertise that they provide CBT? Substitute any form of therapy associated with a salient name and you will grasp the problem. Now, flip the problem using a medical setting model. You may walk into a primary care physician's office and say, "I have a fever and need an antibiotic." The competent physician will first want to take a medical history, perform an examination, and obtain test results. The physician knows that an elevated temperature may result from any number of conditions that will not respond to antibiotic treatment ranging from viral illness to heat stroke. Similarly, a competent psychologist will want to make an assessment before recommending a course of treatment. Thus, a referral from a physician or self-referral of children by their parents should be interpreted as a generic request for treatment, subject to evaluation.

Mental health professionals are licensed to practice in a specific field or to use a specific title in advertising their services. The qualifications evaluated by licensing boards are for generic practice, and only a small percentage of clinicians in psychology seek specialty board certification. Even so, no single specialty board recognized by the American Psychological Association owns a sole claim to CBT. Thus, any licensed practitioner can readily lay claim to providing CBT and will not be challenged unless or until they find themselves called before a licensing board on a competence complaint. Even mildly self-reflective clinicians might consider themselves skilled in CBT based on training with one or two manualized treatment techniques. In reality, such individuals might more reasonably qualify as expert in treating certain conditions, in certain patients, with certain techniques. A broadly trained clinician might choose to approach the care of a patient with an effective treatment that they know well, but that would not qualify as CBT. If the patient improves, does it matter that they believe they received CBT, even if they did not?

The value added to patient care by a skilled experienced psychotherapist is not locked to a specific technique. The skilled clinician will learn through their assessment and discussions with the patient and family what treatments might prove most effective and not use the treatment manual as a text to be slavishly followed. Rather, the clinician will frame reasonable adaptations based on the circumstances, goals, and preferences of the patient and family. For example, a CBT program that addresses dietary control might require modification for an adolescent in an observant Muslim family during Ramadan, when fasting may be expected during daylight hours.

Effective CBT will often require homework or follow through, and when the patient is a child, parents and other family members may need to play a part in adhering to a treatment regimen. The clinician may at times need to address nonadherence, undermining of the treatment plan, or frank refusal to cooperate. These issues will seldom be resolved by reading a treatment manual but will require strong communication and alliance building skills. In some medical circumstances, the therapist may encounter failures to cooperate that qualify as medical neglect, warranting involvement of child protection authorities. For example, a clinician asked to apply CBT to assist an anxious child with insulin-dependent diabetes mellitus may discover that the parents are not providing proper dietary and insulin control to a degree that compromises the child's health. The anxiety may flow from medical instability that will not improve with CBT alone.

Finally, there may be circumstances in which boundary crossings become an issue. When functioning as part of a medical treatment team, a behavioral health practitioner may become privy to information that the patient or family prefers not be widely shared (Hoffman and Koocher 2018). In such circumstances, the practitioner must thread a needle of care in recognizing what must be shared in the electronic record or at team meetings and what confidences can be respected. Other boundary issues may come up if the CBT treatment must optimally extend beyond the medical facility to the home, school, or community as part of an in vivo desensitization or rehearsal treatment model.

Conclusion

While the ethical codes of mental health professionals generally apply well across patient populations, psychological conditions, and treatment techniques, the mix of children, medical settings, and CBT practice raises some unique challenges. In particular, practitioners' clinical competence and consent are the most significant areas of concern. The effects of these issues radiate across varieties of CBT and patient populations. Focusing on them will assure that we treat patients well with highly effective CBT techniques, while striving to cause no harm.

References

Allen, T. M., Wren, A. A., Anderson, L. M., Sabholk, A., & Mauro, C. F. (2018). A group CBT-yoga protocol targeting pain-related and internalizing symptoms in youth. *Clinical Practice in Pediatric Psychology, 6*(1), 7–18. https://doi.org/10.1037/cpp0000206.

Birnie, K. A., Noel, M., Chambers, C. T., Uman, L. S., & Parker, J. A. (2018). Psychological interventions for needle-related procedural pain and distress in children and adolescents. *Cochrane Database of Systematic Reviews.* https://doi.org/10.1002/14651858.CD005179.pub4.

Caporino, N. E., Read, K. L., Shiffrin, N., Settipani, C., Kendall, P. C., Compton, N., & Albano, A. M. (2017). Sleep-related problems and the effects of anxiety treatment in children and adolescents. *Journal of Clinical Child and Adolescent Psychology, 46*(5), 675–685. https://doi.org/10.1080/15374416.2015.1063429.

Ernst, M. M., O'Brien, H. L., & Powers, S. W. (2015). Cognitive-behavioral therapy: How medical providers can increase patient and family openness and access to evidence-based multimodal therapy for pediatric migraine. *Headache: The Journal of Head and Face Pain, 55*(10), 1382–1396. https://doi.org/10.1111/head.12605.

Gola, J. A., Beyda's, R. S., Antonio-Burke, D., Kratz, H. E., & Fingerhut, R. (2016). Ethical considerations in exposure therapy with children. *Cognitive and Behavioral Practice, 23*(2), 184–193. https://doi.org/10.1016/j.cbpra.2015.04.003.

Haman, K. L., & Hollon, S. D. (2009). Ethical considerations for cognitive-behavioral therapists in psychotherapy research trials. *Cognitive and Behavioral Practice, 16*(2), 153–163. https://doi.org/10.1016/j.cbpra.2008.08.005.

Hoffman, J. S., & Koocher, G. P. (2018). Strategies for ethical practice in medical settings. *Practice Innovations, 3*(1), 43–55. https://doi.org/10.1037/pri0000062.

Isaia, A. R., Weinstein, S. M., Shankman, S. A., & West, A. E. (2018). Predictors of dropout in family-based psychosocial treatment for pediatric bipolar disorder: An exploratory study. *Journal of Child and Family Studies, 27*, 1–17. https://doi.org/10.1007/s10826-018-1126-0.

Koocher, G. P. (2005). Behavioral research with children: The Fenfluramine challenge. In E. Kodesh (Ed.), *Learning from cases: Ethics and research with children* (pp. 179–193). New York: Oxford University Press.

Koocher, G. P., & Keith-Spiegel, P. C. (2016). *Ethics in psychology and the mental health professions: Standards and cases* (4th ed.). New York: Oxford University Press.

Law, E. F., Beals-Erickson, S. E., Fisher, E., Lang, E. A., & Palermo, T. M. (2017). Components of effective cognitive-behavioral therapy for pediatric headache: A mixed methods approach. *Clinical Practice in Pediatric Psychology, 5*(4), 376–391. https://doi.org/10.1037/cpp0000216.

Levis, D. J., & Castelda, B. A. (2005). Stampfl's therapist-directed implosive (flooding) therapy. In M. Hersen, J. Rosqvist, A. M. Gross, R. S. Drabman, G. Sugai, & R. Horner (Eds.), *Encyclopedia of behavior modification and cognitive behavior therapy*. Sage Online. https://doi.org/10.4135/9781412950534.n153.

Loades, M. (2015). The cognitive behavioral treatment of depression and low self-esteem in the context of pediatric chronic fatigue syndrome (CFS/ME): A case study. *Journal of Child and Adolescent Psychiatric Nursing, 28*(4), 165–174. https://doi.org/10.1111/jcap.12125.

McGuire, J. F., Wu, M. S., Choy, C., & Piacentini, J. (2018). Editorial perspective: Exposures in cognitive behavior therapy for pediatric obsessive-compulsive disorder: Addressing common clinician concerns. *Journal of Child Psychology and Psychiatry, 59*(6), 714–716. https://doi.org/10.1111/jcpp.12818.

McMurtry, C. M., Tomlinson, R. M., & Genik, L. M. (2017). Cognitive behavioral therapy for anxiety and fear in pediatric pain contexts. *Journal of Cognitive Psychotherapy, 31*(1), 41–56. https://doi.org/10.1891/0889-8391.31.1.41.

Norcross, J. C., Hogan, T., Koocher, G. P., & Maggio, L. A. (2017). *Clinician's guide to evidence-based practices: Mental health and the addictions* (2nd ed.). New York: Oxford University Press.

Olatunji, B. O., Deacon, B. J., & Abramowitz, J. S. (2009). The cruelest cure? Ethical issues in the implementation of exposure-based treatments. *Cognitive and Behavioral Practice, 16*(2), 172–180. https://doi.org/10.1016/j.cbpra.2008.07.003.

Reigada, L. C., Polokowski, A. R., Walder, D., Sigethy, E. M., Benkov, K. J., Bruzzese, J., & Masia Warner, C. (2015). Treatment for comorbid pediatric gastrointestinal and anxiety disorders: A pilot study of a flexible health sensitive cognitive-behavioral therapy program. *Clinical Practice in Pediatric Psychology, 3*(4), 314–326. https://doi.org/10.1037/cpp0000116.

Sookman, D. (2015). Ethical practice of cognitive behavioral therapy. In *The Oxford handbook of psychiatric ethics*. New York: Oxford University Press. https://doi.org/10.1093/oxfordhb/9780198732372.013.35.

Turner, C., O'Gorman, B., Nair, A., & O'Kearney, R. (2018). Moderators and predictors of response to cognitive behavior therapy for pediatric obsessive-compulsive disorder: A systematic review. *Psychiatry Research, 261*, 50–60. https://doi.org/10.1016/j.psychres.2017.12.034.

Emotional Regulation and Pediatric Behavior Health Problems

5

Carisa Parrish, Hannah Fajer, and Alison Papadakis

Case Vignettes

Children and their families experience emotional challenges when faced with health problems. Some health problems are temporary and acute, such as when children are injured, whereas other health problems are more prolonged, such as when children have chronic conditions. There are overlapping and unique aspects to acute and chronic conditions when considering emotion regulation aspects of children's health problems. The case vignettes below were chosen to represent the range of acute and chronic medical treatments and the impact such experiences can have on the emotional lives of children and families.[1]

Acute Vignette (Jack)

In acute health problems, families usually do not expect the medical stress to occur. For example, approximately 120,000 children experience burn injuries each year in the USA that require emergency medical treatment (D'Souza et al. 2009). Many families describe such injuries in their children as among the most stressful experiences and often remark that they have never experienced anything similar. Pediatric burn injuries usually are due to contact with hot objects or spilled food/drink.

Consider 4-year-old Jack: he was home with a babysitter who heated a cup of soup in the microwave. Jack is a typical energetic preschooler who bounced to the table and accidentally hit the edge of the soup bowl, causing it to splash over his chest and legs. He immediately cried out in severe pain. His older sister and babysitter did not know what to do, but pretty quickly, his babysitter took him to the bathroom and showered him with cool water. She called Jack's parents, who rushed home from a nearby restaurant and took him to the local emergency room. At the hospital, Jack was given pain medication, and his chest and legs were scrubbed; his parents watched in horror as the outer layer of his skin peeled off and revealed a large bright pink surface. Jack was crying, and his parents were struggling to remain calm. The nurses and

---

[1] We have removed all identifying information from the vignettes.

C. Parrish (✉)
Division of Child and Adolescent Psychiatry, Department of Psychiatry and Behavioral Sciences, Johns Hopkins University School of Medicine, Baltimore, MD, USA
e-mail: cparris5@jhmi.edu

H. Fajer · A. Papadakis
Department of Psychological and Brain Sciences, Johns Hopkins University, Baltimore, MD, USA

© Springer Nature Switzerland AG 2019
R. D. Friedberg, J. K. Paternostro (eds.), *Handbook of Cognitive Behavioral Therapy for Pediatric Medical Conditions*, Autism and Child Psychopathology Series,
https://doi.org/10.1007/978-3-030-21683-2_5

doctor assured Jack's parents that his pain was managed and that he appeared to only have a partial-thickness or second-degree burn. This news was upsetting, but the medical team explained that Jack would not need surgery, as his skin would likely heal on its own. Jack's mother started crying, as she had not even considered the possibility that surgery might be necessary. Jack's father tried to concentrate as the nurse explained how they would be changing the dressings on Jack's wounds for the next 5 days at home, while Jack sobbed in his mother's arms. He had a hard time imagining how they would be able to handle the dressing changes at home. He could not stand seeing his son cry. He imagined that Jack would continue to be in pain and worried about the emotional impact on his son.

Medical treatment for burns typically involves urgent visit to pediatrician or local burn center, where children's wounds are thoroughly cleaned, dressings applied, and then sent home for regular bandage changes until the injured site has healed. A minority of children require hospitalization or more invasive procedures, such as wound debridement under sedation, surgical excision, or skin grafts. Parents are often involved in medical care, especially as contemporary burn management has shifted primarily to home-based care rather than depending on hospitalization. There are multiple emotional challenges present for children and their families following burn injuries, including management of pain and distress, painful and upsetting medical procedures, and uncertainty of parents regarding their child's likely medical and cosmetic outcome. The course of treatment can range from weeks to months depending on the severity of the injury. For children with more extensive skin surface involvement, rehabilitation may be required to maintain range of motion and functional status. Children's display of pain, distress, and social reintegration, as well as parental anxiety, distress, and guilt, present opportunities for child psychologists and other behavioral health specialists to support optimal emotional adjustment to acute injuries.

Chronic Vignette (Cherish)

With chronic health conditions, children and families are faced with physical symptoms and disorders for months to years. While onset may have been acute or gradual, the chronic condition continues to manifest in ongoing symptoms requiring medical attention. For example, in youth with renal disease, the renals fail to optimally filter an individual's blood. Children may have had worsening renal function due to congenital problems or an abrupt decline and sudden diagnosis of end-stage renal disease. As of 2015, overall prevalence of end-stage renal disease in youth under the age of 22 years was approximately 9600 in the USA (United States Renal Data System 2017). Renal failure requires replacement of renal function over the course of a person's life.

Consider the case of Cherish, an 11-year-old girl whose renal failure was due to obstructive uropathy. She was born with urological difficulties, and her parents knew that eventually she would be classified with end-stage renal disease and ultimately need a kidney transplant. Cherish hated taking her medications; it reminded her that she was different and had to do things that her peers did not. She especially resented her frequent doctor appointments, which usually required blood draws and occasionally identified problems leading to a few nights in the hospital. After a few years, Cherish began receiving dialysis at home, tethered to a pump that prevented her from sleepovers with friends and made her mother nervous to travel away from home. Interactions between Cherish and her mother became strained because Cherish sometimes did not cooperate with her medication routine. Her mother was drained from reminding Cherish every day, several times a day, which medications to take, to stop drinking too much water because her kidneys could not keep up, and her dialysis could not fully manage to filter her blood as her renal functioning further declined. Cherish's mother worried that Cherish's condition would deteriorate before she matched to a donor kidney; she was further concerned that Cherish's emotional and behavioral reactions to the isolation after a transplant would make optimal adherence to her medication schedule difficult and risk the success of the transplant.

Chronic conditions such as end-stage renal disease demonstrate the many sources of emotional stress children and families may encounter with a prolonged medical condition. The range of medical treatments including comprehensive oral medications, fluid management, dialysis, and, ultimately, transplantation are each likely to contribute to acute and persistent stress by repeatedly painful, invasive, and scary medical procedures. Other procedures may not be painful but rather may consume considerable time that disrupts school and social activities for children, and consistent parent work schedules. Home-based peritoneal dialysis usually involves 9 or more hours overnight, and clinic-based hemodialysis typically lasts 3–4 h for 3 days per week. Time-consuming treatments may be endured until more permanent solutions can be accessed (e.g., kidney transplantation). While families may be relieved when transplantation is finally approaching, a new set of emotional challenges emerge in the form of hospitalization, new medications given on a strict timeline, close monitoring for complications that could lead to organ rejection, and months of isolation to prevent infection. While kidney failure may represent a more life-threatening version of chronic conditions, other forms present with similar emotional challenges that are acutely distressing to families (e.g., eczema flares, asthma attacks, gastrointestinal disorders, voiding dysfunction). The emotional ups and downs of the course of medical treatments present many children and families with both chronic and acute stress in dealing with the medical condition and the disruptions caused by the condition and its treatment.

Emotion Regulation and Health Conditions

As can be seen in the above-mentioned examples, children and families experience emotional challenges that are directly and indirectly related to the child's health condition and its treatment. These challenges are present in both acute and chronic conditions. Adherence to medical recommendations challenge children's stress tolerance, and parents often find themselves in the role of nurse and therapist as they provide medical care and emotional comfort to their distressed, physically affected child. It can be difficult to discern whether a child's distress is due to pain, anxiety, or both. Parents feel guilty and often blame themselves for their child's distress. Children feel anxious and may not fully understand why they have to endure ongoing medical treatments. Parents may question the necessity of treatments when children do not easily cooperate and find themselves pleading with medical staff about when the treatment will be finished. Cognitive-behavioral treatments can be employed to address the range of challenges to child and family emotion regulation in medical settings.

Pediatric health problems are often accompanied by emotional challenges for children and their families. Treatment of child health problems often taxes the emotional regulation of the family system, as parents and children cope with stress, physical difficulties, and medical treatment. The Integrative Model of Pediatric Medical Traumatic Stress provides a useful framework for understanding how children and their families are affected by the various aspects of pediatric health conditions (Price et al. 2016). Pediatric medical stress has been defined as "a set of psychological and physiological responses of children and their families to pain, injury, serious illness, medical procedures, and invasive or frightening treatment experiences" (The National Child Traumatic Stress Network 2003a, "Medical Trauma," paragraph 1). This framework details that children and families experience a range of reactions to physical and medical problems that may emerge over multiple time phases, including initial medical events, active medical treatment phase, and post-treatment phase. In this chapter, we focus on describing the role of emotion regulation and its links to pediatric health problems, including interventions to optimize adaptive emotional adjustment to medical and physical difficulties.

Emotion regulation is increasingly recognized as an important component of adaptive psychosocial adjustment to stress. Emotion regulation has been conceptualized as "the processes by which we influence which emotions we have, when we have them, and how we experience and express them" (Gross 2002, p. 282). In the developmental literature, emotion regulation has also been defined as "the extrinsic and intrinsic processes responsible for monitoring, evaluating, and modifying emotional reactions ... to accomplish one's goals" (Thompson 1994, pp. 27–28). Emotion regulation is an important component of psychological and social functioning (Gross and Munoz 1995), making this construct a particularly useful element for understanding children's psychosocial adjustment to health problems. We focus on the emotion regulation of children, as well as the socialization role that parents play.

Emotional Development Milestones

Emotion regulation emerges early in development and matures over time. Displays of specific emotional states (e.g., pain, distress, joy, frustration) emerge in infancy (0–12 months; Honig 2005; Malatesta et al. 1989), and early regulation is typically managed by parent reactions to infant needs (e.g., hunger, sleep, stimulation). Infants display some evidence of self-soothing, such as orienting attention toward and away from desired sources (e.g., Kochanska et al. 2000), but infants are largely dependent on caregivers to reduce distress. The toddler period (12 months–2 years) and increasing language and cognitive skills marks the transition to early childhood, with increased self-awareness and beginnings of self-consciousness emotions (Eisenberg 2000).

During early childhood, children begin to display emotion knowledge and understanding, including identification of emotions, understanding external causes, knowledge of regulation strategies, and presence of conflicting emotions; these skills develop steadily between the ages of 3 and 11 years (Pons et al. 2004). Further, theory of mind and perspective-taking abilities, that emerge during the preschool years (e.g., Lane et al. 2010), lay the groundwork for intentional changes to one's emotional experiences, which is a key feature of emotion regulation. Children's games show their growing awareness that emotions can mislead others during early childhood (e.g., Wimmer and Perner 1983). These cognitive changes have been found to co-occur with children's empathic responses and effective problem-solving during difficult social interactions (Eisenberg et al. 1997). By the end of the preschool period, children begin to understand another's emotions and expressions (Harris et al. 1986, 1987; Harris and Gross 1988). It appears that by 6 years of age, children begin to first demonstrate the ability to discriminate between apparent and real emotions (Gosselin et al. 2002). Differentiating between displayed and felt emotions represents a cognitive skill that likely facilitates the acquisition of particular aspects of emotional understanding.

During middle childhood (ages 5–10 years), children begin to strategically modify their emotional expressions to meet social expectations. The strategic organization of behavior that is associated with conformity to social pressures has been described as reflecting the presence of display rules (Josephs 1994; see also Saarni 1999; Underwood et al. 1992). Display rules appear to reflect social-cultural views of the appropriateness and acceptability of emotional expressivity and, as such, guide one's decisions to display an emotion contingent upon contextual information (Fuchs and Thelen 1988; Gnepp and Hess 1986; Zeman and Shipman 1997).

Children's understanding of and use of display rules increase with age (e.g., Fuchs and Thelen 1988; Gnepp and Hess 1986; Saarni 1979; Underwood et al. 1992; Zeman and Garber 1996; Zeman and Shipman 1996). Older children are more likely to report using display rules to hide emotions than younger children (Gnepp and Hess 1986), but the age effects vary by emotion management method (i.e., facial, verbal, behavioral, or expressive management) and emotion type (Zeman and Garber 1996). Across all age groups, children endorse facial expressive regulation more for anger and sadness than for pain and report behavioral withdrawal during sad situations. Younger children tend to express emotions more freely than older children (Gnepp and Hess 1986;

Underwood et al. 1992); this trend appears to decrease after the fifth grade, with tenth-grade children reporting only slightly more inhibition of emotional displays (Gnepp and Hess 1986). Relatedly, Saarni (1984) has suggested that children begin to be able to dependably use positive substitution during a disappointing situation at approximately 10 years of age. These results suggest that the end of the elementary school years marks an important period in children's development and consolidation of knowledge regarding appropriate display rule use, including guidelines that govern emotional expressivity.

Adolescence is associated with continued development of cognitive and social awareness that promotes further maturation of emotion regulation abilities. From the age of 10 years through the late teen years, brain development supports increased problem-solving, improved appraisal accuracy, and more skills in generating multiple strategies for coping with stress. Adolescents show sensitivity to social contexts and increasingly seek the company and approval of peers over parents. Social role and identity formation shape emotional displays, and adolescents prioritize skillful self-presentation for optimal impression management and relationship formation (Saarni 1999).

In sum, the forms of emotion regulation transform over development (Saarni 1999). In infancy, regulation is largely managed by parents. Emotionally attuned parents manage and provide needs to assist infants and toddlers with the development of self-soothing behaviors. Dyadic regulation is evident by early childhood, as children become more proficient at seeking comfort from caregivers and shifting attention from emotional distress. Young children exhibit emerging skills with intentionally masking emotional displays; by middle childhood and the adolescent period, children are able to strategically display and hide emotions to adapt to a variety of social contexts (e.g., parents, friends, school peers). Adolescents continue to gain practice in altering their emotional experiences and regulating emotional responses to stress. The adolescent period provides extensive practice that gradually leads to more confident regulation, which emerges in concert with neurocognitive changes that promote maturity and independence in coping. Despite their frequent appearance of invulnerability, adolescents benefit from emotional support of parents during stressful times.

Emotion Regulation and Parents

There are several types of cognitive-behavioral parental interventions discussed later in this chapter, all of which are fundamentally rooted in principles of parental socialization of emotion. There are two main ways that parents socialize emotional expression and regulation: operant conditioning and modeling. Through operant conditioning, parents can reward or punish their child's behavior to alter the frequency of that behavior. Therefore, parents can directly shape their child's emotions by noticeably reacting to the way their child experiences and expresses emotions (Eisenberg et al. 1998). Similarly, parents can also impact their child's behavior based on the way they talk about emotion, and the way they themselves express emotion (Eisenberg et al. 1998). This models the expected behavior and emotional expression to children, which they adopt it.

Emotion socialization can take place in a medical setting, and the high emotional intensity associated with injuries, illnesses, and medical procedures may be particularly poignant and influential experiences. Parents' emotional reactions to their child's condition can influence their child's behavior and emotions, and likewise, the way a child responds to their health problem will impact the parental response (Blount et al. 1989). As parents are generally more skilled at emotional regulation than young children, it is critical that they monitor their own emotions, seeking help when needed, to model appropriate emotional responses for their children. Medical staff also must attend to the emotional responses of parents and assist parents in adapting their responses to assist with the child's own emotion regulation. This also emphasizes the importance of parents implementing cognitive-behavioral techniques to help maintain their child's behavior and emotion. Parents who engage in anxiety-enhancing parent behaviors often fail to contribute to their child's cognitive, social, and emotional development (Ginsburg and Schlossberg 2002). Given that the anxiety-enhancing parent behaviors can be due to a combination of the parents' own anxiety and child factors, ensuring maintenance of appropriate emotions and reactions prevents fear and anxiety from spreading between parents and their child (Ginsburg and Schlossberg 2002).

There are multiple factors that influence the emotion-related parenting practices in the context of emotion socialization. These include child, parent, cultural, and contextual factors. Child factors, such as age, gender, and temperament, reflect the fact that socialization is a bi-directional process (Zahn-Waxler 2010). Children's emotions can influence the emotions of their parents, rather than merely the other way around (Zahn-Waxler 2010). Parents also contribute other factors to the socialization process, such as their age, gender, values, and childrearing philosophies (Eisenberg et al. 1998). These variables influence how parents respond to different behaviors from their child. There is also a broader cultural influence on the emotion socialization process. Certain cultures are more accepting of emotional expressivity, and other cultures promote certain emotions and discourage others. This cultural factor interplays with the contextual factor; the competent emotional response is likely to vary by setting (Eisenberg et al. 1998). In the case of a medical context, there are many factors that impact the emotions of a pediatric patient and their family. The stress of illness, injury, and treatment challenges normal emotion regulation abilities, in addition to the need for many families to adjust to a new setting and daily routine. While parents usually have authority over their children at home, they must comply with medical providers, which alters the dynamic between parent and child and forces everyone to adapt. Individual factors and cultural factors will influence the family's ability to accomplish this, while dealing with the anxiety and fear inevitably present in medical settings. When choosing a technique for a cognitive-behavioral intervention, it is important to consider all the different layers of influence to achieve maximum effectiveness of the intervention.

Emotion Regulation and the Cognitive-Behavioral Model

The cognitive-behavioral therapy model targets cognitive and behavioral processes to alter emotional states and mood. Although historically the CBT model focused on cognitive and behavioral processes, more recently, third-wave CBT treatments (e.g., Dialectical Behavior Therapy, Mindfulness-based Cognitive Therapy, Acceptance and Commitment Therapy) have more directly targeted emotional experiences, in part by including emotion observation and acceptance techniques. The CBT model is consistent with theories of emotion regulation, as there are cognitive and behavioral aspects to emotion regulation. For example, James Gross's (1998, 2015) model of emotion regulation outlines five processes that align well with the CBT model. Four processes are defined as antecedent-focused processes, and one strategy is termed response-focused. Antecedent-focused processes include situation selection, situation modification, attentional deployment, and cognitive reappraisal. Antecedent processes are theorized to alter the processes that give rise to emotional experience. In contrast, response modulation (e.g., suppression) focuses on changes to one's emotional responses. These emotional regulatory processes are imagined along a time continuum that spans situation, attention, appraisal, and response. In addition to child self-initiated regulatory efforts, developmental psychologists argue that parents are an important source of regulation support (Diaz and Eisenberg 2015). In our review of CBT interventions to support children's emotion regulation, we will describe both child-focused and parent-implemented CBT approaches to address medical stress and pediatric health conditions.

CBT and Emotion Regulation Focused Interventions

Following from the idea that emotion regulation processes impact different parts of affective experiences (Gross—Situation selection, Situation modification, Attention deployment, Cognitive change, and Response modulation), we describe below different CBT techniques to target these different processes. As we discuss the techniques, we refer to several treatment manuals that contain resources for the techniques. If you would like a description of each manual, please see the annotated bibliography at the end of the chapter. We begin with fundamental emotion regulation skills and then look at those that are antecedent focused, then those that are focused on changing experiences and emotions "in the moment," and then those that are focused on consequence/response processes. Within the target areas/techniques, we describe the target and goal, indications that the target is relevant to a particular case, rationale, some specific interventions, resources for more information, and ways to include parents.

Why Include Parents?

Sometimes parents may feel like it is the therapist's job to "fix" their child and downplay their own role. To provide parents with rationale for their involvement, clinicians can highlight parents' influence on their child's emotional and behavioral development and how that relates to effective medical treatment. Parents have the unique opportunity to teach their children emotion regulation strategies because of their powerful socializing presence in their children's lives. They have more contact with their children and more influence than other adults do. In younger children, clinicians frequently work with the parents to alter their behavior in order to improve their child's emotion regulation. Because young children lack the emotion regulation abilities and emotional competence of adolescents, they are reliant on their parents to help them regulate their emotions and behavior particularly when facing stressful or scary medical treatments.

For example, 4-year-old Jack struggles to remain calm when he is in pain and facing new and frightening burn treatments. As his mother cries, Jack's fear is amplified, so even after his pain is managed, he continues to sob. If his mother was able to model a calm, empathetic demeanor and praise him when he was brave, Jack would likely have been able to better regulate his emotions during his treatment. Even though Cherish is older than Jack, she also struggles to regulate her emotions while frequently taking medications and visiting the hospital. Cherish's mother feels drained and worried about her daughter, and these emotions influence her daily strained interactions with Cherish. If her mother was able to focus on rewarding her daughter's cooperation with her medical regimen, rather than growing frustrated, Cherish would be more likely to tolerate her treatment. In both of these cases, providing Jack's and Cherish's parents with instruction and support would be beneficial for themselves as well as their children's emotional and health outcomes.

While parents can influence children's emotion regulation, clinicians working with parents should be mindful to avoid implying blame for their children's emotional difficulties. Warm acceptance and validation of parents' emotional experiences helps safeguard against parents feeling judged about their own stress reactions and hopefully invites collaboration rather than stoking defensiveness.

Assessment/Functional Analysis

It is important to conduct an initial assessment to determine appropriate treatment targets and then conduct ongoing, regular assessments to determine if interventions are having their intended effect. As a first step of providing emotion regulation targeted intervention, clinicians should use a fundamental CBT functional analysis (also see Chap. 7 of this volume) to identify problem areas that are potential treatment targets, as well as their precipitating and maintaining factors (e.g.,

Southam-Gerow 2016). It is helpful to generate a brief (3–5 item) list of targets of specific, behaviorally operationalized, and potentially changeable problems. For example, Cherish's list might include her cooperation with taking daily medication. Jack's list might include behavioral compliance during changes of his bandages and dressings. With the list in hand, clinicians should look for proximal drivers, factors that occur close in time to the problem behavior (cf. Henggeler et al. 2009). Specifically following the CBT model, clinicians identify antecedents (what happened just before the behavior?) and consequences (what rewards/punishments were provided or not provided, especially taking care to look for negative reinforcement) related to target behaviors. Also as part of the assessment, clinicians should gather information about the contexts and specific situations in which the problem behaviors occur. Factors in these situations include where, with whom, and other conditions the problem behaviors are more likely to be triggered (proximal triggers) or set the general conditions to increase sensitivity to specific triggers (e.g., feeling tired, hungry, and in pain). Distal drivers, that is, factors that occurred in the past but contribute to the problem behavior, may also be important and relevant to case conceptualization. In particular, in a pediatric population, past experiences in medical environments and with previous treatments or procedures may be relevant both as the result of behavioral learning processes (e.g., fear associations with medical settings) and cognitively mediated processes (e.g., beliefs about medical providers). The result of a functional analysis is a solid case conceptualization that focuses the clinician's interventions and selection of specific treatment targets and interventions, of which some options are described below.

Fundamental Emotion Regulation Skills

Emotional Awareness Most interventions to promote emotion regulation begin with promoting patients' recognition of their own and others' emotions. Targeting these fundamental skills is particularly indicated for children who lack an emotional vocabulary or who demonstrate a mismatch between their verbally expressed emotions and their apparent affect. The rationale for this work can be explained to children as multifold: emotions are indicators of what is important to us and it is easier to handle difficult situations and make good choices when we know what we and others are feeling (Southam-Gerow 2016). These interventions typically (1) build children's emotional vocabulary, (2) teach them which bodily and situational cues indicate their own specific emotions and which nonverbal and situational cues indicate others' emotions, (3) introduce a feelings intensity rating system (e.g., a feelings thermometer), and (4) assist children in practicing those skills. There are many resources available for clinicians to teach emotional awareness to children. For example, in *Emotion Regulation in Children and Adolescents: A Practitioner's Guide* (Southam-Gerow 2016), there are several excellent worksheets, games (e.g., charades), and other activities (e.g., imagining directing a movie scene and changing the scene to increase or decrease feeling intensity).

In addition to child-focused emotional awareness interventions, interventions focused on helping parents become more aware of their own emotions and their children's emotions and helping parents to coach their children about emotions may also be indicated. In particular, clinicians may find it helpful to teach parents an emotion tuning process (Havighurst and Harley 2007), which is based in John Gottman's emotion coaching framework (Gottman 1997). Emotion tuning includes a set of skills for parents to become aware of and respond to their children's emotions, instead of missing or dismissing children's emotions or moving to problem-solving too quickly. In emotion tuning, parents tune into their children's emotions by noticing how the child may be feeling, clarifying by asking the child questions about how they feel, reflecting the emotion that they think the child may be feeling, asking the child to locate their emotion in their body, empathizing with the child, and exploring the emotion. This process is difficult for many parents, especially those who were socialized to believe that emotions are signs of weakness or things to gotten over quickly. For example, Cherish's mother might take note that Cherish's brow furrows at the mention of her next medication; she could consider inquiring whether Cherish feels frustrated about taking her medication. Cherish's mother could emphasize and validate Cherish by stating that her frustration makes sense, rather than rushing to scold her for her lack of cooperation.

Gottman's book for parents (1997) is a helpful resource for parents to learn more about this process. The *Tuning into Kids* manual (Havighurst and Harley 2007) has exercises and videos that clinicians can use to help parents explore their own experience of being parented and their beliefs about emotions, as well as role-play exercises to enhance parents' skills and self-efficacy. When parents tune into their children's emotions and children feeling better understood, often there is a natural progression into a problem-solving process to address the issue underlying the emotion (limit setting, identifying goals, generating solutions, evaluating solutions, and selecting a solution; Gottman 1997). Once a child experiences emotional validation from his or her parent, it often facilitates an openness toward problem-solving, whereas starting too quickly with problem-solving sometimes inadvertently intensifies a child's feelings and creates resistance.

Emotional Understanding Beyond identifying emotions and their intensity, there is another set of skills related to understanding emotions and how they work that can be useful treatment targets. In order for children to be able to change or modulate their emotions, they need to understand that emotions are rooted in our biological reactions, have triggers that are both external (e.g., a medical situation) and internal (e.g., our beliefs and values that are often based on our past experiences), can co-occur (e.g., we can feel sad and angry simultaneously), and can be changed or hidden (cf. Southam-Gerow 2016). Most children build this understanding and skills naturally as they develop cognitively and socially, but focused conversations on these topics are indicated if children are missing pieces of understanding. Further, many children, especially those earlier in development, attribute their emotions to solely external triggers (e.g., "I am mad at mom because she hurts me when she changes my bandages"). Conversations about how emotions work (e.g., that they can have internal triggers too like "I am mad at mom because it is important to me to have control over where we sit when we change my bandages") facilitate children's motivation to learn other CBT skills such as cognitive reappraisal (e.g., "When mom cleans my skin, she is helping it to get better"). Like with emotional awareness, there are many resources available for clinicians to teach emotional understanding to children. For pediatric patients, the trigger card game, which involves children earning points for generating triggers (external and internal) for emotions on a set of cards, could be adapted to focus on medically related emotions and triggers (see book by Southam-Gerow 2016). This manual also has excellent psychoeducational content for children about the psychophysiology of fear/anxiety/worry, sadness, anger, and happiness.

Antecedent-Focused Treatment Targets and Intervention

Antecedent-focused treatment targets and interventions are designed to assist children prevent emotion dysregulation. Treatment targets include internal and external triggers for emotion dysregulation.

Prevention: Meeting Basic Needs Like adults, children have increased sensitivity to emotional alarms when their basic needs are not met. Most parents notice that their children are more likely to have emotional and behavioral meltdowns when they are tired or hungry, but they may not prioritize basic needs such as good sleep hygiene, healthy eating, and physical activity for their children (or themselves) when facing medical challenges. Further, medical challenges often disrupt normal family routines, and parents and children may need help with figuring out how to adapt their normal routines or establish new ones. Explicit focus on prevention through meeting basic needs may be indicated in children who have many emotional meltdowns and for those who do not have good eating, sleeping, and activity routines. Child-focused interventions can include teaching children about how not having our physical needs met can set the stage for dysregulation due to external triggers. Also, encouraging children to "Think about your body. What is it telling you that it needs right now?" can help them to tune into their basic needs. Then clinicians can work with children about how to ask for help in meeting those needs more proactively. Parent-focused interventions are often important as well. Clinicians can work with parents to map out schedules to meet their own and their children's needs, maintaining their normal routines as much as possible to provide stability. Especially for parents whose own routines have been affected by a child's illness, clinicians can help parents to prioritize their own basic needs, not only to help reduce their own emotional reactivity but also to model good self-care for their children.

Parents can also build medical interventions into the family's normal routine as much as possible. For example, some children require daily medications. Tying the medications to other parts of a daily routine such as bathing or brushing teeth can increase regimen compliance because they are less likely to be forgotten, and also, clinicians and parents can talk to children about how such routines are about taking care of our bodies and about how the addition of the medication is just extension of the self-care routine that their particular bodies need. Building routines and cognitively tying medical routines to other self-care routines can help to prevent emotion dysregulation, such as anger, centered on having to do such medical interventions.

Prevention: Increasing Self-Efficacy Another strategy to prevent emotion dysregulation is to encourage children to engage in activities that boost their self-efficacy. By doing things that they are good at, children feel better about themselves, which helps them to better handle triggers for negative feelings (Southam-Gerow 2016). This strategy may be indicated if a patient does not have enough self-efficacy building activities or if those activities have been disrupted by his or her medical condition. Activity selection and behavioral activation modules can be borrowed from depression treatment manuals (e.g., Chorpita and Weisz 2009; Curry et al. 2005). Particularly with chronic medical patients, such activities may be important to help them to develop more fully the aspects of their self-concepts that do not involve their illness. For example, Cherish might benefit from learning how many kids see themselves as different, even kids without a medical condition. Use of a positive reward system might help reduce her noncompliance in taking her prescribed medications, thus reducing her mother's use of repeated requests, and ultimately improve their interactions and relationship. Cherish's improved medication adherence may then reduce her distress related to being "different" and improve her self-concept. For our younger patient Jack, parents' use of differential attention could prevent unintentional reinforcement of avoidance behavior related to dressing changes or bath time, thus shortening the overall length of the feared situation and reducing the amount of distress Jack could experience. As a result, he may habituate more quickly, be receptive to the notion that he is brave, and develop a self-concept that includes being able to tolerate scary, painful situations.

Situation Selection Another antecedent-focused treatment is situation selection, which is defined as approaching or avoiding a setting, experience, or circumstance in order to prevent emotional dysregulation when it can be anticipated (Gross 1998). It is frequently applied in daily life: people choose to avoid people they dislike and participate in activities they find pleasurable. However, situation selection must be utilized carefully in medical settings. When appropriate, a patient can choose between variations of a treatment and who is responsible for their care. That being said, patients should not avoid their medical procedures entirely, even if they are unpleasant. While this avoidance of treatment may lead to temporary relief, it will likely result in long-term negative health consequences. The negative reinforcement of this avoidance and fears about procedures can further increase patient fears and resistance to the medical regimen. For this reason, situation selection ought to be decided with the help of others, including medical professionals, therapists when applicable, and well-informed parents. In the case of Jack, the 4-year-old burn patient, he could choose to remove his bedroom mirror, to avoid being upset by the sight of his injuries. In this example, Jack still receives the treatment he requires, but he is able to select the variation of the treatment that is most conducive to his own emotional well-being.

Situation Modification While situation selection is sometimes possible before an emotion-provoking situation occurs, this is not always the case. Sometimes patients encounter situations that evoke negative emotional reactions, but a modification of the situation can alter the emotional impact and encourage emotion regulation (Gross 1998). Situation modification is sometimes also referred to as problem-focused coping (Lazarus and Folkman 1984) or primary control (Rothbaum 1982). Below we will address several more specific methods of situation modification that can be applied to a pediatric medical setting.

Pain Management. Many medical conditions and procedures involve pain, and many young children do not receive adequate pain management (cf. Blount et al. 2006; Howard 2003), often because it is difficult for providers to assess pain in young children (cf. Brown et al. 2018). Inadequate pain management can negatively affect future pain experiences, compliance, and health outcomes (Taddio et al. 1995, 1997; Brown et al. 2014; Miller et al. 2011). Attending to pain when choosing procedures and managing pain with appropriate pharmacological methods are important to assist children with emotion regulation (also see Chap. 14 of this volume). Beyond those situation-modifying techniques, parent-focused interventions can be efficacious. Parental state anxiety during children's medical procedures is associated with child distress during and after procedures (Bernard and Cohen 2006; Racine et al. 2016), and parental and child distress is likely bidirectional, with each influencing increased distress in the other (Blount et al. 1989). Providing parents with strategies to coach their children in pain management techniques (such as distraction, described below) during procedures can increase their own self-efficacy and reduce their procedural anxiety and the child's anxiety and pain (Kain et al. 2007; Manne et al. 1990). These parental interventions are likely most effective when timed to occur before the first procedures if there will be recurring procedures to prevent negative expectations based on an initial bad experience (Brown et al. 2018). It should be noted that these psychological approaches to pain management are used in conjunction with medications as recommended by the medical team.

Provide and Ask for Choices. In many medical situations, there are few options for a child to modify the situation to assist with emotion regulation. For example, if a child requires a medical procedure (e.g., a blood draw), the child and the caregiver cannot change the broad situation. Especially in acute care settings, children often report feeling a lack of control over what is happening to them (Salmela et al. 2011; Salter and Stallard 2004), which is likely to drive stronger emotional responses. Medical providers and parents can give children some control and choices within what is medically indicated. Further, patients and parents can ask and advocate for choice within what is medically necessary. For example, children can be provided choice of color of medical gown, which body part to examine first (e.g., right ear or left ear), sitting with a parent or not, or holding a much-loved stuffed animal or not. Jack could elect to help remove his own bandages, and Cherish could choose to look away from injections she receives. Providing such choice in the middle of painful or distressing symptoms or procedures can mitigate the traumatic nature of those experiences (Blount et al. 2003; Krauss et al. 2016).

Soothing Truth Telling, Not Global Reassurances. When children are distressed about medical issues and procedures, clinicians and parents naturally want to provide emotional reassurance (cf. Kassam-Adams and Butler 2017). They often provide global reassurances like "You're okay," "Everything will be okay," "It won't hurt much," or "Don't worry." However, these types of verbal reassurances from parents and clinicians during procedures can have the opposite effect and instead have been shown to exacerbate the child's pain and distress (Blount et al. 2003; Chorney et al. 2013). Instead, except perhaps in the most extreme circumstances, clinicians and parents can view medical situations as opportunities to build trust with the children by providing them with accurate information presented in a soothing, empathic manner. For example, a parent could tell the child that the vaccination will hurt, but that it will be over quickly. Building trust in the clinician–patient or child–parent relationship can facilitate children turning to caregivers for information, reassurance, and help managing challenging or painful situations, ultimately resulting in better health outcomes.

Attentional Deployment Attentional deployment techniques involve changing the child's attentional focus; typically, these techniques are loosely grouped under the classifications of distraction, concentration, and rumination. Distraction, concentration, and mindfulness techniques can be helpful, in part by preventing or interrupting rumination, which is a repetitive thought pattern that is focused on feelings and their consequences. Rumination is associated with internalizing symptoms such as depression or anxiety because people can get trapped in a cycle of negative thoughts (Nolen-Hoeksema et al. 1993; Nolen-Hoeksema 2000, 2001). In the medical context, rumination can also lead to avoidance of a procedure, excessive reassurance seeking from parents, or other escape behaviors (Weinstock and Whisman 2006).

Distraction shifts focus away from an unpleasant stimulus and concentration absorbs cognitive resources to create a self-sustaining state (Gross 1998). Of these categories of attentional deployment techniques, distraction is the most widely applied to pediatric medical settings; however, there is also support for the use of concentration and mindfulness and interventions to avoid rumination in pediatric medical populations.

Distraction. The goal of distraction is to keep the child focused on something other than the distressing medical procedure. For Jack, this could mean drawing his focus away from his initial chest scrub as his affected skin peels off, while for Cherish, distraction could be used to help her endure her frequent blood draws. There is a wide range of distraction techniques that medical staff or parents can choose to use with the child. Distraction can be classified as either active or passive: active distraction encourages the child's involvement in an activity, while passive distraction requires the child to remain still and observe an activity or stimulus (Koller and Goldman 2012). The nature of the medical procedure dictates whether active or passive distraction should be used.

Examples of active distraction include interactive toys, video games, virtual reality, guided imagery, and controlled breathing (Koller and Goldman 2012). These techniques require different levels of guidance; while medical professionals or parents need only provide toys or video games, techniques like guided imagery and controlled breathing require continued assistance. For guided imagery, the child is led through gradual muscle relaxation and encouraged to let their mind wander to something pleasant and peaceful (Koller and Goldman 2012). Controlled breathing also produces relaxation; patients deliberately pace their breathing to remain calm (Koller and Goldman 2012). Parents or medical professionals can aid the child in breathing exercises by breathing slowly themselves and then encouraging the child to join them.

Passive distraction techniques often consist of auditory or audiovisual stimulation because those require no interaction by the patient (Koller and Goldman 2012). For example, children can listen to music or watch television if a procedure permits. Little additional assistance is required for passive distraction techniques, but parents can work with their child's doctors to provide the technology. They can also draw their child's attention to the music or television as a way of reinforcing this emotion regulation strategy.

These distraction techniques can be applied to a wide variety of pediatric populations. For example, distraction is effective for pediatric cancer patients, who must undergo many painful, uncomfortable, or distressing procedures throughout the course of their treatment. When children play video games during chemotherapy, it can reduce their nausea and anxiety (Redd et al. 1987). Exploring a virtual world with a virtual reality headset can also reduce distress and improve coping during a port access procedure (Wolitzky et al. 2005). Distraction is also effective for children receiving immunizations, IV insertions, or other venipunctures. Live music during needle insertions can decrease behavioral distress, and giving children an assortment of distracting toys during venipuncture can decrease a child's fear (Malone 1996; Cavender et al. 2004). Distraction mechanisms, such as a handheld video game, can additionally decrease pediatric preoperative anxiety (Patel et al. 2006).

While there are many different distraction techniques that can be used for many different pediatric populations, it is important that the technique is compatible with the medical procedure, and accepted by the patient, parents, and doctors. The distraction technique must only require interaction when the child is capable of such, and it is best if it is noninvasive and inexpensive. Whichever technique is selected, parents must remember to encourage their child's participation, to reinforce adaptive emotion regulation rather than maladaptive focus on physical symptoms. This can at times be challenging for parents. Especially when their child is suffering or complaining, it can be natural to offer the child sympathy as a comfort. However, a study by Walker et al. (2006) found that in children with abdominal pain, parental conversation to distract the child from their discomfort decreased the child's complaints compared to parental sympathy and attention alone. Sympathetic statements such as "I know it hurts, but you'll be okay soon" draws the child's attention to their discomfort and reinforces complaints of pain with parental attention (Walker et al. 2006). When parents engage in distraction techniques with their child, they are instead reinforcing their child's management of their behavior in spite of pain.

Concentration. Concentration requires the child's attention to be centered on a particular thought or activity. This can be considered an internal form of situation selection, as the patient chooses what mental space they wish to occupy during a medical procedure (Gross 1998). Concentration can be combined with distraction to make the distraction more effective during an unpleasant situation, as it draws more cognitive resources away from a potential trigger of emotional dysregulation.

Mindfulness. Mindfulness is described as "paying attention in a particular way: on purpose, in the present moment, and non-judgmentally" (Kabat-Zinn 1994, p. 4). Mindfulness-based interventions are designed to improve self-regulation through increased acceptance and self-awareness (e.g., of pain or anger about being ill) and decreased emotional reactivity, cognitive rumination, and avoidance (Baer 2003). In contrast to CBT approaches that are designed to change cognitions and behaviors to improve emotional experience, mindfulness-based approaches teach individuals how to observe those experiences without reacting to them in a habitual or maladaptive way. In adults, it has been demonstrated to alleviate mental and physical health symptoms for patients with cancer, cardiovascular disease, chronic pain, depression, and anxiety disorders (for a review, see Gotnik et al. 2015). Empirical support for its use in children is more limited but suggests that mindfulness-based interventions are feasible and beneficial (Semple et al. 2010). Mindfulness meditation practices may be particularly indicated for children for whom stress is an exacerbating or maintaining factor in dysfunctional somatic problems (e.g., atopic dermatitis, diffuse pain without clear physiological origin), and simple mindfulness meditation practice scripts involving attention to breath and bodily sensations and designed for a pediatric population are available (e.g., Perry-Parrish and Sibinga 2014). For further description of mindfulness-based approaches in this book, see Chaps. 9 and 10 of this volume.

Parental Differential Attention One of the most powerful cognitive-behavioral techniques that parents can implement to facilitate their child's behavioral cooperation is differential attention. Differential attention techniques involve parents providing their child with positive attention when they are behaving appropriately and ignoring them when they are misbehaving (McMahon and Forehand 2003). This follows from the operant conditioning principle of positive reinforcement to increase the frequency of behavior, and negative punishment to decrease the frequency of behavior (Kazdin 2008). There are several skills parents deploy to practice differential attention. One skill is attends. Attends is a form of positive attention in which the parent provides an ongoing narration of their child's behavior or activity (McMahon and Forehand 2003). The two basic types of attends are those that describe overt behavior, and those that indicate desired prosocial behavior (McMahon and Forehand 2003). Parents can also use the skill of rewards. Like attends, this is a positive reinforcement skill, in which the parent uses praise, physical affection, or tangible items to show approval and increase likelihood of the desired behavior occurring (McMahon and Forehand 2003). Lastly, parents can ignore their child to decrease inappropriate behavior. This technique is used in place of positive punishment such as verbal reprimanding, and it lasts until the extinction of the unwanted behavior (Kazdin 2008). Ignoring should be combined with positive attention, such as attends or rewards, in order to increase the desirable behaviors while simultaneously decreasing the incompatible undesirable behaviors (McMahon and Forehand 2003). This combination of positive attention and ignoring comprises differential attention (McMahon and Forehand 2003). Additional resources for clinicians and parents can be found in *Helping the Noncompliant Child* (McMahon and Forehand 2003) and *The Kazdin Method for Parenting the Defiant Child* (Kazdin 2008).

For example, if Jack became emotionally overwhelmed during a frightening medical procedure, like his first time receiving dressings and bandages, he might throw a tantrum to avoid the medical procedure. While his parents naturally would want to comfort him by providing attention and sympathy, this positively reinforces the tantrum and avoidant behavior. Similarly, if the dressing and bandaging was delayed due to the tantrum, this would negatively reinforce the tantrum. Instead, Jack's parents should ignore the tantrum until Jack calms down and regulates his emotions more successfully. Once he manages his emotions through the medical procedure, his parents can provide attention and support to reinforce that coping behavior.

Differential attention is frequently considered as an intervention for oppositional children, but it can additionally be applied to pediatric medical populations. Noncompliance is a common problem for children with acute and chronic illnesses, so positive attention and ignoring can also be used to increase adherence to a medical regimen while decreasing emotional or behavioral opposition (McMahon and Forehand 2003). Although sometimes adaptations are required to assist the parent or the child with medical issues, this emotional compliance makes treating the child far easier (McMahon and Forehand 2003). For this reason, parental intervention into the child's behavioral and emotional self-regulation is key to ensuring that the care regimen is implemented successfully.

Response Processes

In some instances, a child is in a state of emotional dysregulation and the situation cannot be modified. In these cases, the treatment targets are instead the child's emotional responses and cognitions. Both response modulation and cognitive reappraisal are examples of techniques that target response processes because they occur late in the emotion generative process.

Response Modulation Response modulation can occur after the child is already responding emotionally to a situation, and it involves altering the physiological, experiential, or behavioral responses (Gross 1998). To lessen physiological responses and negative experiential components, the child can be given a medication to lessen their symptoms or taught relaxation techniques (Gross 1998). Exposure and desensitization techniques can also be used to help the child habituate to their discomfort, so they are more capable of regulating their emotions.

Exposure Therapies. For children who have an established fear or anxiety association with medical procedures or cues, anxiety exposure therapy techniques, such as those described in the *Coping Cat* manuals (Kendall et al. 2002; Kendall and Hedtke 2006) may be helpful. For example, if Jack displayed a fear of returning to normal bathing in the tub after his burn injury, a desensitization approach could involve having him play in the tub with his clothes on, then with a basin of water and bath toys, in the tub with a small amount of water, and so on, until the normal bathing routine is approximated with the typical amount of water with minimal fear and until typical compliance is observed. Exposure therapies are typically paired with positive reinforcement to optimize compliance (also see Chaps. 7 and 8 of this volume).

Cognitive Change People are constantly evaluating their perceived situation, and this evaluation elicits an emotional response. Cognitive change requires a reappraisal of that evaluation, in order to alter the emotional response (Gross 1998). There are several ways to modify cognitive evaluations. One that is particularly applicable to pediatric medical populations is cognitive reframing. When the child is feeling upset over a perceived failure or deficiency, they can shift their thinking so that the failure is perceived as a success by another standard. For example, Cherish feels upset that her medication regimen makes her different from the other children. To improve her mood and help her medication compliance, she could see her medication and dialysis regimen as proof that she is strong and brave and able to overcome a difficult life obstacle. Cognitive reframing can also help parents and children to sidestep power struggles. For example, in the case of Jake, he and his parents may find themselves angry with one another about bandage changes. He may feel angry that his parents' changing the bandages causes pain, and they may feel angry at his lack of compliance. A therapist could help them to reframe and see themselves as "on the same team" fighting against the problem of his pain. This type of reframing to externalize the problem can open them up to problem-solving ways to give Jack some control and lessen his pain (also see Chaps. 7 and 8 of this volume).

Cognitive reframing can be difficult for children to accomplish on their own. Parents, therapists, or medical professionals can guide children through these changes in thinking by both encouraging it and modeling it themselves. Similarly, when children are feeling angry, adults can help coach them on how to best regulate their emotions.

Emotion Coaching Anger. It is difficult for parents to use emotional coaching in the moment when children express intense anger, especially when the expression is through angry behavior (e.g., whining, complaining, tantrums, throwing things, screaming). Once a child has calmed down by letting off steam or through soothing, parents can help the child to separate their feelings of anger from their angry behaviors and to examine other emotions that may underlie the angry feelings (Havighurst and Harley 2007). For example, Cherish might get angry, scream at her mother, and throw things at home when she learns her friends are having a sleepover that she cannot attend. Once Cherish is calmer, her mother can validate Cherish's feelings of anger, while simultaneously setting behavioral limits, and then help Cherish to articulate underlying emotions of frustration, disappointment, and sadness of missing out. With those emotions identified, they can brainstorm ways for Cherish to connect with her friends through another activity.

Summary

Consideration of emotion regulation and its links to pediatric health and coping provide a useful approach to supporting children and their families experiencing medical stress. Cognitive-behavioral approaches are well suited to target improvements in emotion regulation. Adaptive emotion regulation likely supports adjustment to acute and chronic health conditions and may lead to better health outcomes in youth. CBT approaches provide support to children as well as support for parents and siblings, as the emotional landscape of the family influences children's emotional reactions. In addition to well-established CBT approaches, mindfulness-based interventions offer another technique to support the emotion regulation of youth. In summary, it is important to consider emotion regulation as a key facet to develop in youth facing medical conditions.

Annotated Bibliography of Resources

Emotion Regulation in Children and Adolescents: A Practitioner's Guide (Southam-Gerow 2016).

This manual is designed in the form of modules that can be used together or individually as needed. The target population is children through adolescents with a wide range of mental health diagnoses. The modules target emotion awareness, emotion understanding, antecedent-management techniques, emotional expression, and cognitive reappraisal skills. The manual includes many exercises, activities, and handouts.

Coping Cat and the C.A.T Project (Kendall et al. 2002; Kendall and Hedtke 2006).

These treatment manuals and workbooks use a CBT approach to treat anxiety in 7- to 13-year-old (*Coping Cat*) and 14- to17-year-old (*C.A.T* Project) children. The treatment includes components on psychoeducation for children and families, recognizing and understanding emotional and physical reactions to anxiety, exposure tasks, relaxation techniques, and developing plans for effective coping.

Helping the Noncompliant Child (McMahon and Forehand 2003).

This manual includes instructions for clinicians, in addition to handouts for parents, based on the Helping the Noncompliant Child (HNC) program. It is designed primarily for 3- to 8-year-old children, and it includes sections about implementing the program in specific populations, including pediatrics.

The Kazdin Method for Parenting the Defiant Child (Kazdin 2008).

This book includes cognitive-behavioral strategies for increasing compliance in children. It is designed as a parent handbook, and it includes tips and techniques for working with very young children, school-aged children, and preadolescents.

Defiant Child (Barkley 2013).

This manual is designed to enable clinicians to teach parents how to manage their noncompliant child. This program has been developed over the course of several decades, and it is one of the best-known manuals for improving oppositional behavior.

Incredible Years (Webster-Stratton 2011).

This book promotes parenting strategies and teaching methods that facilitate children's social and emotional competence across a range of settings. *Incredible Years* outlines group training programs for parents, teachers, and children, with the long-term goal of preventing conduct problems in vulnerable youth populations.

Raising an Emotionally Intelligent Child: The Heart of Parenting (Gottman 1997).

This book is targeted at parents. It describes five steps of emotion coaching: awareness of children's emotions, recognizing emotion as an opportunity for intimacy and teaching, listening empathically and validating children's feelings, helping children to label emotions verbally, and while helping children problem solve. It includes specific strategies and suggestions for how to modify based on the child's age.

Tuning in to Kids: Emotionally Intelligent Parenting (Havighurst and Harley 2007).

This program is designed as a parent education program that draws heavily on Gottman's work on parent emotion coaching. The program is designed as a parent education program for parents of preschool children and was designed to be delivered in a group format. The manual contains lesson plans with activities, handouts, and homework for six sessions, which address naming emotions, parents' emotional understanding, and problem-solving and coaching children's fears, worries, and anger.

References

Baer, R. A. (2003). Mindfulness training as a clinical intervention: A conceptual and empirical review. *Clinical Psychology: Science and Practice, 10,* 125–143. https://doi.org/10.1093/clipsy.bpg015.

Barkley, R. A. (2013). *Defiant children: A Clinician's manual for assessment and parent training* (3rd ed.). New York, NY: Guildford Press.

Bernard, R. S., & Cohen, L. L. (2006). Parent anxiety and infant pain during pediatric immunizations. *Journal of Clinical Psychology in Medical Settings, 13,* 285–290. https://doi.org/10.1007/s10880-006-9027-6.

Blount, R. L., Corbin, S., Sturges, J., Wolfe, V., Prater, J., & James, L. (1989). The relationship between adults' behavior and child coping and distress during BMA/LP procedures: A sequential analysis. *Behavior Therapy, 20,* 585–601. https://doi.org/10.1016/S00057894(89)80136-4.

Blount, R. L., Piira, T., & Cohen, L. L. (2003). Management of pediatric pain and distress due to medical procedures. In M. C. Roberts (Ed.), *Handbook of pediatric psychology* (pp. 216–233). New York, NY: Guilford Press.

Blount, R. L., Piira, T., Cohen, L. L., & Cheng, P. S. (2006). Pediatric procedural pain. *Behavior Modification, 30,* 24–49. https://doi.org/10.1177/0145445505282438.

Brown, N. J., Kimble, R. M., Gramotnev, G., Rodger, S., & Cuttle, L. (2014). Predictors of re-epithelialization in pediatric burn. *Burns, 40,* 751–758. https://doi.org/10.1016/j.burns.2013.09.027.

Brown, E. A., DeYoung, A., Kimble, R., & Kenardy, J. (2018). Review of parent's influence on pediatric procedural distress and recovery. *Clinical Child and Family Psychology Review, 21,* 224–245. https://doi.org/10.1007/s10567-017-0252-3.

Cavender, K., Goff, M. D., Hollon, E. C., & Guzzetta, C. E. (2004). Parents' positioning and distracting children during venipuncture. *Journal of Holistic Nursing, 22,* 32–56. https://doi.org/10.1177/0898010104263306.

Chorney, J. M., Tan, E. T., & Kain, Z. N. (2013). Adult-child interactions in the postanesthesia care unit: Behavior matters. Perioperative medicine, 118, 834–841. https://doi.org/10.1097/ALN.0b013e31827e501b.

Chorpita, B. F., & Weisz, J. R. (2009). *MATCH-ADTC: Modular approach to therapy for children with anxiety, depression, trauma, or conduct problems.* Satellite Beach, FL: PracticeWise.

Curry, J. F., Wells, K. C., Brent, D. A., Clarke, G. N., Rohde, P., Albano, A. M., Reinecke, M. A., Benazon, N., March, J. S., et al. (2005). *Treatment for adolescents with depression study (TADS): Cognitive behavioral therapy manual.* Durham, NC: Duke University Medical Center.

D'Souza, A. L., Nelson, N. G., & McKenzie, L. B. (2009). Pediatric burn injuries treated in US emergency departments between 1990 and 2006. *Pediatrics, 124,* 1424–1430. https://doi.org/10.1542/peds.2008-2802.

Diaz, A., & Eisenberg, N. (2015). The process of emotion regulation is different from individual differences in emotion regulation: Conceptual arguments and a focus on individual differences. *Psychological Inquiry, 26,* 37–47. https://doi.org/10.1080/1047840X.2015.959094.

Eisenberg, N. (2000). Emotion, regulation, and moral development. *Annual Review of Psychology, 51,* 665–697. https://doi.org/10.1146/51.1.665.

Eisenberg, N., Murphy, B. C., & Shepard, S. A. (1997). The development of empathetic accuracy. In W. Ickes (Ed.), *Empathetic accuracy* (pp. 73–116). New York, NY: Guilford Press.

Eisenberg, N., Cumberland, A., & Spinrad, T. L. (1998). Parental socialization of emotion. *Psychological Inquiry, 9,* 241–273.

Fuchs, D., & Thelen, M. H. (1988). Children's expected interpersonal consequences of communicating their affective state and reported likelihood of expression. *Child Development, 59,* 1314–1322. https://doi.org/10.2307/1130494.

Ginsburg, G. S., & Schlossberg, M. C. (2002). Family-based treatment of childhood anxiety disorders. *International Review of Psychiatry, 14,* 143–154. https://doi.org/10.1080/09540260220132662.

Gnepp, J., & Hess, D. L. R. (1986). Children's understanding of verbal and facial display rules. *Developmental Psychology, 22,* 103–108. https://doi.org/10.1037/0012-1649.22.1.103.

Gosselin, P., Warren, M., & Diotte, M. (2002). Motivation to hide emotion and children's understanding of the distinction between real and apparent emotions. *Journal of Genetic Psychology, 163,* 479–495. https://doi.org/10.1080/00221320209598697.

Gotnik, R. A., Chu, P., Busschbach, J. J., Benson, H., Fricchione, G. L., & Hunink, M. G. (2015). Standardized mindfulness-based interventions in healthcare: An overview of systematic reviews and meta-analyses of RCTs. *PLoS One, 10*, e0124344. https://doi.org/10.1371/journal.pone.0124344.

Gottman, J. (1997). *Raising an emotionally intelligent child*. New York, NY: Simon & Schuster.

Gross, J. J., & Munoz, R. F.(1995). Emotion regulation and mental health. *Clinical Psychology: Science and Practice, 2*, 151–164. https://doi.org/10.1111/j.1468-2850.1995.tb00036.x.

Gross, J. J. (2015) Emotion regulation: Current status and future prospects. *Psychological Inquiry, 26*, 1–27. https://doi.org/10.1080/1047840X.2014.940781.

Gross, J. J. (1998). The emerging field of emotion regulation: An integrative review. *Review of General Psychology, 2*, 271–299.

Gross, J. J. (2002). Emotion regulation: Affective, cognitive, and social consequences. *Psychophysiology, 39*, 281–291. https://doi.org/10.1017/S0048577201393198.

Harris, P., & Gross, D. (1988). Children's understanding of real and apparent emotion. In J. Astington, P. Harris, & D. Olson (Eds.), *Developing theories of mind* (pp. 295–314). New York, NY: Cambridge University Press.

Harris, P., Donnelly, K., Guz, G., & Pitt-Watson, R. (1986). Children's understanding of the distinction between real and apparent emotion. *Child Development, 57*, 895–909. https://doi.org/10.2307/1130366.

Harris, P., Olthof, T., Meerum Terwogt, M., & Hardman, C. (1987). Children's knowledge of the situations that provoke emotion. *International Journal of Behavioral Development, 10*, 319–344. https://doi.org/10.1177/016502548701000304.

Havighurst, S. S., & Harley, A. (2007). *Tuning into kids: Emotionally intelligent parenting: Program manual* (3rd ed.). Melbourne: University of Melbourne.

Henggeler, S. W., Schoenwald, S. K., Borduin, C. M., Rowland, M. D., & Cunningham, P. B. (2009). *Multisystemic therapy for antisocial behavior in children and adolescents* (2nd ed.). New York, NY: Guilford Press.

Honig, A. S. (2005). Emotional milestones and their link to learning: The ability to form secure attachments during early childhood promotes a lifetime of emotional health. *Scholastic Early Childhood Today, 20*, 30–31.

Howard, R. F. (2003). Current status of pain management in children. *Journal of the American Medical Association, 290*, 2464–2469. https://doi.org/10.1001/jama.290.18.2464.

Josephs, I. (1994). Display rule behavior and understanding in preschool children. *Journal of Nonverbal Behavior, 18*, 301–326.

Kabat-Zinn, J. (1994). *Wherever you go, there you are*. New York, NY: Hyperion.

Kain, Z. N., Caldwell-Andrews, A. A., Mayes, L. C., Weinberg, M. E., Wang, S. M., MacLaren, J. E., et al. (2007). Family-centered preparation for surgery improves perioperative outcomes in children: A randomized controlled trial. *Anesthesiology, 106*, 65–74.

Kassam-Adams, N., & Butler, L. (2017). What do clinicians caring for children need to know about pediatric medical traumatic stress and the ethics of trauma-informed approaches? *AMA Journal of Ethics, 19*, 793–801. https://doi.org/10.1001/journalofethics.2017.19.8.pfor1-1708.

Kazdin, A. E. (2008). *The Kazdin method for parenting the defiant child*. New York, NY: Houghton Mifflin Harcourt.

Kendall, P. C., & Hedtke, K. A. (2006). *Cognitive-behavioral therapy for anxious children: Therapist manual* (3rd ed.). Ardmore, PA: Workbook Publishing.

Kendall, P. C., Choudhury, M., Hudson, J., & Webb, A. (2002). *"The C.a.T. project" manual for the cognitive-behavioral treatment of anxious adolescents*. Ardmore, PA: Workbook Publishing.

Kochanska, G., Murray, K., & Harlan, E. (2000). Effortful control in early childhood: Continuity and change, antecedents, and implications for social development. *Developmental Psychology, 36*, 220–232.

Koller, D., & Goldman, R. D. (2012). Distraction techniques for children undergoing procedures: A critical review of pediatric research. *Journal of Pediatric Nursing, 27*, 652–681. https://doi.org/10.1542/peds.2017-3318.

Krauss, B. S., Krauss, B. A., & Green, S. M. (2016). Managing procedural anxiety in children. *New England Journal of Medicine, 374*, e19–e19.

Lane, J., Wellman, H., Olson, S., LaBounty, J., & Kerr, D. (2010). Theory of mind and emotion understanding predict moral development in early childhood. *British Journal of Developmental Psychology, 28*, 871–889. https://doi.org/10.1348/026151009X483056.

Lazarus, R. S., & Folkman, S. (1984). *The handbook of behavioral medicine*. New York, NY: Guilford Press.

Malatesta, C., Culver, C., Tesman, J. R., & Shepard, B. (1989). The development of emotion expression during the first two years of life. *Monographs of the Society for Research in Child Development, 54*, 1–136. https://doi.org/10.2307/1166153.

Malone, A. B. (1996). The effects of live music on the distress of pediatric patients receiving intravenous starts, venipunctures, injections, and heel sticks. *Journal of Music Therapy, 33*, 19–33. https://doi.org/10.1093/jmt/33.1.19.

Manne, S., Redd, W., Jacobsen, P., Gorfinkle, K., Schorr, O., & Rapkin, B. (1990). Behavioral intervention to reduce child and parent distress during venipuncture. *Journal of Consulting and Clinical Psychology, 58*, 565–572.

McMahon, R. J., & Forehand, R. L. (2003). *Helping the noncompliant child: Family-based treatment for oppositional behavior* (2nd ed.). New York, NY: Guildford Press.

Miller, K., Rodger, S., Kipping, B., & Kimble, R. M. (2011). A novel technology approach to pain management in children with burns: A prospective randomized controlled trial. *Burns, 37*, 395–405. https://doi.org/10.1016/j.burns.2010.12.008.

Nolen-Hoeksema, S. (2000). The role of rumination in depressive disorders and mixed anxiety/depressive symptoms. *Journal of Abnormal Psychology, 109*, 504–511. https://doi.org/10.1037/10021-843X.109.3.504.

Nolen-Hoeksema, S. (2001). Gender differences in depression. *Current Directions in Psychological Science, 10*, 173–175. https://doi.org/10.1007/s00406-002-0381-6.

Nolen-Hoeksema, S., Morrow, J., & Fredrickson, B. (1993). Response styles and the duration of episodes of depressed mood. *Journal of Abnormal Psychology, 102*, 20–28.

Patel, A., Schieble, T., Davidson, M., Tran, M. C. J., Schoenberg, C., Delphin, E., et al. (2006). Distraction with a hand-held video game reduces pediatric preoperative anxiety. *Pediatric Anesthesia, 16*, 1019–1027. https://doi.org/10.1111/j.1460-9592.2006.01914.x.

Perry-Parrish, C. K., & Sibinga, E. M. S. (2014). Mindfulness meditation for children. In R. D. Anbar (Ed.), *Functional symptoms in pediatric disease: A clinical guide* (pp. 343–352). New York, NY: Springer.

Pons, F., Harris, P. L., & de Rosnay, M. (2004). Emotion comprehension between 3 and 11 years: Developmental periods and hierarchical organization. *European Journal of Developmental Psychology, 1*, 127–152. https://doi.org/10.1080/17405620344000022.

Price, J., Kassam-Adams, N., Alderfer, M. A., Christofferson, J., & Kazak, A. E. (2016). Systematic review: A reevaluation and update of the integrative (trajectory) model of pediatric medical traumatic stress. *Journal of Pediatric Psychology, 41*, 86–97. https://doi.org/10.1093/jpepsy/jsv074.

Racine, N. M., Pillai Riddell, R., Khan, M., Calic, M., Taddio, A., & Tablon, P. (2016). Systematic review: Predisposing, precipitating, perpetuating, and present factors predicting anticipatory distress to painful medical procedures in children. *Journal of Pediatric Psychology, 41*, 159–181. https://doi.org/10.1093/jpepsy/jsv076.

Redd, W. H., Jacobsen, P. B., Die-Trill, M., Dermatis, H., McEvoy, M., & Holland, J. C. (1987). Cognitive/attentional distraction in the control of conditioned nausea in pediatric cancer patients receiving chemotherapy. *Journal of Consulting and Clinical Psychology, 55*, 391–395. https://doi.org/10.1037/0022-006X.55.3.391.

Rothbaum, F. (1982). Changing the world and changing the self: A two-process model of perceived control. *Journal of Personality and Social Psychology, 42*, 5–37.

Saarni, C. (1979). Children's understanding of display rules for expressive behavior. *Developmental Psychology, 15*, 424–429. https://doi.org/10.1037/0012-1649.15.4.424.

Saarni, C. (1984). An observational study of children's attempts to monitor their expressive behavior. *Child Development, 55*, 1504–1513.

Saarni, C. (1999). *The development of emotional competence*. New York, NY: Guilford Press.

Salmela, M., Aronen, E. T., & Salanterä, S. (2011). The experience of hospital-related fears of 4- to 6-year-old children. *Child: Care, Health and Development, 37*, 719–726. https://doi.org/10.1111/j.1365-2214.2010.01171.x.

Salter, E., & Stallard, P. (2004). Young people's experience of emergency medical services as road traffic accident victims: A pilot qualitative study. *Journal of Child Health Care, 8*, 301–311. https://doi.org/10.1177/1367493504047320.

Semple, R. J., Lee, J., Rosa, D., & Miller, L. F. (2010). A randomized control trial of mindfulness-based cognitive therapy for children: Promoting mindful attention to enhance social-emotional resiliency in children. *Journal of Child and Family Studies, 19*, 218–229. https://doi.org/10.1007/s10826-009-9301-y.

Southam-Gerow, M. A. (2016). *Emotion regulation in children and adolescents: A Practitioner's guide*. New York, NY: Guilford Press.

Taddio, A., Goldbach, M., Ipp, M., Stevens, B., & Koren, G. (1995). Effect of neonatal circumcision on pain responses during vaccination in boys. *Lancet, 345*, 291–292.

Taddio, A., Katz, J., Ilersich, A. L., & Koren, G. (1997). Effect of neonatal circumcision on pain response during subsequent routine vaccination. *Lancet, 349*, 599–603.

The National Child Traumatic Stress Network. (2003a, September). *Definition of medical traumatic stress*. Paper presented at the Medical Traumatic Stress Working Group meeting, Philadelphia, PA.

Thompson, R. A. (1994). Emotion regulation: A theme in search of definition. In N. A. Fox (Ed.), *The development of emotion regulation: Behavioral and biological considerations: Vol. 59. Monographs for the Society for Research in Child Development* (pp. 25–52). https://doi.org/10.1111/1540-5834.ep9502132762.

Underwood, M. K., Coie, J. D., & Herbsman, C. R. (1992). Display rules for anger and aggression in school-age children. *Child Development, 63*, 366–380. https://doi.org/10.1111/j.1467-8624.1992.tb01633.x.

United States Renal Data System. (2017). *Chapter 7: End-stage renal disease among children, adolescents, and young adults*. Retrieved August 24, 2018, from https://www.usrds.org/2017/view/v2_07.aspx

Walker, L. S., Williams, S. E., Smith, C. A., Garber, J., Van Slyke, D. A., & Lipani, T. A. (2006). Parent attention versus distraction: Impact on symptom complaints by children with and without chronic functional abdominal pain. *International Association for the Study of Pain, 122*, 43–52. https://doi.org/10.1016/j.pain.2005.12.020.

Webster-Stratton, C. (2011). *The incredible years: Parents, teachers, and children's training series*. Seattle, WA: Incredible Years.

Weinstock, & Whisman. (2006). Rumination and excessive reassurance-seeking in depression: A cognitive-interpersonal integration. *Cognitive Therapy and Research, 30*, 333–342. https://doi.org/10.1007/s10608-006-9004-2.

Wimmer, H., & Perner, J. (1983). Beliefs about beliefs: Representation and constraining function of wrong beliefs in young children's understanding of deception. *Cognition, 13,* 103–128. https://doi.org/10.1016/0010-0277(83)90004-5.

Wolitzky, K., Fivush, R., Zimand, E., Hodges, L., & Rothbaum, B. O. (2005). Effectiveness of virtual reality distraction during a painful medical procedure in pediatric oncology patients. *Psychology and Health, 20,* 817–824. https://doi.org/10.1080/14768320500143339.

Zahn-Waxler, C. (2010). Socialization of emotion: Who influences whom and how? In A. K. Root & S. Denham (Eds.), *The role of gender in the socialization of emotion: Key concepts and critical issues: Vol. 128. New directions for child and adolescent development* (pp. 101–109). San Francisco, CA: Jossey-Bass.

Zeman, J., & Garber, J. (1996). Display rules for anger, sadness, and pain: It depends on who is watching. *Child Development, 67,* 957–973. https://doi.org/10.1111/1467-8624.ep9704150177.

Zeman, J., & Shipman, K. (1996). Children's expression of negative affect: Reasons and methods. *Developmental Psychology, 32,* 842–849. https://doi.org/10.1111/1467-8624.ep9704150177.

Zeman, J., & Shipman, K. (1997). Social-contextual influences on expectancies for managing anger and sadness: The transition from middle childhood to adolescence. *Developmental Psychology, 33,* 917–924. https://doi.org/10.1037/0012-1649.33.6.917.

Motivational Interviewing

Kathryn Jeter, Stephen Gillaspy, and Thad R. Leffingwell

Introduction

Pediatric psychologists often ask patients to make behavior changes to support or protect health. This may include adhering to medical advice or complex treatment regimens and protective health habits, like physical activity or reducing substance misuse. Intuitive motivational strategies, such as persuasion or warning of dangers, are often ineffective and resistance to change is a common clinical challenge. Motivational interviewing (MI) is a brief intervention strategy for overcoming resistance and eliciting motivation for behavior change attempts.

The History of Motivational Interviewing (MI)

The technical and theoretical origins of MI are derived from the client-centered counseling strategies promoted by Carl Rogers as well as classic social psychology theories such as those of cognitive consistency (Festinger 1962) and psychological reactance (Brehm 1966). The earliest clinical application of the method that would later develop into MI appeared in the literature in *The Drinker's Check-up,* which employed nonjudgmental, client-centered attending skills in conjunction with a review of assessment feedback (Miller et al. 1988). Following this early work, William Miller continued to advance this method and established a collaborative relationship with Stephen Rollnick, which lead to the publication of the first book fully describing the MI approach in 1991 (Miller and Rollnick 1991).

After Miller and Rollnick developed their clinical and research foundation, applications of MI were directed almost exclusively on addressing the misuse of psychoactive substances, such as alcohol and drug dependence. Their focus on the field of addiction is further illustrated in the subtitle of the seminal MI book, *"Preparing People to Change Addictive Behaviors"* (Miller and Rollnick 1991). Within the course of behavior change, MI aims to address ambivalence. Ambivalence to change is almost universal for individuals struggling with addiction and is often expressed as resistance.

Following early empirical successes within addiction, researchers in other domains started to utilize and investigate MI in alternative contexts including healthcare (Rollnick et al. 2008), health promotion (Resnicow and Rollnick 2011), and

K. Jeter · S. Gillaspy (✉)
Section of General and Community Pediatrics,
University of Oklahoma Health Sciences Center,
Oklahoma City, OK, USA
e-mail: Stephen-Gillaspy@ouhsc.edu

T. R. Leffingwell
Department of Psychology, Oklahoma State University, Stillwater, OK, USA

mental health (Arkowitz and Westra 2004). Similarly, research also started examining the use of MI with different populations and with both adults and adolescents (Jensen et al. 2011; Cushing et al. 2014). Mounting empirical evidence supporting the use of MI to target a wide range of behaviors has transformed the reputation of MI from an addictions intervention to one that is universal. This updated conceptualization of MI was depicted in the subtitle of the second book by Miller and Rollnick (2002), "*Preparing People for Change.*" At present, MI is widely acknowledged as a clinically useful tool for promoting a variety of behavior changes.

Resistance to Change

It is well established that individuals commonly resist professional attempts to initiate behavior change, and changing personal habits is notoriously difficult, even when maintaining the status quo is known to be unhealthy or is actively causing harm. The transtheoretical model posits that individuals may be in the pre-action stages, such as pre-contemplation (not considering change) or contemplation (recognizing need or desire to change but not ready to commit), for months or years (Prochaska et al. 1992). The stage of contemplation is characterized by inconsistent motivation and ambivalence about change. During this stage, a person may acknowledge their need or want to change, while another part of themselves prefers and supports the status quo. The predilection for maintaining the status quo can result from various factors such as a lack of confidence about the likelihood of making successful change, alternative priorities that are currently valued higher, or a preference for immediate rewards in comparison to long-term benefits that are prone to delays or probability discounting (Bickel et al. 2014). Within the MI framework, these individuals can be conceptualized as *stuck* in ambivalence. Therefore, the ultimate goal of the MI encounter is to help people get *unstuck* and progress to making and sustaining important changes in their behavior.

How Patients Talk About Change

Conversations about behavior change are by nature focused on whether the status quo (or current habits) shall continue or change in favor of alternative more adaptive alternatives. During discussions about making a behavior change, patient language can generally be thought of as falling within one of two different forms—*change talk* or *sustain talk*. Change talk is characterized by any expressions that support or promote change. This may include concern about the status quo, worry or apprehension about future risks, thoughts of potential ways to make successful change, or clearly stated intent to change. In comparison, sustain talk is defined as any statements that support or defend the target behavior, such as describing advantages of sustaining the status quo, belittling or minimizing the need for change, verifying barriers to change, or expressing hopelessness about the likelihood of making successful behavior change.

The language that people use when discussing behavior change is an important aspect of MI, and the theoretical framework of MI incorporates essential positions related to patient language. Foremost, MI suggests that the language a patient uses when discussing change is more powerful and has a greater impact on subsequent behavior in comparison to the provider's language. Consequently, MI minimizes common provider-centered strategies that include the provision of education, warning of dangers, attempts at direct persuasion, or dispensing of professional advice. These interventions tend to increase expressions of *sustain talk* as they put the patient in the position of defending the status quo. Additionally, the MI model posits that when people hear themselves articulating more *change talk* and less *sustain talk*, they are more likely to make attempts at behavior change. In their *Theory of Motivational Interviewing,* Miller and Rose (2009) suggested that an individual is more predisposed to feel and/or voice commitment to change as the frequency of *change talk* increases and the frequency of *sustain talk* decreases during an MI conversation. Additionally, their commitment to change is more likely to be supported by a sense of intrinsic motivation. As a result, the central aim throughout an MI encounters to increase the frequency and/or intensity of *change talk* and decrease the frequency and/or intensity of *sustain talk* in order to develop intrinsic motivation and coax a patient toward change.

The Style and Spirit of MI

MI is frequently explained as having a *"style and spirit"* in addition to a collection of proscribed conversational strategies and suggested techniques. The style and spirit of MI are often depicted as the attitude or worldview embraced by the MI provider. Instead of focusing on behaviors that the MI provider is supposed to "do," the style and spirit of MI relate to how the provider should "be" during MI interactions. The style and spirit of MI are often depicted as the "music" or "melody" of MI, as it is these aspects that give MI its pace and feeling, while the skills and strategies of MI are considered the "lyrics."

During its early development, the spirit of MI was portrayed as characterized by three key features (Miller and Rollnick 1991, 2002). First, MI ought to encompass a spirit of *collaboration*. Conversations between the provider and the patient should involve a mutual balance and sharing of power, rather than a "one up, one down" quality. The MI provider should actively avoid assuming the expert role and rather attempt to cultivate a sense of equal partnership while exploring the subject of behavior change. Second, MI should be *evocative* in that the most valued viewpoint in the discussion is that of the patient. Meaningful change is more likely to occur as a result of the patient persuading his or her own self in comparison to the opinions or persuasion of the provider. Consequently, it is imperative for MI providers to behave in ways that foster and evoke the patient's participation and side of the discussion. Last, MI should be *autonomy-supportive*. During the MI encounter, the patient will ideally develop a sense of autonomy and agency, instead of facing attempts to control or restrict personal choice (e.g., "you must..."). This facet of MI decreases the impact of psychological reactance and increases the probability that the patient may rise above ambivalence/reactance and decide to make needed changes.

Miller and Rollnick (2003) recently expanded upon these major features of the spirit of MI. While the facets of collaborative partnership and evocation endure, autonomy support has been incorporated into the broader concept of *acceptance*. Autonomy-support is considered to be one facet of acceptance. Acceptance also incorporates a fundamental belief in the *absolute worth* of the person. The MI provider is encouraged to use *empathy* and *affirmation* and to actively seek to identify and promote the patient's strengths. Finally, *compassion* was added as an essential characteristic of the spirit of MI. *Compassion* denotes the deliberate application of MI in order to achieve what is best for the patient rather than the provider.

Skills and Strategies of MI

In addition to the style and spirit, MI also consists of several prescribed and proscribed strategies to achieve competence in the practice of MI. These essential strategies characterize the *microskills* wherein the spirit of MI is transformed into practice and serve the purpose of enacting the spirit. Use of these MI skills during MI conversations has been demonstrated to promote more positive outcomes (Moyers et al. 2005; Magill et al. 2014). Throughout the interaction, the MI provider's objective is to strategically and intentionally employ active listening skills to evoke and cultivate *change talk* and diminish any *sustain talk* from the patient. The provider should avoid dispensing advice, providing education, or attempting persuasion. These strategies tend to make the conversation *provider-centered* and may have the opposite effects upon client language than MI. Four foundational microskills are encouraged during MI interactions to evoke *change talk*. Commonly represented by the mnemonic acronym OARS, these microskills include asking open-ended questions, providing affirmation, using accurate reflections, and delivering regular summaries.

Open-Ended Questions Providers often rely on short-reply questions to gather information during clinical encounters. Although these closed-ended questions are necessary at times, MI encourages the use of *open-ended questions,* which are unstructured questions that do not provoke a suggested response. This type of questioning takes a nonjudgmental stance, which allows an individual to explore the problem area of focus. In comparison to closed-ended questions that result in short-answers, o*pen-ended questions* place the patient in a more active role and encouraged responses that provide additional information and details.

"How have you been doing since your last visit?"
"What has been the biggest challenge for you lately in managing your daughter's asthma?"
"What do you feel gets in the way of taking your medications?"
"How well do you feel that your family does at communicating about your health?"

Questions such as these invite a more meaningful response that may reveal internal thoughts, feelings, or understanding of the topic.

Affirmation Another important microskill in MI is the use of *affirmations*, or statements that focus on the patient's strengths, personal qualities, or efforts to change. While compliments typically start with "I" statements and confer an implicit evaluation or judgment (e.g., "I think you truly care about your health."), MI encourages providers to employ "you" statements (e.g., "You truly care about your health and are trying your best to make changes, even though it's been challenging."). *Affirmations* are valuable for helping to develop a strong positive relationship. Affirming statements can also help to decrease defensiveness, which is common during interactions about health behavior changes. Additionally, many families who seek professional help for health behavior change have already made attempts to change without success. As a result, they often experience demoralization and lack self-efficacy. In these cases, affirming statements can be used strategically to bolster a patient's self-efficacy.

"Tina's BMI (Body Mass Index) is down today! Tell me about the great changes your family has made since your last visit."
(*Affirmation, Open-ended question*)

"You are someone who values your independence and works hard to not rely on others."
(*Affirmation about personal quality*)

"You have managed to keep checking your blood sugar, even with all of these stressors during final's week at school. Impressive!"
(*Affirmation about effort*)

Reflective Listening The use of reflections and reflective listening is often considered to be the principal skill that MI is built upon (Rosengren 2018). Reflections may seem deceptively straightforward at the first glance, but the intentional use of reflections within MI often takes a great deal of practice to master. This strategy involves listening attentively and making statements in response that communicate your understanding of the message. Reflections can range from simple to complex. Simple, surface-level reflections involve restating the patient's statement with minimal expansion, while deeper complex reflections go beyond what the patient said and attempt to elucidate even greater meaning.

Parent: "I want my son to get more physical activity. I'm worried that he will be at risk for health problems if things don't change at home. But he just wants to play video games all day and gets angry when I suggest we go outside."
Provider: "You want him to be more active but it's hard to get him moving."
(S*imple reflection*)
OR
Provider: "On the one hand, you don't like being the bad guy and enforcing limits, but on the other hand, you truly care about his health and want him to be more active. (*Complex reflection of ambivalence*).

When used correctly, complex reflections can provide new information about a patient's feelings and attitudes. MI encourages providers to use varying levels of reflections to support *change talk*.

Summaries The use of summaries is the fourth microskill that is encouraged during MI interactions. This particular skill represents a more detailed and specialized form of reflection in which the provider organizes and selectively reflects back information from throughout the encounter. Summaries are an effective way to piece together important information from earlier conversations or visits and then present it back in a cohesive manner.

Provider: "Let me make sure I'm hearing you right: You're here today because your physician asked you to come and your mom brought you to the visit. You're not particularly interested in figuring out ways to improve your asthma, and you're a little overwhelmed at the thought of having to do anything else to care for your health. Is that about right?"

Additional Strategies Another highly effective technique encouraged in MI is the use scaled questions or *readiness rulers* (Rollnick et al. 2008). Providers may wish to assess various change qualities using a 0–10 scale during an MI encounter, such as readiness to make change, confidence in the ability to change, or the importance of making change. For example,

Provider: "How ready do you think that you are to start eating healthier today, on a scale from 0 to 10, with zero meaning 'not interested at all' and ten meaning 'totally committed'?"
Patient: "Maybe a six."

While the initial responses to these questions offer a valuable and rapid estimate of the constructs of interest, these questions are particularly lucrative if additional follow-up questions are then asked. The answers awarded to that inquiry would in all likelihood manifest in the form of *change talk*.

Provider: "Ok, somewhere around the middle. Why did you choose six, and not one or two?"
Patient: "I don't know. Even though I really like fast food, I don't want to lose all of the progress that I've made. I like being able to try on clothes at the store."
Provider: "What do you think it would take to move you from a six to an eight?"
Patient: "I would need to feel more support."
Provider: "More support. What would that look like to you?"
Patient: "I guess I would want my siblings to not eat fast food in front of me. Or even better, for them to try to make healthier choices with me. It would feel more doable if I'm not the only one."

This approach consistently evokes indispensable *change talk* into the conversation. Scaled questions are a simple but effective strategy and, as such, are commonly recommended in brief and specialized adaptations of MI that will be discussed later in this chapter.

Two additional strategies are crucial to the competent practice of MI—*rolling with resistance* and *developing discrepancies*. Consistent with its foundation in person-centered interactions, MI providers should avoid argumentation and confrontation in response to a patient's ambivalence and resistance. These proscribed strategies are counterproductive, mainly because they have a tendency to *increase* the frequency and intensity of *sustain talk*. Therefore, an alternative strategy, *rolling with resistance*, is recommended for responding, given its tendency to diminish *sustain talk* or, preferably, bring to mind the "other side of the coin" of *change talk*. MI contains several detailed strategies for rolling with resistance such as the practice of reflective listening strategies but also the use of reframes and statements that emphasize personal choice and autonomy, among others.

Patient: "I know you want me to take the pills every day but I can't remember and don't like the way they make me feel." (*Sustain talk*).

Provider: "You're not so sure that the pills are really worth the side effects" (R*eflection*).

OR

Provider: "The pills cause some side effects you don't like, and you are willing to pay the price of flare-ups to avoid those." (*Reframe*).

OR

Provider: "Whether you take those pills or not and control this illness is ultimately up to you. No one can make that decision for you." (*Emphasize autonomy*).

The strategy of *developing discrepancy* is rooted in theories of cognitive consistency and dissonance, which theorize that individuals strive for consistency between their attitudes and actions (Festinger 1962). As people confront with their own inconsistencies, they are faced with an uncomfortable sense of dissonance and are therefore motivated to change their behavior to alleviate the discrepancy. In other words, when an individual faces and perceives their behavior as inconsistent with a strongly valued attitude or belief, that individual can be expected to modify their behavior to align more clearly with their own attitude or belief. Consequently, the MI provider should constantly be taking note of ways that the status quo may be incongruent with the individual's personal values, goals, or another aspect of his or herself-image. If discrepancies of this kind are identified and propagated, they are likely to progress the person in the direction of change. For example, when working with an individual to target alcohol use, an MI practitioner may say, "you seem like kind of person who truly values your own independence, but at the same time you just feel like your dependent on those beers. In a way, you don't choose to drink them—they choose you."

Four Processes

In the latest edition of *Motivational Interviewing*, Miller and Rollnick (2013) formally introduced a concept known as the *four processes* of MI. Although the four processes describe the opening, middle, and conclusion of an MI encounter, they do not always proceed in a linear fashion. The four processes are defined as *engaging, focusing, evoking,* and *planning*. The first step in an MI encounter, engaging, involves developing rapport and a relationship with the patient, which provides the basic foundation for proceeding. Focusing is considered the process of narrowing the agenda of the conversation down to one, or even a few, of the most important target behaviors to discuss. Evoking is the method that most people may know as the "meat" of the MI conversation. Evoking consists of an intentional conversation about the target behavior, which emphasizes evoking and developing change talk while minimizing resistance. The concluding practice of planning comprises the transition from *whether* or not change should or will happen to *how* a change may happen. This process possibly will include plans to simply come back to the issue if now is not an ideal time to change, or may involve developing a detailed plan for change.

The Case of Joey: A Clinical Example[1]

The following will demonstrate how a provider can proficiently use MI skills and strategies to move a patient toward change. Consider the following clinical example: *Joey is a 16-year-old who was diagnosed with type 1 diabetes at 6 years old. He was referred by his endocrinologist to a pediatric psychologist due to longstanding issues with adherence. Joey's A1c (a lab test that provides an average blood glucose over the last 90 days) was greater than 14%, although his target goal is 7.5% or below. Joey struggles to monitor his blood glucose consistently and often does not give his insulin as prescribed. As a result, Joey's parents frequently ask him about*

---

[1]This is a confabulated clinical example that is loosely based upon an aggregate of provider–patient interactions. All case examples in this chapter are fictitious and intended to illustrate a sampling of MI techniques.

his diabetes care and remind him that he needs to do better, which Joey (like most teenagers) perceives as nagging.

Provider: "Hi Joey. Your physician is concerned about your diabetes care and wanted me to meet with you today. Is it okay if we spend some time today talking about your health? (*Requesting Permission*).
Joey: "Um, I guess. I'm already here."
Provider: "Can you tell me a little about what part of managing diabetes is the easiest for you, and what part is the most challenging?" (*Open-Ended Question*).
Joey: "My A1c is always high, and I am really bad about checking my blood sugar. I am pretty good at remembering to give my insulin when I should. And I try to check my blood sugar, but I like almost I never do it more than once a day.
Provider: "You do try to take care of your diabetes, and you're great at being consistent with your insulin but checking is harder." (*Simple Reflection*).
Father: "Joey knows that he needs to monitor his blood sugar at least four times a day. We constantly remind him to check, and he tells us that he did. But then we come to his doctor's office and learn that he's only checked a handful of times over the last few weeks. He's been lying to us all the time."
Joey: "I haven't lied every time! Sometimes I actually do check when you tell me too. But you constantly nag at me about diabetes. That's all I hear about."
Provider: "Your parents are really worried about the way your take care of your diabetes. You check maybe once a day, but you don't really see the big deal. It's not like you worry about your health or notice any problems even though your A1c is high. (*Amplified Reflection*).
Joey: "No. I mean, I do get headaches more often. And I'm tired all the time. I know I'd probably have more energy if I took care of my diabetes better and actually checked my blood sugar." (*Change Talk*).
Provider: "Was there a time when it was easier for your to check your blood sugar more often?" (*Open-Ended Question*).
Joey: "Yeah, when my parents were doing it for me and watching me when I was young."
Father: "That was definitely when it was easier!"
Joey: "And when I had to go to the school nurse's office to check my blood sugar before lunch and P.E."
Provider: "It sounds like you had a lot of success when you had support and someone holding you accountable at school and at home. Now you're the only one in charge of it, and it's overwhelming to keep up with it. You feel like you try, but it hasn't been enough and your parents end up nagging you. Your family is pretty worried about your health, and even you have noticed some things when your A1c is high that you don't like either, like headaches and just feeling tired all the time." (*Summary*).
Joey: "Yeah, I know I really do need to work on it. I am going to try to check more often. At least twice a day." (*Change Talk*).
Provider: "It sounds like you've already put some thought into what might help you succeed." (*Transition to Planning*).
Father: "Would it be helpful if we start watching you check your blood sugar again like we did when you were younger or would that make it worse?"
Joey: "No, I think it might actually help. I'd feel like we were working on it as a team again. Maybe we could talk to the school nurse, and I can start checking in her office again too."

Evidence Base for Motivational Interviewing

The development and dissemination of MI occurred alongside the age of evidence-based practice. Consequently, rigorous research has been conducted on MI from its very inception. To date, hundreds of randomized clinical trials and several meta-analyses have examined the efficacy of MI. Taken together, the data overwhelmingly support the use of MI for a number of behaviors, including but not limited to alcohol (Burke et al. 2003), tobacco (Heckman et al. 2010), obesity (Armstrong et al. 2011), and gambling (Yakovenko et al. 2015). MI has also been found to be efficacious as an adjunct for the treatment of psychological disorders (Arkowitz et al. 2015). Effect sizes for MI interventions are reliable but small to moderate in size (Lundahl et al. 2010). However, that is unsurprising, given the brief nature of the many MI interventions, sometimes as little as a few minutes in duration (Lundahl et al. 2010; Rubak et al. 2005). As a result, MI is considered a cost-effective intervention, particularly when considering that meaningful change can often be achieved in one or a few brief sessions.

Adherence

Outside the realm of alcohol, tobacco, and substance abuse, MI has become increasingly welcomed within healthcare as an invaluable asset for addressing patient adherence. Adherence can be conceptualized as the "active, voluntary, and collaborative involvement of the patient in a mutually acceptable course of behavior to produce a therapeutic result" (Delamater 2006; Meichenbaum and Turk 1987, pp. 19–39; see also Chap. 25 of this volume). In the United States, it has been estimated that around half of all medical patients do not take their medications as prescribed by their healthcare provider (Sabaté 2003). In addition, approximately 33–69% of all medication-related hospitalizations are thought to be related to poor adherence. Suboptimal adherence to medication treatment regimens can result in worsened health outcomes and increases the risk of mortality. It also contributes to the overutilization of healthcare resources, resulting in substantial societal and financial burdens (McDonnell and Jacobs 2002). Given the deleterious impact of poor adherence, healthcare providers are increasingly looking to behavioral interventions, particularly MI, to help motivate patients to adhere to treatment recommendations.

Pediatric Health Behaviors

MI has been used to address a variety of pediatric health behaviors, including but not limited to accident prevention (Barkin et al. 2008), AIDS (Naar-King et al. 2006, 2009a, b; Robertson et al. 2006; Schmiege et al. 2009), asthma (Borrelli et al. 2010; Chan et al. 2005; Halterman et al. 2011a, b; Seid et al. 2012), calcium intake (Manarino 2007), dental health (Freudenthal and Bowen 2010; Harrison et al. 2007; Ismail et al. 2011; Weinstein et al. 2006), infant health (Taveras et al. 2011; Wilhelm et al. 2006), obesity (Ball et al. 2011; Black et al. 2010; Davis et al. 2011; Flattum et al. 2011; Neumark-Sztainer et al. 2010; Obarzanek et al. 2001; Olson et al. 2008; Resnicow et al. 2005; Wilson et al. 2002), risky sexual behaviors (Barnet et al. 2009; Kiene and Barta 2006), sleep (Cain et al. 2011), and type 1 diabetes (Channon et al. 2003, 2007; Viner et al. 2003; Wang et al. 2010).

Given the extensive breadth of MI literature for pediatric health behaviors, a full review of the literature is beyond the scope of this chapter. For a more comprehensive list of MI research for pediatric health behaviors, the authors encourage that readers examine recent meta-analyses (Borelli et al. 2015; Gayes and Steele 2014; Cushing et al. 2014). Therefore, the following section will focus on MI interventions for specific pediatric health conditions that have the largest and most robust evidence base.

Asthma As one of the most widespread chronic medical conditions in youth, asthma is associated with significant morbidity in childhood and places a substantial burden on the healthcare system (see also Chap. 22 of this volume). Asthma guidelines recommend that individuals with persistent asthma utilize a daily controller medication, use a peak flow to monitor lung function, avoid asthma triggers, and utilize a rescue inhaler as needed (Becker and Abrams 2017). Although the range of effective treatments available implies that asthma symptoms can be well controlled in most patients, asthma remains poorly controlled in the large majority of individuals (Slejko et al. 2014). In order to achieve asthma control, youth and families must engage in a number of health maintenance behaviors, such as avoiding smoke exposure, adhering to inhaled corticosteroid medications, and minimizing exposure to know triggers. Unfortunately, many patients and families are not adherent to asthma treatment regimens (Bender et al. 2000; McQuaid et al. 2003).

Given the numerous health behaviors needed to obtain optimal asthma control, several studies have examined the role of MI in pediatric asthma outcomes. Findings from a recent meta-analysis indicate that asthma is one of the most common pediatric health populations to utilize MI interventions (Gayes and Steele 2014). MI has been used as a core component in innovative interventions to improve asthma in pediatric populations, such as those using group-based and text messaging interventions. One research study by Seid et al. (2012) conducted an intervention for teens with asthma that included two brief in-person sessions that consisted of asthma education and a combination of brief MI and problem-solving skills training. Participants then received 1 month of tailored text messages to improve the adolescents' asthma self-management. Results from this study found improvements in both asthma symptoms and health-related quality of life with medium to large effect sizes (Seid et al. 2012). Another novel study by Halterman and colleagues (2011a, b) examined an intervention that used a combination of directly observed therapy of preventative medications by school nurses followed by three MI sessions (one in-home, two via telephone) to improve adolescent motivation for medication adherence and support adolescents in transitioning to independent preventive medication use. Findings demonstrated improvements in teen-reported variables including asthma symptoms, motivation to take preventative medications, less physical activity limitation, and decreased use of rescue medications (Halterman et al. 2011a). Interventions using MI to improve pediatric asthma generally target adherence to asthma treatment regimens and parental smoking cessation. While some MI interventions in pediatric asthma have focused on the youth (Halterman et al. 2011a; Riekert et al. 2011; Seid et al. 2012), other studies have focused intervention efforts on the parent (Borrelli et al. 2010) or a combination of parent and child (Halterman et al. 2011b). Research has also examined the use of MI as part of a larger intervention to eliminate or reduce passive smoke exposure in children at risk for asthma (Hutchinson et al. 2013). In general, MI has been shown to be an effective intervention in youth with asthma. The effect size for MI for asthma was found to be moderate ($g = 0.444$; 95% CI 0.454, 0.435) in a meta-analysis on MI in pediatric health behavior (Gayes and Steele 2014).

Pediatric Obesity Pediatric obesity is a significant public health epidemic with serious immediate and long-term consequences (see also Chap. 23 of this volume). Roughly one-third of US youth are considered to be overweight or obese (Ogden et al. 2014). Being overweight or obese during childhood may be associated with a heightened risk for a number of additional concerns including behavior problems, depression, peer victimization, poor self-esteem, hypertension, type 2 diabetes, liver disease, and sleep apnea (BeLue et al. 2009; Young-Hyman et al. 2006). In addition to immediate negative outcomes, pediatric obesity often exhibits a chronic negative trajectory when left untreated and is likely to persist into adulthood, producing a lifetime of increased healthcare costs and an increased risk for various medical and psychological comorbidities (Finkelstein et al. 2014; Kiess et al. 2001). Interventions to improve pediatric obesity and address related comorbidities are challenging and often encounter difficulties engaging families in making health behavior changes.

A growing body of research has utilized MI to address pediatric obesity. While some research has utilized MI as a standalone intervention, other studies have used MI as a precursor for subsequent behavioral interventions. Pediatric obesity interventions utilizing MI have also differed in regard to which family members participated in the intervention, with some studies intervening with youth only (Ball et al. 2011; Black et al. 2010; Davis et al. 2011; Flattum et al. 2011; Neumark-Sztainer et al. 2010; Obarzanek et al. 2001; Olson et al. 2008; Resnicow et al. 2005; Wilson et al. 2002), parents only (Schwartz et al. 2007; Taveras et al. 2011), or with both child and parent as a family (Bean et al. 2015; MacDonell et al. 2012). Additionally, research using MI has been used to address a variety of behaviors including increasing fruit/vegetable intake and physical activity and decreasing screen time. A recent meta-analysis on MI in pediatric health behavior by Gayes and Steele (2014) found obesity to be the most common target of MI interventions with a small effect size. More recently, the BMI^2 research trial demonstrated that overweight children who received family-based MI from their pediatrician along with nutritional counseling had significantly improved BMI percentiles across 2 years in comparison to overweight children who received treatment as usual (Resnicow et al. 2015). Overall, studies examining the use of MI for pediatric obesity are promising but have shown some mixed results, likely due to the heterogeneous nature of this body of research.

Type 1 Diabetes The management of type 1 diabetes (T1D) requires that individuals engage in various daily health behaviors such as frequent blood glucose monitoring, regular carbohydrate counting, and consistent administration of short-acting and long-acting insulin (see also Chap. 21 of this volume). An extensive line of scientific evidence shows that maintaining optimal glycemic control, often measured by hemoglobin A1c (HbA1c), improves proximal and distal health outcomes for individuals with T1D. However, the majority of children and adolescents with T1D have an HbA1c above the recommended target, which is commonly related to poor adherence to diabetes treatment regimens (Springer et al. 2006). For example, research from the T1D Exchange Clinic Registry demonstrated that only 17–23% of patients under the age of 18 and 14% of young adults (ages 18–25) had an A1c within the recommended target range (Miller et al. 2015). Consistently, an international comparison of respective registries from 19 countries found that only 8.9%–49.5% of adolescents and young adults (ages 15–24) had an HbA1c at or under the recommended target range (Mcknight et al. 2015).

Taking into consideration the challenging nature of diabetes treatment regimens, a number of studies have examined the benefits of MI to improve adherence in youth with T1D. MI interventions in youth with T1D have been predominately group-based interventions (Channon et al. 2003, 2007; Viner et al. 2003; Wang et al. 2010). A group intervention by Wang et al. (2010) found structured diabetes education to be more effective than MI. Channon et al. (2007) compared group-based MI to a control support group for adolescents with T1D and their parents. In contrast, they found significant improvements in HbA1c for the MI group immediately following the intervention and at 24 months post-intervention. Another study by Channon et al. (2003) examined the preliminary effectiveness of a structured group-based MI intervention for adolescents with T1D. Findings revealed reductions in HbA1c during and after the intervention as well as decreased fear of hypoglycemia and improvements in reported ease of managing diabetes. Another study by Viner et al. (2003) examined a motivational enhancement and solution-focused group intervention in adolescents with T1D and found significant improvements in HbA1c in comparison to a control group. Meta-analysis results on the use of MI in pediatric health behaviors found that MI interventions for those with T1D demonstrated the largest overall effect size. However, these results should be interpreted with caution as there was a significant discrepancy between intervention results.

Given the extensive evidence base supporting the use of MI for a number of health behaviors, it is unsurprising that MI has been increasingly incorporated into medical practice guidelines. MI has been recommended by the American Academy of Pediatrics (AAP) in the treatment of detrimental health behaviors such as obesity, tobacco, and alcohol (Barlow and The Expert Committee 2007; Committee on Environmental Health, Committee on Substance Abuse, Committee on Adolescence,, and Committee on Native American Child 2009; Committee on Substance Abuse 2010). MI was also included as part of recommended behavioral interventions for the comprehensive treatment of obesity in practice guidelines established by the American Association of Clinical Endocrinologists and American College of Endocrinology (Garvey et al. 2016). The basic tenets of MI are also included in the clinical practice guidelines for addressing tobacco use and dependence, which were developed by the U.S. Public Health Service (Tobacco Use and Dependence Guideline Panel 2008). Similarly, the core principles of MI are incorporated into the nationally and federally sponsored alcohol intervention program known as Screening, Brief Intervention, and Referral to Treatment (SBIRT; Babor et al. 2007).

Intervention Characteristics

There are likely a number of factors that influence the effectiveness of MI interventions in pediatric health behavior change. Within the literature on MI interventions for pediatric health behavior change, there exists a great deal of variability between study intervention characteristics. Interventions commonly vary in regard to who participates in treatment: child only, parent only, or child and parent. Additionally, interventions may be conducted on an individual format or within a group setting. MI may be delivered as alone or as part of a multicomponent treatment. The following section will review moderator findings from recent meta-analyses on the use of MI in pediatric health (Borelli et al. 2015; Gayes and Steele 2014). However, results from any meta-analysis should be interpreted with caution given that these moderator findings are not derived experimentally (Rosenthal and DiMatteo 2001). We hope that by reviewing these findings, future research can be developed to experimentally evaluate these proposed causal mechanisms.

Session Characteristics

Much of the research examines the effectiveness of MI delivered in a group setting. Group interventions are popular, as they have the distinct advantage of being economical; however, little research has examined the impact of how MI delivered in a group setting versus an individual setting may impact change talk and sustain talk, or how change talk within the group may impact each participants' personal behaviors. Results from the meta-analysis by Gayes and Steele (2014) found individual and group MI interventions to be comparable in terms of effectiveness, although they found that individual MI sessions demonstrated a larger degree of variability in effectiveness (Gayes and Steele 2014). Interestingly, interventions using a combination of individual and group interventions were not found to be effective in comparison (Gayes and Steele 2014).

Participant Characteristics

Despite the well-established benefits of MI in adults, the efficacy of MI in school-age children remains unclear. Younger children may not have the developmental abilities to formulate long-term goals or awareness of the ambivalence between long-term goals and their current health behaviors; thus, youth may not exhibit the same degree of benefits from MI interventions. Given these concerns, the vast majority of MI literature focuses on promoting change in adolescents. During this critical developmental period, youth must learn to navigate competing demands, develop their personal identity, expand their autonomy, and cultivate independence from caregivers. These goals correspond well with the brief, supportive, and autonomy-based nature of MI.

The target of MI is another common variable in interventions to improve pediatric health behaviors. In general, MI interventions can target the youth alone, the parent alone, the parent and youth separately but concurrently, or the family unit as a whole. Gayes and Steele (2014) categorized interventions as child only, parent only, or both parent and child. Their results demonstrated that all participant variations were effective. However, interventions that focused on both the parent and the child were considerably more effective at improving pediatric health outcomes.

In their systematic review and meta-analysis, Borelli et al. (2015) examined parent focused versus parent–child dyad focused interventions using MI for a wide range of health behaviors. Results revealed that over half of MI interventions were delivered to the parent alone (52%), while a much smaller number of interventions targeted the child with ancillary involvement from the parent (12%) or the parent–child dyad (8%). The additional 28% of studies utilized a combination of participant targets (e.g., focused on parent–child dyad in addition to group intervention). Overall, their findings demonstrated in relation to comparison groups, MI interventions that involved parents were associated with significant positive changes in a number of pediatric health behaviors, such as improving oral health management, making healthier dietary choices, increasing physical activity, limiting access to screen time, reducing duration of screen time, smoking cessation, reducing body mass index, improving household smoking restrictions, and decreasing rates of dental caries (Borelli et al. 2015).

Taken together, these findings suggest that parent involvement is an important part of MI interventions for pediatric health behaviors. However, it remains unclear what level of parent involvement is best suited for promoting pediatric health behavior changes. Outside of the MI literature, family-focused interventions have demonstrated significant and longstanding improvements in various health domains such as obesity (Epstein et al. 2007). Interventions that target the family unit rather than the parent or the child individually may be more successful. These interventions may be more likely to impact all members of the family rather than just the targeted child, making it easier for the targeted child to make and maintain health behavior changes. In general, the research shows that MI interventions that involve parents appear to be more effective, but the degree of parent involvement necessary to elucidate the best outcomes is still unknown.

Intervention Dose

The dose of MI that is necessary to achieve meaningful behavior change in the majority of patients is an important factor to consider when investigating the use of MI in pediatric health behaviors. Based on treatment fidelity guidelines by the National Institutes of Health Behavior Change Consortium, treatment dose can be thought of as a culmination of the "length of intervention contact, number of contacts, and frequency of contacts" (Bellg et al. 2004). Generalized research on the effects of psychological interventions suggests that higher effect sizes are associated with a stronger treatment dose (Shadish et al. 2000). The adult MI literature suggests that there is a significant dose response for MI interventions, with higher treatment doses leading to more positive intervention outcomes (Burke et al. 2003; Lundahl et al. 2010; Rubak et al. 2005). However, MI interventions in pediatric health suggest the opposite holds true. Two recent meta-analyses found that MI produced small yet significant effect sizes across a range of pediatric health behaviors and lasted, on average, only four to five sessions (Cushing et al. 2014; Gayes and Steele 2014). Unfortunately, these studies do not take into consideration the length of intervention contact (e.g., total minutes of MI) or frequency of contacts (e.g., number of in person or telephone MI sessions). Additional research will be necessary to ascertain the ideal MI treatment dose. Nonetheless, these comparable findings suggest that additional MI sessions are likely not necessary to achieve meaningful change in pediatric health behaviors.

Standalone Versus Complimentary Intervention

In its early conception, MI was initially developed as a patient-centered counseling style with the goal of helping an individual change their behavior by progressing them to a higher-level stage of change. Although originally developed as a standalone intervention, MI has been increasingly conceptualized as a preparative, complementary intervention to promote health behavior change. The adult MI literature has shown relatively high effect sizes when MI is used as a preparative intervention, even for "treatment as usual" control groups (Brown and Miller 1993; Daley et al. 1998). In the pediatric literature, MI has been utilized as both a standalone treatment and a part of a multicomponent intervention, commonly paired with cognitive behavior therapy. When comparing 18 studies that utilized MI as a standalone intervention with 19 studies that utilized MI in conjunction with other treatment components, Gayes and Steele (2014) found that research findings on MI as a standalone intervention were not significantly different from findings that used MI as part of a larger intervention, although descriptively MI-only interventions typically showed larger effect sizes. When delivered as a standalone treatment, MI has the benefit of being able to produce meaningful change with limited need for additional resources. When delivered as part of a multicomponent intervention, MI can be deployed to address multiple domains in addition to motivation in order to improve outcomes. It will be important for future research to replicate these findings to determine if MI delivered as a standalone intervention is an effective and sufficient treatment option.

Applications and Adaptations of Motivational Interviewing

In its rigorous form, MI interventions involve a principle-driven approach that depends on the proficiency of the provider to recognize proper targets for MI and intertwine MI strategies with other interventions as needed depending on needs of the particular patient or presenting concern. However, real-world settings have demanded replicable interventions for specific problematic behaviors (e.g., alcohol misuse) or intervention settings (e.g., primary care) that are relatively straightforward and easy to disseminate. As a result, there have been several efforts to create detailed MI-based treatment and intervention models.

Motivational Enhancement Therapy (MET) is one illustration of an MI-based treatment. MET was initially designed and evaluated as a component of a large multisite clinical trial of interventions for alcohol abuse and dependence known as Project MATCH (Miller et al. 1992). Developed as a brief intervention, MET consisted of four treatment sessions that utilized the basic principles of MI. Similar to the initial Drinker's Check-up (Miller et al. 1988) and preliminary versions of MI, the MI conversation in MET occurred in the context of the provider reviewing with the patient his or her results from a comprehensive clinical assessment, mainly in the first two sessions. In the latter two sessions, which were spread out by a few weeks, the practitioner would utilize MI principles to foster motivation and progress toward change.

Further adaptations of MI have endeavored to produce simplified models of targeted intervention, which could be more readily disseminated to providers with a range of skills and experience. One such example comes from the Surgeon General's influential document *Treating Tobacco Dependence* (Tobacco Use and Dependence Guideline Panel 2008), which encouraged the "5 As" model of brief intervention. This model was created specifically so that it could be implemented by different healthcare providers during each and every encounter with a patient who uses tobacco (Tobacco Use and Dependence Guideline Panel 2008). The five As are as follows: (1) *Assess* every patient for tobacco use, and for those who are current users, proceed to (2) *Advise* quitting with concise, personalized feedback, (3) *Assess* the patient's readiness to attempt quitting and motivate those who are not currently ready, (4) *Assist* those attempting to quit by offering guidance, prescriptions, or referrals, and (5) *Arrange* for follow-up to discuss at later visits. The strategies and techniques suggested for assessing readiness to change and cultivating motivation in patients basically describe the practice of MI. Along the same lines, a similar model of brief intervention grounded in MI, is Screening, Brief Intervention, and Referral to Treatment (SBIRT; Babor et al. 2007). SBIRT was created primarily to be utilized in hectic hospital emergency departments to tackle patients whose alcohol or drug use may have played a part in their illness or injury. The brief intervention component of SBIRT is fundamentally MI.

Training in MI

Although some may mistakenly view MI as a simple intervention, the reality is that MI is a complicated clinical intervention that requires sufficient training to achieve mastery. MI is developed within the field of psychology; however, a large body of evidence has established that MI can be effectively delivered in a competent manner by a variety of health professionals including medical and social service providers (Madson et al. 2009). In fact, training in MI is often incorporated into the standard education of students attending nursing school, medical school, and pharmacy school. Within the field of pediatric psychology, it has been suggested training in MI should be included in competency-based training and considered part of best training practices in pediatric psychology (Gillaspy et al. 2015). However, a single or brief series of trainings or workshops is unlikely to provide sufficient training so that providers may achieve and maintain effectiveness at the practice of MI. Sustained competency in the provision of MI usually requires intensive training that includes performance feedback followed by ongoing coaching and supervision (Schwalbe et al. 2014; see www.motivationalinterviewing.org for extensive resources on training in MI).

Conclusions

MI is an invaluable evidence-based approach designed to resolve overcome resistance, resolve ambivalence, and support patients in making progress toward healthy behavior changes. Considering the extensive range of health behaviors that it can be used to address shape, applications of MI possess a high degree of clinical utility. Furthermore, this approach can be learned and integrated into common practice by healthcare providers of varied educational backgrounds, and it can be applied to numerous health behaviors. In summary, the utilization of MI to support health behavior change in pediatric populations is accumulating rapidly, and findings in this area of research are promising.

References

Arkowitz, H., & Westra, H. A. (2004). Integrating motivational interviewing and cognitive behavioral therapy in the treatment of depression and anxiety. *Journal of Cognitive Psychotherapy, 18*, 337–360. https://doi.org/10.1891/jcop.18.4.337.63998.

Arkowitz, H. M., R, W., & Rollnick, S. (2015). *Motivational interviewing in the treatment of psychological problems*. New York: Guilford.

Armstrong, M. J., Mottershead, T. A., Ronksley, P. E., Sigal, R. J., Campbell, T. S., & Hemmelgarn, B. R. (2011). Motivational interviewing to improve weight loss in overweight and/or obese patients: A systematic review and meta-analysis of randomized controlled trials. *Obesity Reviews, 12*(9), 709–723.

Babor, T. F., McRee, B. G., Kassebaum, P. A., Grimaldi, P. L., Ahmed, K., & Bray, J. (2007). Screening, brief intervention, and referral to treatment (SBIRT): Toward a public health approach to the management of substance abuse. *Substance Abuse, 28*, 7–30.

Ball, G. D. C., Mackenzie-Rife, K. A., Newton, M. S., Alloway, C. A., Slack, J. M., Plotnikoff, R. C., et al. (2011). One-on-one lifestyle coaching for managing adolescent obesity: Findings from a pilot, randomized controlled trial in a real-world, clinical setting. *Paediatrics & Child Health, 16*, 345–350.

Barkin, S. L., Finch, S. A., Ip, E. H., Scheindlin, B., Craig, J. A., Steffes, J., et al. (2008). Is office-based counseling about media use, timeouts, and firearm storage effective? Results from a cluster-randomized, controlled trial. *Pediatrics, 122*, e15–e25.

Barlow, S. E., & the Expert Committee. (2007). Expert committee recommendations regarding the prevention, assessment, and treatment of child and adolescent overweight and obesity: Summary report. *Pediatrics, 120*, S164–S192. https://doi.org/10.1542/peds.2007-2329C.

Barnet, B., Liu, J., DeVoe, M., Duggan, A. K., Gold, M. A., & Pecukonis, E. (2009). Motivational intervention to reduce rapid subsequent births to adolescent mothers: A community-based randomized trial. *Annals of Family Medicine, 7*(5), 436–445.

Bean, M. K., Powell, P., Quinoy, A., Ingersoll, K., Wickham, E. P., III, & Mazzeo, S. E. (2015).

Motivational interviewing targeting diet and physical activity improves adherence to paediatric obesity treatment: Results from the MI values randomized controlled trial. *Pediatric Obesity, 10*(2), 118–125.

Becker, A. B., & Abrams, E. M. (2017). Asthma guidelines: The global initiative for asthma in relation to national guidelines. *Current Opinion in Allergy and Clinical Immunology, 17*, 99–103.

Bellg, A. J., Borrelli, B., Resnick, B., Hecht, J., Minicucci, D. S., Ory, M., et al. (2004). Enhancing treatment fidelity in health behavior change studies: Best practices and recommendations from the NIH behavior change consortium. *Health Psychology, 23*, 443.

BeLue, R., Francis, L. A., & Colaco, B. (2009). Mental health problems and overweight in a nationally representative sample of adolescents: Effects of race and ethnicity. *Pediatrics, 123*, 697–702.

Bender, B., Wamboldt, F., O'Connor, S. L., Rand, C., Szefler, S., Milgrom, H., et al. (2000). Measurement of children's asthma medication adherence by self-report, mother report, canister weight, and Doser CT. *Annals of Allergy, Asthma & Immunology, 85*(5), 416–421.

Bickel, W. K., Johnson, M. W., Koffarnus, M. N., MacKillop, J., & Murphy, J. G. (2014). The behavioral economics of substance use disorders: Reinforcement pathologies and their repair. *Annual Review of Clinical Psychology, 10*, 641–677. https://doi.org/10.1146/annurev-clinpsy-032813-153724.

Black, M. M., Hager, E. R., Le, K., Anliker, J., Arteaga, S. S., DiClemente, C., et al. (2010). Challenge! Health promotion/obesity prevention mentorship model among urban, black adolescents. *Pediatrics, 126*, 280–288.

Borelli, B., Tooley, E. M., & Scott-Sheldon, L. A. J. (2015). Motivational interviewing for parent-child health interventions: A systematic review and meta-analysis. *Pediatric Dentistry, 37*, 254–265.

Borrelli, B., McQuaid, E. L., Novak, S. P., & Hammond, S. K. (2010). Motivating Latino caregivers of children with asthma to quit smoking: A randomized trial. *Journal of Consulting and Clinical Psychology, 78*(1), 34–43.

Brehm, J. W. (1966). *A theory of psychological reactance*. Oxford: Academic Press.

Brown, J. M., & Miller, W. R. (1993). Impact of motivational interviewing on participation and outcome in residential alcoholism treatment. *Psychology of Addictive Behaviors, 7*, 211.

Burke, B. L., Arkowitz, H., & Menchola, M. (2003). The efficacy of motivational interviewing: A meta-analysis of controlled clinical trials. *Journal of Consulting and Clinical Psychology, 71*, 843–861. https://doi.org/10.1037/0022-006X.71.5.843.

Cain, N., Gradisar, M., & Moseley, L. (2011). A motivational school-based intervention for adolescent sleep problems. *Sleep Medicine, 12*, 246–251.

Chan, S. S. C., Lam, T. H., Salili, F., Leung, G. M., Wong, D. C. N., Botelho, R. J., et al. (2005). A randomized controlled trial of an individualized motivational intervention on smoking cessation for parents of sick children: A pilot study. *Applied Nursing Research, 18*, 178–181.

Channon, S., Smith, V. J., & Gregory, J. W. (2003). A pilot study of motivational interviewing in adolescents with diabetes. *Archives of Disease in Childhood, 88*, 680–683.

Channon, S. J., Huws-Thomas, M. V., Rollnick, S., Hood, K., Cannings-John, R. L., Rogers, C., et al. (2007). A multicenter randomized controlled trial of motivational interviewing in teenagers with diabetes. *Diabetes Care, 30*(6), 1390–1395.

Committee on Environmental Health, Committee on Substance Abuse, Committee on Adolescence, & Committee on Native American Child. (2009). From the American Academy of Pediatrics: Policy statement—Tobacco use: A pediatric disease. *Pediatrics, 124*, 1474–1487.

Committee on Substance Abuse. (2010). Alcohol use by youth and adolescents: A pediatric concern. *Pediatrics, 125*, 1078–1087. https://doi.org/10.1542/peds.2010-0438.

Cushing, C. C., Jensen, C. D., Miller, M. B., & Leffingwell, T. R. (2014). Meta-analysis of motivational interviewing for adolescent health behavior: Efficacy beyond substance use. *Journal of Consulting and Clinical Psychology, 82*(6), 1212.

Daley, D. C., Salloum, I. M., Zuckoff, A., Kirisci, L., & Thase, M. E. (1998). Increasing treatment adherence among outpatients with depression and cocaine dependence: Results of a pilot study. *American Journal of Psychiatry, 155*, 1611–1613.

Davis, J. N., Gyllenhammer, L. E., Vanni, A. A., Meija, M., Tung, A., Schroeder, E. T., et al. (2011). Startup circuit training program reduces metabolic risk in Latino adolescents. *Medicine and Science in Sports and Exercise, 43*(11), 2195–2203.

Delamater, A. M. (2006). Improving Patient Adherence. *Clinical Diabetes, 24*, 71–77.

Epstein, L. H., Paluch, R. A., Roemmich, J. N., & Beecher, M. D. (2007). Family-based obesity treatment, then and now: Twenty-five years of pediatric obesity treatment. *Health Psychology, 26*, 381.

Festinger, L. (1962). *A theory of cognitive dissonance* (Vol. 2). Stanford, CA: Stanford University Press.

Finkelstein, E. A., Graham, W. C. K., & Malhotra, R. (2014). Lifetime direct medical costs of childhood obesity. *Pediatrics, 133*, 854.

Flattum, C., Friend, S., Story, M., & Neumark-Sztainer, D. (2011). Evaluation of an individualized counseling approach as part of a multicomponent school-based program to prevent weight-related problems among adolescent girls. *Journal of the American Dietetic Association, 111*(8), 1218–1223.

Freudenthal, J. J., & Bowen, D. M. (2010). Motivational interviewing to decrease parental risk related behaviors for early childhood caries. *Journal of Dental Hygiene, 84*(1), 28–33.

Garvey, W. T., Mechanick, J. I., Brett, E. M., Garber, A. J., Hurley, D. L., Jastreboff, A. M., et al. (2016).

American Association of Clinical Endocrinologists and American College of Endocrinology comprehensive clinical practice guidelines for medical care of patients with obesity. *Endocrine Practice, 22*(s3), 1–203.

Gayes, L. A., & Steele, R. G. (2014). A meta-analysis of motivational interviewing interventions for pediatric health behavior change. *Journal of Consulting and Clinical Psychology, 82*(3), 521.

Gillaspy, S. R., Litzenburg, C. C., Leffingwell, T. R., & Miller, M. B. (2015). Training in motivational interviewing as a best training practice in pediatric psychology: Relationship to core competencies. *Clinical Practice in Pediatric Psychology, 3*(3), 225.

Halterman, J. S., Riekert, K., Bayer, A., Fagnano, M., Tremblay, P., Blaakman, S., et al. (2011a). A pilot study to enhance preventive asthma care among urban adolescents with asthma. *Journal of Asthma, 48*(5), 523–530.

Halterman, J. S., Szilagyi, P. G., Fisher, S. G., Fagnano, M., Tremblay, P., Conn, K. M., et al. (2011b). Randomized controlled trial to improve care for urban children with asthma. *Archives of Pediatrics & Adolescent Medicine, 165*(3), 262–268.

Harrison, R., Benton, T., Everson-Stewart, S., & Weinstein, P. (2007). Effect of motivational interviewing on rates of early childhood caries: A randomized trial. *Pediatric Dentistry, 29*(1), 16–22.

Heckman, C. J., Egleston, B. L., & Hofmann, M. T. (2010). Efficacy of motivational interviewing for smoking cessation: A systematic review and meta-analysis. *Tobacco Control, 19*(5), 410–416.

Hutchinson, S. G., Mesters, I., van Breukelen, G., Muris, J. W., Feron, F. J., Hammond, S. K., et al. (2013). A motivational interviewing intervention to PREvent PAssive Smoke Exposure (PREPASE) in children with a high risk of asthma: Design of a randomised controlled trial. *BMC Public Health, 13*(1), 177.

Ismail, A. I., Ondersma, S., Jedele, J. M. W., Little, R. J., & Lepkowski, J. M. (2011). Evaluation of a brief tailored motivational intervention to prevent early childhood caries. *Community Dentistry and Oral Epidemiology, 39*, 433–448.

Jensen, C. D., Cushing, C. C., Aylward, B. S., Craig, J. T., Sorell, D. M., & Steele, R. G. (2011). Effectiveness of motivational interviewing interventions for adolescent substance use behavior change: A meta-analytic review. *Journal of Consulting and Clinical Psychology, 79*(4), 433.

Kiene, S. M., & Barta, W. D. (2006). A brief individualized computer-delivered sexual risk reduction intervention increases HIV/AIDS preventive behavior. *Journal of Adolescent Health, 39*(3), 404–410.

Kiess, W., Galler, A., Reich, A., Müller, G., Kapellen, T., Deutscher, J., ... & Kratzsch, J. (2001). Clinical aspects of obesity in childhood and adolescence. *Obesity reviews, 2*, 29–36.

Lundahl, B. W., Kunz, C., Brownell, C., Tollefson, D., & Burke, B. L. (2010). A meta-analysis of motivational interviewing: Twenty-five years of empirical studies. *Research on Social Work Practice, 20*, 137–160.

Madson, M. B., Loignon, A. C., & Lane, C. (2009). Training in motivational interviewing: A systematic review. *Journal of Substance Abuse Treatment, 36*, 101–109.

Magill, M., Gaume, J., Apodaca, T. R., Walthers, J., Mastroleo, N. R., Borsari, B., et al. (2014). The technical hypothesis of motivational interviewing: A meta-analysis of MI's key causal model. *Journal of Consulting and Clinical Psychology, 82*, 973.

Manarino, M. (2007). *A motivational interviewing technique to improve calcium intake among adolescent girls*. Retrieved from ProQuest dissertations and theses.

McDonnell, P. J., & Jacobs, M. R. (2002). Hospital admissions resulting from preventable adverse drug reactions. *Annals of Pharmacotherapy, 36*, 1331–1336.

MacDonell, K., Brogan, K., Naar-King, S., Ellis, D., & Marshall, S. (2012). A pilot study of motivational interviewing targeting weight-related behaviors in overweight or obese African American adolescents. *Journal of Adolescent Health, 50*, 201–203.

McKnight, J. A., Wild, S. H., Lamb, M. J. E., Cooper, M. N., Jones, T. W., Davis, E. A., et al. (2015). Glycaemic control of type 1 diabetes in clinical practice early in the 21st century: An international comparison. *Diabetic Medicine, 32*, 1036–1050.

McQuaid, E. L., Kopel, S. J., Klein, R. B., & Fritz, G. K. (2003). Medication adherence in pediatric asthma: Reasoning, responsibility, and behavior. *Journal of Pediatric Psychology, 28*, 323–333.

Meichenbaum, D., & Turk, D. C. (1987). Facilitating treatment adherence. In D. Meichenbaum & D. C. Turk (Eds.), *Treatment adherence: Terminology, incidence and conceptualisation* (pp. 19–39). New York: Plenum Press.

Miller, W. R., & Rollnick, S. (1991). *Motivational interviewing: Preparing people to change addictive behavior*. New York: Guilford Press.

Miller, W. R., Zweben, A., DiClemente, C. C., & Rychtarik, R. G. (1992). Motivational enhancement therapy manual. Rockville, MD: National Institute on Alcohol Abuse and Alcoholism.

Miller, W. R., & Rollnick, S. (2002). *Motivational interviewing: Helping people change* (2nd ed.). New York: Guilford Press.

Miller, W. R., & Rollnick, S. (2013). *Motivational interviewing: Helping people change* (3rd ed). New York: Guilford Press.

Miller, W. R., & Rose, G. S. (2009). Toward a theory of motivational interviewing. *American Psychologist, 64*, 527.

Miller, W. R., Sovereign, R. G., & Krege, B. (1988). Motivational interviewing with problem drinkers: II. The Drinker's check-up as a preventive intervention. *Behavioural and Cognitive Psychotherapy, 16*, 251–268.

Miller, K. M., Foster, N. C., Beck, R. W., Bergenstal, R. M., DuBose, S. N., DiMeglio, L. A., et al. (2015). Current state of type 1 diabetes treatment in the US: Updated data from the T1D exchange clinic registry. *Diabetes Care, 38*, 971–978.

Moyers, T. B., Miller, W. R., & Hendrickson, S. M. (2005). How does motivational interviewing work? Therapist interpersonal skill predicts client involvement within motivational interviewing sessions. *Journal of Consulting and Clinical Psychology, 73*, 590.

Naar-King, S., Wright, K., Parsons, J. T., Frey, M., Templin, T., Lam, P., et al. (2006). Healthy choices: Motivational enhancement therapy for health risk behaviors in HIV positive youth. *AIDS Education and Prevention, 18*, 1–11.

Naar-King, S., Outlaw, A., Green-Jones, M., Wright, K., & Parsons, J. T. (2009a). Motivational interviewing by peer outreach workers: A pilot randomized clinical trial to retain adolescents and young adults in HIV care. *AIDS Care, 21*, 868–873.

Naar-King, S., Parsons, J. T., Murphy, D. A., Chen, X., Harris, R., & Belzer, M. E. (2009b). Improving health outcomes for youth living with the human immunodeficiency virus. *Archives of Pediatrics & Adolescent Medicine, 163*, 1092–1098.

Neumark-Sztainer, D. R., Friend, S. E., Flattum, C. F., Hannan, P. J., Story, M. T., Bauer, K., et al. (2010). New moves-preventing weight-related problems in adolescent girls. *American Journal of Preventive Medicine, 39*, 421–432.

Obarzanek, E., Kimm, S. Y. S., Barton, B. A., Van Horn, L., Kwiterovich, P. ⊙., Simons Morton, D. G., et al. (2001). Long-term safety and efficacy of a cholesterol-lowering diet in children with elevated low-density lipoprotein cholesterol: Seven-year results of the dietary intervention study in children (DISC). *Pediatrics, 107*, 256–264.

Ogden, C. L., Carroll, M. D., Kit, B. K., & Flegal, K. M. (2014). Prevalence of childhood and adult obesity in the United States, 2011-2012. *JAMA, 311*, 806–814.

Olson, A. L., Gaffney, C. A., Lee, P. W., & Starr, P. (2008). Changing adolescent health behaviors: The healthy teens counseling approach. *American Journal of Preventive Medicine, 35*(5S), S359–S364.

Prochaska, J. O., DiClemente, C. C., & Norcross, J. C. (1992). In search of how people change: Applications to addictive behaviors. *American Psychologist, 47*(9), 1102.

Resnicow, K., & Rollnick, S. (2011). *Handbook of motivational counseling: Goal-based approaches to assessment and intervention with addiction and other problems*. Hoboken, NJ: Wiley.

Resnicow, K., Taylor, R., Baskin, M., & McCarty, F. (2005). Results of Go Girls: A weight control program for overweight African-American adolescent females. *Obesity Research, 13*, 1739–1748.

Resnicow, K., McMaster, F., Bocian, A., Harris, D., Zhou, Y., Snetselaar, L., et al. (2015). Motivational interviewing and dietary counseling for obesity in primary care: An RCT. *Pediatrics, 135*, 649–657.

Riekert, K. A., Borrelli, B., Bilderback, A., & Rand, C. S. (2011). The development of a motivational interviewing intervention to promote medication adherence among inner-city, African-American adolescents with asthma. *Patient Education and Counseling, 82*, 117–122.

Robertson, A. A., Stein, J. A., & Baird-Thomas, C. (2006). Gender differences in the prediction of condom use among incarcerated juvenile offenders: testing the information-motivation-behavior skills (IMB) model. *Journal of Adolescent Health, 38*, 18–25.

Rollnick, S., Miller, W. R., Butler, C. C., & Aloia, M. S. (2008). *Motivational interviewing in health care: Helping patients change behavior*. New York: Guilford Press.

Rosengren, D. B. (2018). *Building motivational interviewing skills: A practitioner workbook* (2nd ed.). New York: Guilford Press.

Rosenthal, R., & DiMatteo, M. R. (2001). Meta-analysis: Recent developments in quantitative methods for literature reviews. *Annual Review of Psychology, 52*, 59–82.

Rubak, S., Sandbæk, A., Lauritzen, T., & Christensen, B. (2005). Motivational interviewing: A systematic review and meta-analysis. *British Journal of General Practice, 55*, 305–312.

Sabaté, E. (2003). *Adherence to long-term therapies: Evidence for action*. Geneva: World Health Organization.

Schmiege, S. J., Broaddus, M. R., Levin, M., & Bryan, A. D. (2009). Randomized trial of group interventions to reduce HIV/STD risk and change theoretical mediators among detained adolescents. *Journal of Consulting and Clinical Psychology, 77*, 38–50.

Schwartz, R. P., Hamre, R., Dietz, W. H., Wasserman, R. C., Slora, E. J., Myers, E. F., ... Resnicow, K. A. (2007). Office-based motivational interviewing to prevent childhood obesity. *Archives of Pediatric & Adolescent Medicine, 161*, 495–501.

Schwalbe, C. S., Oh, H. Y., & Zweben, A. (2014). Sustaining motivational interviewing: A meta-analysis of training studies. *Addiction, 109*, 1287–1294.

Seid, M., D'Amico, E. J., Varni, J. W., Munafo, J. K., Britto, M. T., Kercsmar, C. M., et al. (2012). The in vivo adherence intervention for at risk adolescents with asthma: Report of a randomized pilot trial. *Journal of Pediatric Psychology, 37*, 390–403.

Shadish, W. R., Navarro, A. M., Matt, G. E., & Phillips, G. (2000). The effects of psychological therapies under clinically representative conditions: A meta-analysis. *Psychological Bulletin, 126*, 512.

Slejko, J. F., Ghushchyan, V. H., Sucher, B., Globe, D. R., Lin, S. L., Globe, G., et al. (2014). Asthma control in the United States, 2008-2010: Indicators of poor asthma control. *Journal of Allergy and Clinical Immunology, 133*(6), 1579–1587.

Springer, D., Dziura, J., Tamborlane, W. V., Steffen, A. T., Ahern, J. H., Vincent, M., et al. (2006). Optimal control of type 1 diabetes mellitus in youth receiving intensive treatment. *The Journal of Pediatrics, 149*, 227–232.

Taveras, E. M., Blackburn, K., Gillman, M. W., Haines, J., McDonald, J., Price, S., et al. (2011). First steps for mommy and me: A pilot intervention to improve nutrition and physical activity behaviors of postpartum mothers and their infants. *Maternal and Child Health Journal, 15*, 1217–1227.

Tobacco Use and Dependence Guideline Panel. (2008). A clinical practice guideline for treating tobacco use and dependence: 2008 update: A US public health service report. *American Journal of Preventive Medicine, 35*(2), 158.

Viner, R. M., Christie, D., Taylor, V., & Hey, S. (2003). Motivational/solution-focused intervention improves HbA1C in adolescents with type 1 diabetes: A pilot study. *Diabetes Medicine, 20*, 739–742.

Wang, Y., Nakronezny, P. A., Stewart, S. M., Edwards, D., Mackenzie, M., & White, P. C. (2010). A randomized controlled trial comparing motivational interviewing in education to structured diabetes education in teens with type 1 diabetes. *Diabetes Care, 33*, 1741–1743.

Weinstein, P., Harrison, R., & Benton, T. (2006). Motivating mothers to prevent caries. *Journal of the American Dental Association, 137*, 789–793.

Wilhelm, S. L., Stephans, M. B. F., Hertzog, M., Rodehorst, T. K. C., & Gardner, P. (2006). Motivational interviewing to promote sustained breastfeeding. *Journal of Obstetric, Gynecologic, and Neonatal Nursing, 35*, 340–348.

Wilson, D. K., Friend, R., Teasley, N., Green, S., Reaves, I. L., & Sica, D. A. (2002). Motivational versus social cognitive interventions for promoting fruit and vegetable intake and physical activity in African American adolescents. *Annals of Behavioral Medicine, 24*, 310–319.

Yakovenko, I., Quigley, L., Hemmelgarn, B. R., Hodgins, D. C., & Ronksley, P. (2015). The efficacy of motivational interviewing for disordered gambling: Systematic review and meta-analysis. *Addictive Behaviors, 43*, 72–82.

Young-Hyman, D., Tanofsky-Kraff, M., Yanovski, S. Z., Keil, M., Cohen, M. L., Peyrot, M., & Yanovski, J. A. (2006). Psychological status and weight-related distress in overweight or at-risk-for-overweight children. *Obesity, 14*, 2249–2258.

Cognitive Behavioral Therapy with Youth: Essential Foundations and Elementary Practices

7

Robert D. Friedberg and Jennifer K. Paternostro

Introduction

Cognitive behavioral therapy (CBT) for children represents one of the most widely researched and popular approaches to treatment. The model has grown from upstart status to mainstream standard. Multiple randomized clinical trials, meta-analyses, systematic reviews, clinical case studies, and texts document efficacy and effectiveness in various settings with different populations. Bookshelves are stocked with many workbooks and manuals. Clearly, CBT is a success story. This chapter begins with a brief overview of the theoretical and empirical foundations of CBT with youth. In particular, work with behavioral problems, depression, and anxiety is reviewed. A modular approach to CBT is explained. Finally, a confabulated case example is presented to illustrate salient points.

R. D. Friedberg (✉)
Child Emphasis Area, Palo Alto University, Palo Alto, CA, USA
e-mail: rfriedberg@paloaltou.edu

J. K. Paternostro
Division of Developmental and Behavioral Pediatrics, Stead Family Department of Pediatrics, University of Iowa Stead Family Children's Hospital, Iowa City, IA, USA

Theoretical Foundations and Empirical Status

Learning theory (classical conditioning, operant conditioning, and social learning theory) and informational processing paradigms are foundational elements in CBT (Friedberg and Thordarson 2018). Classical conditioning is deeply embedded within treatment protocols for anxiety spectrum problems, and operant concepts dominate the landscape in parent training/behavior management models. Self-efficacy (Bandura 1977), a fundamental social learning theory construct, pervades multiple CBT interventions.

Ancient philosophers realized that people are not solely disturbed by adverse events but also by their subjective appraisals (Beck et al. 1979). While this perspective is not new, operationalizing and empirically studying individuals' cognitive interpretations and their connection to emotional distress is a scientific advance. Cognition is categorized into cognitive products (automatic thoughts), cognitive processes (cognitive distortions), and cognitive structures (Beck 1976; Ingram and Kendall 1986). The content-specificity hypothesis (CSH: Beck 1976; Cho and Telch 2005; Ghahramanlou-Holloway et al. 2007; Jolly 1993; Lamberton and Oei 2008) identifies different cognitive features. The CSH states that different mood states are associated unique

Table 7.1 Hot cognitive content

Mood state	Cognitive content
Depression	Negative view of self Negative view of others/experiences Negative view of the future
Anxiety	Overestimation of the probability of danger (e.g., confusing possibility with probability) Overestimation of the magnitude of the danger (catastrophizing) Ignoring rescue factors Neglect coping skills
Panic	Catastrophic misinterpretation of normal bodily sensations
Social anxiety	Fear of negative evaluation
Anger	Hostile attributional bias (e.g., confusing deliberate with accidental) Negative labeling of others Violation of personal rules Pervasive sense of unfairness

thought patterns. Table 7.1 lists the different types of thoughts linked to distinct mood states.

CBT has been identified as a well-established treatment for symptomatic reduction of a variety of psychiatric symptoms (Flessner and Piacentini 2017; Weisz and Kazdin 2017). Contemporary clinical researchers are propelling CBT with youth in exciting directions. Kendall and his colleagues own a long record of applying CBT to a wide range of internalizing and externalizing disorders (Kendall 2012; Kendall and Finch 1976; Kendall and Hedtke 2006; Kendall and Braswell 1985; Kendall et al. 2010). Most notably, the Coping Cat program for anxious youth is widely supported and applied in multiple settings (Beidas et al. 2008; Kendall et al. 2008). Kolko and Perrin (2014) commented that Coping Cat is particularly well suited to work in integrated pediatric behavioral health care (IPBHC) settings.

Chorpita, Weisz, and their teams are advancing the field with a modular approach to CBT (Chorpita and Daleiden 2009; Chorpita and Weisz 2009; Weisz et al. 2015). Rather than relying on multiple discrete disorder manuals, modular CBT extracts the most robust common intervention strategies found in empirically supported protocols and groups them into conceptual categories. Bearman and Weisz (2015) cogently argued that modular approaches serve parsimony while avoiding reductionism. mCBT fits well within IPBHC settings because there is an emphasis on time-efficient treatment, comorbidity, and transdiagnostic processes (Arora et al. 2016, 2017; Kolko and Perrin 2014; Wissow et al. 2008, 2016).

Developmental, emotional, and behavioral problems are disproportionately higher in youth with chronic health conditions (Blackman and Conaway 2013). Disruptive behavior disorders, depression, and anxiety disorders are conditions seen frequently in pediatric settings (Kolko and Perrin 2014). Moreover, these problems often co-occur with medical conditions. The research on the effectiveness of CBT as a treatment for a range of psychological conditions is clear. The following section briefly reviews the literature on the empirical status of CBT for disruptive behavior problems, depression, and anxiety.

Disruptive Behavior Disorders

There are several well-established and probably efficacious treatments for youth with disruptive behaviors. Lochman et al. (2017) reported that Parent Management Training-Oregon Model (PMTO: Forgatch and Gewirtz 2017) was well established for youth. Comer et al. (2013) recommended programs that employ a primary behavioral focus such as Parent-Child Interaction Therapy (PCIT: Zisser-Nathanson et al. 2017), Incredible Years (Webster-Stratton and Reid 2017), Helping the Non-Compliant Child (McMahon and Forehand 2003), and Triple P-Positive Parenting Program (Sanders 2012).

McCart and Sheidow (2016) confirmed that Multi-Systemic Therapy (MST: Henggeler et al. 2009) was a well-established approach. MST is a family-based intervention that targets justice-involved youth with a history of serious offenses (McCart and Sheidow 2016). MST draws from Bronfenbrenner's (1979) social ecological model and commonly offers intensive 24/7 services. In their review, Lochman et al. (2017) noted that Problem-Solving Therapy (PST: Kazdin 2017) was effective for patients with disruptive behaviors. Finally, Coping Power demonstrated reductions in aggression, substance abuse problems, and delinquency (Lochman et al. 2008, 2017).

Several of these empirically supported protocols have been adapted for the pediatric primary care settings (Berkout and Gross 2013). Berkovits et al. (2010) adapted Parent-Child Interaction Training to the primary care setting (PC-PCIT). They delivered PCIT in four 90-min weekly sessions. The results showed decreased behavioral difficulties, improved discipline tactics, and increased parental self-efficacy. The Incredible Years protocol has been applied in the pediatric primary care setting with promising outcomes (Lavigne et al. 2008a, b; McMenamy et al. 2011). The MATCH-ADTC platform which aggregates techniques from these discrete protocols recommends praise, active ignoring, giving effective commands, delivering rewards, and implementing time-out as well as other response cost procedures (Chorpita and Weisz 2009; Weisz and Chorpita 2012).

Depression

Major depressive disorder is one of the most prevalent mental health disorders among children and adolescents. The literature on evidence-based treatments for adolescents with depressive disorders distinctly identifies CBT and its variants as a well-established intervention with large effect sizes across treatment formats (Chorpita et al. 2011; Weersing et al. 2017). The Treatment for Adolescents with Depression Study (TADS 2003, 2004, 2005, 2007) concluded that the combination of psychotropic medication and CBT intervention yielded robust response rates of 73% at week 12, 85% at week 18, and 86% at week 36. Further, the addition of CBT to medication therapy was found to enhance the safety of medication (TADS 2007).

Weersing et al. (2017) conducted a systematic review of 42 randomized controlled trials of evidence-based treatments for children and adolescents with depression. They found that individual and group CBT reached well-established criteria for treating depression. CBT was considered a possibly efficacious intervention for children below 13 years. Although the approach did not reach the threshold for a well-established treatment for young children with depression, CBT nonetheless surpassed alternative treatment modalities such as psychodynamic therapy and family-based intervention (Weersing et al. 2017). Psychoeducation, target monitoring, pleasant/activity scheduling, relaxation, problem-solving, and cognitive restructuring are the best practices culled from these studies by MATCH-ADTC (Chorpita and Weisz 2009; Weisz and Chorpita 2012).

Youth with chronic health conditions experience higher rates of depression adding more layers of complexity to treatment (Szigethy et al. 2014; Verhoof et al. 2013). When compared to treatment as usual in a primary care setting, youth with depression who received brief CBT intervention had a greater number of symptom-free days and better quality of life (Dickerson et al. 2018). Dickerson and colleagues also found that CBT was more cost-effective at 24-month follow-up. Further, a randomized efficacy trial comparing CBT and supportive nondirective therapy (SNDT) in depressed youth with inflammatory bowel disease (IBD) discovered a greater reduction in IBD activity in youth who received CBT intervention (Szigethy et al. 2014).

Anxiety Spectrum

The prevalence of anxiety disorders in children and adolescents is remarkably high, with recent estimates of approximately 6.5% for youth of age 6–18 years (Polanczyk et al. 2015). Furthermore, nearly 33% of community-based adolescents and approximately 50% of clinically referred youth meet diagnostic criteria for at least one anxiety disorder (Hammerness et al. 2008). Additionally, anxiety is considered a gateway disorder to other conditions (Weems and Silverman 2013). Similar to depression, anxiety spectrum disorders are also frequently co-morbid with pediatric medical conditions (Pao and Bosk 2011). The literature on evidence-based treatment for anxiety disorders undoubtedly supports the use of cognitive and behavioral interventions (Bennett et al. 2016; Crowe and McKay 2017; Higa-McMillan et al. 2016). Young patients receiving proper CBT experienced a three to seven times greater likelihood of improvement than control groups (Bennett et al. 2016). Higa-McMillan et al. (2016) identified CBT, exposure, modeling, CBT with parents, psychoeducation, and CBT plus medication as well-established treatments for youth with anxiety disorders. CBT in conjunction with exposure-based intervention demonstrated large effect sizes, sustainability of effects at 1 year of follow-up, and included advanced empirical support. Moreover, CBT interventions are effective with diverse patients and treatment modalities as well as in various therapeutic settings (Higa-McMillan et al. 2016). Additionally, CBT is the first-line approach in the treatment of pediatric OCD and was found superior to medication alone and combined medication and CBT (Freeman et al. 2014). Psychoeducation, construction of hierarchies, and exposure are the key common elements to treating anxiety spectrum disorders (Chorpita and Weisz 2009; Weisz and Chorpita 2012).

Although the standard treatment for CBT intervention ranges from 10 to 15 sessions, health care settings are not always afforded the flexibility to implement a prolonged treatment approach. Therefore, over the last several years, efforts to tailor CBT intervention to the health care setting expanded. Stepped-care frameworks for the delivery of CBT aim to find a balance between cost and time savings, and effective intervention in pediatric populations (Kendall et al. 2016). Rapee et al. (2017) concluded that a stepped-care approach targeting youth with anxiety disorders resulted in treatment efficacy similar to traditional best practices. Finally, Ginsburg and her team (2016) evaluated a brief pediatrician-delivered CBT. The core components included psychoeducation, exposure, cognitive restructuring, problem-solving, relapse prevention, and anxiety-focused parent training. They found the brief intervention in a pediatric setting resulted in decreased symptomology, perceived disease burden, and functional impairment.

Modular CBT

Contemporary CBT with youth is trending toward modular approaches (Chorpita and Weisz 2009; Nangle et al. 2016). The common elements embedded in the modules are considered golden nuggets (Friedberg and Thordarson 2018). These powerful core practices can be packaged into five broad categories (psychoeducation, target monitoring, basic behavioral tasks, cognitive restructuring, and exposure/experiments), resulting in a condensed and concentrated approach to treatment (Friedberg et al. 2009, 2011).

Psychoeducation

Psychoeducation is the procedural platform that launches mCBT. It prepares young patients for treatment by providing information about their presenting problems, treatment methods, and the course of therapy. Patient education works to place youngsters and their families on the same page as their clinical providers. Moreover, there are a variety of functions served by psychoeducation including increased motivation, reducing stigma, help-seeking, self-empowerment, objectification of illness, and reducing stigma (Fristad 2006; Wesseley et al. 2008). Psychoeducation may be delivered through verbal instruction, pamphlets, books, audio recordings, videos, Internet sites, and other media.

Target Monitoring

Target monitoring is similar to a clinical positioning device and consequently guides treatment by evaluating progress toward goals (Chorpita 2014). There are multiple ways to accomplish target monitoring including use of standardized symptom scales and measures of functional improvement. Further, regular and reliable chronicling of treatment progress and process represents measurement-based care (Bickman 2008; Bickman et al. 2011; Scott and Lewis 2015). Various authors (Gondek et al. 2016; Jensen-Doss et al. 2018) attest to the many advantages

MBC offers, including faster recovery times, more symptom improvement, and better clinician judgment.

Symptom Scales Administering standard symptom scales to patients is a familiar practice for many clinicians. Symptom scales typically involve patients and their caretakers completing checklists assessing presence, frequency, intensity, and/or duration of problems. Table 7.2 lists several recommended symptom scales. Additionally, readers may wish to review Beidas et al. (2015) excellent compendium of free, brief, reliable, and valid measures. Finally, Table 7.2 lists many additional symptom inventories.

Idiographic Methods Idiographic target measures are personalized and developed especially for individual young patients. These personalized metrics include functional analyses, behavior logs, and thought diaries. Completing a functional analysis is a vital component of target monitoring. Often, this is referred to the A (Antecedent) B (Behavior), C (Consequence) model. A functional analysis involves determining the antecedents (cues, triggers, etc.) and consequences (positive reinforcers, negative reinforcers, response cost, and punishers) to the presenting complaint. B in the model refers to the presenting complaint or problem. Essentially, CBT clinicians position the presenting problems via a functional analysis. Figure 7.1 demonstrates the way in which the relationship between antecedents, behavioral responses, and consequences helps clinicians properly locate problem areas.

Table 7.2 Recommended target metrics

Target focus	Measure	Reference
Broad symptoms	Pediatric symptom checklist (PSC-17) Brief problem checklist	Gardner et al. (1999) and Chorpita et al. (2010)
Depression	Children's depression Inventory-2 Beck depression Inventory-2	Kovacs (2010) and Beck (1996)
Hopelessness	Beck hopelessness scale Children's hopelessness scale	Beck (1978) and Kazdin et al. (1986)
Anxiety	Multi-dimensional anxiety scale for Children-2 Screen for child anxiety related emotional disorders	March (2013) and Birmaher et al. (1997)
Social anxiety	Social phobia and anxiety inventory for children-SPAI-C	Beidel et al. (1995)
Generalized anxiety	Penn State Children's worry questionnaire	Chorpita et al. (1997)
OCD	Children's Yale-Brown obsessive-compulsive scale (CY-BOCS) Parent (PR) and self-report (SR) report form	Storch et al. (2006)
ADHD	Vanderbilt ADHD rating scale SNAP-IV	Wolraich et al. (2003) and Swanson et al. (1983)
Disruptive behavior disorders	Eyberg child behavior inventory (ECBI)	Eyberg and Ross (1978)

Behavior logs typically involve frequency counts of relevant actions. Contextual parameters (where, when, who, etc.) are also frequently recorded. Behavior logs are quite simple to complete and can be easily personalized. There are a variety of free premade charts available online (https://www.freeprintablebehaviorcharts.com).

Completing thought diaries capture cognitive components to emotional distressing situations. For readers who are unfamiliar with thought diaries, they include three columns specifying the triggering situation, emotional reaction, and cognitive reappraisal (Fig. 7.2). There are several important points to keep in mind when building a thought diary with young patients. The first broad rule to remember is that completing a thought diary is not an innate skill. Young patients need to be taught how to do it! Second, descriptions of situations should be objective statements about activating events and free from embedded judgments and conclusions. Therefore, check to make

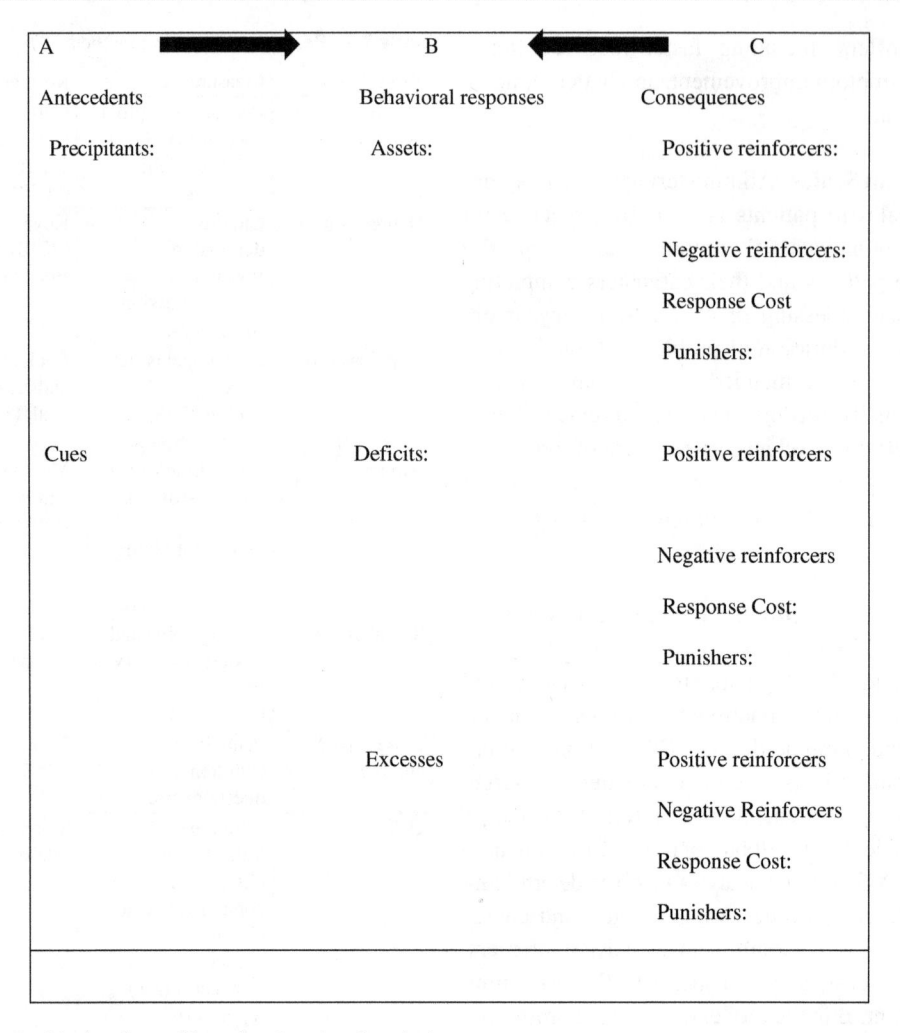

A	B	C
Antecedents	Behavioral responses	Consequences
Precipitants:	Assets:	Positive reinforcers:
		Negative reinforcers:
		Response Cost
		Punishers:
Cues	Deficits:	Positive reinforcers
		Negative reinforcers
		Response Cost:
		Punishers:
	Excesses	Positive reinforcers
		Negative Reinforcers
		Response Cost:
		Punishers:

Fig. 7.1 Positioning the problem via a functional analysis

Situation	Feeling	Thought	Distortion	New coping thought	Re-rate Feeling

Fig. 7.2 Typical thought diary

sure there are no automatic thoughts rooted in the situation column. Next, the feeling column records only emotions and like the situation (column), no automatic thoughts should reside there. The thought category is the place to note cognitive content. The essential issue is catching automatic thoughts that are "hot cognitions." Hot cognitions refer thoughts associated with emotional arousal and align according to content-specificity hypothesis (Table 7.1). Finally, identifying and labeling cognitive distortions is an advanced type of target monitoring.

Basic Behavioral Tasks

Basic behavioral tasks include widely used procedures such as pleasant activity scheduling (PAS), behavioral activation (BA), relaxation, contingency contracting, and social skills training. These skill-based techniques are employed early and often in treatment. Pleasant activity scheduling and behavioral activation typically target withdrawal, avoidance, and lack of positive reinforcement. Young patients with medical conditions and co-existing depressive symptoms may benefit from mobilizing effects of BA and PAS. Patients with peer problems often profit from social skills intervention. Basic behavioral tasks are commonly used in parent training interventions.

Cognitive Restructuring

Cognitive interventions may be divided into two broad categories such as cognitive restructuring and rational analysis. Cognitive restructuring methods emphasize changing distressing and unproductive thought content as well as problem-solving. Rational analysis procedures are more sophisticated and nuanced interventions, which target illogical and faulty reasoning patterns. Problem-solving, pros/cons lists, and self-instructional methods are considered cognitive restructuring techniques. Tests of evidence, reattribution, and decatastrophizing are common approaches to rational analysis.

There are many different problem-solving models. However, there are commonalities among all of these paradigms (Chorpita and Weisz 2009; Nangle et al. 2016). First, definitions of problems should be operationalized and measurable (Nezu and Nezu 1989). Second, problem-solving approaches include a brainstorming component where positive/negative and short-term/long-term consequences of each strategy are evaluated. Based on this analysis, the most productive option is chosen and implemented. Finally, efforts toward better problem resolution are rewarded.

Coping counter-thoughts are produced via cognitive restructuring. Similar to problem-solving, there are multiple ways to conduct cognitive restructuring, yet there are similarities between the divergent approaches. Coping thoughts should explicitly address stressors recorded in the event/situation column located on a thought diary. Friedberg et al. (2001) recommended that therapists should take care that young patients' coping thoughts are not platitudinous or Pollyannish. The coping thoughts should be believable and accurate but not completely positive (Padesky 1993). Additionally, decreased emotional distress should accompany the counter-thought. Finally, cognitive restructuring includes a problem-solving strategy or action plan (Kendall and Suveg 2006). We have constructed a RAIN mnemonic (Fig. 7.3) to help clinicians recall these points. Coping thoughts should be realistic (R), accurate (A), impactful resulting in a reduction of emotional distress (I), and necessary (N) including an action plan.

For example, Thought 5-O is a new cognitive restructuring method that can engage young patients in re-engineering their beliefs. The procedure is based on the slang reference to police (e.g., 5-O) and teaches youth to patrol their thinking, identify suspect assumptions (e.g., distortions), and then correct the skewed interpretation. The Thought 5-O worksheet asks the patient to record the event, feeling, thought, suspect, and a 5-O alternative. Figure 7.4 shows a sample completed Thought 5-O diary. Fortunately, the literature is replete with a host of child friendly workbooks and exercises that

R: Make the new thought REALISTIC

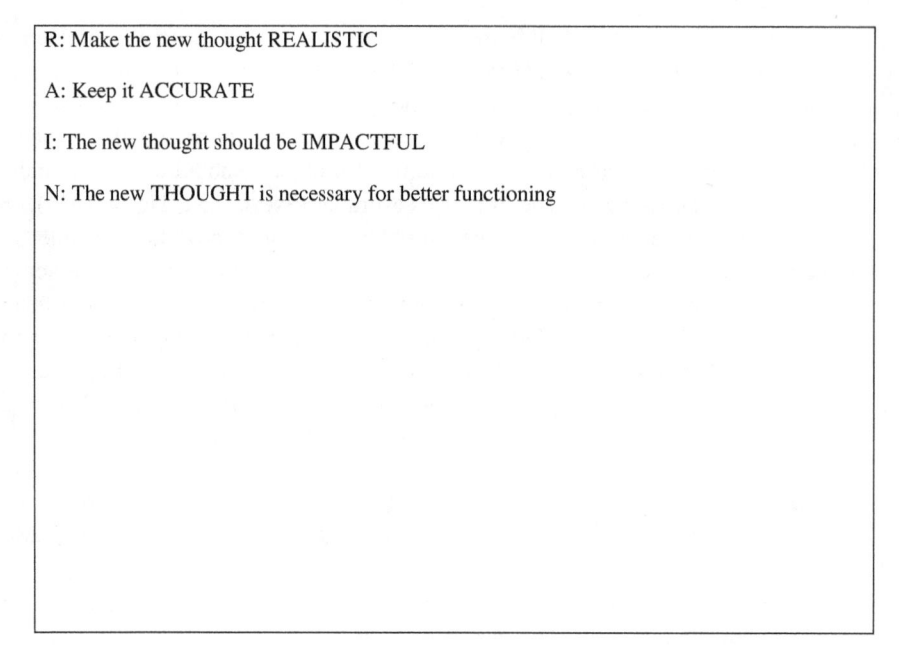

A: Keep it ACCURATE

I: The new thought should be IMPACTFUL

N: The new THOUGHT is necessary for better functioning

Fig. 7.3 Make it RAIN

makes cognitive restructuring accessible to young patients (Friedberg and McClure 2015; Friedberg et al. 2001, 2009; Kendall and Hedtke 2006; Stallard 2002).

Rational analysis techniques focus on logical reasoning. Tests of evidence, reattribution, and decatastrophizing each has common rubrics (Beck 2011). Tests of evidence include interventions such as examining facts confirming and disconfirming beliefs. Reattribution is fueled by the search for alternate meanings (e.g., What's another way of explaining____? What's another way of looking at _____). Decatastrophizing works to decrease young patients' exaggeration of the magnitude of the danger, overestimation of the probability of the threat, and neglect of coping strategies. (e.g., What is the worst that could happen? What is the likelihood? What is the best that could happen? How likely? If the worst thing happens, how can you cope?, etc.).

Exposures and Experiments

Bandura (1977) emphasized that "performance accomplishments provide the most dependable source of efficacy expectations because they are based on one's own personal experiences (p. 81)." Exposures and experiments (E/E) stand as an essential module. In this stage of treatment, young patients demonstrate they can execute their coping skills in emotionally evocative situations. Simply, experiential learning opportunities characterize E/E. Patients fortify their coping skills by approaching various stressors and adversities.

Effective exposures and experiments contribute to many propitious outcomes including increased sense of emotional control (Kollman et al. 2009), attitudinal changes (Moses and Barlow 2006; Rosqvist 2008), and new learning (Craske and Mystowski 2006). We recommend that E/E are collaboratively designed (Ginsburg and Kingery 2007), emotionally poignant (Hannesdottir and Ollendick 2007), and artfully crafted (Kendall et al. 2006; Peterman et al. 2015).

There are several general principles for implementing behavioral exposures and experiments (Friedberg et al. 2009; Kendall et al. 2006; Peterman et al. 2015; Wells 1997). Once is never enough when it comes to exposures and experiments. E/Es need to be repeated and prolonged. Additionally, E/E should also be comprehensive

Situation	Feeling	Thought	Suspect	5-O correction
Friend got picked for Student Council and I didn't	Sad (8)	I'm a loser. I don't count.	All or none thinking	Not being picked for student council and my friend making it does not mean I am loser or don't count. She is good at some things and I am good at other things.
Going to the 1st soccer team meeting	Worried (8)	I won't know anyone. The other kids will think I am too lame for this team. No one will talk to me and they will laugh at me behind my back. It's going to be awful	Catastrophizing Emotional reasoning	This is just my scared feelings talking. I don't know for sure what will happen. I might feel freaky but it probably won't be awful.

Fig. 7.4 Thought 5–0

and incorporate the physiological, emotional, cognitive, behavioral, and contextual elements of the avoided circumstance. Finally, E/Es need to be systematically processed (Wells 1997). Patients make predictions about the experience, conduct the experiment, and subsequently interpret findings. In this way, a conceptual anchor is forged.

Case Example

Parker[1] was a 9-year-old child who presented with a variety of anxious symptoms. She experienced many generalized worries, which she found to be uncontrollable. The worries included concerns about doing poorly in school, losing friends, getting sick, her best friend being deported, parents becoming injured in car accidents, nuclear war, and food shortages. Further, she also complained of difficulties initiating and maintaining sleep through the night. Painful stomach aches and headaches accompanied these worries. Consequently, her family sought treatment from her pediatrician as well as specialty evaluation through pediatric gastroenterology and neurology clinics. Her pediatrician and specialty physician concluded that the symptoms were "functional" and exacerbated by "stress reactions." Subsequently, she was seen by a clinical psychologist who completed an initial evaluation. After the evaluation, Parker and her family began a course of mCBT.

Psychoeducation

Treatment began with psychoeducation. The clinician explained the biopsychosocial model (Engel 1977) and CBT. CBT was explained through an experiential exercise applying a familiar visual illusion that is used in the Universal Protocol for Children (UP-C; Ehrenreich-May et al. 2018). Furthermore, Parker's mother and father were encouraged to read *Freeing Your Child from Anxiety* (Chansky 2004) as a supplemental parenting resource.

Target Monitoring

In order to create a baseline, several target metrics were obtained. At the initial evaluation, Parker and her parents completed the Screen for Child Anxiety and Related Emotional Disturbances (SCARED; Birmaher et al. 1997). Both the parent and child version indicated an elevated level of anxiety especially in generalized worries. Additionally, Parker and her parents created an anxiety hierarchy using Subjective Units of Distress (SUDS) (Fig. 7.5).

Basic Behavioral Tasks

Due to Parker's autonomic hyperarousal and somatic complaints, relaxation training was introduced. Relaxation training was initiated with Parker learning to breathe diaphragmatically by blowing soap bubbles in the air. Once the controlled breathing was acquired, she practiced the technique for 20 min in session and was invited to try the relaxation two times daily at home.

Cognitive Restructuring

Similar to most children with anxiety related problems, her symptoms were fundamentally associated with fears of loss of control (Chorpita and Barlow 1998). Consequently, the skewed beliefs regarding control were targeted by several cognitive interventions. More specifically, the therapist and Parker completed the Master of Disaster exercise (Friedberg et al. 2009). Parker disclosed that letting go of any control was intolerable and would lead to disasters. Socratic questioning embedded in the Master of Disaster worksheet targeted her catastrophic thinking (e.g., How sure are you that the disaster will happen? What convinces you? Has the disaster even happen before? How did you handle it? If you have a plan to handle your disaster, how bad can it be? How in control of things are you? etc.).

---

[1] Parker is a confabulated case based on combinations of patients treated.

Fear/Worry	Subjective Unit of Distress (SUDS) (1-10)
Parents Injured	10
Poor School performance	9
Friend Being Deported	8
Nuclear war	6
Food Shortages	6

Fig. 7.5 Parker's hierarchy

Further, Parker felt certain that control was the solution, when, in fact, it was the problem. Accordingly, the Chinese Finger Trap exercise (Friedberg et al. 2009; Hayes et al. 1999) was used to prime Parker for graduated exposures and experiments. In the Chinese Finger Trap, the young patient inserts her two fore-fingers into each end of a woven tube. The trap tightens if the person tries to pull away. In order to escape, the patient has to "give in" or surrender by pushing into the trap.

Exposures and Experiments

Several direct exposures to Parker's specific worries followed. To address fears of nuclear war, friends being deported, and worldwide food shortages, Parker repeatedly read newspapers and watched TV news at home and in-session. Further, Parker took several "pop" quizzes during her therapy sessions to address her school performance fears. Finally, she engaged in multiple imaginal exposures where she visualized her parents being injured.

Conclusion

CBT offers clinicians a unified theoretical framework and authoritative empirical support for multiple procedures. The approach is robust and flexible, which enables application to diverse populations and settings. New developments in the field identify powerful modular components within the treatment paradigm. In summary, clinicians' confidence in CBT processes and procedures is well founded.

References

Arora, P. G., Stephan, S. H., Becker, K. D., & Wissow, L. (2016). Psychosocial interventions for use in pediatric primary care: An examination of providers' perspectives. *Families, Systems & Health, 34*(4), 414–423.

Arora, P. G., Godoy, L., & Hodgkinson, S. (2017). Serving the underserved: Cultural considerations in behavioral health integration in pediatric primary care. *Professional Psychology: Research and Practice, 48*, 139–148.

Bandura, A. (1977). *Social learning theory*. Englewood Cliffs, NJ: Prentice-Hall.

Bearman, S. K., & Weisz, J. R. (2015). Review: Comprehensive treatments for youth co-morbidity: Evidence guided approaches to a complicated problem. *Child and Adolescent Mental Health, 20*, 131–141.

Beck, A. T. (1976). *Cognitive therapy and the emotional disorders*. New York, NY: International University Press.

Beck, A. T. (1978). *Beck hopelessness scale*. San Antonio, TX: Psychological Corporation.

Beck, A. T. (1996). *Beck depression inventory–II*. San Antonio, TX: Psychological Corporation.

Beck, J. S. (2011). *Cognitive behavior therapy: The basics and beyond* (2nd ed.). New York, NY: Guilford.

Beck, A. T., Rush, A. J., Shaw, B. F., & Emery, G. (1979). *Cognitive therapy of depression*. New York, NY: Guilford Press.

Beidas, R. S., Podell, J. L., & Kendall, P. C. (2008). Cognitive-behavioral treatment for child and adolescent anxiety: The coping cat program. In C. W. LeCroy (Ed.), *Handbook of evidence-based treatment* manuals for children and adolescents (pp. 405–430). New York, NY: Oxford Press.

Beidas, R. S., Stewart, R. E., Walsh, L., Lucas, S., Downey, M. M., Jackson, K., et al. (2015). Free, brief, and validated: Standardized instruments for low-resource mental health settings. *Cognitive and Behavioral Practice, 22*, 5–19.

Beidel, D. C., Turner, S. M., & Morris, T. L. (1995). A new inventory to assess childhood social anxiety and phobia: The social phobia and anxiety inventory for children. *Psychological Assessment, 7*, 73–79.

Bennett, K., Manassis, K., Duda, S., Bagnell, A., Bernstein, G. A., Garland, E. J., et al. (2016). Treating child and adolescent anxiety effectively: Overview of systematic reviews. *Clinical Psychology Review, 50*, 80–94.

Berkout, O. V., & Gross, A. M. (2013). Externalizing behavior challenges within primary care settings. *Aggression and Violent Behavior, 18*, 491–495.

Berkovits, M. D., O'Brien, K. A., Carter, C. C., & Eyberg, S. M. (2010). Early identification and intervention: A comparison of two abbreviated versions of parent-child interaction therapy. *Behavior Therapy, 41*, 375–387.

Bickman, L. (2008). A measurement feedback system is necessary to improve mental health outcomes. *Journal of the American Academy of Child and Adolescent Psychiatry, 47*, 1114–1119.

Bickman, L., Kelley, S. D., Breda, C., de Andrade, A. R., & Riemer, M. (2011). Effects of routine feedback to clinicians on mental health outcomes of youths: Results of a randomized trial. *Psychiatric Services, 60*, 1423–1429.

Birmaher, B., Khetarpal, S., Brent, D. A., Cully, M., Balach, L., Kaufman, J., et al. (1997). The screen for child anxiety related emotional disorders (SCARED): Scale construction and psychometric characteristics. *Journal of the American Academy of Child and Adolescent Psychiatry, 36*, 545–553.

Blackman, J. A., & Conaway, M. R. (2013). Developmental, emotional and behavioral co-morbidities across the chronic health condition spectrum. *Journal of Pediatric Rehabilitation Medicine, 6*, 63–71.

Bronfenbrenner, U. (1979). Contexts of child rearing: Problems and prospects. *American Psychologist, 34*(10), 844–850.

Chansky, T. E. (2004). *Freeing your child from anxiety*. New York, NY: Three Rivers Press.

Cho, Y., & Telch, M. J. (2005). Testing the cognitive content-specificity hypothesis of social anxiety and depression: An application of structural equation modeling. *Cognitive Therapy and Research, 29*, 399–416.

Chorpita, B. F. (2014, June). *Putting more evidence in evidence-based practice*. Los Angeles, CA: Keynote address delivered at the National Resource Council of the National Academies.

Chorpita, B. F., & Barlow, D. H. (1998). The development of anxiety: The role of control in the early environment. *Psychological Bulletin, 124*, 3–21.

Chorpita, B. F., & Daleiden, E. L. (2009). Mapping evidence-based treatments for children and adolescents: Applications of the distillation and matching model to 615 treatments from 322 randomized trials. *Journal of Consulting and Clinical Psychology, 77*, 566–577.

Chorpita, B. F., & Weisz, J. R. (2009). *Modular approach to treatment for children with anxiety, depression, trauma, and conduct problems (MATCH-ADTC)*. Satellite Beach, CA: Practicewise.

Chorpita, B. F., Tracey, S. A., Brown, T. A., Collica, T. J., & Barlow, D. H. (1997). Assessment of worry in children and adolescents: An adaptation of the Penn State worry questionnaire. *Behaviour Research and Therapy, 35*, 569–581.

Chorpita, B. F., Reise, S., Weisz, J. R., Grubbs, K., Becker, K. D., & Krull, J. L. (2010). Evaluation of the brief problem checklist: Child and caregiver interviews to measure clinical progress. *Journal of Consulting and Clinical Psychology, 78*(4), 526–536.

Chorpita, B. F., Daleiden, E. L., Ebesutani, C., Young, J., Becker, K. D., Nakamura, B. J., et al. (2011). Evidence-based treatments for children and adolescents: An updated review of indicators of efficacy and effectiveness. *Clinical Psychology: Science and Practice, 18*(2), 154–172.

Comer, J. S., Chow, C., Chan, P. T., Cooper-Vince, C., & Wilson, L. A. S. (2013). Psychosocial treatment efficacy for disruptive behavioral problems in young children. *Journal of the American Academy of Child and Adolescent Psychiatry, 52*, 26–36.

Craske, M. G., & Mystowski, J. L. (2006). Exposure therapy and extinction: Clinical studies). In M. G. Craske, D. Hermans, & D. Vansteenwagen (Eds.), *Fear and learning from basic processes to clinical implications* (pp. 217–233). Washington, DC: American Psychological Association.

Crowe, K., & Mckay, D. (2017). Efficacy of cognitive-behavioral therapy for childhood anxiety and depression. *Journal of Anxiety Disorders, 49*, 76–87.

Dickerson, J. F., Lynch, F. L., Leo, M. C., DeBar, L. L., Pearson, J., & Clarke, G. N. (2018). Cost-effectiveness of cognitive behavioral therapy for depressed youth declining antidepressants. *Pediatrics, 141*(2), 1–9.

Ehrenreich-May, J., Kennedy, S. M., Sherman, J. A., Bilek, E. L., Buzzella, B. A., Bennett, S. M., et al. (2018). *Unified protocols for transdiagnostic treatment of emotional disorders in children and adolescents*. New York, NY: Oxford.

Engel, G. (1977). The need for a new medical model: A challenge for biomedicine. *Science, 196*, 129–136.

Eyberg, S. M., & Ross, A. W. (1978). Assessment of child behavior problems: The validation of a new inventory. *Journal of Clinical Child Psychology, 7*, 113–116.

Flessner, C. A., & Piacentini, J. C. (Eds.). (2017). *Clinical handbook of psychological disorders in children and adolescents: A step-by-step manual*. New York, NY: Guilford.

Forgatch, M. S., & Gewirtz, A. H. (2017). The evolution of the Oregon model of parent management training; an intervention for anti-social behavior in children and adolescents. In J. R. Weisz & A. E. Kazdin (Eds.), *Evidence-based psychotherapies for children and adolescents* (3rd ed., pp. 85–102). New York, NY: Guilford.

Freeman, J., Garcia, A., Frank, H., Benito, K., Conelea, C., Walther, M., et al. (2014). Evidence base update for psychosocial treatments for pediatric obsessive-compulsive disorder. *Journal of Clinical Child & Adolescent Psychology, 43*(1), 7–26.

Friedberg, R. D., & McClure, J. M. (2015). *Clinical practice of cognitive therapy with children and adolescents: The nuts and bolts* (2nd ed.). New York, NY: Guilford.

Friedberg, R. D., & Thordarson, M. A. (2018). Cognitive behavioral therapy. In J. Matson (Ed.), *Handbook of child psychopathology and developmental disabilities treatment* (pp. 43–62). New York, NY: Springer.

Friedberg, R. D., Friedberg, B. A., & Friedberg, R. J. (2001). *Therapeutic exercises for children*. Sarasota, FL: Professional Resource Press.

Friedberg, R. D., McClure, J. M., & Garcia, J. H. (2009). *Cognitive therapy techniques for children and adolescents*. New York, NY: Guilford.

Friedberg, R. D., Gorman, A. A., Hollar-Wilt, L., Biuckians, A., & Murray, M. (2011). *Cognitive behavioral therapy for busy child psychiatrists and other mental health professionals*. New York, NY: Routledge.

Fristad, M. A. (2006). Psychoeduation treatment for school-age children with bipolar disorder. *Development and Psychopathology, 18*, 1289–1306.

Gardner, W., Murphy, M., Childs, G., Kelleher, K., Pagano, M., McInerny, T. K., et al. (1999). The PSC-17: A brief pediatric symptom checklist with psychosocial problem subscales: A report from PROS and ASPN. *Ambulatory Child Health, 5*(3), 225–236.

Ghahramanlou-Holloway, M., Wenzel, A., Lou, K., & Beck, A. T. (2007). Differentiating cognitive content between depressed and anxious outpatients. *Cognitive Behavior Therapy, 36*, 170–178.

Ginsburg, G. S., & Kingery, J. N. (2007). Evidence-based practice for childhood anxiety disorders. *Journal of Contemporary Psychotherapy, 37*, 123–132.

Ginsburg, G. S., Drake, K. L., Winegrad, H., Fothergill, K., & Wissow, L. (2016). An open-trial of the anxiety action plan (AxAP): A brief pediatrician-delivered intervention for anxious youth. *Child & Youth Care Forum, 45*, 19–32.

Gondek, D., Edbrooke-Childs, J., Fink, E., Deighton, J., & Wolpert, M. (2016). Feedback from outcome measures and treatment effectiveness, treatment efficiency, and collaborative practice: A systematic review. *Administration and Policy in Mental Health and Mental Health Services Research, 43*, 325–343.

Hammerness, P., Harpold, T., Petty, C., Menard, C., Zar-Kessler, C., & Biederman, J. (2008). Characterizing non-OCD anxiety disorders in psychiatrically referred children and adolescents. *Journal of Affective Disorders, 105*, 213–219.

Hannesdottir, D. K., & Ollendick, T. H. (2007). The role of emotion regulation in the treatment of anxiety disorders. *Clinical Child and Family Psychology Review, 10*, 275–293.

Hayes, S. C., Strosahl, K. D., & Wilson, K. G. (1999). *Acceptance and commitment therapy*. New York, NY: Guilford.

Henggeler, S. W., Schoenwald, S. K., Borduin, C. M., Rowland, M. D., & Cunningham, P. B. (2009). *Multisystemic therapy for antisocial behavior in children and adolescents*. New York, NY: Guilford.

Higa-McMillan, C. K., Francis, S. E., Rith-Najarian, L., & Chorpita, B. F. (2016). Evidence base update: 50 years of research on treatment for child and adolescent anxiety. *Journal of Clinical Child & Adolescent Psychology, 45*(2), 91–113.

Ingram, R. E., & Kendall, P. C. (1986). Cognitive clinical psychology: Implications of an information processing perspective. In R. E. Ingram (Ed.), *Information processing approaches to clinical psychology* (pp. 3–21). Orlando, FL: Academic Press.

Jensen-Doss, A., Haimes, E. M. B., Smith, A. M., Lyon, A. R., Lewis, C. C., Stanick, C. F., et al. (2018). Monitoring treatment progress and providing feedback is viewed favorably but rarely used in practice. *Administration and Policy in Mental Health Services and Research, 45*, 48–61.

Jolly, J. B. (1993). A multi-method test of the cognitive content-specificity hypothesis in young adolescents. *Journal of Anxiety Disorders, 7*, 223–233.

Kazdin, A. E. (2017). Parent management training and problem-solving skills training for child and adolescent conduct problems. In J. R. Weisz & A. E. Kazdin (Eds.), *Evidence-based psychotherapies for children and adolescents* (3rd ed., pp. 142–158). New York, NY: Guilford.

Kazdin, A. E., Rodgers, A., & Colbus, D. (1986). The hopelessness scale for children: Psychometric characteristics and concurrent validity. *Journal of Consulting and Clinical Psychology, 54*, 241–245.

Kendall, P. C. (2012). Anxiety disorders in youth. In P. C. Kendall (Ed.), *Child and adolescent therapy* (4th ed., pp. 143–187). New York, NY: Guilford Press.

Kendall, P. C., & Braswell, L. (1985). *Cognitive behavioral therapy for impulsive children*. New York, NY: Guilford Press.

Kendall, P. C., & Finch, A. J. (1976). A cognitive-behavioral treatment for impulsive control: A controlled study. *Journal of Consulting and Clinical Psychology, 44*, 852–857.

Kendall, P. C., & Hedtke, K. A. (2006). *Coping cat workbook*. Ardmore, PA: Workbook Publishing.

Kendall, P. C., & Suveg, C. (2006). Treating anxiety disorders in youth. In P. C. Kendall (Ed.), *Child and adolescent therapy: Cognitive behavioral procedures* (3rd ed., pp. 243–294). New York, NY: Guilford.

Kendall, P. C., Robin, J. A., Hedtke, K. A., Suveg, C., Flannery-Schroeder, E., & Gosch, E. (2006). Considering CBT with anxious youth? Think exposures. *Cognitive and Behavioral Practice, 12*(1), 136–148.

Kendall, P. C., Hudson, J. L., Gosch, E. A., Flannery-Schroeder, E., & Suveg, C. (2008). Cognitive-behavioral therapy for anxiety disordered youth: A randomized clinical trial evaluating child and family modalities. *Journal of Consulting and Clinical Psychology, 76*, 282–287.

Kendall, P. C., Furr, J. M., & Podell, J. L. (2010). Child-focused treatment of anxiety. In J. R. Weisz & A. E. Kazdin (Eds.), *Evidence-based psychotherapies for children and adolescents* (2nd ed., pp. 45–60). New York, NY: Guilford Press.

Kendall, P. C., Makeover, H., Swan, A., Carper, M. M., Mercado, R., Kagan, E., et al. (2016). What steps to take? How to approach concerning anxiety in youth. *Clinical Psychology: Science and Practice, 23*, 211–229.

Kolko, D. J., & Perrin, E. (2014). The integration of behavioral health interventions in children's health care: Services, science and suggestions. *Journal of Clinical Child and Adolescent Psychology, 43*, 216–228.

Kollman, D. M., Brown, T. A., & Barlow, D. H. (2009). The construct validity of acceptance: A multitrait-multimethod investigation. *Behavior Therapy, 40*, 205–218.

Kovacs, M. (2010). *The children's depression inventory-2 manual*. North Tonawanda, NY: Multi-Health Systems.

Lamberton, A., & Oei, T. P. (2008). A test of the cognitive content specificity hypothesis in depression and anxiety. *Journal of Behavior Therapy and Experimental Psychiatry, 39*(1), 23–31.

Lavigne, J. V., LeBailly, S. A., Gouze, S. A., Cicchetti, C., Arend, R., et al. (2008a). Predictor and moderator effects in the treatment of oppositional defiant disorder in primary care. *Journal of Pediatric Psychology, 33*, 462–472.

Lavigne, J. V., LeBailly, S. A., Gouze, K. R., Cicchetti, C., Pochyly, J., Arend, R., et al. (2008b). Treating oppositional defiant disorders in primary care: A comparison of three models. *Journal of Pediatric Psychology, 33*(5), 449–461.

Lochman, J. E., Wells, K. C., & Lenhart, L. (2008). *Coping power child group program: Facilitators guide*. New York, NY: Oxford Press.

Lochman, J. E., Boxmeyer, C., Powell, N., Dillon, C., & Kassing, F. (2017). Disruptive behavior disorders. In C. A. Flessner & J. C. Piacentini (Eds.), *Clinical handbook of psychological disorders in children and adolescents: A step-by-step manual* (pp. 299–328). New York, NY: Guilford.

March, J. S. (2013). *The multidimensional anxiety scale for children* (2nd ed.). Toronto, ON: Multi-Health Systems.

McCart, M. R., & Sheidow, A. J. (2016). Evidence-based psychosocial treatments for adolescents with disruptive behavior. *Journal of Clinical Child & Adolescent Psychology, 45*(5), 529–563.

McMahon, R. J., & Forehand, R. L. (2003). *Helping the non-compliant child* (2nd ed.). New York, NY: Guilford.

McMenamy, J., Sheldrick, R. C., & Perrin, E. C. (2011). Early intervention in pediatric offices for emerging disruptive behavior in toddlers. *Journal of Pediatric Health Care, 25*, 77–86.

Moses, E. B., & Barlow, D. H. (2006). A new unified approach for emotional disorders based on emotion science. *Current Directions in Psychological Science, 15*, 146–150.

Nangle, D. W., Hansen, D. J., Grover, R. L., Kingery, J. N., & Suveg, C. (2016). *Treating internalizing disorders in children and adolescents: Core techniques and strategies*. New York, NY: Guilford.

Nezu, A. M., & Nezu, C. M. (1989). Clinical decision-making in the practice of behavior therapy. In A. M. Nezu & C. M. Nezu (Eds.), *Clinical decision-making in behavior therapy* (pp. 57–113). Champaign, IL: Research Press.

Padesky, C. A. (1993, September). *Socratic questioning: Changing minds or guiding discovery?* London: Keynote address delivered at the European Congress of Behavioral and Cognitive Therapies.

Pao, M., & Bosk, A. (2011). Anxiety in medically ill children/adolescence. *Depression and Anxiety, 28*, 40–49.

Peterman, J. B., Read, K. L., Wei, C., & Kendall, P. C. (2015). The art of exposure: Putting science into practice. *Cognitive and Behavioral Practice, 22*(3), 379–392.

Polanczyk, G. F., Salum, G. A., Sugaya, L. S., Caye, A., & Rohde, L. A. (2015). Annual research review: A meta-analysis of the worldwide prevalence of mental disorders in children and adolescents. *The Journal of Child Psychology and Psychiatry, 56*(3), 345–365.

Rapee, R. M., Lyneham, H. J., Wuthrich, V., Chatterton, M. L., Hudson, J. L., Kangas, M., et al. (2017). Comparison of stepped care delivery against a single, empirically validated cognitive-behavioral therapy program for youth with anxiety. *Journal of the American Academy of Child and Adolescent Psychiatry, 56*, 841–848.

Rosqvist, J. (2008). *Exposure treatment for anxiety disorders*. New York, NY: Routledge.

Sanders, M. R. (2012). Development, evaluation, and multi-national dissemination of the Triple P-Positive Parenting Program. *Annual Review of Clinical Psychology, 8*, 1–35.

Scott, K., & Lewis, C. C. (2015). Using measurement based care to enhance any treatment. *Cognitive and Behavioral Practice, 22*, 49–59.

Stallard, P. C. (2002). *Think good, feel good: A cognitive behavioural workbook for children and young people*. Chichester: Wiley.

Storch, E. A., Murphy, T. K., Adkins, J. W., Lewin, A. B., Geffken, G. R., Johns, N., et al. (2006). The Children's Yale-Brown obsessive-compulsive scale: Psychometric properties of child and parent-report formats. *Journal of Anxiety Disorders, 20*, 1055–1070.

Swanson, J. M., Sandman, C. A., Deutsch, C. K., & Baren, M. (1983). Methylphenidate hydrochloride given with or before breakfast: I. Behavioral, cognitive, and electrophysiologic effects. *Pediatrics, 72*, 49–55.

Szigethy, E., Bujoreanu, S. I., Youk, A. O., Weisz, J., Benhayon, D., Fairclough, D., et al. (2014). Randomized efficacy trial of two psychotherapies for depression in youth with inflammatory bowel disease. *Journal of the American Academy of Child & Adolescent Psychiatry, 53*(7), 726–735.

Treatment for Adolescents with Depression Study (TADS) Team. (2003). Treatment for adolescents with depression study: Rationale, design, and methods. *Journal of the American Academy of Child and Adolescent Psychiatry, 42*, 531–542.

Treatment for Adolescents with Depression Study (TADS) Team. (2004). Fluoxetine, cognitive behavioral therapy, and their combination of for adolescents with depression. *Journal of the American Medical Association, 292*, 807–820.

Treatment for Adolescents with Depression Study (TADS) Team. (2005). The treatment for adolescents with depression study (TADS): Demographic and clinical characteristics. *Journal of the American Academy of Child and Adolescent Psychiatry, 44*, 28–40.

Treatment for Adolescents with Depression Study (TADS) Team. (2007). Treatment for adolescents with depression study: Long-term effectiveness and safety outcomes. *Archives of General Psychiatry, 64*, 1132–1143.

Verhoof, E., Maurice-Stam, H., Heymans, H., & Grootenhuis, M. (2013). Health-related quality of life, anxiety and depression in young adults with disability benefits due to childhood-onset somatic conditions. *Child and Adolescent Psychiatry and Mental Health, 7*(12), 1–9.

Webster-Stratton, C., & Reid, M. J. (2017). The incredible years parents, teachers, and children training series: A multi-faceted treatment approach for young children. In J. R. Weisz & A. E. Kazdin (Eds.), *Evidence-based psychotherapies for children and adolescents* (3rd ed., pp. 122–142). New York, NY: Guilford.

Weems, C. F., & Silverman, W. K. (2013). Anxiety disorders. In T. P. Beauchaine & S. P. Hinshaw (Eds.), *Child and adolescent psychopathology* (2nd ed., pp. 513–542). New York, NY: Wiley.

Weersing, V. R., Jeffreys, M., Do, M.-C. T., Schwartz, K. T. G., & Bolano, C. (2017). Evidence based update of psychosocial treatments for child and adolescent depression. *Journal of Clinical Child & Adolescent Psychology, 46*(1), 11–43.

Weisz, J. R., & Chorpita, B. F. (2012). "Mod Squad" for youth psychotherapy: Restructuring evidence based treatment for clinical practice. In P. C. Kendall (Ed.), *Child and adolescent therapy: Cognitive-behavioral procedures* (pp. 379–397). New York, NY: Guilford.

Weisz, J. R., & Kazdin, A. E. (Eds.). (2017). *Evidence-based psychotherapies for children and adolescents* (3rd. ed.). New York, NY: Guilford.

Weisz, J. R., Krumholz, L. S., Santucci, L., Thomassin, K., & Ng, M. Y. (2015). Shrinking the gap between research and practice: Tailoring and testing youth psychotherapies in clinical care contexts. *Annual Review of Clinical Psychology, 11*, 39–63.

Wells, A. (1997). *Cognitive therapy of anxiety disorders: A practice manual and conceptual guide*. New York, NY: Wiley.

Wesseley, S., Bryant, R. A., Greenberg, N., Earnshaw, M., Sharpley, J., & Hughes, J. H. (2008). Does psychoeducation help prevent post-traumatic psychological distress? *Psychiatry: Interpersonal and Biological Processes, 71*, 287–302.

Wissow, L. S., Anthony, B., Brown, J., DosReis, S., Gadomski, A., Ginsburg, G., et al. (2008). A common factors approach to improving the mental health capacity of primary pediatric care. *Administration and Policy in Mental Health and Mental Health Services Research, 35*, 305–318.

Wissow, L. S., van Ginneken, N., Chandra, J., & Rahman, A. (2016). Integrating children's mental health into primary care. *Pediatric Clinics of North America, 63*, 97–113.

Wolraich, M. L., Lambert, W., Doffing, M. A., Bickman, L., Simmons, T., & Worley, K. (2003). Psychometric properties of the Vanderbilt ADHD diagnostic parent rating scale in a referred population. *Journal of Pediatric Psychology, 28*, 559–568.

Zisser-Nathanson, A. R., Herschell, A. D., & Eyberg, S. M. (2017). Parent-child interaction therapy and the treatment of disruptive behavior disorders. In J. R. Weisz & A. E. Kazdin (Eds.), *Evidence-based psychotherapies for children and adolescents* (3rd ed., pp. 103–121). New York, NY: Guilford.

Necessary Adaptations to CBT with Pediatric Patients

Corinne Catarozoli, Lara Brodzinsky, Christina G. Salley, Samantha P. Miller, Becky H. Lois, and Johanna L. Carpenter

Introduction

Working with a child or adolescent who has been diagnosed with a medical illness can sometimes feel daunting, particularly for a mental health clinician who has not worked in a pediatric setting or has little familiarity with that particular illness or condition. The tendency may even be to refer out to a "specialist" in the area, with the assumption that specific training is required to work with this population. On the contrary, clinicians practicing CBT can "tweak" what they already know to fit medical issues as the presenting problem.

A substantial evidence base has been established supporting the use of CBT protocols with medically compromised children, and the impact of these treatments on both physical and mental health outcomes is compelling (Pao and Bosk 2011; Powers et al. 2005). Within medical settings (e.g., outpatient medical specialty clinic, inpatient medical unit, ICU, and primary care), CBT shows promise for treatment targets such as anxiety, depression, pain, and somatic symptoms, as well as adherence to medical regimens and the unique challenges faced by families and staff during all phases of treatment, including palliative care (Pao and Bosk 2011; Stanger et al. 2013; Allen et al. 2006). While a CBT provider working in a medical environment will find numerous similarities to traditional outpatient treatment, there are some key distinctions to the overall therapeutic frame and specific intervention strategies that should be considered. First, medical settings are fast-paced, and disease status can shift quickly. Thus, pediatric psychologists must be able to flexibly apply CBT interventions to best fit the current circumstances and illness profile. Frequency, length, and timing of sessions tend to be more fluid and are often dependent on medical procedures, current physical symptoms, or other factors outside of the control of both clinician and patient, and it is not uncommon for

C. Catarozoli (✉)
Weill Cornell Medicine, New York, NY, USA
e-mail: cos2006@med.cornell.edu

L. Brodzinsky · B. H. Lois
Department of Child and Adolescent Psychiatry, Child Study Center, Hassenfeld Children's Hospital at NYU Langone, New York, NY, USA

C. G. Salley
Department of Child and Adolescent Psychiatry, NYU School of Medicine and Hassenfeld Children's Hospital at NYU Langone, New York, NY, USA

S. P. Miller
Dell Children's Medical Center Chronic Disease Program, Dell Medical Group, University of Texas at Austin, Austin, TX, USA

Johanna L. Carpenter
Division of Behavioral Health, Nemours/A.I. duPont Hospital for Children and Sidney Kimmel Medical College, Thomas Jefferson University, Wilmington, DE, USA

these to change with little warning. Treatment plans may similarly need to be altered to fit disease progression or new illness symptoms, and CBT providers may need to pivot and change course from the plan as these dynamics shift.

A major difference when working in pediatric medical settings is the nature of the referral source. Instead of seeing patients who are self-referred or brought in by parents for distressing symptoms, children are almost exclusively referred by the medical team. Families may have limited knowledge or understanding about a referral in advance, and psychology services may not always be readily welcomed. Patients or parents may react with confusion, hostility, or defensiveness when they are told that their doctor believes psychological factors are contributing to medical symptoms or other difficulties. Additionally, there may be conflict between the family and medical team regarding the referral reason, and the pediatric psychologist is then in the position of diplomatically navigating these differences of opinion. Part of the initial role of a psychologist is thus to gently provide a rationale for CBT interventions in the context of medical illness and promoting buy-in for the family. Given that most patients are flagged and referred by medical staff who have identified some challenge that has arisen related to the illness, the role of a pediatric psychologist in a medical setting encompasses both clinician and consultant. Consultation, which may be an unfamiliar task to CBT providers, is typically brief and limited in scope. Assessment and intervention are restricted to just that which is relevant to the illness or referral question. The consultation model can at times feel foreign to clinicians who are accustomed to comprehensive evaluations and treatment plans that span multiple domains (i.e., school, family, social settings).

Some of the most concrete differences of practicing in a medical setting include aspects of the physical environment. Oftentimes, physical privacy during sessions is limited as best, as treatment may be conducted bedside with roommates nearby and nursing staff periodically checking in, or in an open clinic while children are actively receiving treatment. Confidentiality is similarly limited in the sense that information disclosed by a patient may be relayed back to the medical team in service of answering a referral question. Even electronic documentation may be more available for a wider range of medical providers to view than a more protected mental health note. These limitations should be made clear up front, so patients understand that all parties are openly communicating.

CBT Model in Pediatrics

The foundational aspects of CBT—the connection between one's thoughts, feelings, and behaviors—are completely applicable to youth facing medical conditions. For instance, a teen with a diagnosis of cancer and an upcoming chemotherapy appointment may think to himself/herself, "what's the point of going through this awful treatment? I'm not going to get better," which may result in feelings of hopelessness, anger, and fear, and then lead to avoidant behavior such as refusing to talk during treatments or even skipping them altogether.

The major difference in the cognitive triangle (see Fig. 8.1), when one thinks about intervention, comes into play when we consider challenging this youth's thoughts about not getting better and corresponding feelings of hopelessness. These thoughts and feelings may in fact be realistic and require acceptance, rather than a change-oriented strategy such as problem-solving or cognitive restructuring. Similarly, youth with health challenges may incorporate somatic symptoms into the "feelings" picture of the cognitive triangle. Youth may share feelings of fatigue, medication regimen "burn out," nausea, stress, and pain as steady states that act as secondary emotions to the primary feeling of numbness or helplessness. For these reasons, specific CBT skills such as exposure, relaxation, and radical acceptance may be particularly beneficial to youth with medical illness.

Several CBT approaches, including adaptations to Dialectical Behavior Therapy, Acceptance and Commitment Therapy, and Parent–Child Interaction Therapy, may aid in the management

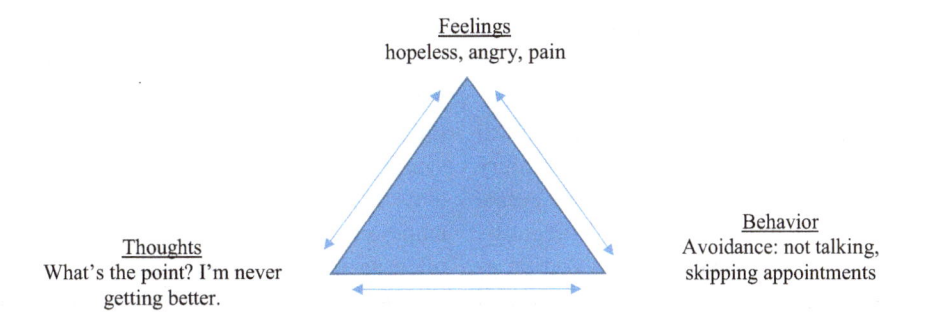

Fig. 8.1 The CBT model in pediatrics

Feelings
hopeless, angry, pain

Thoughts
What's the point? I'm never getting better.

Behavior
Avoidance: not talking, skipping appointments

of complex dynamics that can emerge within the context of coping with a medical condition or parenting a child with illness. Common techniques utilized in these CBT approaches mirror their use in traditional settings, with key distinctions that should be considered to improve "goodness-of-fit." These distinctions will be discussed in depth throughout this chapter.

Understanding Behavioral Health Symptoms from a CBT Framework

Among the current trends in pediatrics are patient-centered care, which suggests that treatment plans should be developed in collaboration with patients and address patient-directed goals (Eichner and Johnson 2018); as well as the concept of patient-centered medical homes where both physical and behavioral health issues can be addressed (Asarnow et al. 2015). As such, physicians are referring their medical patients for behavioral health treatment at an increasing rate. When pediatric patients present for behavioral health treatment, they often arrive with physical complaints such as pain, nausea, vomiting, and fatigue, as well as other distressing symptoms that are directly related to medical treatments, procedures, and/or changes in lifestyle that result from their illness or condition. In many cases, it may be premature to begin the discussion about these symptom presentations from a traditional CBT framework without first connecting the dots between psychological and physical functioning. Introducing the mind–body connection and providing education on the role of stress in symptom formation and maintenance can provide a common language for case conceptualization and treatment planning, as well as a helpful bridge toward introducing CBT.

The Mind–Body Connection

In general, the mind–body connection suggests that one's psychological functioning (thoughts, feelings, and behaviors) is directly linked to physical functioning. In mind–body medicine, the two are seen as functioning not separately but as a unit, where thoughts and emotions directly influence the body and vice versa (Selhub 2007). This concept is quite simple and can be easily explained to pediatric patients of all ages while using developmentally appropriate language, props, and examples. In session, a child, adolescent and/or parent might be asked to think of something pleasurable and take note of how their body feels. Likewise, they could also be asked to think of something stressful that recently happened and take note of how their body feels, then participate in deep breathing exercises and take note of any changes in how their body feels. The latter exercise can be used to exemplify the bidirectional pathway through which the mind and body communicate. It also is an example of how stress impacts both the mind and the body and presents an opportunity for pediatric patients and their families to share their own examples of stress, particularly as it relates to the child or adolescent's medical condition.

Stress Within the Context of Medical Conditions

Kazak et al. (2006) and later Price et al. (2016) discuss the effects of medical illness and injury within the context of traumatic stress. The events leading up to diagnosis, the time of diagnosis itself, the projected treatment course, and prognosis can all act as sources of both acute and chronic stress. Additionally, the range of preexisting experiences and patients' developmental levels, as well as family system changes also influences their response to medical stress. Presenting this model to pediatric patients and families can serve to further validate and normalize their experience of stress within context. It then leads to a conversation about the biological effects of psychological stress and vice versa that may stem from their experiences.

The Stress Response

By providing psychoeducation that mirrors familiar CBT protocols, therapists can use the analogies of the "gas pedal" and "brake" to explain how the sympathetic and parasympathetic nervous systems work to "rev us up" and "calm us down." Talking through the "fight or flight" stress response and how it applies to pediatric patients' experiences begin to bridge the gap between theoretical and personal by connecting the dots within their mind–body experience For example, in the case of a child presenting with abdominal pain, clinicians can explain that the stress response, or "gas pedal," which might be triggered by a stomach ache, results in increased blood pressure and muscle tension, leading to mood changes (i.e., irritability, fear), and hypervigilance to the sensation of abdominal pain.

As the behavioral health expert, psychologists can then introduce the foundational aspects of CBT as a framework for applying evidence-based interventions that address these presenting problems. In the case of the child presenting with abdominal pain, the therapist can explain that a relaxation response, or "brakes," can be triggered by goal-directed behaviors such as deep breathing, progressive muscle relaxation, guided imagery, biofeedback, and hypnosis (Kibby et al. 1998). Presenting these and other relaxation training techniques as a way to activate the parasympathetic nervous system and decrease symptoms helps pediatric patients and families feel empowered to effect some change within what is often an uncontrollable situation. It also opens the door to further cognitive and behavioral interventions.

Intervention Adaptations: Behavior Management

In the pediatric setting, behavioral problems are a common reason for referral to a pediatric psychologist. The presenting behavioral issue might be what a child or adolescent is doing (e.g., engaging in oppositional or disruptive behavior that interferes with medical care) or not doing (e.g., avoiding physical exertion in the context of chronic pain). Specific examples of "doing" behaviors include pulling out IVs or PICC lines; becoming physically and/or verbally aggressive prior to, or during, medical procedures; refusing to follow directions or cooperate in physical or occupational therapy; and generally engaging in noncompliant, combative, and/or attention-seeking behavior toward medical staff and/or caregivers. "Not doing" behaviors include failing to adhere to medical regimens that have been prescribed in the context of chronic conditions (such as diabetes or cystic fibrosis) and avoidance of school or other daily activities due to concern about triggering pain or other physical symptoms (e.g., vomiting, seizures). It is not uncommon for children and adolescents to exhibit behaviors from both general categories.

Conceptualizing the Function of Behaviors of Concern

Regardless of the form that the specific presenting behavior takes, it is important to consider the hypothesized function of the behavior, as well as the forces that have shaped and maintained the behavior in question. Certainly, some of the behaviors listed above could reflect learned patterns of disruptive behavior that have been inadvertently reinforced by environmental responses, perhaps coupled with variables such as the child's strong-willed temperament, desire to be in control, and/or low frustration tolerance. This would suggest the need for parent behavioral management training approaches, such as Parent-Child Interaction Therapy (PCIT; McNeil and Hembree-Kigin 2010) or Parent Management Training (PMT; Kazdin et al. 2005). Alternatively, for many of the behaviors described above, the function could be to avoid/delay an aversive stimulus (e.g., medical procedure, IV/PICC line) or to otherwise reduce or avoid anxiety (e.g., by not working through pain or discomfort). This could suggest underlying needle phobia, other procedural anxiety, illness or pain anxiety, and/or symptoms of posttraumatic stress—and ultimately point to the need for the treatment plan to include anxiety or trauma-informed treatment (including exposure therapy; Pao and Bosk 2011), and/or interventions to manage procedural discomfort (e.g., Boerner et al. 2014). Nonadherence behaviors are particularly multifaceted and could indicate family-level interventions utilizing problem-solving skills training (Carpenter et al. 2014; Wysocki et al. 2006), individual interventions targeting emotional conditions, and/or procedural anxiety interventions. Table 8.1 shows behavioral interventions that are commonly used in the medical setting or in the context of pediatric medical conditions.

Considerations for Behavioral Interventions in the Medical Setting

Parental and caregiver factors are essential to consider when implementing behavioral strategies in the pediatric setting. Caregiver responses to a child's illness or hospitalization can vary widely (Pinquart 2013) but may include overprotective, hypervigilant, or permissive parenting approaches (Carey et al. 2002; Holmbeck et al. 2002). For example, caregivers may be less likely to set limits or behavioral contingencies with

Table 8.1 Common behavioral strategies in pediatric settings

Noncompliant/oppositional behavior
- Parent training (PCIT, PMT) (training caregivers to increase warmth/positivity and use adaptive behavior management strategies)
- Reward/positive reinforcement systems (reinforcing desired behaviors using specific praise and/or token economy)

Consider: Incorporating medical play and praising appropriate medical behaviors

Nonadherence
- Problem-solving skills (e.g., behavioral family systems therapy)
- Apps or technology use to stay on track with medical tasks

Consider: Shaping ultimate adherence goal by setting approximations of this larger goal

Procedural anxiety and/or pain/illness anxiety
- Behavioral distraction (e.g., playing videogames, watching TV)
- Progressive muscle relaxation (systematically tensing, holding, and releasing muscles)
- Diaphragmatic breathing (abdominal breathing method that involves breathing down into the diaphragm to promote optimal gas exchange and relaxation)
- Reward/positive reinforcement systems (reinforcing desired behaviors using specific praise and/or token economy)
- Positive practice (e.g., rehearsing steps leading up to medical procedure)
- Graded hierarchical exposure (facing real or imagined anxiety-provoking stimuli that have been rank-ordered by difficulty)
- Modeling (e.g., viewing videos of other children or teens with medical conditions who describe their illness coping)

Consider: Personal history of caregiver, increasing opportunities for child/teen's perceived control, reducing uncertainty, incorporating medical play

PCIT parent-child interaction therapy; *PMT* parent management training

their child if they perceive their child to be fragile or to need special allowances due to his/her medical condition. Furthermore, caregivers may reject interventions that appear not to take into consideration their child's health history and condition. Thus, clinicians must be particularly sensitive and diplomatic when working with permissive caregivers to change their parenting behavior. It can sometimes be helpful to discuss parent training as a way to help strengthen their child's personal resources (e.g., self-esteem) by giving him/her clear opportunities to be successful, rather than as a way to improve their child's behavior (which may be tolerable to caregivers). Another approach to help achieve buy-in from permissive caregivers can be to link parent training interventions to their child's physical health. Parents who are not overly concerned about their child's general compliance may be concerned about his/her adherence with medical tasks at home. Interventions such as PCIT may need to be tailored to incorporate medical play in order to build positive medical coping behaviors (Bagner et al. 2004).

Similar challenges can arise when designing behavioral interventions to overcome anxiety or pain avoidance responses, as caregivers' instinct to protect their child from distress may interfere with the goals of the intervention. Clinicians must be cognizant of caregivers' own anxiety about their child's distress levels, as well as caregivers' personal history of needle fears, pain, or other somatic conditions, which can affect their perceptions of, and support for, the behavioral intervention. Exposure treatment, which involves facing either imagined or actual anxiety-provoking stimuli, must always be very carefully planned to gradually increase the level of difficulty and to begin at a level that guarantees success (Kendall et al. 2005). Physical activity engagement would also be considered exposure for patients with activity avoidance secondary to pain anxiety. In discussing exposure with families, it is often helpful to frame exposures as exercises to "retrain" or "rewire" the body (or brain, or the nervous system).

In addition, when addressing procedural and/or pain/illness anxiety, it is recommended that efforts also be made to target the child's sense of certainty/predictability and perceived control, given linkages between these constructs and psychological adjustment among children with chronic illness (e.g., Mullins et al. 2007). This can be achieved by allowing the child to control as many aspects of the procedure as possible and setting up an established procedural routine during exposures (perhaps posted as a schedule). This new routine can then be rehearsed to help it become automatic for the child. If available, collaboration with Child Life Specialists is also highly desirable in order to provide the child with the opportunity for medical play, which has been associated with improved anxiety and distress tolerance (Moore et al. 2015). Also, with the availability of videos of peer models with various health conditions (e.g., through The Coping Club website http://copingclub.com/), it is possible for children and teens to watch brief videos of peers demonstrating different behavioral strategies to promote relaxation (Ernst 2011).

A final consideration when implementing behavioral interventions in pediatric populations is the importance of slowly shaping new health behaviors such as medical task completion behaviors. This approach often runs counter to medical team preferences, as intermediate goals may be set that do not reflect optimal disease management practices. Yet, the gradual approach is crucial for patient engagement and buy-in, as well as to establish initial successes and form long-term habits. Problem-solving-focused interventions, used most prominently in patients with type 1 diabetes (e.g., Carpenter et al. 2014; Wysocki et al. 2006), can be applied to help youth and their family members to focus on well-defined and achievable goals, as well as to brainstorm solutions to better integrate medical tasks into their daily lives. Adolescents frequently prefer applications and other forms of technology to help them to remember or communicate about medical tasks. It should be noted that caregivers of older youth and adolescents presenting with adherence challenges frequently express considerable stress and frustration about their child's inconsistent adherence. By focusing on practical, manageable goals and steps to achieve those adherence goals, it is often possible to redirect caregivers' frustration into solution identification.

Intervention Adaptations: Cognitive Approaches

The way in which children and their families think about their illness experience has been found to be an important component of their adjustment. Factors such as hope (Jamieson et al. 2014; Maikranz et al. 2007; Santos et al. 2015) and optimism (Chahal et al. 2017; Mannix et al. 2009) have been associated with better functioning or reported as useful for adaptive coping among children with health conditions. Other benefits have also been identified. For example, hope has been linked to better treatment adherence (Van Allen et al. 2016), and cognitive processes such as rumination, sense-making, and benefit-finding are found to underlie post-traumatic growth among children with serious medical conditions (Picoraro et al. 2014).

Models of stress and coping also highlight the importance of cognitive coping efforts in buffering the challenging aspects of pediatric illness and its management. Compas et al. (2012) reviewed the literature on child and adolescent coping with illness and noted that two models of coping (Connor-Smith et al. 2000; Walker et al. 1997) have been applied to pediatric illness. They distinguish between primary control coping (i.e., interactions with others and the environment) and secondary control coping "which includes efforts to adapt to stress through reappraisal, positive thinking, acceptance, or distraction" (Compas et al. 2012, p. 6). Thus, the use of CBT to address maladaptive cognitions arising in children with health issues is supported by the premise that cognitive coping processes can contribute to positive functioning in the context of pediatric illness. It is further supported by literature suggesting that clinical intervention designed to enhance benefit-finding, hope, or optimism can be utilized in pediatric medical populations (Hilliard et al. 2012; Van Allen et al. 2016. Examples of cognitions shared by pediatric populations are listed in Table 8.2.

It has long been accepted that a child's illness affects the entire family. The thought processes of parents are particularly relevant when therapists are addressing cognitions in their pediatric

Table 8.2 Common child and adolescent cognitions related to illness

Domain	Thought
Pain/symptoms/procedures	It's going to hurt!
	I have too much pain to do what I enjoy (school, soccer)
Diagnosis	Why me? This is unfair. I don't deserve this
	This illness makes me weird/different
Treatment	Medicine makes me feel worse. It can't be helping
	Missing a dose of medicine here and there isn't a big deal
Prognosis	My treatment doesn't matter, I'm not going to die anyway
	The doctors have given up on me
Social life/leisure time	I can't do anything I want to do anymore
	Everyone is moving on with their lives and I'm left behind
Family dynamics	My parents are always on my back. I have no privacy
	My sister can do whatever she wants and I can't

patients. Parents are not only emotionally affected by the child's illness but also required to serve an active role in the management of their child's condition. Given their integral role, parents' own maladaptive thoughts can be disruptive through direct transmission to the child (the child adopts the parents' negative views on the condition or its treatment), conflict with the child's medical providers (the parent struggles to communicate effectively with the child's medical team), or poor communication (medical information is inaccurately explained). Thus, therapists working with children in these settings often work closely with parents to address their unhelpful thoughts when they impact the child's adjustment or course of treatment.

Difficult thoughts will undoubtedly arise when children are diagnosed with a medical condition given the initial shock and disruption to their "normal" life. Distressing cognitions often appear out of these major life shifts and, for many, are a normative response in the course of their adaptation to living with a chronic health issue. Near the time of diagnosis, distressing cognitions will represent early reactions to the diagnosis and may reflect the child's attempts to understand the illness, learn and manage treatment demands, and navigate complicated health systems, while simultaneously making sense of how and why this happened to them. During this early period, distressing cognitions can be expected given the lack of experience and knowledge of the condition and may include distortions such as catastrophizing (*this is the end of a normal life*) but may also be the result of misunderstanding (*this new diet means I'll never be able to eat good food again*). Other thoughts may be an adoption of their parents' negative beliefs surrounding the condition gleaned directly through parents' comments (*our lives will never be the same*) or through observed behaviors (parent engaging in conflict with medical team).

At the time of diagnosis, it is normal for children and parents to desire an understanding of how and why this happened to them. Children may wonder if they did something to cause the illness or think, *"This is unfair. I don't deserve this"* while parents may feel guilty, *"I should have seen the signs that my child was ill and acted sooner"* or expect the worst, *"Things will only get harder from here."* Therapists working with families during this phase can address many of these negative thoughts by normalizing the difficulty of adjusting to the illness and reassuring them that many families have the same concerns. Providing families with accurate information regarding the diagnosis and treatment expectations is important to clarifying any misconceptions that may cause undue distress. Some parents may be able to clearly articulate their fears, while others may experience mental images that they struggle to put into words. Parents can be prompted by "what thought or image comes to mind when you think of what things might be like for your son over the next week (or month, three months, a year)." Here, therapists can provide accurate information through the use of clinical tools (e.g., treatment "road maps" provided by medical team outlining treatment plan) and expertise from medical providers while encouraging flexible thinking by asking, "are there other possible outcomes." Addressing parental anxiety early on should not be underestimated as a powerful tool to assist with children's adjustment. Children and adolescents can engage similarly in this process. Even very young children can identify what they worry may happen to them through drawing or play.

Treatment for medical conditions arising in childhood may be time limited if curative or lifelong for chronic conditions. How children and family perceive the treatment or lifestyle changes (e.g., dietary changes) can impact their overall adjustment and may also affect their adherence to necessary recommendations. Negative thoughts regarding treatment recommendations are not surprising given the possibility of side effects, burden on the family to integrate the treatment into their lives, and the fact that the required treatment differentiates the child from their healthy peers. Children may report negative thoughts regarding their treatments, such as *"This medicine does more harm than good,"* and parents may express similar apprehensions.

Behavioral challenges and parent–child conflict may arise when a child has negative views of their treatment if it results in battles surrounding cooperation in taking medicine or adhering to other treatments. While parents may report this conflict to their child's doctors, other times, their concerns or negative perceptions regarding treatment recommendations may go unspoken. These unspoken thoughts or family secrets may become apparent if there is evidence of obvious poor treatment adherence but can also go unaddressed for sometime. Families may not be forthcoming to their treatment providers with these views as they may attempt to avoid conflict with the doctors recommending the treatments, worry about ramifications of bringing up these concerns, or embarrassment. In their clinician–consultant role, pediatric psychologists are tasked to work with families to identify these unhelpful views so that they can be addressed.

Difficulty coping with pain or other physical symptoms (e.g., nausea, fatigue) or distress surrounding procedures may be exacerbated by cognitions related to these realities of treatment. For example, many children experience some degree of pain throughout their treatment, and this can be from brief interventions such as finger pricks for blood draws to lingering pain while recovering from major surgeries. Intrusive thoughts about symptoms (*I can't eat or I'll throw up*) and exaggeration (*This pain will never end*) are unhelpful. Coaching the child to use positive self-talk strategies (*I can do this*) or reframe into a more helpful thought (*This is an important step toward getting better*) can be useful. Restructuring to more accurate, nuanced, and balanced thoughts that acknowledge the temporary nature of various physical symptoms (*The pain can be managed with medication*) can also ameliorate distress. One approach to addressing expectations and beliefs about symptoms may be asking the patient (with parental participation if developmentally appropriate) to complete a record of activities and symptom severity over the course of several days. Together, the therapist and patient can then examine fluctuations in the symptoms while also identifying activities that may ease symptoms (e.g., distraction) or be a problematic trigger (e.g., engaging in too many physical activities that day). Reviewing these charts with the patient's medical provider (with or without the patient present) may add other important insight or solutions to symptom management. With this compilation of data, therapists can engage in the patient in exercises to challenge extreme expectations about their symptoms and also problem solve practical approaches to ameliorate symptoms (e.g., relaxation, use of medication). Therapists may also work with patients to calibrate their ratings of symptoms. For example, medical providers may be concerned if a patient is frequently reporting their pain to be a "9 or 10" out 10. The patient may also be distressed that they are having the "maximum" amount of pain possible. Provide the patient with examples of what a 1, 5, and 10 might mean (e.g., a 10 means the pain is so bad you will have to be admitted to the hospital). Keep explanations developmentally appropriate and relevant to the illness.

Other negative thoughts associated with symptoms of anxiety and depression in pediatric health populations may stem from real or perceived changes in relationships (peers or family) and leisure time. Children may worry if others will perceive them as a "freak" (*No one understands what I am going through*) or experience isolation (*It's depressing to be around me*). They may be concerned with how they differ from other children (*My sister has it so easy*). They may be struggling to cope with changes in physical abilities that impact their involvement in activities (*I can't keep up in soccer anymore; I can't do anything fun*).

Therapists working with ill children are tasked to help children identify their unhelpful thoughts. As noted above, sometimes distressing thoughts are the result of a poor understanding of the illness and its course and may be addressed through further education with the family. Involving various providers from the multidisciplinary team (doctors, nurses, and social workers) is often a useful tool for addressing these issues as they can each speak from their expertise. Other upsetting thoughts will be accurate, but unhelpful if they become the object of pre-occupation (*This medicine tastes disgusting; I can't play baseball anymore*). Distraction or replacing negative thoughts with positive self-talk (*I will get through this; I am strong*) can be used to combat rehearsal of some distressing thoughts. Other accurate, but upsetting thoughts, may be addressed by exploring if there are any positive aspects to the issue (*This medicine is disgusting but it's helping my body; I can't play baseball but I can be the team manager*). Identifying black-and-white thinking and introducing a more nuanced perspective can decrease distress.

Difficult emotions will certainly arise when facing negative thoughts regarding prognosis. Children with chronic health issues may have to tackle the notion that "it's always going to be this way" or that "no matter what I do I'll still be sick." Those with poor prognoses may be burdened by thoughts surrounding the life-limiting nature of their disease (*I won't get to graduate with my friends; I'm afraid to die; My parents are going to be all alone; What happens when someone dies?*). These thoughts tend to be a poor fit for traditional cognitive restructuring as exercises such as evidence-finding and de-catastrophizing are clearly inappropriate.

Cognitive behavioral therapists thus find themselves in unchartered territory when facing these thoughts as they may reflect devastating realities. To address these difficult thoughts and the feelings accompanying them, pediatric psychologists can support families in talking about these issues together. Frequently, family members are independently thinking about these topics but fearful to start a conversation. Children, especially older adolescents, may be thinking about death but do not want to broach the subject for fear that it will upset their parents, whereas parents often worry that if they speak about death, their child will think they are giving up on them. Open, honest, and developmentally appropriate communication is key. Families may be surprised to find that some children and adolescents want to be involved in planning and making decisions as they approach the end-of-life (e.g., important people or objects they want near them, how symptoms are managed) or what may take place at services following their death. Clinical tools such as "Voicing my Choices" or "My Wishes" can aid in these conversations. The purpose of these tools (found at https://fivewishes.org/Home) is to aid families and clinicians in their conversations with the child about how he/she would like to be cared for physically and emotionally as he/she becomes more ill. This is one way that children and adolescents can be empowered and included in discussions about advance care planning.

Some children may experience relief merely by knowing they have a trusted adult with whom they can share these thoughts. Misconceptions about death can be clarified if they are distressing. In some cases, parents may provide reassurance to their child *(There are people we love in heaven already and you will not be alone there; We will miss you but our love will always keep us connected)* or use spiritual or religious beliefs to give comfort. It may also be appropriate to provide reassurance surrounding issues that can be controlled or predicted in these situations such as telling the child that they will not be in pain or alone at the time of death. Use of bibliotherapy can be helpful for families as many will struggle to find the words to use on their own. Books such as *"Lifetimes: The beautiful way to explain death to children"* (Mellonie and Ingpen 1983) and *"The Invisible String"* (Karst and Lew-Vriethoff 2018) are just some options for supporting conversations about the understanding death as part of the natural cycle of life as well as the infinite connection between loved ones, even after death.

Intervention Adaptations: Family Dynamics

Despite the significant variation in medical treatment regimes for different chronic diseases, the impact of chronic disease on families is broadly similar. The stressor of managing a chronic disease resembles other chronic stressors by disrupting family functioning in the domains of organization, cohesion, communication, affective environment, and problem-solving (Alderfer et al. 2008). McClellan and Cohen (2007) found that families coping with the most common pediatric chronic illnesses (i.e., cystic fibrosis, juvenile rheumatoid arthritis, type 1 diabetes, asthma, hemophilia, and sickle cell disease) demonstrated low family cohesion, poor communication, high parenting stress, and negative affect. Greater parenting stress appears unrelated to illness severity and duration. Parenting stress is associated with greater parental responsibility and a decrease in experiencing competence and control in the parenting role (Cousino and Hazen 2013; Golfenshtein et al. 2016).

Regardless of illness, disease management can entail tremendous restrictions on a family's daily routine and inflict significant financial burden associated with the hospitalizations, medications, and routine medical appointments (U.S. Department of Health and Human Services 2013). Parents are often sleep deprived and miss work due to appointments or hospital stays; ill children as well as healthy siblings also miss school and other milestones or events (McCann et al. 2015). In these circumstances, parents of children with chronic conditions and disability can experience high levels of anger, anxiety, and depression (Cohen et al. 2010). In addition, meta-analysis reviews of the literature suggest a significant negative effect for having a sibling with a chronic illness (Vermaes et al. 2012). The literature further suggests that a key factor in sibling wellness is the amount of parental attention diverted away from siblings and instead focused on the chronic disease (McMahon et al. 2001).

The transition to disease self-management during adolescence and young adulthood is a critical issue for families and may magnify weaknesses in family functioning. Parents are often uncertain how to reconcile protecting their child against the negative effects of medical nonadherence and facilitating the development of autonomy around the medical regime (Akre and Suris 2014; Swallow et al. 2011). If the disease or its management routines have been a source of conflict within the home or a source of embarrassment for the child, children may have difficulty assuming responsibility. Thus, the function of parental involvement in the medical regime must be assessed like any other behavior that may affect disease outcome.

Poor family functioning can compromise medical treatment adherence and thus risk inferior treatment outcomes (McGoldrick et al. 2011). Parental cognitions and distress stemming from a child's chronic illness can lead to parents' increased attention on a child's somatic symptoms and a tendency to excuse their child from certain responsibilities. These well-intentioned, albeit overprotective, parental behaviors have been associated with greater functional disability, reinforced belief of self-inadequacy, negative emotions including anxiety and depression, and poorer emotion regulation (Van Slyke and Walker 2006) and provide an excellent starting place for intervention.

Specific Strategies for Cognitive Behavioral Therapy-Based Family Work

The child's attachment to and relationship quality with caregivers are critical factors to assess when selecting interventions. When children experience pain or emotional distress, attachment-seeking behaviors often increase. A nurturing parent–child relationship can be a beneficial support system that buffers against the stress of living with a chronic disease. Parallel child- and parent-sessions focused on primary control and secondary control coping strategies (as described above) can allow for parents to coach their child in the use of more adaptive coping strategies (Compas et al. 2012). Furthermore, parents who develop a repertoire of their own effective coping strategies can subsequently model more adaptive coping mechanisms for youth. Parental modeling of coping skills has proven to be especially beneficial for adolescents who are preparing to enter adulthood and assume greater personal responsibility for the management of their chronic illness (Kieckhefer et al. 2009).

As described earlier, parent's cognitions play a role in their child's functioning and may need to be addressed by the pediatric psychologist. Common maladaptive cognitions include externalized attributions (attributing both illness and recovery solely to external factors often beyond one's control) and perceived guilt/burden (e.g., a child's guilt about financial burden of medical costs or family stress). Also, parents experience guilt for not being able to "do enough," about genetics, or replaying moments of the past (Carter and Threlkeld 2012). A novel psychosocial intervention, Mastering Each New Direction (MEND; Distelberg et al. 2018), utilizes narratives to help parents and children challenge myths and dysfunctional beliefs about the child's chronic illness. The MEND program has been delivered in integrated behavioral health medical settings. Families attend the program three times per week for 3 hours, which includes peer group, multifamily, and individual therapy. MEND uses language as a primary agent of change. How families talk about chronic illness and illness management is predictive of their coping. In the beginning of the treatment, the MEND therapist assesses the language and coping processes used by the patient and family members in order to better understand the family's meanings and subsequent behaviors related to coping with the illness. The therapist makes special note of how parent and child responses are interdependent, addresses family stress, and helps co-author a more adaptive narrative.

Other CBT-based family work involves parent training designed to help caregivers develop the complex parenting skills needed to provide sufficient support to their chronically ill child. A novel attachment-based psychosocial intervention for pediatric chronic illness, Mother-Child-Disease Triangle (MCDT), combines elements of CBT with trauma-focused CBT (Jensen et al. 2014) while working toward enhancement of the caregiver–child relationship (Dehghani-Arani et al. 2018). Although grounded in attachment theory, much of the psychoeducational material used in treatment sessions mirrors CBT and TF-CBT. There is the added emphasis of improving the mother–child attachment and using expressive therapies like art. The first three sessions of MCDT, conducted individually with the caregiver, involve (1) modifying the caregiver's cognitions about self, the disease, and child; (2) understanding how past negative emotional experiences from medical events have influenced the relationship with child; and (3) developing play therapy skills and the caregiver's ability for emotional attunement. The next three sessions are conducted individually with the child and involve (1) modifying the child's cognitions about himself/herself, the disease, and his/her caregivers; (2) understanding how past negative emotional experiences from medical events have influenced the relationship with his/her caregiver; and (3) helping the child learn to make effective requests and appropriately express his/her needs and feelings. The final three sessions involve conjoint sessions, whereby caregiver and child are able to test their skills through role-play and receive feedback from the therapist. The techniques used in these sessions are dialectic and Socratic conversation, cognitive and emotional modification, psychoeducation, and role-play.

Limitations to CBT with Pediatric Patients

Despite the many applications for CBT with pediatric patients discussed in this chapter, there remain instances when CBT interventions are limited in what they can reasonably accomplish, or may even be outright inappropriate. A common pitfall when working with pediatric patients is relying solely on traditional change-based CBT approaches, particularly given that there is often a realistic component to these emotions. Anxiety, despair, or pain may in fact be completely normative reactions to dealing with an acute or chronic illness. Worries about health, prognosis, and even life expectancy are often well founded. Attempting to outright challenge these cognitions not only is unlikely to be successful but can also be extremely invalidating to the child and family. Posing questions such as, "What's the worst-case scenario?", "How likely is that to happen?", and "How terrible would it be if it happened?" is clearly contraindicated in many of these scenarios. A therapist also will not fare well by using the traditional approach of correcting a child's overestimation of risk and underestimation of their ability to cope, particularly when risk is objectively high and the potential negative outcomes are devastating. Instead, a reasonable goal may be to acknowledge the truth and generate a synthesis between the reality of disease risk and the patient's strengths. A pediatric psychologist may work to introduce slightly more nuance to an anxious or hopeless thought, but changing it outright is likely not a reasonable goal.

Given that CBT tends to be an active, change-based, problem-solving approach to managing negative emotions or problematic behavior, it is understandable that a CBT therapist may have the urge to jump in and fix issues that arise in the medical setting and may receive pressure from medical providers to do so. However, children dealing with illnesses often face problems that cannot be solved and situations that are objectively dire. In these cases, a CBT therapist needs to change course. The importance of bearing witness to a child's experience should not be underestimated. Sitting, listening, and watching are incredibly potent approaches. CBT therapists new to this concept often feel ineffective or as though they are not doing enough. Redefining what is considered therapeutic in situations with no easy solution may alleviate these concerns and help pediatric psychologists acknowledge the value in their presence.

In sum, CBT as an approach is extremely relevant for pediatric populations in addressing anxiety, pain, and distress related to medical conditions. Clinicians should take care to make tweaks to traditional CBT interventions to improve goodness-of-fit for this group. Incorporating physical symptoms into the CBT conceptualization is imperative to best understand a patient's presentation, and discussion of the pain-stress connection is helpful to provide a rationale for this approach. A variety of behavioral, cognitive, and family-focused techniques can be used to engage children with medical illness, and these should be implemented flexibly to account for changing disease status and concurrent medical treatment. CBT clinicians need not learn a whole new approach when working with children with medical illness but instead adapt and reframe what they already know.

References

Akre, C., & Suris, J. C. (2014). From controlling to letting go: What are the psychosocial needs of parents of adolescents with a chronic illness? *Health Education Research, 29*(5), 764–772.

Alderfer, M. A., Fiese, B. H., Gold, J. I., Cutuli, J. J., Holmbeck, G. N., Goldbeck, L., et al. (2008). Evidence-based assessment in pediatric psychology: Family measures. *Journal of Pediatric Psychology, 33*(9), 1046–1061.

Allen, L. A., Woolfolk, R. L., & Escobar, J. I. (2006). Cognitive-behavioral therapy for somatization disorder: A randomized controlled trial. *Archives of Internal Medicine, 166*(14), 1512–1518.

Asarnow, J. R., Kolko, D. J., Miranda, J., & Kazak, A. E. (2015). The pediatric patient-centered medical home: Innovative models for improving behavioral health. *American Psychologist, 72*(1), 13–27.

Bagner, D. M., Fernandez, M. A., & Eyberg, S. M. (2004). Parent-child interaction therapy and chronic illness: A case study. *Journal of Clinical Psychology in Medical Settings, 11*, 1–6.

Boerner, K. E., Gillespie, J. M., McLaughlin, E. N., Kuttner, L., & Chambers, C. T. (2014). Implementation of evidence-based psychological interventions for pediatric needle pain. *Clinical Practice in Pediatric Psychology, 2*, 224–235.

Carey, L. K., Nicholson, B. C., & Fox, R. A. (2002). Maternal factors related to parenting young children with congenital heart disease. *Journal of Pediatric Nursing, 17*, 174–183.

Carpenter, J. L., Price, J. E. W., Cohen, M. J., Shoe, K. M., & Pendley, J. S. (2014). Multifamily group problem-solving intervention for adherence challenges in pediatric insulin-dependent diabetes. *Clinical Practice in Pediatric Psychology, 2*, 101–115.

Carter, B. D., & Threlkeld, B. M. (2012). Psychosocial perspectives in the treatment of pediatric chronic pain. *Pediatric Rheumatology, 10*(1), 15.

Chahal, N., Jelen, A., Rush, J., Manlhiot, C., Boydell, K. M., Sananes, R., et al. (2017). Kawasaki disease with coronary artery aneurysms: Psychosocial impact on parents and children. *Journal of Pediatric Health Care, 31*(4), 459–469. https://doi.org/10.1016/j.pedhc.2016.11.007.

Cohen, L. L., Vowles, K. E., & Eccleston, C. (2010). The impact of adolescent chronic pain on functioning: Disentangling the complex role of anxiety. *The Journal of Pain, 11*(11), 1039–1046.

Compas, B. E., Jaser, S. S., Dunn, M., & Rodriguez, E. M. (2012). Coping with chronic illness in childhood and adolescence. *Annual Review of Clinical Psychology, 8*, 455–480. https://doi.org/10.1146/annurev-clinpsy-032511-143108.

Connor-Smith, J. K., Compas, B. E., Wadsworth, M. E., Thomsen, A. H., & Saltzman, H. (2000). Responses to stress in adolescence: Measurement of coping and involuntary stress responses. *Journal of Consulting and Clinical Psychology, 68*(6), 976–992.

Cousino, M. K., & Hazen, R. A. (2013). Parenting stress among caregivers of children with chronic illness: A systematic review. *Journal of Pediatric Psychology, 38*(8), 809–828.

Dehghani-Arani, F., Besharat, M. A., Fitton, V. A., & Aghamohammadi, A. (2018). Efficacy of an attachment-based intervention model on health indices in children with chronic disease and their mothers. *Administration and Policy in Mental Health and Mental Health Services Research, 45*, 900–910.

Distelberg, B., Tapanes, D., Emerson, N. D., Brown, W. N., Vaswani, D., Williams-Reade, J., et al. (2018). Prospective pilot study of the mastering each new direction psychosocial family systems program for pediatric chronic illness. *Family Process, 57*(1), 83–99.

Eichner, J. M., & Johnson, B. H. (2018). Patient and family centered care and the pediatrician's role: American Academy of Pediatrics policy statement. *Pediatrics, 129*(2), 394–404.

Ernst, M. (2011). The Coping Club: A new user-generated resource for children with pain and other medical conditions [website review]. *Pediatric Pain Letter, 13*(2), 1–4.

Golfenshtein, N., Srulovici, E., & Deatrick, J. (2016). Interventions for reducing parenting stress in families with pediatric conditions: An integrative review. *Journal of Family Nursing, 22*(4), 460–492.

Hilliard, M. E., Harris, M. A., & Weissberg-Benchell, J. (2012). Diabetes resilience: A model of risk and protection in type 1 diabetes. *Current Diabetes Reports, 12*(6), 739–748.

Holmbeck, G. N., Johnson, S. Z., Wills, K. E., McKernon, W., Rose, B., Erklin, S., et al. (2002). Observed and perceived parental overprotection in relation to psychosocial adjustment in preadolescents with a physical disability: The mediational role of behavioral autonomy. *Journal of Consulting and Clinical Psychology, 70*, 96–110.

Jamieson, N., Fitzgerald, D., Singh-Grewal, D., Hanson, C., Craig, J. C., & Tong, A. (2014). Children's experiences of cystic fibrosis: A systematic review of qualitative studies. *Pediatrics, 133*(6), e1683–e1697.

Jensen, T. K., Holt, T., Ormhaug, S. M., Egeland, K., Granly, L., Hoaas, L. C., et al. (2014). A randomized effectiveness study comparing trauma-focused cognitive behavioral therapy with therapy as usual for youth. *Journal of Clinical Child & Adolescent Psychology, 43*(3), 356–369.

Karst, P., & Lew-Vriethoff, J. (2018). *The invisible string*. New York: Little, Brown.

Kazak, A. E., Kassam-Adams, N., Schneider, S., Zelikovsky, N., Alderfer, M. A., & Rourke, M. (2006). An integrative model of pediatric medical traumatic stress. *Journal of Pediatric Psychology, 31*(4), 343–355.

Kazdin, A. E., Marciano, P. L., & Whitley, M. K. (2005). The therapeutic alliance in cognitive- behavioral treatment of children referred for oppositional, aggressive, and antisocial behavior. *Journal of Consulting and Clinical Psychology, 73*(4), 726.

Kendall, P. C., Robin, J. A., Hedtke, K. A., Suveg, C., Flannery-Schroeder, E., & Gosch, E. (2005). Considering CBT with anxious youth? Think exposures. *Cognitive and Behavioral Practice, 12*(1), 136–148.

Kibby, M. Y., Tyc, V. L., & Mulhern, R. K. (1998). Effectiveness of psychological intervention for children and adolescents with chronic medical illness: A meta-analysis. *Clinical Psychology Review, 18*(1), 103–117.

Kieckhefer, G. M., Trahms, C. M., Churchill, S., & Simpson, J. N. (2009). Measuring parent-child shared management of chronic illness. *Pediatric Nursing, 35*(2), 101–108.

Maikranz, J. M., Steele, R. G., Dreyer, M. L., Stratman, A. C., & Bovaird, J. A. (2007). The relationship of hope and illness-related uncertainty to emotional adjustment and adherence among pediatric renal and liver transplant recipients. *Journal of Pediatric Psychology, 32*(5), 571–581.

Mannix, M. M., Feldman, J. M., & Moody, K. (2009). Optimism and health-related quality of life in adolescents with cancer. *Child: Health, Care and Development, 35*(4), 482–488. https://doi.org/10.1111/j.1365-2214.2008.00934.x.

McCann, D., Bull, R., & Winzenberg, T. (2015). Sleep deprivation in parents caring for children with complex needs at home: A mixed methods systematic review. *Journal of Family Nursing, 21*(1), 86–118.

McClellan, C. B., & Cohen, L. L. (2007). Family functioning in children with chronic illness compared with healthy controls: A critical review. *The Journal of Pediatrics, 150*(3), 221–223.

McGoldrick, M., Carter, B., & Garcia-Preto, N. (2011). *The expanded family life cycle: Individual, family, and social perspectives*. Boston: Allyn and Bacon. Google Scholar.

McMahon, M. A., Noll, R. B., Michaud, L. J., & Johnson, J. C. (2001). Sibling adjustment to pediatric traumatic brain injury: A case-controlled pilot study. *The Journal of Head Trauma Rehabilitation, 16*(6), 587–594.

McNeil, C. B., & Hembree-Kigin, T. L. (2010). *Parent-child interaction therapy*. Berlin: Springer Science & Business Media.

Mellonie, B., & Ingpen, R. (1983). *Lifetimes: A beautiful way to explain death to children*. New York: Bantam Books.

Moore, E. R., Bennett, K., Dietrich, M. S., & Wells, N. (2015). The effect of directed medical play on young children's pain and distress during burn wound care. *Journal of Pediatric Health Care, 29*, 265–273.

Mullins, L. L., Wolfe-Christensen, C., Hoff Pai, A. L., Carpentier, M. Y., Gillaspy, S., Cheek, J., et al. (2007). The relationship of parental overprotection, perceived child vulnerability, and parenting stress to uncertainty in youth with chronic illness. *Journal of Pediatric Psychology, 32*(8), 973–982.

Pao, M., & Bosk, A. (2011). Anxiety in medically ill children/adolescents. *Depression and Anxiety, 28*(1), 40–49.

Picoraro, J. A., Womer, J. W., Kazak, A. E., & Feudtner, C. (2014). Posttraumatic growth in parents and pediatric patients. *Journal of Palliative Medicine, 17*(2), 209–218.

Pinquart, M. (2013). Do the parent–child relationship and parenting behaviors differ between families with a child with and without chronic illness? A meta-analysis. *Journal of Pediatric Psychology, 38*, 708–721.

Powers, S. W., Jones, J. S., & Jones, B. A. (2005). Behavioral and cognitive-behavioral interventions with pediatric populations. *Clinical Child Psychology and Psychiatry, 10*(1), 65–77.

Price, J., Kassam-Adams, N., Alderfer, M. A., Christofferson, J., & Kazak, A. E. (2016). Systematic review: A reevaluation and update of the integrative (trajectory) model of pediatric medical traumatic stress. *Journal of Pediatric Psychology, 41*(1), 86–97.

Santos, S., Crespo, C., Canavarro, C., & Kazak, A. E. (2015). Family rituals and quality of life in children with cancer and their parents: The role of family cohesion and hope. *Journal of Pediatric Psychology, 40*(7), 664–671.

Selhub, E. (2007). Mind-body medicine for treating depression. *Alternative & Complementary Therapies, 2*, 4–9.

Stanger, C., Ryan, S. R., Delhey, L. M., Thrailkill, K., Zhongze, L., Zhigang, L., et al. (2013). A multicomponent motivational intervention to improve adherence among adolescents with poorly controlled type 1 diabetes: A pilot study. *Journal of Pediatric Psychology, 38*(6), 629–637.

Swallow, V., Lambert, H., Santacroce, S., & MacFadyen, A. (2011). Fathers and mothers developing skills in managing children's long-term medical conditions: How do their qualitative accounts compare? *Child: Care, Health and Development, 37*(4), 512–523.

U.S. Department of Health and Human Services. (2013). *Health resources and services administration, Maternal and Child Health Bureau (The National Survey of Children with Special Health Care Needs Chartbook 2009–2010)*. Rockville, MD: U.S. Department of Health and Human Services.

Van Allen, J., Steele, R. G., Nelson, M. B., Peugh, J., Egan, A., Clements, M., et al. (2016). A longitudinal examination of hope and optimism and their role in type 1 diabetes in youths. *Journal of Pediatric Psychology, 41*(7), 741–749.

Van Slyke, D. A., & Walker, L. S. (2006). Mothers' responses to children's pain. *The Clinical Journal of Pain, 22*(4), 387–391.

Vermaes, I. P., van Susante, A. M., & van Bakel, H. J. (2012). Psychological functioning of siblings in families of children with chronic health conditions: A meta-analysis. *Journal of Pediatric Psychology, 37*(2), 166–184.

Walker, L. S., Smith, C. A., Garber, J., & Van Slyke, D. A. (1997). Development and validation of the pain response inventory for children. *Psychological Assessment, 9*(4), 392–405.

Wysocki, T., Harris, M. A., Buckloh, L. M., Mertlich, D., Lochrie, A. S., Taylor, A., et al. (2006). Effects of behavioral family systems therapy for diabetes on adolescents' family relationships, treatment adherence, and metabolic control. *Journal of Pediatric Psychology, 31*, 928–938.

DBT for Multi-Problem Adolescents

Alec L. Miller and Casey T. O'Brien

Introduction

Dialectical Behavior Therapy (DBT, Linehan 1993a, b), originally developed by Marsha Linehan, transformed the field of Psychology and Cognitive Behavior Therapy as the first evidence-based treatment for suicidal behavior and Borderline Personality Disorder (BPD). Building off of a dialectical worldview that considers reality as consisting of polar opposites, DBT balances the change-oriented strategies of behaviorism and cognitive therapy with acceptance-based interventions adapted from Eastern philosophy, leaders, and contemplative practices. It simultaneously pushes patients to achieve their goals through lasting behavioral changes, while also understanding patients as they are and validating the difficulty that arises when trying to make this change.

This balance of acceptance and change strategies helped to create a compassionate and effective treatment program for patients with high-risk behaviors and multiple-treatment failures. The treatment program includes individual therapy, skills training, skills phone coaching, and consultation team for providers (Linehan 1993a, b). It has become the treatment of choice for multi-problem, chronically suicidal and self-injurious adults, and has since expanded transdiagnostically and to younger age ranges (Miller et al. 2007; Ritschel et al. 2013).

Recent national comorbidity studies have found that adolescent suicide is the second and third leading cause of death among 15- to 24-year-olds and 10- to 14-year-olds, respectively, with rates trending upwards over the last decade (Center for Disease Control (CDC) 2015). Among the 9th–12th grades nationwide, 18% have seriously contemplated attempting suicide, 14.6% have made a plan, and 8.6% attempted suicide (CDC 2015). Additional studies within community samples have found that 15–30% of adolescents engage in non-suicidal self-injury (NSSI; Miller and Smith 2008). Despite the high incidence and prevalence of adolescent suicidality and NSSI behaviors, no comprehensive evidence-based treatments for suicidal adolescents existed prior to DBT's expansion to adolescents (Rathus et al. 2017).

In the 1990s, Alec Miller and Jill Rathus set out to develop a treatment to begin addressing the problem of adolescent suicidality. Given DBT's effectiveness treating adult suicidality, they began by implementing Linehan's adult program within an inner city outpatient clinic (Miller et al. 1997). While maintaining the adult program's core structure, treatment targets, and theoretical underpinnings, Miller and Rathus incorporated

A. L. Miller (✉) · C. T. O'Brien
Cognitive and Behavioral Consultants, LLP
(Westchester & Manhattan), White Plains, NY, USA
e-mail: amiller@cbc-psychology.com

client feedback, clinical observation, and literature on adolescent development, adapting the program in order to address the unique development and environmental needs associated with multi-problem youth (Miller et al. 1997; Rathus and Miller 2002). A multi-family skills group format was created so both teens and parents were taught skills together, a new family-based skill module was added, family therapy sessions were included, phone coaching was also offered to parents, and secondary adolescent-family treatment targets were identified. Research studies have since established this DBT program for adolescents (DBT-A) as being an effective treatment for suicidal, multi-problem teens and their families (Goldstein et al. 2015; McCauley et al. 2018; Mehlum et al. 2014, 2016; Rathus and Miller 2002).

This chapter provides an overview of the theories, modes, functions, and interventions of DBT-A, with a special emphasis on the biosocial theory and the role of families in treatment. It is intended to complement the DBT Adaptations with Pediatric Patients chapter in this book by providing an overview of standard, outpatient DBT-A. As such, adaptations to other settings are first reviewed, and differences between when and how to use DBT-A versus DBT-CMI are noted. Research and outcome studies are summarized, and a clinical vignette is included to highlight the application of DBT-A for an adolescent with multiple high-risk behaviors and a chronic medical condition.

Adaptations to Cross-Disciplinary Settings

Medical Settings

DBT-A has not only expanded into multiple mental health treatment settings (Ritschel et al. 2013), but adaptations for school and medical settings have also become popular in recent years. Becky Lois, Alec Miller, and colleagues created DBT Adapted for Adolescents with Chronic Medical Illnesses (DBT-CMI, Hashim et al. 2013; Lois and Miller 2017) after noticing the prevalence of medical non-adherence behaviors within pediatric populations and the detrimental impact of these behaviors on treatment effectiveness and health.

DBT-CMI combines the theoretical underpinnings, stylistic strategies, and many skills of DBT-A with research on factors that contribute to high rates of adolescent medical non-adherence. In addition to adapting the treatment structure to fewer sessions, teaching skills within individual and family sessions rather than in a skills group and providing booster sessions, DBT-CMI has adjusted treatment targets so that medical non-adherence behaviors are the highest treatment priority. It also includes new secondary targets specific to adolescents with chronic medical illnesses, including emotion dysregulation and avoidance, social pressures, shift of illness responsibility, and denial/invincibility.

Both DBT-CMI and DBT-A primarily target behaviors that put a teen's life at risk. However, DBT-CMI has medical non-adherence as the primary risk behavior while DBT-A focuses on any life-threatening behaviors (e.g., suicidal behaviors, NSSI, homicidal behaviors). In addition, DBT-CMI is designed for pediatric medical populations while DBT-A is intended for psychological and psychiatric outpatient populations. Because of these differences, DBT-CMI would be the treatment of choice if medical non-adherence was the only life-threatening behavior present along with an absence of multiple psychiatric diagnoses. Instead, if an adolescent presented with multiple psychological problems and had risk behaviors in areas other than medical non-adherence, we believe DBT-A would be a better fit. For more information on DBT-CMI and directly addressing medical non-adherence, please see Chap. 10.

School Settings

With growing concern about mental health within school-aged populations, two different types of DBT programs have begun to be implemented in schools. As a secondary or tertiary prevention intervention for a targeted/selective group of high-risk or high-need students, the comprehensive DBT-A program, including individual therapy, skills group, coaching, and consultation team, is adapted to fit the school setting and schedule (Miller et al. Under review). Preliminary studies on these "Comprehensive School-Based DBT" programs have found that DBT not only reduces the number of disciplinary incidents at schools (e.g., referrals to assistant principals, detentions, suspensions; Catucci 2011) but is also associated with improvements in psychosocial and academic functioning (Dadd 2016; Mazza and Hanson 2015).

The second form of school-based DBT is a universal intervention where DBT skills are taught to all students within a general education setting. This program, called Skills Training for Emotional Problem Solving for Adolescents (STEPS-A; Mazza et al. 2016), takes the DBT skills and principles and adjusts the format of skills teaching to better fit an academic setting by creating thirty 42-min lesson plans and skills learning tests. It acts as a primary prevention model and can be used by schools to meet social-emotional curriculum needs.

Theoretical Foundations and Conceptualization

DBT-A treats "multi-problem youth" who experience emotional and behavioral dysregulation that often manifest as multiple psychiatric diagnoses leading to impairment in many areas of functioning. Problems may include NSSI, suicidal behaviors, alcohol and drug use, risky sexual behaviors, disordered eating, medically dangerous medication non-adherence, physical fighting, and other harmful behaviors. DBT can also be useful for youth who have less severe problems, such as experimental drinking and drug use, chronic interpersonal difficulties, suicidal ideation without history of attempts, dysregulated anger, frequent family conflict, school refusal, and frequent impulsive behaviors.

Biosocial Theory

Conceptualizing the development of this chronic emotional and behavioral dysregulation relies on the "biosocial theory." Developed by Linehan (1993a), the biosocial theory proposes a transaction between (1) a biological vulnerability to emotion dysregulation and (2) an invalidating environment, which over time leads to pervasive emotional dysregulation and the potential development of BPD.

Biological Vulnerability According to the biosocial theory, the biological vulnerability to emotion dysregulation includes three components: emotional sensitivity, emotional reactivity, and a slow return to baseline. Emotional sensitivity refers to experiencing distinctive changes in emotions and related physiological sensations in response to relatively subtle changes in cues and includes having an emotional resting state that is slightly higher than an individual without this biological vulnerability. Metaphorically, emotional sensitivity looks like a pot of water on a stove that starts boiling at 80° rather than 70° and increases by 10° even when only 1° of heat is added.

Emotional reactivity is defined as experiencing quick, intense changes in emotions and physiological sensations, taking only 1 min to boil rather than 10 min to achieve a simmer. A slow return to baseline captures taking longer for an individual's emotions and physiological sensations to return to resting state, leaving them more vulnerable to reacting to additional triggers for a longer period of time. Using the same metaphor, a slow return to baseline would look like the pot of water needing 2 h to return to room temperature instead of 30 min, making it easier for the pot to boil again when new heat is added. Added to this biological vulnerability of emotional sensitivity, reactivity, and a slow return to baseline is not having the capability to modulate emotions; these adolescents lack the skills needed to redirect attention and shift behavior in non-mood-dependent ways.

Invalidating Environment An invalidating environment is defined as the tendency of people in a person's life to pervasively dismiss, negate, punish, or respond erratically to the person's internal experiences. Through words, behaviors, and/or cultural messages, invalidating environments communicate to the person that what the person is thinking, feeling, or doing is wrong or inaccurate. This pervasive invalidation can at times seem intentional, such as traumatic experiences related to neglect, abuse, or bullying. However, invalidation often can be unintentional and can even stem from well-meaning actions, such as when a parent is trying to comfort a teen and says, "You are okay. Don't worry. You will just do better next time." To a teen that is feeling sad about losing the soccer game and worried about not making the team next year, this statement that is intended to comfort, can actually be invalidating because the statement dismisses the teen's sad and worried feelings. Teens may also experience social exclusion or non-inclusive cultural messages that lead to a chronic sense of being different (e.g., an LGBTQ adolescent experiencing the hetero-normative culture as highly invalidating). For teens, an invalidating environment can be composed of a variety of individuals including parents, siblings, extended family, peers, teachers, coaches, other school personnel, and even healthcare professionals.

Invalidating environments can be invalidating in many ways. They can indiscriminately reject emotional experiences or attribute them to unacceptable personality characteristics such as "over-reactivity," "manipulation," "attention-seeking," "wanting drama," or an inability to see things realistically (e.g., "Stop worrying! It's not a big deal. You're just being dramatic."). Invalidating environments can be intolerant of emotional displays (e.g., "Put a smile on your face. Don't ruin this for your sister"), and/or intermittently reinforce emotional escalation by providing soothing responses, accommodations, or expanded limits only after the teen escalates. For example, in response to a teen saying "I wasn't invited to my classmate's party. I want to stay home today," the parent initially responds with "That doesn't matter. You need to go to school." However, when the teen escalates to saying "I'm just going to kill myself. I have no friends," the parent responds differently with "Maybe we should stay home together today." Last, invalidating environments can also oversimplify the ease of problem-solving (e.g., "*Just study more next time and you'll do fine.*").

Individuals in an invalidating environment do not receive effective instruction on how to regulate emotions. Instead, maladaptive learning can occur as individuals learn that they cannot trust their own thoughts or feelings of situations, leading to self-invalidation, basing their reactions on cues from others, which leads to confusion about identity, goals, and values. Teens may learn that "emotions are bad," that they need to heighten their emotional displays of distress in order to have their distress "heard" by others or to oscillate between emotional inhibition (keeping it all in) and extreme emotional displays. They may also learn to form unrealistic goals or expectations of themselves and others.

Transaction It is important to highlight that biological vulnerability and invalidating environments do not occur within separate vacuums. Instead, each side transacts with the other, adversely shaping each other over time. A teen with extreme emotional vulnerability may inadvertently elicit invalidation from their environment; the emotional reactivity can make it difficult for a teen to effectively communicate how they are feeling, leaving the environment more vulnerable to being invalidating (e.g., an anxious student shows up late to class and is too embarrassed to share that he is feeling nervous about giving a class presentation, so the teacher criticizes him for being late and disrupting the class). Or, a highly invalidating environment might transact with low emotional vulnerability, leading to heightened levels of emotional sensitivity and reactivity (e.g., a coach that constantly blames players, highlights and labels failures, criticizes breaks as weaknesses, and shames emotional displays or injuries makes a player cry after every practice and refuse to attend games).

Unlike an interactional model that details how biology and environment can combine together to lead to an outcome, the transactional model includes how the biological vulnerability can exacerbate the environment to become more invalidating and how an invalidating environment can exacerbate a teen's biological vulnerability. Biological emotional vulnerability and invalidating environment are not only variables in the equation but also outcomes.

Behaviorism

In addition to the Biosocial Theory, Behavioral Principles and Learning Theory have also influenced DBT's conceptualization and treatment. As shown in Fig. 9.1, an individual can experience intense emotional distress related to an internal or external cue (emotion dysregulation), which in turn naturally leads to an urge to avoid or reduce the distress. Problem behaviors, such as suicidal thinking, NSSI, and binge eating, often stem from this urge to reduce distress as these behaviors actually lead to a short-term reduction in distress. This short-term relief or reduction in distress maintains the behavior through a negative reinforcement cycle. However, because the behaviors do not actually change the cue that initially triggered the distress, they are problematic in the long term, leading to more shame or more punishment by the environment. That increase in shame and punishment can then lead to more frequent and more intense internal and external cues that are distressing. Thus, DBT views problematic behaviors both as consequences of emotion dysregulation and as attempts to regulate intense emotions.

For example, in response to an external stimulus of needing to get a medical test and an internal stimulus of thinking "they will tell me something is terribly wrong," an individual might experience intense fear (emotional distress). They then might act on the urge to refuse to attend the doctor's appointments, serving the function to avoid the distress associated with medical tests. This refusal is actually effective at reducing emotional distress in the short term because the feared situation is avoided (relief). However, it can end up causing more problems in the long term, as the problem of needing the medical test does not actually get solved and avoidance behaviors get negatively reinforced. This then leads to increases in emotion dysregulation over time.

NSSI and suicidality follow a similar negative reinforcement pattern (Klonsky et al. 2015). Due to neurobiological mechanisms, NSSI can actually lead to the temporary reduction of intense emotions or numbness (Groschwitz and Plener

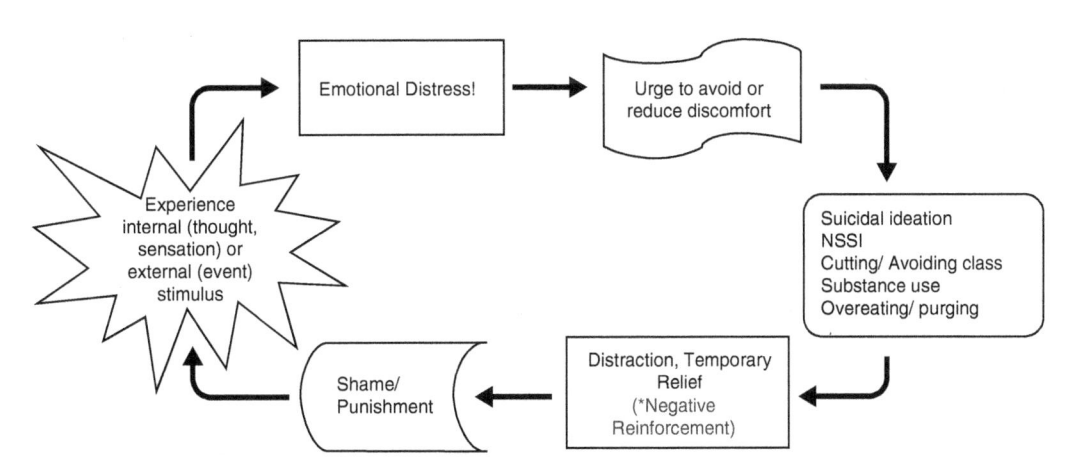

Fig. 9.1 Negative reinforcement cycle displaying how problem behaviors are both a consequence of emotion dysregulation and an attempt to control emotion dysregulation

2012). However, in the long term, it can increase emotion dysregulation and is associated with increased risk of suicidal actions (Burke et al. 2015; Klonsky et al. 2015).

Dialectics

A dialectical worldview considers reality as consisting of polar opposites, and the tension between these opposites is necessary to develop a synthesis (Linehan 1993a). Through this dialectical philosophy, DBT assumes that there is no absolute truth and contradictions can co-exist, two opposing ideas can both be true.

Dialectics are a cornerstone of DBT and are woven throughout all components of treatment (Linehan 1993a). The biosocial theory uses dialectics to inform the transactional model. DBT assumptions balance that (a) people are doing the best they can, and at the same time, (b) people need to do better, try harder, and be more motivated to change. DBT skills and strategies balance the core dialectic of acceptance and change; some strategies are intended to increase self-acceptance (e.g., mindfulness and validation), while others are intended to achieve behavior change (e.g., problem-solving and reinforcement).

Treatment Stages

DBT considers treatment as progressing through five stages. Each stage has different targets and its own overarching treatment goal. Table 9.1 details the primary treatment goals for each stage. Transitioning from one stage to another is dependent on the type, severity, and complexity of problem behaviors. Pretreatment typically lasts for a few weeks, and because stage 1 includes the skills group, it requires at least a 6-month commitment.

Table 9.1 DBT-A treatment stages and goals

Treatment stage	Goal
Pre-treatment	Orient and commitment to treatment; agree upon goals
Stage 1	Attain basic capacities, establish safety, increase behavioral control
Stage 2	Increase non-anguished emotional experiencing; reduce traumatic stress; treat comorbid conditions
Stage 3	Increase self-respect, achieve individual goals, address normal problems in living
Stage 4	Find freedom and joy

Adapted from Alec L. Miller, Jill H. Rathus, and Marsha M. Linehan, *Dialectical Behavior Therapy with Suicidal Adolescents*, p. 45, Table 3.1 © Guilford Press, 2007, with permission

Treatment Functions, Modes, and Strategies

Because problematic behaviors are conceptualized as both maladaptive problem-solving solutions to emotion dysregulation and a consequence of emotion dysregulation, DBT focuses on replacing problematic behaviors with skillful ones through five treatment functions: (1) increase motivation for treatment and change, (2) increase capabilities, (3) generalize capabilities to all settings, (4) structure the environment to motivate and reinforce adaptive behaviors, and (5) provide support to providers to maintain provider effectiveness and skills and reduce provider burnout.

Each mode of the DBT-A program addresses one or more of these treatment functions. As mentioned above, the four primary modes of standard DBT include weekly individual sessions, skills training group, between-session phone coaching, and a clinician consultation team. For DBT-A, families are incorporated into the skills training group, becoming a multi-family skills group (MFSG) that includes both teens and their parents/caregivers. Because families are a key component of the teen's environment, family sessions act as a fifth mode of

9 DBT for Multi-Problem Adolescents

Table 9.2 Treatment modes and functions of DBT-A

Modes of treatment	Associated treatment functions
Individual psychotherapy	1. Increase motivation 2. Increase capabilities 3. Generalize capabilities
Multi-family skills training group	2. Increase capabilities
Inter-session phone coaching	3. Generalize capabilities
Consultation team	5. Maintain provider effectiveness and skills and reduce provider burnout
Family sessions	3. Generalize capabilities 4. Structure the environment
Parent training	4. Structure the environment
Ancillary treatments (Pharmacotherapy) (Consulting with school staff)	4. Structure the environment

Adapted from Alec L. Miller, Jill H. Rathus, and Marsha M. Linehan, *Dialectical Behavior Therapy with Suicidal Adolescents*, p. 72, Table 4.1 © Guilford Press, 2007, with permission

Table 9.3 Hierarchy of primary treatment targets for individual and group sessions in Stage 1 of DBT-A treatment

Individual DBT sessions	Multi-family skills group sessions

1. Decreasing life-threatening behaviors
  (a) Suicidal/homicidal crisis behaviors
  (b) Suicide attempts
  (c) NSSI
  (d) Suicidal ideation or communication
2. Decreasing therapy-interfering behaviors
  (a) By the adolescent
  (b) By the therapist
  (c) By participating family members
3. Decreasing quality-of-life-interfering behaviors
  (a) High-risk, impulsive behaviors
  (b) Dysfunctional interpersonal interactions
  (c) Substance abuse-related behaviors
  (d) School problems
4. Increasing behavioral skills
	1. Decreasing behaviors likely to destroy therapy
	2. Increasing skill acquisition, strengthening, and generalization
	  (a) Core mindfulness skills
	  (b) Interpersonal effectiveness
	  (c) Emotion regulation
	  (d) Distress tolerance
	  (e) Walking the middle path
	3. Decreasing therapy-interfering behaviors

Adapted from Alec L. Miller, Jill H. Rathus, and Marsha M. Linehan, *Dialectical Behavior Therapy with Suicidal Adolescents*, p. 45, Table 3.1 and p. 47, Table 3.2 © Guilford Press, 2007, with permission

DBT-A treatment, being scheduled as needed or added as a regular (weekly, bi-weekly, monthly) session. Within DBT-A, parents also receive between-session phone coaching and can schedule parent consultation sessions. Table 9.2 provides and overviews how each mode of DBT-A addresses one or more of the five different treatment functions.

Individual Psychotherapy

The primary function of individual therapy is to increase and maintain client motivation. Although individual sessions also help to enhance the patient's capabilities and generalize skills to different settings, these functions are primarily met in skills group and phone coaching, respectively. The clinician's primary responsibilities within individual therapy include assessing the patient's problem behaviors and skill deficits, orienting the patient and family to treatment components, building commitment to treatment and change, problem-solving how to address problem behaviors and deficits, and organizing the other modes of treatments to maintain effectiveness. To this latter responsibility, the individual clinician often acts as the "quarterback" of the patient's treatment.

Target Hierarchy and Diary Cards Because DBT is intended to treat multi-problem patients, clinicians use a "target hierarchy" to provide an overarching framework that specifies a priority order for what behaviors are targeted in treatment (see Table 9.3; Miller et al. 2007). In collaboration with the patient, the clinician individualizes this target hierarchy by identifying patient-specific behaviors, emotions, urges, and thought patterns that are the focus of treatment. There are often a number of targets that fall within quality-of-life-interfering behaviors, so the clinician and patient often build a sub-hierarchy within this area to provide a priority order for quality-of-life-interfering behaviors.

The target hierarchy also acts as the road map within session, with any life-threatening behaviors addressed first in session, followed by therapy-interfering behaviors and then quality-of-life-interfering behaviors (behavioral skill development generally gets addressed within the skills group). The patient and clinician also use the target hierarchy to modify a "diary card" to include individualized targets. A dairy card is a self-monitoring chart that patients complete between sessions to track their specific behavioral targets, emotions, and skills use. The clinician supports the patient in completing the dairy card daily and reviews it at the beginning of each session. Information from the diary card is used to create the session's agenda.

Core Strategies Building off of the core dialectic acceptance and change, DBT clinicians rely on a balance of validation and problem-solving interventions within individual sessions. Validation strategies are acceptance-based strategies and communicate warmth, build the relationship, or highlight how the patient's experience is understood or normative. Validation interventions can be helpful at reducing the emotional intensity of the interaction and supporting a person to stay in the conversation. They can range from actively listening or reflecting back what the patient is saying, to explaining how the patient's emotions make sense given their history or the situation. "Radical Genuineness" by the clinician is also a form of validation in which the clinician treats the patient with equality and does not "fragilize" them (e.g., treating the patient as fragile or incapable). When using validation, it is important to validate the valid, not the invalid. For example, if a teen becomes upset that parent did not let them go to a party and then punches a hole in the wall, the clinician should validate the disappointment or frustration but should not validate the physical aggression.

The counterbalance to validation's acceptance-based intervention is problem-solving strategies. Problem-solving strategies are change oriented and use interventions from traditional Cognitive Behavioral Therapy. They include skills training, exposures, and cognitive modification, as well as contingency management strategies including positive and negative reinforcement, shaping, extinction, and punishment.

Problem-solving within DBT will often first begin with completing a "Behavior Chain Analysis" to better understand factors that contributed to the patient experiencing an urge, emotion, or thought, or engaging in a target behavior. Behavioral Chain Analyses include describing the vulnerabilities that contributed to a patient responding to a situation in a particular way, such as history of trauma or disrupted sleep the night prior. The prompting event, or the trigger, is identified as well as the "links," or moment-to-moment emotions, thoughts, urges, actions, and situational changes that occurred in response to the prompting event and lead to the target behavior. The immediate and long-term consequences following the target behavior are also discussed in order to better understand factors that maintain the target behavior or contribute to continued difficulties. After completing a Behavioral Chain Analysis, a Solution Analysis is conducted during which the clinician and patient identify different skills or problem-solving solutions that can address each piece of the chain or key links in the chain.

Orienting and Commitment Strategies Although initial DBT-A sessions focus heavily on orienting and commitment strategies, these strategies are also used throughout treatment to maintain motivation and commitment to skills use and behavior change. Orienting includes providing a rationale for DBT by linking the teen's problem behaviors to their goals and the DBT skills. Orienting also includes explaining the DBT framework including MFSG, confidentiality limits between teens and parents, diary cards, consultation team, and phone coaching. For teens that explain they are only in treatment because "my parents are making me," an informal orienting and commitment strategy includes asking "how can we help get your parents off your back?" and explaining how DBT can support them in gaining more trust, freedom, and privacy.

DBT commitment strategies are used with both teens and parents and include identifying pros and cons of entering treatment versus keeping things as they are, playing devil's advocate to prompt the patient to argue on behalf of engaging in treatment or using a skill, and connecting current commitment to past commitments (e.g., "you've come to sessions on time every week for the past month, and because of that, I believe we can also get you to group on time next week"). Foot-in-the-door and door-in-the-face are two additional commitment building strategies in which the clinician either gains commitment to a "small" step and then builds off of that "small" commitment to motivate the patient towards a large goal (e.g., "if you can commitment to one week of group, how about one full module?"), or initially asking for an overly large step, making it easier for the patient to commit to a second, more realistic step (e.g., Clinician: "Can you commit to no cutting for 6 months?" Pt: "No." Clinician: "Okay. What about 3 months instead?").

A final commitment strategy that we have found to be very helpful with teens and often get taught to parents within parent consultation sessions is called freedom to choose/absences of alternatives. This strategy provides the teen with two natural choices, highlighting the natural consequences of each choice and allowing the teen to make a genuine choice of which path they choose. For example, for a teen that is refusing to take a necessary antibiotic, a clinician or parent could explain "you could choose not to take the antibiotic and then the painful infection could come back with more medical tests needed, or you could choose to take the antibiotic and we can help you tolerate the possible stomach ache. It is your choice."

Stylistic Strategies of Clinician Communication Reciprocal Communication, which is more acceptance-based, includes mirroring the patient, taking the patient seriously, and treating their concerns with the utmost importance. It is validating as the clinician acts as an authentic person within the exchange through "self-involving self disclosure" (explaining how the patient's behavior affects you) as well as sharing of relevant personal stories that validate the patient's experience.

On the other hand, irreverence, which is change-oriented communication, is responding to the patient's statement in an unexpected, offbeat manner in order to gain the attention of an emotionally dysregulated teen. For example, if a teen said "I think it's best for me to stay home today because I will get a concussion if I faint at school," an irreverent response could be "let's figure out how you can always wear a helmet." Irreverence is not sarcasm, which mocks or conveys contempt, and instead is extending the patient's statement to another logical conclusion, throwing the patient off-balance to facilitate changing towards a new perspective. Because irreverence tends to be a different style from what teens are used to from other adults, it is a key technique when working with teens and can help strengthen the clinician–client relationship.

Dialectical Strategies In addition to constantly balancing the core dialectic of acceptance and change, DBT clinicians use additional dialectical strategies within individual sessions to highlight dialectical tensions, or extreme positions, and work towards a synthesis or a "middle path." There are eight dialectical treatment strategies in DBT including (1) metaphors, (2) entering the paradox, (3) devil's advocate, (4) extending, (5) activating the client's wise mind, (6) allowing natural change, (7) making lemonade out of lemons, and (8) assessing dialectically by asking "what is being left out?" (Linehan 1993a). As modeled throughout this chapter, metaphors are a particularly useful strategy when working with adolescents and families, as they highlight key concepts in a more interesting and relatable manner. They can also be used to reframe conflict and dialectical tensions, making it easier to move towards a synthesis between polarized family members.

Case Management Strategies There are two different types of case management strategies: Consultation-to-the-patient and consultation-to-the-environment. With consultation-to-the-patient, the clinician acts as a consultant to the patient to teach them how to be their own advocate and use skills to change their environment. Because teens build mastery and learn ways to effectively shape their own environment, consultation-to-the-patient is generally the more preferred intervention over consultation-to-the-environment because intervening for the teen may inadvertently reinforce passivity, dependence, and the unfortunate idea that they are unable to do it on their own.

However, at times when the patient has unsuccessfully and repeatedly tried to shape their environment, when the environment may be too powerful for a teen to influence, such as with a school system, or when the lack of environmental change leaves too high of a risk, such as when friends are encouraging risk behaviors, consultation-to-the-environment may be preferred. With consultation-to-the-environment, the clinician intervenes directly to change the environment and, if possible, it is recommended that the teen be involved in the consultation in order to model effective skill use.

Family and Parent Session

Family sessions support the function of structuring the environment and promoting skills generalization. They can be scheduled as regular sessions (weekly, bi-weekly, or monthly), in addition to the weekly individual sessions, supporting the practice skills together as a family, or on an as-needed basis. Situations when an as-needed family session would be particularly helpful include instances when parents are needed to participate in a crisis plan, a crisis unexpectedly arises between family members and problem-solving is needed, a key link of the teen's target behavior is frequent invalidation by a family member or family conflict, or contingencies within the home are reinforcing maladaptive behavior or punishing adaptive behavior. Mindfulness skills, particularly non-judgmentally observing and describing feelings, and Walking the Middle Path skills, including validation and dialectics, are often used within family session to reduce family conflict and improve understanding of each other's perspectives.

It is important the clinicians conducting family sessions hold a dialectical stance, within which all perspectives can be true at the same time and focus on reducing invalidation and increasing validation between family members. Clinicians can also conduct "family behavioral chain analyses" that include two or more overlapping behavior chain analyses of teen and parent behaviors. These can help with assessment and understanding of the transaction between the behaviors of each family and can lead to the family problem-solving together. Because the clinician tends to be the teen's individual clinician, it is important to orient teens and parents to the limits of confidentiality between individual and family sessions.

Regular parent consultation sessions can also be incorporated to a teen's treatment plan, and can be particularly helpful in cases where parents need additional support in using contingency management, structuring the home environment, or navigating crisis situations. A clinician different from the individual clinician would conduct these sessions because parenting goals can often be in conflict with the teen's goals. Parent sessions often focus on behavior management strategies, including building and troubleshooting behavior management plans to reinforce adaptive behavior and ignore maladaptive behavior. They can also include problem-solving how parents can use distress tolerance skills to reduce their own emotional dysregulation and despair that they may experience in response to their teen's dysregulated behavior. Similar to family sessions, Walking the Middle Path skills are also a primary focus of these sessions, with parents benefiting from role-playing how to evaluate what is valid about the teen's emotions, thoughts, and behaviors.

Multi-Family Skills Group

DBT-A skills are taught in a multi-family format with both teens and parents attending together. Although other formats are available (teen only, concurrent teen and parent groups, etc.), the multi-family format is recommended because it allows for a more dialectical experience within which both the parents and teen share their experience of using skills, offers a supportive network, and can enhance family motivation (Rathus et al. 2017). Additionally, both of the Randomized Clinical Trials (RCTs) on DBT-A have used the MFSG format (See "Review of Empirical Evidence" below).

The MFSG curriculum covers five different modules of skills over 24 weeks, namely Mindfulness, Emotion Regulation, Distress Tolerance, Interpersonal Effectiveness, and Walking the Middle Path. As detailed in Table 9.4, each skill module addresses one of five different problem areas common for multi-problem teens and their families. The Walking the Middle Path module is specific to DBT-A and includes teaching the concepts of dialectics and validation, two concepts that support families in reframing family conflict and improving ability to understand another family member's perspective.

Skills groups are usually led by two clinicians, each with differing responsibilities; at any given time, one clinician focuses primarily on teaching the skills while the other clinician focuses on behavior management and providing alternative explanations and examples of skills. In addition to handouts, clinicians will often use metaphors, practice activities (e.g., each skill group begins with a mindfulness practice), role-playing, psychoeducation, and modeling to teach the skills. Modeling can include both the clinicians using the skill in group or sharing a personal story about how they used the skill outside of the group. When using a personal story, it is important that the story includes only a brief explanation of struggle so that success through the skills is highlighted in order to instill hope.

Homework is also a large component of the skills group with the first half of each group session focused on reviewing and troubleshooting homework. Homework activities include practicing a specific skill or set of skills prior to the next session, writing about it through the use of a worksheet, and sharing about it during the homework review portion of group. If a group member has difficulty completing the homework, then clinicians' focus on briefly problem-solving how they can complete the homework going forward. Homework is considered to be an essential part of the skills group because practicing the skills throughout the week has been correlated with achieving treatment goals (Mehlum et al. 2014; Rathus and Miller 2015).

Target Hierarchy for Skills Group Because skills groups primarily serve the function to improve individual and family capabilities, they have a different target hierarchy than individual sessions (see Table 9.3). Unlike individual sessions, group leaders will often ignore individual therapy-interfering behaviors (e.g., doodling; head down) in order to prioritize teaching skills, as long as the behaviors do not reach the level of group-destroying behaviors, or a level that would inhibit others from learning the skills or the leader from teaching. This difference in target hierarchy helps ensure that the focus of skills group remains on the teaching and learning of skills.

Phone Coaching

Once patients are fully committed to DBT and begin to learn skills, they are oriented to phone coaching. Teens are encouraged to call their clinician between sessions when in distress for in-vivo support on using skills prior to engaging in problem behaviors. It is the main generalization tool used within DBT and calls focus on short-term problem-solving to reduce distress in the moment. If the teen is unwilling or unable to use skills to maintain safety even with coaching, then phone coaching can also turn into crisis intervention during which other family members might become part of the phone calls to maintain safety. Another function of phone coaching is to provide an opportunity for teens and clinicians to repair

Table 9.4 Overview of DBT-A's five problem areas and corresponding skills module

Problem area	DBT skills modules and skills
Reduced awareness and focus; confusion about self Not always aware of what you are feeling, why you get upset, or what your goals are, and/or having trouble staying focused	**Core mindfulness skills** "Wise Mind" (States of Mind) "What Skills" (Observe, Describe, Participate) "How Skills" (Don't Judge, One-Mindful, Do What Works)
Emotion dysregulation Fast, intense mood changes with little control and/or steady negative emotional state; mood-dependent behaviors	**Emotion regulation skills** "Model of Emotions" "ABC PLEASE" "The Wave Skill" "Check the Facts" "Opposite Action"
Interpersonal problem Pattern of difficulty keeping relationships steady, getting what you want, keeping self-respect, loneliness	**Interpersonal effectiveness skills** "GIVE" "DEARMAN" "FAST" "Factors to Consider" "THINK"
Impulsivity Acting without thinking it all through; escaping or avoiding emotional experiences	**Distress tolerance skills** "Distract with Wise Mind ACCEPTS" "Self-Soothe with Six Senses" "IMPROVE the Moment" "Pros & Cons" "TIPP" "Radical Acceptance" "Willingness"
Teenager and family challenges Extreme thinking, feeling and acting; absence of flexibility; difficulty navigating family conflict or effectively influencing others' behaviors	**Walking the middle path** "Dialectic Thinking & Acting" "Dialectical Dilemmas" "Validation of Self" "Validation of Others" "Increasing Positive Behaviors" "Decreasing Unwanted Behaviors"

Reprinted from Jill H. Rathus and Alec L. Miller, *DBT Skills Manual for Adolescents*, p. 15, Table 1.6 © Guilford Press, 2015, with permission

their relationship so that neither has to wait until the next session to resolve the problem. Last, phone coaching can be used to share good news between sessions. This helps break the relationship between clinician attention and support occurring solely when there is suicidal or maladaptive behavior and helps maintain both clinician and patient treatment motivation.

Because it was observed that parents could also benefit from phone coaching to support their skills generalization, parent phone coaching was added into the DBT-A program. Parents are assigned a phone coach, usually a skills group leader that is different than the teen's individual clinician, or their parenting clinician. Separating coaching in this way helps to maintain trust between teen and clinician and allow for coaching focused on parenting goals that may differ from teen goals. Unlike teen phone coaching, parent phone coaching focuses on skills generalization during times of distress and does not include repairing the relationship function.

Consultation Team

An essential component of DBT is the weekly consultation team within which DBT clinicians can receive support from each other. Acting as "therapy to the clinicians," the consultation team aims to reduce clinician burn out and maintain motivation to engage in the challenging task of working with multi-problem adolescents and their families. It also helps enhance clinician capabilities and ensure fidelity to the treatment model. Each weekly team meeting begins with a mindfulness practice and includes clinicians requesting consultation on specific situations or patients. Items are addressed in a hierarchy similar to that used within individual sessions (i.e., life-threatening behaviors addressed first) and strategies that serve as "consultation-to-the-provider" are generally preferred over "consultation-to-the-environment." Depending on the specific consultation request, teams can provide validation, empathy building, problem assessment, problem-solving, and/or clinician skills training as a form of feedback.

Review of Empirical Evidence

DBT-A's efficacy at treating multi-problem youth has been well supported by research. Since 2002 when Rathus and Miller published their initial, quasi-experimental outcome data indicating DBT-A's effectiveness, three RCTs have been completed, each done by a different research group, establishing DBT-A as a well-established Empirically Supported Treatment for suicidal adolescents (Goldstein et al. 2015; McCauley et al. 2018; Mehlum et al. 2014, 2016). Numerous open and quasi-experimental trials have also indicated DBT-A's application for a variety of adolescent presentations including bipolar disorder (Goldstein et al. 2015), externalizing disorders (Marco et al. 2013), eating disorders (Fischer and Peterson 2015; Safer et al. 2007; Salbach-Andrae et al. 2009), school refusal (Chu et al. 2014), and trichotillomania (Welch and Kim 2012), as well as treatment settings including residential (Sunseri 2004), long-term inpatient (McDonell et al. 2010), school (Mazza et al. 2016; Perepletchikova et al. 2011), and children's hospitals (Lois and Miller 2017).

Mehlum et al. (2014) conducted a seminal RCT in Olso, Norway, with 77 adolescents who had recent and repetitive NSSI behaviors and at least three BPD symptoms. They compared 19 weeks of comprehensive outpatient DBT-A (weekly individual sessions, MFSG, phone coaching, consultation team) to Enhanced Usual Care, which consisted of at least weekly individual CBT or psychodynamic sessions and as-needed family or phone sessions. Patients receiving DBT-A experienced significant reductions in NSSI episodes, suicidal ideation, and depressive symptoms, as well as reductions in hopelessness and BPD symptoms, with large effect sizes. On the other hand, patients receiving EUC only experienced significant reductions in depressive symptoms, with small effect sizes. Both treatment conditions had good treatment retention with low use of emergency services. Overall, DBT-A was found to be superior to EUC at reducing NSSI, suicidality, and depression.

At a 1-year follow-up, Mehlum et al. (2016) found that DBT-A remained superior to EUC in long-term reduction of NSSI. The differences in reduction of suicidal ideation, depression, hopelessness, and BPD symptoms between treatment conditions did not persist through 1-year post treatment. However, this was because patients in the EUC condition experienced significant reductions in these areas from post-treatment to 1-year follow-up, causing them to "catch up" with patients in the DBT-A condition. As such, Mehlum and colleagues concluded that DBT-A leads to a stronger long-term reduction of NSSI and may contribute to a more rapid recovery of suicidality, depression, and BPD symptoms.

McCauley et al. (2018) have also completed a large, multi-site RCT comparing comprehensive DBT to a control treatment condition of weekly individual and group supportive therapy (IGST) over 6 months for adolescents with recent and repeated suicidal behaviors and at least three BPD symptoms. The DBT condition used the adult DBT manual with modifications so that the skills were taught in a MFSG format and both parents and teens received phone coaching. They found significant advantages for DBT on all primary outcomes including suicide attempts, NSSI, and self-harm (suicide attempts and NSSI combined), as well as higher treatment completion rates. Similar to Melhum and colleagues (2016), rates of self-harm continued to decrease through 1-year follow-up, with no statistically significant differences between groups at that time as the IGST condition "caught up" to the DBT condition.

Clinical Vignette

Jane[1] was a 17-year-old Hispanic female diagnosed with Major Depressive Disorder, Generalized Anxiety Disorder, Social Anxiety Disorder, and Alcohol Use Disorder. At intake, she presented with an intermittently depressed and irritable mood, chronic passive suicidal ideation ("things would be easier if I wasn't here"), low self-esteem, and NSSI. She also experienced daily and distressing worries about academic performance, family health, and interpersonal relationships and significant worry about feeling embarrassed during class, parties, dances, and sporting events, using alcohol as a way to attend parties without anxiety. Although not meeting criteria for an Eating Disorder, Jane would also engage in disordered eating behaviors including restricting food when feeling depressed or anxious and adjusting insulin levels to accommodate.

Jane lived with her married, biological parents in an urban environment. Her two older sisters had moved away to attend college. Her parents reported concerns about frequent arguments, irritability, Jane locking self in her bathroom to self-harm, coming home drunk and past curfew, and worsening grades. Although Jane generally received As and Bs, taking primarily high honors classes, her grades had worsened to primarily Bs and one C within the year prior to starting treatment. She explained that these worsening grades were due to missing classes that she thought were "pointless."

Medically, Jane had a history of type 1 diabetes mellitus (T1DM). She and her parents reported that since the age of 12, Jane had effectively, independently managed her insulin levels, adhering to doctor's recommendations. However, the T1DM complicated the risk behaviors discussed at intake: (1) NSSI cuts required closer monitoring due to higher risk of infection, (2) Jane's alcohol use had required emergency attention for both alcohol poisoning and blood sugar levels, (3) Jane would adjust insulin levels to accommodate binge drinking or restricted eating behaviors, (4) Jane was more vulnerable to emotion dysregulation and anxiety-like physiological symptoms when blood sugar levels were high or low.

Prior to DBT, Jane had previously attended weekly "talk" therapy for 1.5 years, which also included monthly family sessions with the same clinician. Both Jane and her parents explained that they did not find the therapy helpful at changing Jane behaviors, although they found the monthly family sessions helpful in better understanding each other's perspectives. Jane was also followed up by a psychiatrist, who referred her to DBT, and was prescribed 20 mg of Fluoxetine that was reported to be partially helpful in reducing the intensity of irritability and depression.

Course of Treatment

During pretreatment stage, Jane shared that she did not want treatment but was willing to participate in DBT. Commitment strategies were used to strengthen this commitment by connecting DBT's skills and family involvement in treatment to her goal "to get my parents off my back." Jane was oriented to the DBT-A's five problem areas and she endorsed difficulties in all areas. The individualized target hierarchy displayed in Fig. 9.2 was also collaboratively developed.

Initial treatment sessions also focused on orienting Jane and her parents to the comprehensive DBT program including weekly individual therapy and diary card, weekly 2-h MFSG, 24/7 skills coaching for Jane, 24/7 skills coaching for her parents with a group leader, and as-needed family sessions. The clinician also consulted with Jane's medical doctors, including her endocrinologist to better understand history of medical adherence behaviors and impact of non-adherence.

Both Jane and her parents agreed to participate in the comprehensive program and because

---

[1]This vignette has been fully deidentified with portions confabulated to maintain confidentiality.

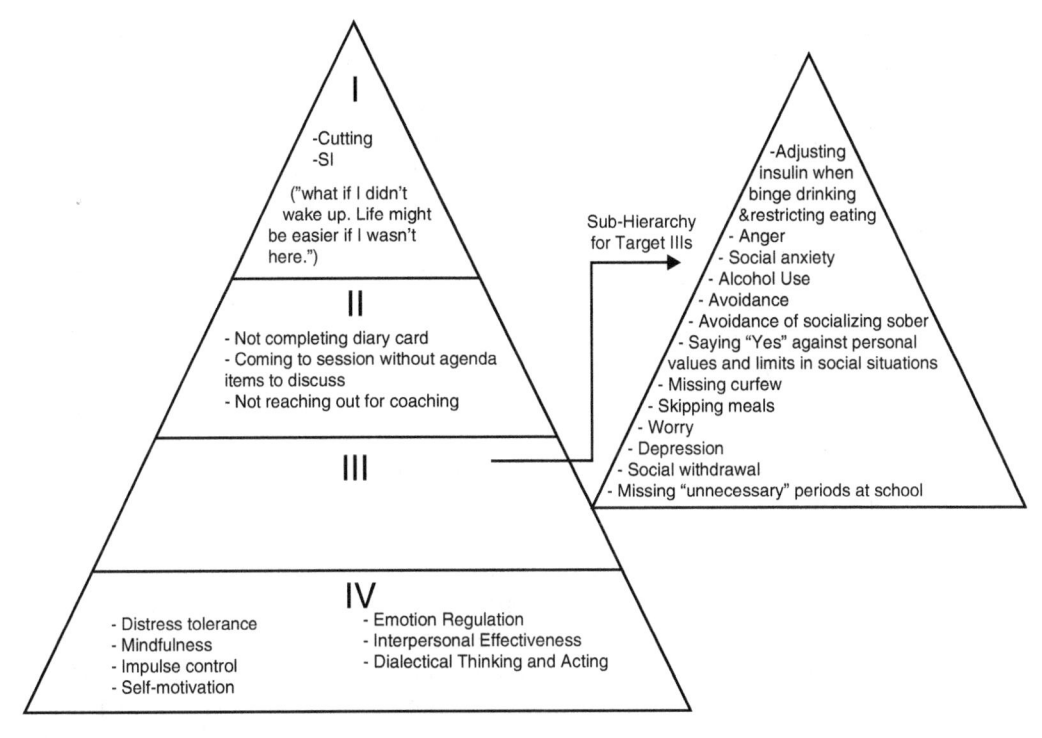

Fig. 9.2 Jane's individualized hierarchy of treatment targets

Jane was initially participating only to satisfy her parents' request, the commitment strategy of devil's advocate was used to strengthen her individual commitment to the program. This helped her identify additional life worth living goals to "feeling more in control over how I feel, feel more comfortable in social situations, and have less family arguments" and connect these goals to participation in the program. Additionally, Jane would often forget to bring her diary card completed to session, and the commitment strategies of foot-in-the-door and pros and cons were used by initially asking her to complete it once a week before session, then asking to complete it daily, and creating the pros and cons of "tracking emotions daily" versus "continuing with status quo."

Chain analyses of Jane's NSSI and SI indicated that it was serving an emotion regulation function, helping her to feel calmer after feeling angry following an argument with her parents or after feeling shame in relation to an interpersonal interaction within which she agreed to do something that was against her personal values. Both anger and shame were identified as key links in her chains. Solution analyses focused on identifying distress tolerance and emotion regulation skills to reduce these emotions in a more effective and safer way and reaching out for coaching any time anger or shame reached 3 out of 5 or higher. Drinking and restricting eating behaviors were found to serve a similar emotion regulation function through chain analyses as she often used drinking as a way to reduce anxiety in social situations and restricting to increase a sense of control when feeling overwhelmed, worried, or depressed. In addition to solution analyses focused on emotion regulation and distress tolerance skills, exposures were completed as a way to reduce vulnerabilities to anxiety-provoking situations.

Family sessions were also conducted with Jane's individual clinician as a way to problem solve the family conflict that often acted as the trigger to anger and consequently risk behavior. Within family sessions, Jane practiced communicating her feelings, goals, and needs to her parents through her words by focusing on the Observe and Describe mindfulness skills. Parents focused on initially validating these more accurate expressions of her feelings and goals before problem-solving. These both helped the parents to understand the triggers and function of her behaviors and acted as a natural reinforcer to skillful behavior; the more Jane felt validated, the more she shared openly with her parents. Additional reinforcers that parents could provide were also identified, such as an extended curfew on weekend if Jane attended all school the week prior and completed all test-prep activities by 1:00 p.m. on Saturday. Last, Jane's parents met twice with their parent coach for parenting sessions focused on developing a plan on how to respond to Jane when she shares an urge to self-harm or has self-harmed.

Treatment Outcomes

Outcomes after 6 months of DBT included cessation of cutting and suicidal ideation, reduction of NSSI urges from 4 s and 5 s (out of 5) twice a week to 3 s about once a month, consistent completion of diary card and even independently creating an electronic diary card, increased proactive agenda setting, and calling for coaching with communication of a specific goal for the call. As indicated by ratings on the dairy card, Jane experienced decreased frequency and intensity of anger and worry, decreased frequency of depressive symptoms, increased monitoring of drinking behaviors that led to a reduction in the amount and frequency of alcohol use, increased attending social activities sober, absence of restricted eating behaviors with reduction of urges to restrict from 4, on average, to 2 about once a week, and increased use of skills to act in accordance with personal values. Additionally, school attendance and grades improved, and Jane's insulin pump and endocrinologist both indicated an absence of any medical non-adherence behaviors for 4 months. Family conflict reduced significantly from about two to three arguments per week to about one, less intense argument per month.

Parents and Jane also reported improved openness and validation between each other contributing to a reported improved relationship. Following the 6 months, Jane and her parents agreed to continue with weekly individual sessions with family sessions about once every 2 months in order to maintain gains, increase life satisfaction, and increase independently living skills including increasing Jane's ability to self-monitor and navigate medical appointments as a way to prepare for Jane to successfully launch off to college.

Conclusion

While keeping the core structure, theoretical underpinnings, treatment assumptions, and strategies the same, DBT-A's inclusion of families within the skills groups, phone coaching, parent consultation sessions, and family sessions has not only helped to address the unique developmental demands of working with adolescents, but has also been well received by parents. During graduations from MFSG, parents routinely highlight that, despite their initial hesitation in being part of the skills group, they find the family involvement within the DBT-A program invaluable; they share that they not only have new and more effective strategies to support their children in achieving their goals, but they also feel more confident in navigating stress that can naturally arise when parenting emotionally dysregulated teens.

Although initially developed for multi-problem, suicidal adolescents, DBT-A's conceptualization that problem behaviors are both an outcome of, and an attempt to regulate, underlying emotion dysregulation has lent itself well to generalizing the treatment across diagnoses and settings. Research has begun to encourage DBT-A as a transdiagnostic treatment effective within multiple types of clinical, medical, and school settings. When creating a DBT program, it is recommended that clinicians begin by first adopting the comprehensive DBT-A program and then adapt it from there to fit population and setting needs. We hope that this chapter has helped to increase understanding of how to implement, develop, and refer to DBT programs for adolescents.

References

Burke, T. A., Hamilton, J. L., Abramson, L. Y., & Alloy, L. B. (2015). Non-suicidal self-injury prospectively predicts interpersonal stressful life events and depressive symptoms among adolescent girls. *Psychiatric Research, 228,* 416–424.

Catucci, D. (2011). Dialectical behavior therapy with multi-problem adolescents in school setting. *New York School Psychologist Newsletter.* Retrieved July 14, 2018, from http://nyasp.org/newsletters/news2011fall.pdf

Center for Disease Control (CDC). (2015). Youth risk behavior surveillance—United States, 2015. *Morbidity and Mortality Weekly Report, 65*(SS-6), 1–174.

Chu, B. C., Rizvi, S. L., Zendegui, E. A., & Bonavitacola, L. (2014). Dialectical behavior therapy for school refusal: Treatment development and incorporation of web-based coaching. *Cognitive and Behavioral Practice, 22,* 317. https://doi.org/10.1016/j.cbpra.2014.08.002.

Dadd, A. C. (2016). The effectiveness of dialectical behavior therapy in treating multiproblem adolescents in a school setting (Doctoral dissertation). *ProQuest Dissertations Publishing.* ProQuest Number: 10000744.

Fischer, S., & Peterson, C. (2015). Dialectical behavior therapy for adolescent binge eating, purging, suicidal behavior, and non-suicidal self-injury: A pilot study. *Psychotherapy, 52*(1), 78–92.

Goldstein, T. R., Fersch-Podrat, R. K., Rivera, M., Axelson, D. A., Merranko, J., Yu, H., et al. (2015). Dialectical behavior therapy for adolescents with bipolar disorder: Results from a pilot randomized trial. *Journal of Child and Adolescent Psychopharmacology, 25*(2), 140–149.

Groschwitz, R. C., & Plener, P. L. (2012). The neurobiology of non-suicidal self-injury (NSSI): A review. *Suicidology Online, 3,* 24–32.

Hashim, R., Vadnais, M., & Miller, A. L. (2013). Improving adherence in adolescent chronic kidney disease: A DBT feasibility trial. *Clinical Practice in Pediatric Psychology, 1,* 369–379.

Klonsky, E. D., Glenn, C. R., Styer, D. M., Olino, T. M., & Washburn, J. J. (2015). The functions of nonsuicidal self-injury: Converging evidence for a two-factor structure. *Child and Adolescent Psychiatry and Mental Health, 9*(44), 1–9.

Linehan, M. M. (1993a). *Cognitive-behavioral treatment of borderline personality disorder.* New York, NY: Guildford Press.

Linehan, M. M. (1993b). *Skills training manual for treating borderline personality disorder.* New York, NY: Guilford Press.

Lois, R. H., & Miller, A. L. (2017). Stopping the non-adherence cycle: The clinical and theoretical basis for dialectical behavior therapy adapted for adolescents with chronic medical illness (DBT-CMI). *Cognitive and Behavioral Practice, 25*(1), 32–43.

Marco, J. H., Garcia-Palacios, A., & Botella, C. (2013). Dialectical behavioural therapy for oppositional defiant disorder in adolescents: A case series. *Psicothema, 25*(2), 158–163.

Mazza J. J., & Hanson, J. (2015). *DBT in schools.* Presented at the Convention of the National Association of School Psychologists (NASP), Orlando, FL.

Mazza, J. J., Dexter-Mazza, E. T., Miller, A. L., Rathus, J. H., & Murphy, H. E. (2016). *DBT skills training in schools: The skills training for emotional problem solving for adolescents (DBT STEPS-A).* New York, NY: Guilford Press.

McCauley, E., Berk, M. S., Asarnow, J. R., Adrian, M., Cohen, J., Korslund, K., et al. (2018). Efficacy of dialectical behavior therapy for adolescents at high risk for suicide: A randomized clinical trial. *JAMA Psychiatry, 75,* 777. https://doi.org/10.1001/jamapsychiatry.2018.1109.

McDonell, M. G., Tarantino, J., Dubose, A. P., Matestic, P., Steinmetz, K., Galbreath, H., et al. (2010). A pilot evaluation of dialectical behavioral therapy in adolescent long-term inpatient care. *Child and Adolescent Mental Health, 15*(4), 193–196.

Mehlum, L., Tormoen, A., Ramberg, M., Haga, E., Diep, L., Laberg, S., et al. (2014). Dialectical behavior therapy for adolescents with recent and repeated self-harming behavior-first randomized controlled trial. *Journal of the American Academy of Child and Adolescent Psychiatry, 53,* 1082–1091.

Mehlum, L., Ramberg, M., Tormoen, A. J., Haga, E., Diep, L. M., Stanley, B. H., et al. (2016). Dialectical behavior therapy compared with enhanced usual care for adolescents with repeated suicidal and self-harming behavior: Outcomes over a 1-year follow-up. *Journal of the American Academy of Child and Adolescent Psychiatry, 55,* 295–300.

Miller, A. L., & Smith, H. L. (2008). Adolescent non-suicidal self-injurious behavior: The latest epidemic to assess and treat. *Applied and Preventive Psychology, 12,* 178–188.

Miller, A. L., Rathus, J. H., Linehan, M. M., Wetzler, S., & Leigh, E. (1997). Dialectical behavior therapy adapted for suicidal adolescents. *Journal of Practical Psychiatry and Behavioral Health, 3,* 78–86.

Miller, A. L., Rathus, J. H., & Linehan, M. M. (2007). *Dialectical behavior therapy with suicidal adolescents.* New York, NY: Guilford Press.

Miller, A. L., Mazza, J. J., Dexter-Mazza, E., Graling, K., Gerardi, N., & Rathus, J. H. (Under review). *Delivering comprehensive DBT in schools.*

Perepletchikova, F., Axelrod, S., Kaufman, J., Rounsville, B., Douglas-Palumberi, H., & Miller, A. L. (2011). Adapting dialectical behavior therapy for children: Towards a new research agenda for childhood suicidality and self-harm behaviors. *Child and Adolescent Mental Health, 16,* 116–121.

Rathus, J. H., & Miller, A. L. (2002). Dialectical behavior therapy adapted for suicidal adolescents. *Suicide & Life-Threatening Behavior, 32*(2), 146–157.

Rathus, J. H., & Miller, A. L. (2015). *DBT skills manual for adolescents*. New York, NY: Guilford Press.

Rathus, J. H., Miller, A. L., & Bonavitacola, L. (2017). DBT with adolescents. In M. A. Swales (Ed.), *The Oxford handbook of dialectical behaviour therapy*. https://doi.org/10.1093/oxfordhb/9780198758723.013.18.

Ritschel, L., Miller, A. L., & Taylor, V. (2013). DBT with multi-diagnostic youth). In J. Ehrenreich-May & B. Chu (Eds.), *Transdiagnostic mechanisms and treatment for youth psychopathology* (pp. 203–232). New York, NY: Guilford Press.

Safer, D. L., Lock, J., & Couturier, J. L. (2007). Dialectical behavior therapy modified for adolescent binge eating disorder: A case report. *Cognitive and Behavioral Practice, 14*, 157–167.

Salbach-Andrae, H., Schneider, N., Seifert, K., Pfeiffer, E., Lenz, K., Lehmkuhl, U., et al. (2009). Short-term outcome of anorexia nervosa in adolescents after inpatient treatment: A prospective study. *European Child & Adolescent Psychiatry, 18*(11), 701–704.

Sunseri, P. A. (2004). Preliminary outcomes on the use of dialectical behavior therapy to reduce hospitalization among adolescents in residential care. *Residential Treatment for Children & Youth, 21*(4), 59–76.

Welch, S. S., & Kim, J. (2012). DBT-enhanced cognitive behavioral therapy for adolescent trichotillomania: An adolescent case study. *Cognitive and Behavioral Practice, 19*(3), 483–493.

DBT Adaptations with Pediatric Patients

10

Becky H. Lois, Vincent P. Corcoran, and Alec L. Miller

Brief Review of DBT

Dialectical Behavior Therapy (DBT), the first evidence-based treatment for suicidal adults diagnosed with borderline personality disorder, has since been adapted for multi-problem youth with various mental and medical disorders. In Chap. 9 of this volume, Miller and O'Brien provide a detailed review of DBT for multi-problem adolescents. In brief while DBT originated as an outpatient treatment, it has since been adapted for adolescents in inpatient, residential, forensic, school, and medical settings (Miller et al. 2007; Rathus and Miller 2015).

DBT balances acceptance strategies originally adapted from eastern meditative practices and western contemplative practices with change strategies that have evolved from cognitive-behavioral therapy and systemic approaches.

DBT has become identified as a compassionate and effective treatment program for patients with high-risk behaviors, multiple-treatment failures, and/or previously considered too challenging to treat. The standard outpatient DBT treatment program includes individual therapy, skills training, skills phone coaching, and consultation team for providers (Linehan 1993a, b). It has become the treatment of choice for multi-problem, chronically suicidal, and self-injurious adults and has since expanded trans-diagnostically and to younger age ranges (Miller et al. 2007; Ritschel et al. 2013). Below, we describe the adaptation of DBT for youth diagnosed with chronic medical illnesses.

Life with a Chronic Medical Illness (CMI)

Living with a chronic medical illness (CMI) can be difficult; managing symptoms, receiving ongoing treatment, and handling financial costs while trying to maintain a sensible quality of life can feel like an enormous burden to the individual (Sav et al. 2013). A chronic medical illness can be defined as a disability interfering with "normal" life and/or demanding treatment for ≥3 months during a 1-year period (Westbom and Kornfält 1987). Furthermore, the majority of CMIs are considered noncommunicable diseases

B. H. Lois (✉)
Department of Child and Adolescent Psychiatry, Hassenfeld Children's Hospital at NYU Langone, Child Study Center, New York, NY, USA
e-mail: Becky.Lois@nyulangone.org

V. P. Corcoran
Clinical Psychology Doctoral Program, Graduate School for Arts and Sciences, Fordham University, Bronx, NY, USA

A. L. Miller
Cognitive and Behavioral Consultants, LLP (Westchester and Manhattan), White Plains, NY, USA

(NCDs), meaning they do not result from an infectious agent but emerge from complex interactions between genes, physiology, environment, and behavior (World Health Organization 2018). These include cardiovascular diseases, chronic respiratory diseases, cancers, obesity, diabetes, and other autoimmune disorders (World Health Organization 2018; Center for Disease Control 2018). In 2012, approximately half of all adults in the United States were living with a CMI, and one in four adults were living with two or more of such conditions (Ward et al. 2014). Given their complex nature, the onset of a CMI may leave an individual feeling a mix of emotions, perhaps anger stemming from the thought that developing the illness was largely out of their control, or even guilt for believing they did not do enough to prevent onset. Nonetheless, given the often-slow progression and long duration of CMIs, a profound lifestyle shift is often required to address symptoms, prevent further medical complication, and improve prognosis (Phillips et al. 2016; Sav et al. 2013). Therefore, most if not all, CMIs require a degree of self-management on behalf of the patient. Self-management often includes a range of behaviors that include but are not limited to, taking medications, showing up to routine medical appointments, and following certain dietary restrictions (Phillips et al. 2016; Sav et al. 2013). Understandably, because of these new demands placed on the individual, non-adherence to recommended treatment guidelines is not uncommon. However, reducing the occurrence of non-adherent behaviors is of utmost importance because of their connection to poor patient outcome and higher health care costs (van Dulmen et al. 2007; Kravitz and Melnikow 2004). However, while non-adherence-focused interventions with adult populations have been demonstrated to be effective (Adriaanse et al. 2013; Gregg et al. 2007), less is known about promoting adherent behaviors and reducing health care costs in pediatric populations via psychological intervention (McGrady and Hommel 2013).

Youth Living with a Chronic Medical Illness (CMI): Non-adherence Amplified

In the case of youth living with CMIs, the issue of non-adherence becomes of even greater concern. While estimates of chronic conditions in childhood and adolescence range from 16 to 25%, research also indicates that a majority are non-adherent to their medical regimen (Compas et al. 2012; McGrady and Hommel 2013). When taking into consideration the complexities of youth development, an understanding of why it can be especially difficult to live with a CMI during these formative years emerges. Youth living with a CMI engage in health risk behaviors to the same extent or even more so than their peers, leaving them at a "double disadvantage" in regard to health outcomes (Sawyer et al. 2007). Additionally, youth face many challenges that are specific to their illness and stage of life, such as complicated medical regimens, frequent school absences and medical hospitalizations, and physical symptoms such as pain or functional limitation (Butz 2006; Graves et al. 2010; Kahana et al. 2008). As a result, these youth often report feelings of "differentness," stigma, and isolation from their peers; conflict with family members around illness management behaviors (e.g., arguments about taking medication, injecting insulin, following dietary restrictions); and mental health issues such as depression, anxiety, and PTSD as much as four times that as their healthy same-aged peers (Weersing et al. 2012; Patel et al. 2010; Katon 2003).

Given all of these challenges, many youths do not follow their prescribed medical regimens in order to "get a break" and a period of "normalcy" from a life that can otherwise feel burdensome and overwhelming. For some, this behavior can be transient, experimental, or inadvertent. For others, it can become chronic and problematic. Youth with chronic patterns of non-adherence may have a tendency to engage in this avoidance behavior as their primary method of coping when faced with illness-related reminders. For example, a teen with diabetes may elect to go out after school with friends and eat pizza, without stopping to count carbs or administer insulin to cover and correct high blood sugar (see Fig. 10.1). Skipping these steps can feel "freeing" in the moment, allowing the teen to enjoy time with his or her friends without having to think about their diabetes as a part of the picture. Many youth will discuss a feeling of relief after engaging in this behavior, especially when experiencing their illness as a burden or obstacle to normalcy in an already stressful existence. This feeling of relief is *negatively reinforcing*, providing an escape from the often-intense and aversive emotional experience of confronting the reality of one's medical condition and responsibilities. The avoidance is maintained by the corresponding relief, a cycle that can be incredibly difficult to break without conscious effort and motivation.

Another factor that often leads to the above-mentioned pattern of avoidance is a struggle with acceptance of illness and/or rejection of the reality of the illness. One can easily imagine how thoughts such as "why me" and "this isn't fair" can directly impact a child's ability to fully incorporate his or her medical condition into daily life. With many chronic illnesses, there are aspects that cannot be controlled or changed. Therefore, approaches that solely prioritize problem-solving may be perceived as invalidating. For instance, some conditions lead to deterioration no matter what you do or do not do. At the same time, there are behaviors that lend themselves well to change-based strategies, such as the need to create a predictable schedule around medication dosing and challenging thoughts that are not in line with one's goals for improved medical outcomes. Therefore, balancing illness acceptance with increased self-regulatory behaviors (e.g., self-management of the chronic illness) appears crucial to more positive outcomes in youth living with CMIs.

DBT and Non-adherence as a Systems Issue

One cognitive behavioral treatment that is uniquely positioned to address the co-occurring duality of acceptance and behavior change is dialectical behavior therapy (DBT). With an explicit focus on therapy-interfering behaviors and validation of emotional experiences, DBT provides a strong framework from which to target medical non-adherence. Therapist and patients can work collaboratively to tackle the negative reinforcement cycle, acknowledging that they will inevitably experience the environmental triggers and reminders of illness. When these triggers arise, therapist and patient can together validate corresponding thoughts and feelings and still consider engaging in more effective behavior rather than avoidance.

Youth living with CMIs and corresponding behavioral challenges are often labeled as

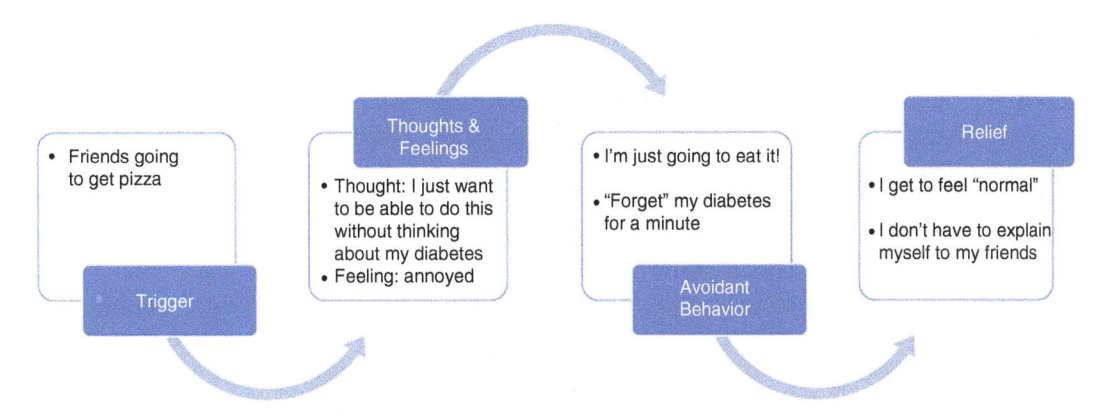

Fig. 10.1 Negative reinforcement cycle of avoidance in CMI

"problematic" or "difficult" as a result of medical providers' and teams' frustration with lack of progress or follow through with recommendations. Family members such as parents and caregivers can be the recipients of such labels as well. These dynamics can lead to intense polarization within the system and patient–family–provider interactions that can be fraught with tension and negative judgment. Youth may refuse to engage with their medical provider or under-report any challenges for fear of disappointing their doctor; parents may be quick to blame their child in an effort to "take the heat off" of them due to concerns that they might be perceived as a "bad parent"; doctors may feel hopeless and helpless about any possible improvement with a patient and thus decrease the amount of time spent or "give up" on partnering with the patient and family on other ways to improve outcomes. The tendency is to "zoom in" on the family unit, which often leads to a lack of focus on the larger system that transacts with that family unit.

Within the family unit, there is often significant polarization on the part of the parent and child around responsibility for illness management. DBT frames these polarizations as *dialectical dilemmas*. One such dialectical dilemma from traditional adolescent DBT involves the behavioral extremes of *forcing autonomy* versus *fostering independence* (see Fig. 10.2). Within a family that includes a child with a chronic illness, a parent who forces autonomy may tell their child that it is time for him/her to take full responsibility for taking medication, arranging and going to doctor's appointments, at a time when the child does not feel developmentally or emotionally ready. This dynamic often occurs in families where the parent has been acting as "illness manager" for some time and feels that the child should step in and take over. Youth, in these instances, may also be pushing for autonomy or withdrawing from parental surveillance, which can lead to increased conflict and burn out for both parties and push families further in the direction of polarization.

On the opposite end, parents may push to foster dependence due to concerns that allowing the child or adolescent to "spread his/her wings" will result in poor judgment and decision-making. These parents may have a realistic reason for this concern, particularly if there is a history of medical non-adherence or permission given for the child or adolescent to be more independent only to have the process end in a poor outcome. For example, a parent of a teen with cystic fibrosis may have decided to allow her teen to manage his own chest physiotherapy treatments at the teen's request, without parental supervision, only to find out a few weeks later at a doctor's appointment that the teen was not doing any chest therapy at all. The parent may then push in the direction of fostering dependence due to her own frustration, anxiety, and fear that his/her child will not follow through if left to manage things independently. The outcome of this exchange is often, again, increased conflict and burn out.

To combat the tendency to isolate the family unit as the primary issue in a non-adherence picture, and for the family themselves to become polarized in dialectical dilemmas, it can be helpful to "zoom out" or, in other words, consider how the whole system transacts with the family system (see Fig. 10.3). This allows for a *middle path* consensus on how to best approach the situation given the systems involved and the transactions between them (Miller et al. 2007).

For example, consider Jason, a 16-year-old African American male diagnosed with type 1 diabetes since the age of 8. He comes to his endocrinology appointments with his mother who is working two jobs and feeling overwhelmed by managing Jason's diabetes as well as his three younger siblings at home as a single parent. Jason and his mom have been arguing consistently about his requests to stay out after school with his friends and "hang out," instead of coming home and helping with his siblings. Jason's mom understands Jason's desire to be with his friends, but she also needs his help at home and is worried that she will not be able to keep a close eye on his blood sugars if he is out of the house for too long. She feels she has reason to worry, as a few months ago she reluctantly gave Jason permission to go away for the weekend with his close friend, who was going on a trip with his family. During this trip, Jason only checked his blood sugar about

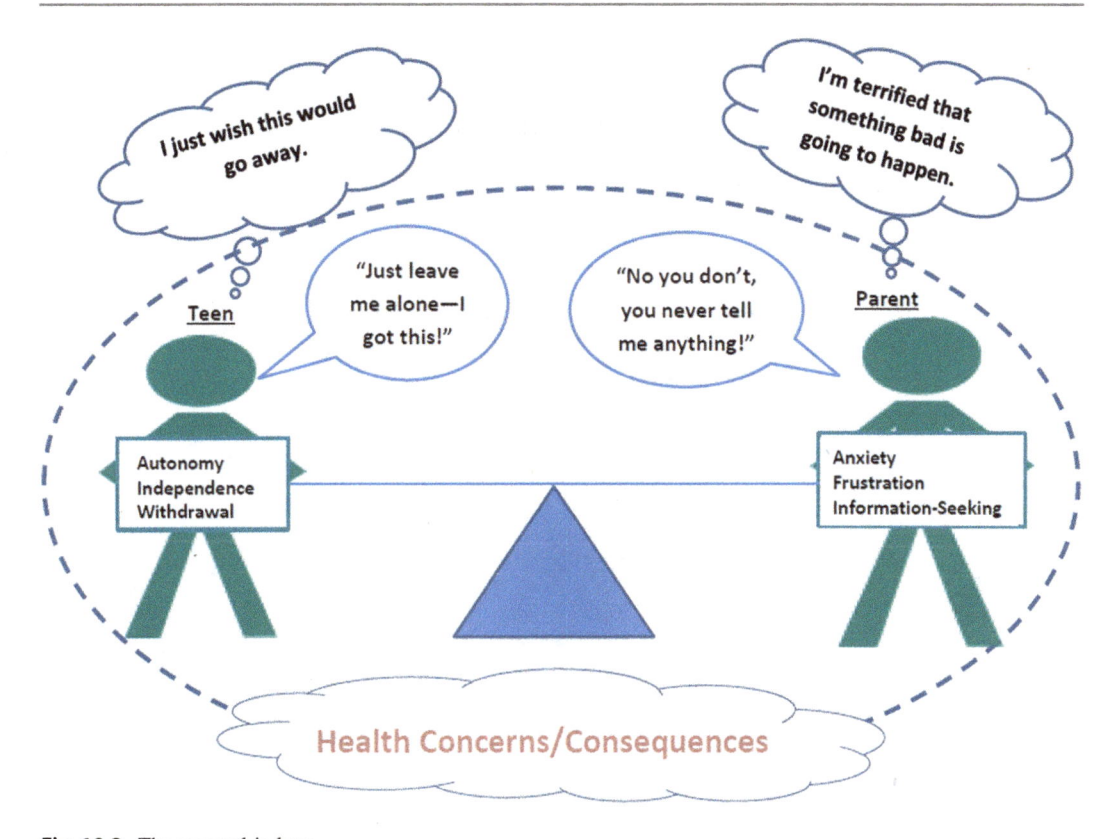

Fig. 10.2 The zoomed-in lens

once a day and did not take any of his short-acting insulin. His mother found out when she snuck a peek at his glucometer and saw only a few checks.

About a week later, Jason and his mom attended an endocrinology appointment, where his doctor informed them that his HbA1c had increased from 10.6 to 11.9 since his last visit. The doctor told Jason that if he continued to minimally manage his diabetes, Jason would eventually lose limbs, go blind, and die. Jason's mother shared that she was doing the best that she could, but that she could not make him take care of himself as "he has a mind of his own." The family was discussed later in the medical team's endocrinology rounds, with the team expressing concerns that Jason's mother was not watching him closely enough or taking her role as his caregiver seriously.

Jason and his mother represent both the dialectical dilemmas that are so common in families with children with chronic health conditions, as well as the layers of complication that come into the picture when additional systems become involved and family resources are low.

DBT for Chronic Medical Conditions (DBT-CMI)

As previously mentioned, the structure and skills contained within DBT may prove uniquely helpful for youth with chronic medical conditions and their families. DBT for Chronic Medical Conditions (DBT-CMI; Lois and Miller 2017; Hashim et al. 2013) is an adaptation of the traditional adolescent DBT protocol, with a focus on targeting medical non-adherence as the primary target in a brief, systems-based treatment approach. Adolescents were particularly selected as the population to target, given the high prevalence rates of medical non-adherence, family conflict, and psychosocial stress during

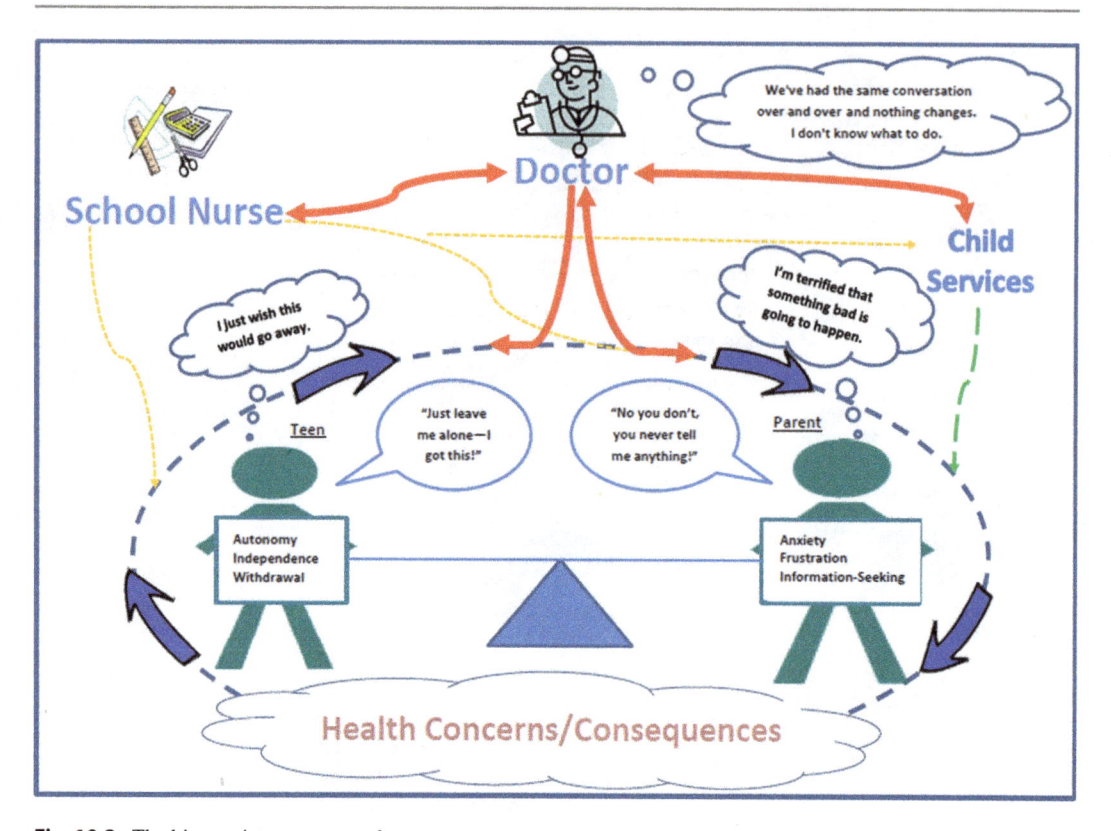

Fig. 10.3 The bigger picture—zoomed-out

this developmental stage (Taddeo et al. 2008). The protocol consists of six weekly individual sessions, three parent/family sessions, and one shared session between the patient and the medical provider, in an effort to address the adjustments required by the whole system to tackle non-adherence as a complex, multi-faceted issue.

As described in Table 10.1, the early sessions of DBT-CMI focus on orientation, commitment, and problem definition and assessment. The therapist expertly weaves orientation to DBT-CMI treatment with assessment of the history of the medical picture together, highlighting and validating how the patient's illness trajectory—diagnosis, the "roller coaster ride" of relapse and remission, changing of medications, doctors, and expectations from peers and family—can sometimes make it feel inevitable that you want to get off the ride. Goals of the patient and caregiver are established early as well, in an effort to "hook" them into treatment and induce motivation to change issues and behaviors that matter to the family system. The therapist also emphasizes the transactions between teen, caregiver, medical team, school, and the subsequent emotions, thoughts, and behaviors that result for all.

Once the teen and family have been oriented to treatment and have set personalized goals both in the short and the long term, the therapist begins to share a nonjudgmental conceptualization of any maladaptive behavior (e.g., non-adherence and avoidance) that tends to occur around illness management. This *negative reinforcement cycle* conceptualization, discussed earlier on in this chapter, is shared with both the teen and the parent in an effort to de-couple the teen's behavior from something that feels intentional and manipulative. The focus is instead on the inevitable triggers the teen experiences in his/her environment, such as doctor's appointments, uncomfortable physical sensations, or reminders to take medications and how these triggers lead

Table 10.1 Session summary of DBT-CMI

Session	Description	Who attends? How long will we meet?
Session 1: Getting to know you; orientation to the program	• Lots of questions! • Helping you to understand what you signed up for and how it might help • Setting goals	• Teen only (ok for parent to join) • 1 h
Session 2: Why is this so hard?	• Helping both of you to understand why managing my medical condition is so tough • Tracking your behavior: Diary card • What do my feelings have to do with it? Mindfulness skills	• Both parent and teen, if possible • 1.5 h (45 min with teen, 45 min with parent)
Session 3: What's getting in my way?	• Reviewing diary card to understand how my thoughts, feelings, and situations around me influence how I manage my medical condition	• Teen only • 45 min–1 h
Session 4: Consultation with medical team (possibly at medical visit); validation	• Invite medical team member to portion of session to clarify anything about your medical condition that's confusing • Information on validation: What it is, what happens when it's not going on, and how to do it! • Introduction to shared pleasant activities	• Both parent and teen, if possible • 1.5 h (45 min with teen, 20 min with parent; 25 min with teen and parent together)
Session 5: Radical acceptance	• How to come to terms with having my medical condition (not to stay stuck being angry or sad about it, so much so that I can't keep moving forward in my life)	• Teen only • 45 min–1 h
Session 6: Wrap up, review, and relapse prevention	• Feedback on your progress! • Review of skills taught: What worked best for the both of you • Setting of short- and long-term goals • Coping ahead: What might get in the way?	• Both parent and teen, if possible • 1.5 h (45 min with teen, 45 min with parent and teen together)
Booster session 1 (1 month after session 6): How's it going?	• Checking in on progress; any stumbling blocks? • Skills review as needed	• Teen only • 45 min–1 h
Booster session 2 (1 month after booster 1): Fine tuning	• Review of goals (both related and unrelated to my medical condition); problem solve as needed	• Teen only • 45 min–1 h

to aversive negative emotional states that make sense and are valid given the situation. The therapist explains that the focus of DBT-CMI is to break the typical flow of these thoughts and behaviors into an automatic response of avoidance—skipping medication, ignoring dietary restrictions, etc.—and instead create a new pathway to more effective coping. Teens are also asked at this point to start self-monitoring their illness behavior, thoughts, and feelings via a DBT-CMI-specific diary card in an effort to increase the teens' mindfulness of patterns in environmental triggers, emotional reactions, and urges to avoid illness-related tasks.

In future sessions, the teen's diary card is reviewed at the start to emphasize its importance and allow the teen and DBT-CMI therapist to work through any episodes of non-adherence or urges to not adhere. The teen and therapist partner on chain behavioral analyses of these events to synthesize understanding of the connection between thoughts, feelings, and subsequent behavior and brainstorm more effective ways of managing similar circumstances in the future. The therapist also takes these opportunities to reinforce effective skill use or shape the beginnings of effective skill use (e.g., the teen was aware of the urge to skip his/her medication and how intense that urge was, but was unable to resist the urge; therapist praises mindful awareness of urges as the first step in behavior change).

The DBT-CMI protocol includes many skills from traditional adolescent DBT, including specific mindfulness, distress tolerance, emotion regulation, and interpersonal effectiveness skills (Rathus and Miller 2015). These skills are interwoven throughout the treatment in a method that is prescriptive to the teen and family's needs and goals and were specifically chosen given their utility in a pediatric population with challenges with illness management. Skills are taught to both the teen and the parent in an effort to reinforce the need for the family system to make adjustments as a whole, rather than the teen being the only person in need of behavior change or skill building. Specific focus is spent on validation, given the typical dynamic between teens and their parents when faced with the chronic stress of illness management. Teens and their parents are taught these skills separately and are then brought together in a DBT-CMI family session to practice them, as they often feel clumsy at first and require encouragement and modeling. The therapist reminds both teen and parent of the tendency to self-invalidate with "should" statements, which can exacerbate feeling of stress and hopelessness in both parties, as well as the tendency to externalize frustration and stress on each other via invalidating statements. These discussions are highly impactful, given the frequency of conflict and emotional intensity that is often seen in teens with illness management issues and their families.

In addition to the joint teen and parent sessions, the therapist also makes it a priority to involve the teen's medical provider in a session focused on skill building and nonjudgmental interaction. Teens and their medical providers may get caught in polarized interactions that are similar to those found at home with their families. Physicians have strong feelings about what needs to happen medically and understandably experience strong reactions when recommendations are not followed. They may be frustrated, fearful, or hopeless about the teen ever understanding the importance of adherence or the consequences of non-adherence. In turn, the teen may feel that his/her medical provider does not understand how hard he/she is trying, and how difficult it is to stay on top of everything all the time. He/she may feel misunderstood, judged, or unfairly blamed without the effective skills to voice his/her position or make lasting behavioral changes. A joint teen-provider session can prove incredibly useful in highlighting these patterns to both parties via a nonjudgmental, validating stance. This allows the physician to learn the same skills as his/her patient and begin to view the teen as someone who is making an effort to change and take accountability. Many physicians who have participated in DBT-CMI with us have shared that this was the first time that they had made eye contact with their patient or heard what was really getting in the way of some of their recommendations. Teens have also shared that they had never really thought of their doctors as "people with feelings," or that they did not realize their doctor cared enough to see them outside of the normal medical visit. These shifts in awareness can lead to subsequent shifts in behavior, both for the teen and for the medical provider.

Toward the end of treatment, the focus shifts toward viewing the teen's life with a medical condition in the long term and the inevitable struggles that will continue to surface. Radical acceptance becomes a key skill in facing these realities more effectively. The teen and parent also engage in a skills review and plan ahead for potential barriers to skill use, with a commitment to help each other stay on track. After the six weekly sessions, the teen and parent attend two booster sessions over 2 months to provide continued review and relapse prevention strategies. Goals for both the teen and the parent are also reviewed for any successes, barriers to success, or adjustment required for ongoing growth.

DBT-CMI Research

DBT-CMI was initially created as a result of a clinical need in pediatric renal transplant candidates, as physicians treating these patients were consulting with psychologists and requesting methods to "fix" medical non-adherence ahead of transplantation. These patients were listed as inactive on a transplant list due to their non-adherence, meaning that the medical team did not feel comfortable transplanting them until their adherence improved. A pilot feasibility trial was conducted utilizing DBT-CMI with seven adolescents with end-stage renal disease who were identified by their medical providers as high risk due to non-adherence. Measures of illness acceptance, quality of life, and depression were conducted pre- and post-treatment. Transplant team reports of adherence, and health improvements were conducted at pre-, mid-, and post-treatment. Significant improvements were evident at post-treatment for depression and adherence, with all seven patients being subsequently activated on the transplant list (Hashim et al. 2013).

Given the success of this initial pilot, a larger study of DBT-CMI in a sample of teens with type 1 diabetes was conducted in order to test the feasibility of the model within a different chronic illness model with hard biomarkers for non-adherence measurement. Fifty adolescents in a busy urban endocrinology clinic were recruited along with their families and randomized into either DBT-CMI or usual care, which consisted of medical follow-up every 1–3 months that included contact with a social worker for support and case management. Adherence was measured by a subjective report as well as through objective medical data (blood glucose meter downloads and HbA1c) and secondary outcomes included depression, quality of life, family conflict, and emotion regulation. The DBT-CMI protocol was expanded to include additional family sessions, as the authors hypothesized that there would be more family conflict and influence in a condition such as diabetes that involves multiple behavioral adjustments and actions throughout the day. Findings indicated significant improvement in depression for those teens enrolled in DBT-CMI, with no significant differences between groups on adherence outcomes (Lois et al. 2019). Exploratory analyses were conducted within the DBT-CMI group, with findings indicating significant improvements in adherence as the weekly sessions progressed but then becoming non-significant at the booster sessions. There was a trend toward adherence improvement as parental involvement in sessions increased.

Clinical Implications from Early Research

While the research examining DBT-CMI is still in its infancy, several findings may point to clinical issues that are relevant to consider. For one, the exploratory analyses from the diabetes trial may indicate the need for a stronger "dose" of treatment, particularly for teens who may not have reached a certain threshold of adherence improvement. These analyses also indicated a trend toward outcome improvement as parents participated in more sessions. Given the systemic nature of the non-adherence problem, it makes sense that increased family involvement may prove useful—particularly in a brief treatment model and with a medical condition that requires active daily participation and management.

The different adherence outcomes in the two pilots are also notable, in that the renal patients in the first trial demonstrated significant improvements when compared to the diabetes sample. This finding may have occurred due to the salient and palpable feeling of accomplishment of being able to receive a kidney transplant, which proved highly motivating to the teens in that sample. Many renal patients reported feeling stigmatized and judged by their medical teams, who had told them their behavior was too problematic to be considered for transplantation. Half of the sample was also on dialysis, which would ideally end post-transplantation and dramatically improve their quality of life. In contrast, in a condition such as diabetes, there is less of a significant and tangible motivator for behavior change because the illness, by its nature, may not change much with time. Adherence improvements may lead to quality-of-life improvements, such as increased energy and decreases in family conflict, but these changes may not feel as substantial or immediate as those found in the kidney sample or other disease conditions where adherence improvements can lead to significant life changes. Thus, when approaching non-adherence issues in treatment it is critically important to consider anything that may be externally motivating to the patient, whether it is linked to the illness or not. For example, a medical provider may not be comfortable starting her patient with diabetes on an insulin pump until she sees some improvements in adherence. If the patient is motivated to receive a pump, it may be helpful to obtain the physician's commitment that at a certain level of improvement she will discuss this option with the patient more readily.

Case Examples

Jessica[1]

To further illustrate DBT-CMI in action, consider Jessica, a 14-year-old Hispanic female with type 1 diabetes. She lives at home in a two-bedroom apartment with her mother, who is a police officer, and two younger siblings ages 8 and 6. Her father left the family when she was 9. Jessica was diagnosed with diabetes when she was 11 after a 2-week-long course of feeling sick, losing weight, and being constantly thirsty and fatigued. She was referred to DBT-CMI by her endocrinologist, who became concerned at Jessica's consistently increasing HbA1c despite her report that she was "doing everything all the time." The physician also indicated that Jessica's mom was "very defensive" and "seemed to have given up" on helping Jessica to manage her behavior.

Early on in treatment, Jessica shared that she felt a great deal of burden and shame when she thought about her diabetes. She reported a belief that she was diagnosed at 11 because she was "acting out a lot" at that age and eating a lot of candy. She also felt uncomfortable managing her diabetes while at school and when around peers. To her knowledge she was the only one in her peer group who had a medical condition that required consistent management throughout the day. Jessica's mother reported high levels of anxiety and stress about Jessica's health and her behavior, sharing at several points that she could barely sleep and worried that her daughter would have a short life due to the decisions she was making today. Jessica would roll her eyes upon hearing this feedback from her mother and regularly told her to "chill" during early sessions.

After the therapist provided psychoeducation on the negative reinforcement cycle of non-adherence and conceptualized Jessica's avoidance pattern as providing relief from intense feelings of shame, Jessica began to discuss her tendency to leave her insulin pump at home. She wanted to "hide" her diabetes from others. Jessica's mother corroborated these occurrences, stating that she would frequently find the pump and other diabetes supplies hidden in Jessica's room. Mom would then have to go to work late to drop off the supplies, which added to her personal stress and subsequent conflict with Jessica. When discussing this behavior, it became apparent that Jessica was choosing to leave her pump at home due to fears that the other students would see it. On days when her mother would catch her and ensure that she was wearing it, Jessica would change her outfits to something baggy so that her pump felt less visible. Regardless, Jessica refused to check her blood sugar while in school or cover for any carbohydrates eaten during her lunch period.

Throughout treatment, Jessica and her mother became more aware of the connection between Jessica's feelings of shame and embarrassment and her tendency to engage in avoidance as a primary strategy. Jessica voiced a desire to change this behavior, as she was aware that her mother's stress and anxiety were leading to her not being able to go out on her own with her friends or establish any trust in the home. Her mother agreed that if Jessica could make some improvements in her adherence, particularly by wearing her insulin pump every day and checking her blood sugar more regularly, she would be more likely to allow Jessica to spend time with her friends outside of school.

---

[1]The name of this client, as well as others mentioned throughout the manuscript, and all identifying information are completely altered and based on multiple clients, and thus, they are composite patients with no true identifying information.

Jessica and her therapist worked through the various DBT-CMI skills, with particular focus on Mindfulness, Opposite Action, and Radical Acceptance (Lois and Miller 2017). Jessica's endocrinologist also attended a DBT-CMI session to talk with her about her concerns regarding the insulin pump's visibility and ways to manage her diabetes without it having to feel so obvious (e.g., how to check blood sugar quickly under the table and in multiple body locations; different areas of the body where it was safe to wear her pump). Jessica was encouraged to ask her doctor questions and use the time to better understand how to make her diabetes regimen work for her.

Jessica was able to successfully implement an opposite action by wearing her pump first under more close-fitting clothing, then changing her pump site to a more noticeable location, to finally placing her pump on her arm while wearing a short-sleeve T-shirt. She noted that these changes elicited reactions from her peers that were anxiety provoking, but tolerable, and that making these changes resulted in significant feelings of accomplishment and pride. Jessica's mother subsequently felt comfortable allowing her more freedoms both inside and outside of the home, which further reinforced and maintained Jessica's behavioral changes and sense of effectiveness. Jessica's mother also made significant improvements in her attempts to outwardly acknowledged Jessica's efforts, particularly given how difficult it had been for her to face her diagnosis in isolation. Jessica, in turn, was able to reinforce her mother for her concerns as a normal reaction given Jessica's history of non-adherence and her mother's daily job of protecting the public as a police officer – it was sometimes difficult for her mother to "turn that off" with Jessica at home.

At the end of treatment, Jessica was successfully wearing her insulin pump to school every day and consistently checking her blood sugar before lunch at the cafeteria table with her friends. She credited opposite action and her mother's willingness to give her more freedom as the primary levers for her behavior change. Her medical provider was pleased with her progress and now approached the medical visit with a focus on partnership with Jessica in an effort to come up with recommendations that felt feasible and likely to be implemented, given Jessica's priorities and concerns.

Joseph

Joseph, a 15-year-old African American male with a diagnosis of end-stage renal disease, was referred to his DBT-CMI therapist due to his medical team's concerns that he was "apathetic" about improving his adherence behavior and becoming activated on the kidney transplant list. Joseph was on dialysis and was currently being home-schooled, as he had missed so many days for his medical treatments. His parents were actively involved in his medical care, but both worked full-time and could not accompany him to his dialysis treatments or many of his medical appointments. Joseph agreed to attend his first DBT-CMI session, but told his medical team that he "wasn't making any promises" about continuing past the first session.

Joseph's DBT-CMI therapist met with him at the first session and prioritized orientation and commitment strategies, given Joseph's reluctance to sign up for treatment. Utilizing a nonjudgmental and validating perspective, Joseph's therapist conveyed her role as separate from his medical providers. She aligned herself with him and his goals, both medical and non-medical. The therapist utilized standard DBT commitment strategies (e.g., freedom to choose, absence of alternatives) to note how coming to DBT-CMI sessions was one more thing for Joseph to do, and at the same time if he chose not to participate it would likely influence his medical providers' stance that he did not care about his health and therefore was not ready to be transplanted. Joseph also reviewed the pros and cons of engaging in DBT-CMI, with particular focus on his goal to go back to school and spend more time with friends – something that would be much more possible post-transplantation than in his current life situation on dialysis. After reviewing his options,

Joseph agreed to participate but continued to be stressed about attending yet another appointment. To accommodate Joseph, his DBT-CMI therapist suggested they meet during his dialysis appointments, which felt more manageable and worth offering once Joseph was able to argue for treatment.

Early sessions with Joseph focused on the negative reinforcement cycle and its impact on his current avoidant behavior, which consisted of missing doses of his medication and coming late to dialysis. Joseph also acknowledged that he often brought inappropriate food to dialysis (e.g., salty McDonald's French fries) because it "got a rise" out of his nurses. He reported feeling like he needed to exert some level of control over his behavior after feeling "forced" to do things throughout his day that were difficult or frustrating to him. He initially shared that he did not take his medication because he was "lazy" but was later able to acknowledge that taking his medication resulted in a reminder that he was sick and not able to do things his friends were doing.

Joseph's parents attended early sessions as well and were eager to learn how to best support him getting activated on the transplant list. His mother reported feelings of sadness and frustration with Joseph, whom she considered to be a "smart boy with the wrong priorities." Joseph's father shared similar frustrations, stating that his son was "old enough to know better." They were responsive to a more nonjudgmental review of his non-adherence that was based on his negative emotions and lack of skillfulness in managing them, rather than an active desire to rebel and make things difficult for all involved.

Throughout treatment, Joseph reported consistent feelings of anger over his medical diagnosis and regimen. He shared that he had been diagnosed at the age of 11 after being superficially stabbed in the arm on the street by a stranger while hanging out with his friends. Joseph reported that he subsequently went to the ER, where labs were drawn and he and his family were notified that he was in kidney failure. It became clear to his DBT-CMI therapist that Joseph believed that the stabbing caused his kidney disease, which led to high levels of anger at the person who had stabbed him and feelings of helplessness at the fact that this had happened to him. His therapist relayed this story to Joseph's renal doctor, who attended the next DBT-CMI session and shared that Joseph's unfortunate stabbing incident had actually led to his early diagnosis and early treatment. Joseph was shocked to hear this news and reported at the end of the session that "maybe all that happened to me was a blessing." His doctor was surprised that Joseph had continued to believe that the stabbing resulted in his kidney disease, as the team had repeatedly shared the realities of his diagnosis; his therapist validated the doctor's experience while also acknowledging that Joseph may not have been ready to hear the information at the time.

Later sessions focused on teaching Joseph and his parents the skills of Wise Mind, validation of self and other, accumulating positive experiences both individually and as a family, and interpersonal effectiveness. They all responded well to role-plays of these skills and acknowledged that validation felt "clumsy" at first, as they were not a "touchy feely" family. Joseph and his parents were encouraged to use language that felt genuine to them (e.g., "it makes sense that you're mad; I would be too") and to stick to the facts when initially having the urge to judge each other's behavior. Joseph was also introduced to radical acceptance as a shift in his typical thinking. He shared that he tended to get angry about what he could not control, rather than see that he had a choice to accept it in order to maximize his focus on where he could be most effective.

Toward the end of treatment, Joseph had become more adherent to his medications and was taking them consistently ahead of his dialysis treatments. He was participating more fully in his medical visits with the team, which reassured them that he would take his post-transplant care more seriously. He reported feeling less of an urge to resist the medical team's recommendations, which he attributed to feeling less angry in general and realizing that "it's better for me to go with the flow and focus on my goals rather than fight at every step."

Conclusion

Youth facing chronic health conditions undergo many challenges, including feelings of isolation, differentness from peers, family conflict, and risk-taking behavior. It is important to view these challenges in the context of a larger system of medical providers, school personnel, family members, peers, and community agencies, all of which have an influence on outcome and require intervention. DBT-CMI shows preliminary promise as a brief, systems-based psychotherapy to target common and potentially high-risk struggles when confronted with chronic illness, such as non-adherence and lack of illness acceptance. Further research is required to better understand any mechanisms for change when using DBT-CMI across and within disease groups.

Diary Card (PUMP)

Week of _____   Filled Out in session Y / N

DAY	BG checks (_/_)	Urges to not check BG (0-5)	Actions (y/n)	Give bolus (_/_)	Urges to not give bolus (0-5)	Actions (y/n)	Happy (0-5)	Shame (0-5)	Anger (0-5)	Fear (0-5)	Sad (0-5)	Pride (0-5)	NOTES (more room on the back)
Monday													
Tuesday													
Wednesday													
Thursday													
Friday													
Saturday													
Sunday													

Tasks to Complete	Completed? (y/n)

Instructions: Circle the days you worked on each skill

Wise mind	Mon	Tues	Wed	Thurs	Fri	Sat	Sun
Observe (just notice what's going on inside)	Mon	Tues	Wed	Thurs	Fri	Sat	Sun
Describe (put words on the experience)	Mon	Tues	Wed	Thurs	Fri	Sat	Sun
Don't judge	Mon	Tues	Wed	Thurs	Fri	Sat	Sun
Identify and label emotions	Mon	Tues	Wed	Thurs	Fri	Sat	Sun
PLEASE (reduce vulnerability to emotion mind)	Mon	Tues	Wed	Thurs	Fri	Sat	Sun
Engaging in pleasant activities	Mon	Tues	Wed	Thurs	Fri	Sat	Sun
Building structure (time, work, play)	Mon	Tues	Wed	Thurs	Fri	Sat	Sun
GIVE (improving the relationship)	Mon	Tues	Wed	Thurs	Fri	Sat	Sun
ACCEPTS (distract)	Mon	Tues	Wed	Thurs	Fri	Sat	Sun
Validate self	Mon	Tues	Wed	Thurs	Fri	Sat	Sun
Think dialectically (non black and white)	Mon	Tues	Wed	Thurs	Fri	Sat	Sun
Radical Acceptance	Mon	Tues	Wed	Thurs	Fri	Sat	Sun

References

Adriaanse, M. A., De Ridder, D. D., & Voorneman, I. (2013). Improving diabetes self-management by mental contrasting. *Psychology & Health, 28*(1), 1–12. https://doi.org/10.1080/08870446.2012.660154.

Butz, A. M. (2006). Evidence-based practice: What is the evidence for medication adherence in children? *Journal of Pediatric Health Care, 20*(5), 338–341. https://doi.org/10.1016/j.pedhc.2006.05.003.

Center for Disease Control. (2018, June 12). *Chronic disease prevention and health promotion*. Retrieved from https://www.cdc.gov/chronicdisease/index.htm

Compas, B. E., Jaser, S. S., Dunn, M. J., & Rodriguez, E. M. (2012). Coping with chronic illness in childhood and adolescence. *Annual Review of Clinical Psychology, 8*, 455–480. https://doi.org/10.1146/annurev-clinpsy-032511-143108.

Graves, M. M., Roberts, M. C., Rapoff, M., & Boyer, A. (2010). The efficacy of adherence interventions for chronically ill children: A meta-analytic review. *Journal of Pediatric Psychology, 35*(4), 368–382. https://doi.org/10.1093/jpepsy/jsp072.

Gregg, J. A., Callaghan, G. M., Hayes, S. C., & Glenn-Lawson, J. L. (2007). Improving diabetes self-management through acceptance, mindfulness, and values: A randomized controlled trial. *Journal of Consulting and Clinical Psychology, 75*(2), 336–343. https://doi.org/10.1037/0022-006X.75.2.336.

Hashim, B. L., Vadnais, M., & Miller, A. L. (2013). Improving adherence in adolescent chronic kidney disease: A DBT feasibility trial. *Clinical Practice in Pediatric Psychology, 1*(4), 396–379.

Kahana, S., Drotar, D., & Frazier, T. (2008). Meta-analysis of psychological interventions to promote adherence to treatment in pediatric chronic health conditions. *Journal of Pediatric Psychology, 33*(6), 590–611. https://doi.org/10.1093/jpepsy/jsm128.

Katon, W. J. (2003). Clinical and health services relationships between major depression, depressive symptoms, and general medical illness. *Biological Psychiatry, 54*(3), 216–226. https://doi.org/10.1016/S0006-3223(03)00273-7.

Kravitz, R. L., & Melnikow, J. (2004). Medical adherence research: Time for a change in direction? *Medical Care, 42*(3), 197–199. https://doi.org/10.1097/01.mlr.0000115957.44388.7c.

Linehan, M. M. (1993a). *Skills training manual for treating borderline personality disorder*. New York: Guilford Press.

Linehan, M. M. (1993b). *Cognitive-behavioral treatment of borderline personality disorder*. New York: Guilford Press.

Lois, B. H., & Miller, A. L. (2017). Stopping the nonadherence cycle: The clinical and theoretical basis for dialectical behavior therapy adapted for adolescents with chronic medical illness (DBT-CMI). *Cognitive and Behavioral Practice, 25*, 32–43.

Lois, B. H., Corcoran, V. P., Catarozzoli, C. R., McGrath, M., Bauman, L. J., & Miller, A. L. (2019). Randomized clinical trial of a brief DBT-based intervention to improve medical adherence in adolescents with type 1 diabetes. Manuscript in preparation.

McGrady, M. E., & Hommel, K. A. (2013). Medication adherence and health care utilization in pediatric chronic illness: A systematic review. *Pediatrics, 132*(4), 730–740. https://doi.org/10.1542/peds.2013-1451.

Miller, A. L., Rathus, J. H., & Linehan, M. M. (2007). *Dialectical behavior therapy with suicidal adolescents*. New York, NY: Guilford Press.

Patel, V., Maj, M., Flisher, A. J., DeSilva, M. J., Koschorke, M., & Prince, M. (2010). Reducing the treatment gap for mental disorders: A WPA survey. *World Psychiatry, 9*, 169–176.

Phillips, L., Cohen, J., Burns, E., Abrams, J., & Renninger, S. (2016). Self-management of chronic illness: The role of 'habit' versus reflective factors in exercise and medication adherence. *Journal of Behavioral Medicine, 39*(6), 1076–1091. https://doi.org/10.1007/s10865-016-9732-z.

Rathus, J. H., & Miller, A. L. (2015). *DBT skills training manual for adolescents*. New York, NY: The Guilford Press.

Ritschel, L. A., Miller, A. L., & Taylor, V. (2013). Dialectical behavior therapy for emotion dysregulation. In J. Ehrenreich-May & B. Chu (Eds.), *Transdiagnostic mechanisms and treatment for youth psychopathology* (pp. 203–232). New York, NY: Guilford Press.

Sav, A., King, M. A., Whitty, J. A., Kendall, E., McMillan, S. S., Kelly, F., et al. (2013). Burden of treatment for chronic illness: A concept analysis and review of the literature. *Health Expectations, 18*, 312–324. https://doi.org/10.1111/hex.12046.

Sawyer, S., Drew, S., & Duncan, R. (2007). Adolescents with chronic disease--the double whammy. *Australian Family Physician, 36*(8), 622–627.

Taddeo, D., Egedy, M., & Frappier, J.-Y. (2008). Adherence to treatment in adolescents. *Paediatrics & Child Health, 13*(1), 19–24.

van Dulmen, S., Sluijs, E., van Dijk, L., de Ridder, D., Heerdink, R., & Bensing, J. (2007). Patient adherence to medical treatment: A review of reviews. *BMC Health Services Research, 7*, 55. https://doi.org/10.1186/1472-6963-7-55.

Ward, B. W., Schiller, J. S., & Goodman, R. A. (2014). Multiple chronic conditions among US adults: A 2012 update. *Preventing Chronic Disease, 11*, E62. https://doi.org/10.5888/pcd11.130389.

Weersing, V. R., Rozenman, M. S., Maher-Bridge, M., & Campo, J. V. (2012). Anxiety, depression, and somatic distress: Developing a transdiagnostic internalizing toolbox for pediatric practice. *Cognitive and Behavioral Practice, 19*, 68–82. https://doi.org/10.1016/j.cbpra.2011.06.002.

Westbom, L., & Kornfält, R. (1987). Chronic illness among children in a total population. An epidemiological study in a Swedish primary health care district. *Scandinavian Journal of Social Medicine, 15*(2), 87–97.

World Health Organization. (2018, June 1). *Noncommunicable diseases*. Retrieved from http://www.who.int/news-room/fact-sheets/detail/noncommunicable-diseases

Pharmacological Interventions

11

Rahil R. Jummani and Jess P. Shatkin

Introduction

Children and adolescents, like their adult counterparts, demonstrate variable susceptibility to the impact of acute and chronic medical conditions. Children are often more severely affected than adults because medical problems may lead to long-term disruptions of not only day-to-day functioning and physical and mental health and well-being, but also the course of their psychosocial development (Bursch and Forgey 2013). Absences from school lead to potential academic delays. Social development may also be hindered as the quality and quantity of peer interactions are compromised. It is not only the underlying biological pathology that is taxing, however. Acute and chronic medical *interventions* may be as traumatizing for youth as the disorders they are meant to evaluate and/or treat.

The diagnosis and treatment of a serious medical condition are stressful (Brosbe et al. 2013).

After a medical diagnosis or injury, feelings of sadness, loneliness, loss, fear, and anxiety are common. Very young patients may be scared and confused throughout the ordeal. Numerous and invasive diagnostic procedures, separation from parents and guardians, imposing equipment, multiple providers, and painful interventions such as injections and surgeries contribute to the stress experience (Rzucidlo and Campbell 2009). Stress-related symptoms in turn may negatively impact physical health outcomes.

There are numerous cases of illness-related and iatrogenic trauma in the literature. For example, studies demonstrate that many child and adolescent heart, kidney, or liver transplant recipients experience notable anxiety, posttraumatic stress disorder (PTSD), or depressive symptoms and/or disruptive behavior during the first-year post-transplant (Bursch and Forgey 2013). A high proportion of youth living with HIV report depression, which increases the morbidity and mortality of the condition. Treatment adherence and quality of life are compromised (Brown et al. 2016).

Cancer diagnosis in adolescence is associated with a high occurrence of mood disorders, especially depression. Suicide attempts have been found to increase up to fourfold over general population levels in these individuals (Park and Rosenstein 2015). Other investigators have found that youth with conditions such as seizure

R. R. Jummani (✉)
Department of Child and Adolescent Psychiatry, Hassenfeld Children's Hospital at NYU Langone, Child Study Center, New York, NY, USA
e-mail: Rahil.Jummani@nyulangone.org

J. P. Shatkin
Department of Child and Adolescent Psychiatry, Child and Adolescent Mental Health Studies (CAMS), NYU College of Arts and Science and Hassenfeld Children's Hospital at NYU Langone, Child Study Center, New York, NY, USA

© Springer Nature Switzerland AG 2019
R. D. Friedberg, J. K. Paternostro (eds.), *Handbook of Cognitive Behavioral Therapy for Pediatric Medical Conditions*, Autism and Child Psychopathology Series,
https://doi.org/10.1007/978-3-030-21683-2_11

disorders or systemic lupus erythematosus (SLE) experience more anxiety and depression than controls. Asthma patients, especially those with severe and acute life-threatening symptoms during the course of their illness, have high levels of PTSD symptoms. Even those undergoing relatively commonplace procedures, such as tonsillectomy, indicate transient depressive symptoms (Bursch and Forgey 2013). Care can and should be provided with an awareness of the stressful nature of acute and chronic medical illnesses and the diagnostic and treatment procedures involved (Rzucidlo and Campbell 2009). Such trauma-informed care may reduce the psychological burden of medical ailments and accompanying interventions.

Despite trauma-informed diagnostic and treatment strategies, coping with a medical condition is often challenging, and youth may manifest notable mental health symptoms, such as disruptive behavior or school problems, or the full presentation of an adjustment disorder, major or persistent depressive disorder, anxiety disorder, and/or acute or post-traumatic stress disorder. Fortunately, we now have a significant evidence base for the treatment of many of these conditions.

Explanation of Specific Medications

Selective Serotonin Reuptake Inhibitors (SSRIs)

Selective serotonin reuptake inhibitors (SSRIs) are considered the first-line pharmacological treatments for anxiety disorders, including generalized, social, and separation anxiety disorder, and obsessive-compulsive disorder (OCD). As will be discussed later, they appear less effective for the treatment of depression, with the exception of fluoxetine, and trauma and stressor-related disorders such as PTSD. The SSRIs studied in youth include citalopram, escitalopram, fluoxetine, fluvoxamine, paroxetine, and sertraline. Their mechanism involves blockade of the serotonin transporter, increasing serotonin at the synapse. Common side effects include agitation, nausea, stomachaches, diarrhea, irritability, paradoxical activation, headaches, and sleep problems. Fluoxetine is FDA-approved for the treatment of depression in children and adolescents and escitalopram for the treatment of depression in adolescents only.

A low SSRI starting dose and slow taper are always prudent, especially when used in anxious youth. For anxiety disorder treatment, starting doses may be lower than the typical dosages suggested in Table 11.1 below.

Serotonin-Norepinephrine Reuptake Inhibitors (SNRIs)

The SNRIs are second-line agents for the treatment of anxiety disorders and depression in children and adolescents. Their mechanism of action involves increasing the availability of both serotonin and norepinephrine at the synapse. The SNRIs studied in youth include venlafaxine and duloxetine. As mentioned in the studies reviewed subsequently in this chapter, they are less efficacious than SSRIs for the treatment of anxiety disorders, and they take longer to work. For depression, venlafaxine appears no more effective than placebo; duloxetine shows promise, but more studies are needed. These agents have even more limited data to support their use in the treatment of PTSD. Common side effects of the SNRIs include nausea, agitation, stomachaches, headaches, and at higher doses, hypertension. Venlafaxine appears to have an increased risk for suicidality compared to placebo and other antidepressants. At this time, duloxetine is the only medication that is FDA-approved for the treatment of generalized anxiety disorder in children and adolescents. Table 11.2 presents generic and brand names, starting daily dosages, and therapeutic daily dosages for SNRIs.

Alpha-2-Agonists

The alpha-2-agonists, clonidine and guanfacine, decrease central norepinephrine release. There is some evidence that they mitigate the

Table 11.1 Selective serotonin reuptake inhibitors (SSRIs)

Generic name	Brand name	Starting daily dose	Therapeutic daily dose
Citalopram	Celexa	10–20 mg	20–40 mg
Escitalopram	Lexapro	5–10 mg	10–30 mg
Fluoxetine	Prozac	10–20 mg	10–60 mg
Fluvoxamine	Luvox	25–50 mg	50–200 mg
Paroxetine	Paxil	10–20 mg	10–60 mg
Sertraline	Zoloft	25–50 mg	25–200 mg

re-experiencing, avoidance, and hyperarousal of PTSD. They have been used to treat hypertension in adults and are also used to reduce tics and attention-deficit/hyperactivity disorder (ADHD) symptoms, primarily impulsivity and hyperactivity, in children and adolescents. Outbursts, aggression, and sleep problems may also respond to these agents. The most common side effect is sedation. Other side effects include irritability, depression, and if rapidly discontinued, rebound hypertension. Heart rate and blood pressure should be monitored during use. Generic and brand names, starting daily dosages, and therapeutic daily dosages for the alpha-2-agonists are listed in Table 11.3.

Alpha-1-Antagonists

Alpha-1-antagonists mitigate the effects of norepinephrine postsynaptically and reduce sympathetic tone. While there are multiple placebo-controlled trials of the alpha-1-antagonist prazosin in adults for the treatment of PTSD symptoms, there are no open-label or placebo-controlled trials in the pediatric population. A small number of case reports are suggestive that the medication may be effective. The starting dose is 1 mg, and the therapeutic dose range is 2–4 mg. Common side effects include hypotension, headache, dizziness, nausea, and sedation.

Beta-Antagonists (Blockers)

Beta-blockers are used to treat hypertension and tremor in adults. They reduce central adrenergic tone and have been used behaviorally in adults, children, and teenagers for the treatment of performance anxiety, aggression, impulsivity, restlessness, self-injurious behavior, and PTSD symptoms. With the exception of the treatment of performance anxiety, the beta-blockers are not first-line psychiatric treatments and are typically used in conjunction with other first- or second-line agents for refractory symptoms. Propranolol crosses the blood–brain barrier and has been used clinically and in research studies with children and adolescents. The starting dose is 10 mg, and therapeutic doses between 40 and 80 mg have been used for PTSD symptoms. Side effects include sedation, nausea, vomiting, constipation, exercise intolerance, diarrhea, vivid dreams, depression, and rarely, hallucinations. Heart rate and blood pressure should be monitored since they may be lowered by beta-blockers. Propranolol should not be used in children with asthma, and it should be used cautiously in those with diabetes.

Second-Generation Antipsychotics

Second-generation antipsychotics are used clinically to treat various disorders and symptoms such as psychosis, mania, mood instability, impulsivity, tics, aggression, agitation, and irritability. They have been studied for the treatment of PTSD symptoms in both adults and children. Adult studies show promise, particularly for reducing intrusive re-experiencing. Limited data support the use of risperidone and quetiapine in improving intrusive, hyperarousal, and avoidance symptoms in children and adolescents. The primary mechanism of action of the second-generation antipsychotics is dopamine (D2) and serotonin (5HT)

Table 11.2 Select serotonin-norepinephrine reuptake inhibitors (SNRIs)

Generic name	Brand name	Starting daily dose	Therapeutic daily dose
Duloxetine	Cymbalta	20–30 mg	30–60 mg
Venlafaxine	Effexor XR	37.5–75 mg	37.5–225 mg

Table 11.3 Alpha-2-agonists

Generic name	Brand name	Starting daily dose	Therapeutic daily dose
Clonidine	Catapres	0.05–0.1 mg	0.1–0.4 mg divided tid-qid
Clonidine extended release	Kapvay	0.1 mg	0.1–0.4 mg divided bid
Guanfacine	Tenex	0.5–1 mg	2–4 mg divided bid-tid
Guanfacine extended release	Intuniv	1 mg	2–4 mg

receptor blockade. Common side effects include weight gain and metabolic problems, drowsiness/sedation, dizziness, nasal congestion, dry mouth, constipation, and blurry vision. Extrapyramidal side effects, including tremor, dystonia, dyskinesia, and akathisia, are more common with first-generation antipsychotics but may also occur. With risperidone, prolactin elevation is also a possibility. Neuroleptic malignant syndrome is a rare but emergent side effect consisting of muscle rigidity, confusion, diaphoresis, hyperthermia, and autonomic instability with fluctuations of heart rate and blood pressure.

When treating with second-generation antipsychotics, weight and metabolic parameters, including fasting glucose and lipid profile, must be monitored along with regular physical assessment for signs of muscle rigidity and tremor. An electrocardiogram is necessary before initiation and during treatment with some agents due to risk of QTc prolongation, which in rare cases can result in sudden death. Table 11.4 presents the generic and brand names, starting daily doses, and therapeutic daily doses for select second-generation antipsychotics.

Antiepileptic Mood Stabilizers

The antiepileptic mood stabilizers are employed clinically to treat various disorders and symptoms, such as seizures, mania, mood instability, impulsivity, aggression, agitation, and irritability. They have been examined in the adult PTSD literature. There are limited data for treating trauma-related symptoms in the pediatric population with carbamazepine and divalproex. The putative mechanism of the anticonvulsant mood stabilizers is a dampening of abnormal neural activity in limbic regions of the brain. Common side effects include drowsiness/sedation, nausea, vomiting, dizziness, and appetite and weight changes. Leukopenia is rare. Hepatitis and pancreatitis are possible with divalproex. Blurred or double vision has also been reported when using higher doses of carbamazepine. When these agents are prescribed, plasma drug levels, hepatic functioning, and blood count must be monitored. The generic and brand names, starting daily doses, and therapeutic doses for select antiepileptic mood stabilizers are listed in Table 11.5.

The Antidepressant Black Box Warning

Many psychiatric conditions, such as depression, PTSD, and severe anxiety, have an inherent risk of suicidality, and suicide is the second leading cause of death in adolescence (Kolves and De Leo 2016). Since the introduction and widespread use of the SSRI and SNRI agents, the trend of suicides has modestly declined, and geographic areas with greater antidepressant prescriptions have experienced lower suicide rates. For example, the rate of suicide in males aged 15–19 years decreased from 17.6 per 100,000 person-years in 1992 to 12.2 per 100,000 person-years in 2002 (Hammad et al. 2006). However, a slight short-term increase in suicidal ideation and behavior in youth has been shown in studies involving SSRI, SNRI, and other antidepressant agents, leading to a black box warning of all antidepressant medications for pediatric use by the FDA in 2004 (Hammad et al. 2006).

A subsequent meta-analysis was published by Hammad and colleagues in 2006 to investigate the relationship between antidepressant medication use and suicidality in children and adolescents; 24 randomized, placebo-controlled trials comprising a total of 4582 participants were included. Nine various antidepressants were utilized in these trials: bupropion, citalopram, fluoxetine, fluvoxamine, mirtazapine, nefazodone, paroxetine, sertraline, and venlafaxine extended release. Four trials had no events in the drug or placebo groups and were therefore not included in the risk ratio analysis of suicidality. There were no completed suicides in any of the remaining 20 trials for which the risk ratio of suicidality was determined. The overall risk ratio for antidepressants in depression trials only was 1.66 (95% CI, 1.02–2.68), and for all indications, it was 1.95 (95% CI, 1.28–2.98). The authors interpreted these findings as indicating that for every 100 patients treated with an antidepressant, one to three patients would be expected to have an increase in suicidality due to short-term treatment with the antidepressant (Hammad et al. 2006).

A second meta-analysis by Bridge and colleagues in 2007 included 27 studies with over 5000 subjects and reported similar findings. They concluded that the benefits of antidepressants appear to be greater than the risk of suicidal ideation/suicide attempt across indications in children and adolescents (Bridge et al. 2007). The period of greatest risk for suicidality with antidepressant use appears to be early in treatment. While the risk is relatively small, it is significant and consistent across studies.

Ironically, reduced rates of antidepressant prescribing in the years immediately following the FDA implemented black box warnings led to an increase in the suicide rate among children and adolescents in the United States (Gibbons et al. 2007). Epidemiologic studies demonstrate an association between increased antidepressant use and lower suicide rates, as well as a correlation between reduced SSRI use and increased suicide rates in youth. Therefore, the risk of suicidality with antidepressant use should not preclude the appropriate prescribing of these critically important life-saving medications. Rather, close monitoring is recommended for all children and adolescents being newly prescribed antidepressants (e.g., weekly in person appointments during the first month of treatment). Certain patient and family characteristics warrant especially close monitoring, including youth with a history of suicidal ideation, intent, plan, or attempt; a family history of suicide; psychiatric comorbidity; pain; limited support and coping skills; and/or impulsivity.

Psychopharmacologic Interventions: The Evidence Base

Mood, anxiety, and trauma and stressor-related disorders have been studied to varying degrees in childhood, adolescence, and adulthood. While it is clear that many of these conditions run in families, and there is a genetic basis for their presentation, it is also apparent that environmental stressors and triggers often herald their presentation or full manifestation. The interplay of genes, environment, and individual vulnerabilities is the subject of ongoing research.

While there are yet to be developed curative treatments in the field of mental health, there are interventions that have been found to be effective in mitigating symptoms and dramatically improving quality of life. These therapies include psychotherapy, especially cognitive behavioral therapy, and medication interventions. Most studies to date demonstrate that while mild manifestations of mood, trauma, or anxiety-based disorders may respond to either psychotherapy or

Table 11.4 Select second-generation antipsychotics

Generic name	Brand name	Starting daily dose	Therapeutic daily dose
Quetiapine	Seroquel; Seroquel XR	25–50 mg, divided bid-tid for immediate release	50–200 mg, divided bid-tid for immediate-release preparation
Risperidone	Risperdal	0.25–0.5 mg	0.5–6 mg, divided qd-bid

Table 11.5 Select antiepileptic mood stabilizers

Generic name	Brand name	Starting daily dose	Therapeutic daily dose
Carbamazepine	Tegretol; Tegretol XR	100–200 mg, divided bid-qid for immediate release and bid for extended release	200–600 mg, divided bid-qid for immediate release and bid for extended release
Divalproex	Depakote; Depakote ER	250–750 mg, divided bid-tid for delayed release and daily for extended release	500–2000 mg, divided bid-tid for delayed release and daily for extended release

psychopharmacology, moderate to severe presentations often require the presence of both for significant symptom relief and quality-of-life improvement (March and Vitiello 2009; Walkup et al. 2008).

Studies have shown that the selective serotonin reuptake inhibitors (SSRIs) are good first-line agents for the treatment of mood and anxiety disorders in children and adolescents when medication is necessary. Their primary mechanism of action is believed to be the blockade of the serotonin transporter, leading to increased synaptic serotonin levels. Medication response rates are comparable to those in adults (March and Vitiello 2009; Walkup et al. 2008). There is also an evidence base for the use of the serotonin-norepinephrine reuptake inhibitors (SNRIs) in children and adolescents as well as in adults. The evidence base for the use of SSRIs and SNRIs in depression and in trauma and stressor-related disorders, such as PTSD, in youth is less substantial than it is for the anxiety disorders. Other agents such as the alpha-agonists and antagonists may hold more promise for PTSD (Connor et al. 2013).

There is little direct evidence for the use of SSRIs, SNRIs, or other agents in youth coping with medical problems. The indications for their use are based solely on research among youth with primary psychiatric conditions without complicating medical illness, as well as studies of adults with medical problems, and clinical experience (Bursch and Forgey 2013). As a result, this chapter will address the current evidence base for the medication management of anxiety, depressive, and PTSD symptoms in childhood and adolescence. Practitioners are advised to consider this evidence when making decisions about utilizing medication for the treatment of these disorders among youth with complicating medical difficulties.

Specific Disorders

Anxiety Disorders

Fear and anxiety are developmentally adaptive processes that are a normal response to environmental stressors and the perception of danger. Normative stranger and separation anxiety peak between 8 and 18 months of age, followed by early childhood and school-aged fears related to specific threats, such as the dark, animals, insects, water, natural disasters, school, harm to self or others, death, germs, and disease. A fear of medical procedures, such as vaccinations and blood draws, is also common. Anxiety in adolescence is characterized typically by fear of negative evaluation and rejection by peers. Developmental anxiety is transient, has a predictable trajectory, and does not cause excessive distress or dysfunction.

Disordered anxiety is distinguished from typical fear and worry by its elevated frequency, intensity, and duration, and obstruction of normative functioning. Avoidance, substantial distress, and somatic manifestations are prominent. Children with intense and persistent fear, shyness, and social withdrawal when faced with unfamiliar settings and people (novelty) are at heightened risk for developing an anxiety disorder. Neuroimaging data demonstrate dysfunction of the prefrontal cortex (PFC), basal ganglia, and amygdala-based circuits. There is a relative decrease in the PFC's ability to modulate the limbic anxiety circuits among individuals with pathological levels of anxiety (Shatkin 2015).

Anxiety disorders are among the most common mental health conditions across the lifespan, often emerging in childhood or adolescence. An estimated 32% of teens meet criteria for an anxiety disorder between the ages of 13 and 18 years (Merikangas et al. 2010). Approximately half of those with anxiety disorders in adulthood first experience pathological anxiety before the age of 11 years (Piacentini et al. 2014). Prevalence estimates in youth vary and are in the range of 5–10%, with females outnumbering males by a ratio of about 2:1. While it is well known that those enduring stressful life events, such as a medical illness, are at increased risk, families and physicians may miss the signs of pathological fear and worry, and a minority of affected youth receives treatment.

Untreated, anxiety takes a significant toll on everything from academic achievement to social engagement. Pathological anxiety is often chronic and highly comorbid with depression, substance use, and suicidality during the adolescent years. Early treatment is effective, and research supports the use of psychotherapy, especially cognitive behavior therapy (CBT) with over 40 positive studies in youth, and medication management. Almost all CBT research trials show efficacy for exposure-based protocols in reducing symptoms and diagnoses (Creswell and Waite 2016).

SSRIs are considered the first-line pharmacological treatments for the anxiety disorders, including generalized, social, and separation anxiety disorders, and the SNRIs have also been shown to be effective treatments for these conditions. There are over 20 trials examining the efficacy of SSRIs and SNRIs for the treatment of anxiety disorders in youth (Creswell and Waite 2016). Given the strong evidence base for these agents, and limited efficacy data for, and concern about the adverse effects of, other medications such as the tricyclic antidepressants (TCAs) and benzodiazepines, the focus here will be on treatment with the SSRIs and SNRIs for anxiety.

Virtually, all treatment trials with SSRI and SNRI medications in youth with anxiety disorder symptoms show superiority over placebo. While the SSRIs have been shown to be most effective for the treatment of anxiety and are considered first-line pharmacological treatments, it is noteworthy that the only medication that is FDA-approved for the treatment of generalized anxiety disorder in patients 7–17 years of age is the SNRI duloxetine.

Fluvoxamine and sertraline have been shown in multicenter trials with children and adolescents to notably reduce anxiety as compared to placebo in separation anxiety disorder, social anxiety disorder, obsessive-compulsive disorder (OCD), and generalized anxiety disorder. Fluvoxamine was examined in an 8-week, double-blind, placebo-controlled study of 128 children and adolescents ages 6–17 years who had not responded to 3 weeks of psychotherapy for an anxiety disorder. The group treated with fluvoxamine showed significant improvement compared to the placebo group. Five children dropped out of treatment in the fluvoxamine group due to adverse events, including sedation, somatic discomfort, or hyperactivity and one child dropped out of treatment in the placebo group due to irritability and insomnia (The Research Unit on Pediatric Psychopharmacology Anxiety Study Group 2001).

The largest single study of childhood anxiety treatment, the Child/Adolescent Anxiety Multimodal Treatment Study (CAMS), involved a 12-week, randomized, double-blind, placebo-controlled trial of 488 children and adolescents ages 7–17 years old with an anxiety disorder. Treatment was pursued with sertraline, 14 sessions of CBT, both sertraline and CBT, or placebo. All intervention arms were superior to placebo, and 81% of the group receiving combination therapy showed significant improvement compared to 60% of the CBT group, 55% of the sertraline group, and 24% of the placebo group. Adverse events, including suicidal and homicidal ideation, were no more frequent in the sertraline group than in the placebo group. No child attempted suicide. There was less insomnia, fatigue, sedation, and restlessness associated with CBT than with sertraline (Walkup et al. 2008). Uncontrolled follow-up at 24 and 36 weeks demonstrated sustained treatment benefits of medication (Piacentini et al. 2014).

The efficacy of fluoxetine for the treatment of separation anxiety disorder, social anxiety disorder, and/or generalized anxiety disorder has also been assessed. In a 12-week, double-blind, placebo-controlled trial of 84 youth 7–17 years old, significantly more participants in the fluoxetine group (61%) were found to be very much or much improved compared to the placebo group (35%) by week 12. Drowsiness, headache, nausea, and abdominal pain occurred more frequently in the fluoxetine arm than in the placebo arm of the study (Birmaher et al. 2003).

The SNRI venlafaxine extended release (ER) was evaluated in an 8-week, double-blind, placebo-controlled trial of 320 children and adolescents ages 6–17 years old with generalized anxiety disorder. Venlafaxine-treated patients improved notably more than those receiving placebo. Anorexia was more commonly experienced in the venlafaxine than the placebo group. One participant treated with venlafaxine withdrew from the trial due to suicidal ideation while another subject treated with placebo withdrew due to a suicide attempt (Rynn et al. 2007).

The safety and efficacy of duloxetine was assessed in a 10-week, randomized, double-blind, placebo-controlled trial of 272 children and adolescents ages 7–17 years old with generalized anxiety disorder. Greater remission of symptoms was observed in the duloxetine group than in the placebo group by week 10. Side effects of nausea, vomiting, anorexia, oropharyngeal pain, dizziness, cough, and palpitations occurred more often in those randomized to duloxetine than to placebo. The rate of treatment-emergent suicidal ideation was equivocal for the two groups, 5.9% for duloxetine, and 5.2% for placebo (Strawn et al. 2015a, b).

Ipser et al. (2010), Uthman and Abdulmalik (2010), and Strawn et al. (2015a, b), each conducted pooled analyses of randomized-controlled trials of SSRIs and SNRIs for the treatment of childhood anxiety disorders, demonstrating their substantial advantage over placebo. Meta-analysis of the extant data by Uthman and Abdulmalik showed that the SSRIs fluvoxamine and paroxetine were more efficacious than the SNRI venlafaxine (Uthman and Abdulmalik 2010).

The most recent meta-analysis by Strawn et al. published in 2018 extracted data from nine randomized, parallel-group, placebo-controlled trials conducted between the years 1997 and 2014 evaluating seven SSRI and SNRI medications in a total of 1673 youth with anxiety disorders. The agents examined in these studies were the SSRIs fluoxetine, fluvoxamine, paroxetine, and sertraline and the SNRIs atomoxetine, venlafaxine, and duloxetine. Statistically significant treatment effects were noted within 2 weeks of starting treatment. By week 6 of treatment, clinically significant differences were detected. SSRIs demonstrated an earlier response and greater efficacy than SNRIs for the treatment of anxiety disorders. Differences were seen as early as week 2, and by week 8, SNRIs showed only 40% of the response rate seen with the SSRIs (Strawn et al. 2018).

In Strawn et al.'s meta-analysis, the use of high-dose SSRI was associated with earlier improvement, but end results appear to be similar for high- or low-dose SSRI intervention in terms of overall response trajectory. By week 12, patients on both high-dose and low-dose SSRI intervention were markedly improved but with much more notable variance seen across studies for the low-dose conditions. The authors believe that more serotonergically selective agents may be more effective for the treatment of anxiety in youth, and they recommend preferentially using SSRIs as first-line agents for the psychopharmacological management of pediatric anxiety disorders (Strawn et al. 2018).

The use of benzodiazepines as first-line agents for the treatment of anxiety in youth is not supported by the research literature. In fact, some youth have a paradoxical response to benzodiazepines, becoming more agitated or disinhibited rather than relaxed or subdued. These agents may be used conservatively when necessary while awaiting a therapeutic response from an SSRI or SNRI that has also been initiated, or as a management strategy for more severe, refractory anxiety.

Depression

Less common in childhood, depression takes a toll during the adolescent years. Prevalence in children is estimated to be approximately 2–3% and climbs to about 8% in teenagers with possibly as many as 20% of all youth experiencing at least one episode of depression by age 18 years (Sakolsky and Birmaher 2012; Varigonda et al. 2015). The disorder impairs academic, family, and social functioning and is associated with recurrent and protracted episodes in adulthood and increased risks of both suicide and substance abuse. Medically compromised youth are especially susceptible to developing a depressive disorder (Bursch and Forgey 2013).

While early intervention is warranted, many depressed youths remain untreated. Evidence-based treatments are available, such as CBT and interpersonal psychotherapy (IPT), and they are highly effective for ameliorating mild to moderate depression. In terms of medication, older tricyclic antidepressants are much less commonly used due to their limited efficacy and notable side effect burden. The SSRIs, followed by SNRIs, have become the primary pharmacological treatments for moderate to severe major depressive disorder (MDD). Fluoxetine is FDA-approved for the treatment of depression in children and adolescents, and escitalopram is approved for the treatment of adolescents only. However, data supporting the medication management of pediatric depression are complicated.

Studies of psychopharmacological interventions for depression in children and adolescents have been plagued by high placebo response rates. The higher placebo response in youth compared to adults may be due to the nature of depression in youth, the therapeutic impact of interactions with study personnel, other research design elements, and/or characteristics of patients and families who enroll in research studies of psychopharmacological treatments for depression. Meta-analyses of the literature demonstrate that fluoxetine has the most favorable risk–benefit profile for the psychopharmacological treatment of depression in children and adolescents (Bursch and Forgey 2013).

The most comprehensive study of depression treatment in youth is the Treatment for Adolescents with Depression Study (TADS), a randomized, placebo-controlled trial evaluating the effectiveness of fluoxetine alone, CBT alone, the combination of fluoxetine and CBT, or placebo for acute (12 weeks) and maintenance (36 weeks) treatment with a naturalistic follow-up period (1 year) in 439 adolescents ages 12–17 years diagnosed with MDD. Over half the sample had at least one other comorbid psychiatric condition (March and Vitiello 2009).

At the end of the acute phase of treatment (12 weeks), the combination of CBT and fluoxetine (response rate 71%) and fluoxetine alone (response rate 61%) were both found to be superior to treatment with CBT alone (response rate 43%) and placebo (response rate 34%). By 18 weeks of treatment, individual interventions trailed behind combination treatment with a response rate of 85% for CBT + fluoxetine and response rates of 69% and 65% for fluoxetine alone and CBT alone, respectively. By the end of the maintenance phase (36 weeks), the three treatment arms had similar response rates: combination treatment had a response rate of 86%, and both fluoxetine and CBT alone demonstrated response rates of 81% (March and Vitiello 2009).

In the TADS study, patients treated with fluoxetine alone were much more likely than those treated with the combination of fluoxetine and CBT, CBT alone, or placebo to report suicidal ideation or experience treatment-related suicidal behavior. Findings suggest that the combination of CBT and fluoxetine is more efficacious than either fluoxetine or CBT alone for the treatment of moderate to severe depression in adolescents (March and Vitiello 2009).

Two other randomized-controlled trials have also demonstrated the efficacy of fluoxetine for the treatment of depression in youth, and studies of other SSRIs have also been pursued. One double-blind, randomized, placebo-controlled trial in 133 children and adolescents spanning 8 weeks compared escitalopram and placebo, finding significantly improved scores in post hoc analysis for adolescents aged 12–17 years but no meaningful difference between escitalopram and placebo in children aged 6–11 years. Headache and abdominal pain were notable side effects in the escitalopram group. Potential suicide-related events were observed in one escitalopram- and two placebo-treated patients. There were no completed suicides (Wagner et al. 2006).

A subsequent 8-week, prospective, randomized, double-blind, placebo-controlled multisite trial with 312 participants examined escitalopram and placebo for the treatment of depression, this time only in adolescents. The response rate was higher for escitalopram (91%) than for placebo, which nonetheless also had a high response rate (76%). Headache, menstrual cramps, insomnia, nausea, and flu-like symptoms were more common in the medication group. The incidence of suicidal ideation was similar for both groups (Emslie et al. 2009).

An 8-week, randomized, double-blind, placebo-controlled study compared the safety and efficacy of citalopram with placebo in the treatment of 174 children and adolescents ages 7–17 years with MDD. The difference in response rate at week 8 between placebo (24%) and citalopram (36%) was statistically significant but of questionable clinical value. Citalopram treatment was reported to be well tolerated. Notable side effects that occurred in either treatment group included rhinitis, nausea, and abdominal pain (Wagner et al. 2004). In a subsequent European, multicenter, double-blind study of 244 adolescents, 13–18 years old, with major depression randomized to treatment with citalopram or placebo, no significant differences in improvement of scores from baseline to week 12 between citalopram and placebo were found. The response rate was 59–61% in both groups (von Knorring et al. 2006).

Sertraline has also been examined for its efficacy in the treatment of depression in youth. Two multicenter randomized, double-blind, placebo-controlled trials were conducted with a total of 376 children and adolescents ages 6–17 years old with MDD. Patients were randomly assigned to receive sertraline or placebo for 10 weeks, and the data from the two trials were pooled a priori as neither trial was significant on its own. Sertraline-treated patients experienced statistically significantly greater improvement than placebo patients, and 69% of sertraline-treated patients compared with 59% of placebo patients were considered responders. Sertraline treatment was generally well tolerated, but diarrhea, vomiting, anorexia, and agitation occurred at least twice as often in the sertraline group as the placebo group (Wagner et al. 2003).

Three randomized, placebo-controlled trials have been conducted evaluating the efficacy of paroxetine for the treatment of depression in youth. No statistically significant differences were observed for paroxetine compared with placebo in any of these trials (Berard et al. 2006; Emslie et al. 2006; Keller et al. 2001).

While there are reported to be statistically higher response rates to medication interventions than to placebo in some of the positive studies above, the frequently high placebo response rates in depression treatment trials reduce the power of these studies to detect a meaningful difference. This high placebo response rate has not been seen in placebo-controlled trials for youth with anxiety or other psychiatric conditions. A meta-analysis of 27 randomized, placebo-controlled, parallel-group trials of antidepressants with 5310 participants younger than 19 years of age was published by Bridge and coworkers in 2007. They concluded that relative to placebo, antidepressants are efficacious for pediatric MDD, OCD, and non-OCD anxiety disorders, with the strongest effects in non-OCD anxiety disorders, intermediate effects in OCD, and more modest effects in MDD (Bridge et al. 2007).

Systematic reviews indicate that prior estimates of SSRI efficacy for the treatment of depression may have been artificially inflated. A recent meta-analysis evaluating the efficacy of SSRIs for the treatment of MDD involved 13 pediatric depression placebo-controlled trials with a total of 3004 patients. Five different SSRIs were assessed in these studies: fluoxetine, paroxetine, sertraline, citalopram, and escitalopram. Treatment gains were found to occur early during the course of intervention, as early as 2 weeks after medication initiation but to be minimal after 4 weeks of medication treatment. Maximizing dosing did not appear to impact the results. All SSRIs examined appeared equally effective and were found to have lower potency for the treatment of depression in children and adolescents compared to adults (Varigonda et al. 2015).

Randomized-controlled trials assessing the safety and efficacy of SNRIs for the treatment of

MDD in children and adolescents have also been pursued. Xu et al. conducted the first meta-analysis of five such trials, published between 1997 and 2014, with a total of 973 patients ages 7–17 years with MDD who were prescribed duloxetine (three trials), venlafaxine extended release (two trials), or placebo. The treatment response to SNRI intervention was not demonstrated to be superior to placebo. More frequent side effects for SNRIs compared to placebo were found including abdominal pain, dizziness, nausea, headache, and nasopharyngitis. Many more patients administered with SNRIs dropped out of these studies due to adverse effects than did those receiving placebo. There was evidence of increased suicide risk for venlafaxine extended release compared to placebo as well (Xu et al. 2016).

A meta-analysis published in 2016 by Cipriani and colleagues involved 34 available randomized, double-blind, placebo-controlled studies conducted between 1986 and 2014 including a total of 5260 children and adolescents enrolled for the acute treatment of MDD. Trials with 14 antidepressant medications were represented: amitriptyline, citalopram, clomipramine, desipramine, duloxetine, escitalopram, fluoxetine, imipramine, mirtazapine, nefazodone, nortriptyline, paroxetine, sertraline, and venlafaxine. Studies included patients with comorbid non-mood psychiatric disorders. Fluoxetine, sertraline, and escitalopram proved to have statistical efficacy greater than placebo for the treatment of depression, but only fluoxetine appeared to be markedly more effective than placebo, with a medium effect size. Fluoxetine was also found to be the best tolerated medication. An analysis of venlafaxine data suggested a concerningly increased risk for suicidal ideation or behavior compared to placebo, and five other antidepressants: fluoxetine, escitalopram, imipramine, duloxetine, and paroxetine (Cipriani et al. 2016).

In light of treatment studies in child and adolescent depression, psychotherapy, such as CBT or IPT, should be the first-line treatment pursued whenever feasible. If not medically contraindicated due to medication interactions or prior lack of response to an adequate trial, fluoxetine should be the first-line psychopharmacological agent pursued when therapy is unavailable, symptoms are refractory to therapy alone, or when combination treatment with CBT is being initiated for moderate to severe depression. More research into safe and effective pharmacological interventions for depression in youth is needed.

Posttraumatic Stress Disorder (PTSD)

A child or adolescent's perception of the severity of his or her medical condition is a consistent predictor of posttraumatic stress disorder (PTSD). The development of PTSD, in turn, has a significant negative impact on an individual's quality of life and ability to recuperate and function in the context of medical illness or injury. Several studies with adolescents have shown that the greater the severity of baseline or ongoing traumatic stress symptoms, the lower the reported quality-of-life measures (Rzucidlo and Campbell 2009). Developmental trajectories of traumatized youth are negatively impacted with developmental arrest or regression in some. Academic and social problems are notable, and comorbid depression, anxiety, impulsivity, aggression, poor emotion regulation, and disruptive behavior are common. There is an increased risk for suicide, self-injury, substance abuse, and criminality among older children and adolescents.

PTSD is currently conceptualized as a constellation of symptoms in various broad domains, including avoidance, intrusive re-experiencing, negative alterations in cognitions and mood, and hyperarousal. Specific target symptoms for intervention also include irritability, angry outbursts, poor concentration, and sleep disturbances. The underlying pathophysiology of PTSD involves changes in catecholamine (dopamine, norepinephrine, and epinephrine) secretion and hypothalamic-pituitary-adrenal (HPA) axis dysregulation. Alterations of other neurotransmitter systems also appear to contribute to the development of symptoms, including serotonin, gamma-aminobutyric acid (GABA), and corticotropin-releasing factor (CRF). Therefore, treatments that attenuate adrenergic responses, decrease dopaminergic activity, and/or increase serotonin availability hold promise.

The first-line treatment for youth with PTSD continues to be psychotherapy, especially trauma-focused CBT, with a focus on ensuring safety, providing psychoeducation, developing coping and behavior management strategies, overcoming avoidance through exposure and use of the trauma narrative, and engaging parents and other family members (Keeshin and Strawn 2014). There is limited data for the use of medications in pediatric PTSD, and psychopharmacologic interventions to date continue to be largely based on data from medication trials in adults with PTSD. Notable pediatric data follow.

SSRIs are considered among the first-line pharmacological interventions for PTSD symptoms in adults with many studies supporting their use. Trials in children and adolescents have been less promising than those in the adult literature. Seedat et al. (2001, 2002) conducted two open-label trials of the safety and tolerability of the SSRI citalopram in youth, first in eight and subsequently in 24 participants with PTSD. Both studies demonstrated improvement in symptoms of re-experiencing, avoidance, and hyperarousal.

The first double-blind placebo-controlled trial of SSRI for pediatric PTSD, conducted by Cohen et al. (2007), examined the use of sertraline or placebo as adjunctive therapy for 24 female patients ages 10–17 years old receiving trauma-focused CBT over 12 weeks. While a medium effect size was associated with sertraline use, the study concluded that there was no notable difference between the sertraline and placebo groups. Because trauma-focused CBT is a potent treatment for PTSD, the difference between the sertraline and placebo arms may have been difficult to detect in this small study. A subsequent, larger multisite placebo-controlled 10-week trial of 131 youth with PTSD, however, also failed to demonstrate a notable difference between sertraline and placebo (Robb et al. 2010).

Given the putative noradrenergic hyperactivity in PTSD, the alpha agonists, guanfacine and clonidine, the alpha antagonist prazosin, and the beta-blocker propranolol have each been studied in alleviating symptoms of the disorder. The alpha-2-agonists decrease central norepinephrine release. A small, 8-week, open-label study evaluating guanfacine extended-release in 19 pediatric patients with comorbid attention-deficit/hyperactivity disorder (ADHD) and PTSD symptoms found the medication to be well tolerated with a decrease in symptoms of re-experiencing, avoidance, and hyperarousal (Connor et al. 2013). Case-series also suggest that guanfacine immediate release may be effective for the treatment of PTSD symptoms in youth, specifically nightmares.

Clonidine immediate release has been shown in case reports to mitigate symptoms of re-experiencing trauma in children, including nightmares, as well as hyperarousal, including hypervigilance, sleep disruption, and exaggerated startle responses. One open-label trial of clonidine immediate release in a day hospital setting in seven treatment refractory children ages 3–6 years demonstrated notable improvement (Harmon and Riggs 1996). Seventeen children with PTSD experienced decreases in trauma-related symptoms in another open-label trial of clonidine (Perry 1994).

Alpha-1-antagonists and centrally acting beta-antagonists mitigate the effects of norepinephrine postsynaptically and reduce sympathetic tone. While there are multiple placebo-controlled trials of the use of prazosin in adults for the treatment of PTSD symptoms, there are no open-label or placebo-controlled trials in the pediatric population. A small number of case reports, however, do suggest that the medication may be effective (Brooks and Strawn 2014).

The beta-blocker propranolol has been studied in youth. One small pilot study of 11 children ages 6–12 years treated with propranolol for PTSD over 4 weeks demonstrated a significant reduction in PTSD symptoms, aggression, and insomnia (Famularo et al. 1988). A more recent pilot study evaluated 10 days of propranolol or placebo administration within 12 h of accidental trauma in 29 children and adolescents aged 10–18 years as secondary prevention for PTSD symptom development. At 6 weeks follow-up, there were no differences in the number of patients meeting full or subthreshold criteria for PTSD in the propranolol versus placebo group (Nugent 2007).

Second-generation antipsychotics are used clinically to treat various disorders and symptoms such as psychosis, mania, tics, mood instability, impulsivity, aggression, agitation, and irritability. Second-generation antipsychotics have been examined in the treatment of PTSD symptoms as well in adults and children. Adult studies show promise, particularly for reducing intrusive re-experiencing, but the data in children and adolescents are limited. Several pediatric case reports of risperidone are found in the literature. In three preschool-aged children with acute stress disorder symptoms, improvement in intrusive, hyperarousal, and avoidance symptoms was reported within the first 2 days of treatment with risperidone (Meighen et al. 2007).

In one small open-label trial of risperidone in 18 youth, 13 experienced a remission of PTSD symptoms; however, comorbid mood disorders were present in many of the participants, suggesting that some of the noted improvement was due to improvement in the co-occurring mood disorder, rather than within the bonafide PTSD symptoms (Horrigan and Barnhill 1999). Finally, a small 6-week open-label study of quetiapine in six adolescents ages 15–17 years old found the medication to be well tolerated and to reduce symptoms of PTSD as well as anxiety, depression, and anger (Stathis et al. 2005).

The antiepileptic mood stabilizers have been examined in the adult PTSD literature as well and have limited data in the pediatric population. In one open-label study of youth ages 8–17 years old with PTSD receiving residential treatment, carbamazepine titrated to serum levels of 10–11.5 μg/mL, led to symptom resolution in 22 of the 28 treated patients and symptom reduction in the remaining six patients. Carbamazepine was well tolerated with no reported side effects. Patients were discharged to community care on their remission doses of carbamazepine (Looff et al. 1995). In a pilot trial of 12 adolescent males 15–17 years old with comorbid PTSD and conduct disorder, high-dose or low-dose divalproex was randomly administered. The intervention was well tolerated, and those who received high-dose divalproex experienced clinical improvement (Steiner et al. 2007).

There are no notable clinical trials supporting the use of benzodiazepines for the treatment of PTSD in youth. Benzodiazepines used during acute traumas, such as medical procedures, may in fact potentiate trauma symptoms and make recovery after trauma exposure more difficult (Zohar et al. 2011). They furthermore increase the risk of delirium, interfere with normal sleep, may cause paradoxical agitation and disinhibition in youth, and have the potential to be abused or lead to dependence (Bursch and Forgey 2013).

While evidence for the use of SSRI and SNRI medications for the treatment of PTSD alone or in combination with other evidence-based interventions such as trauma-focused CBT is limited, given the comorbidity of the disorder with depression and anxiety, the use of SSRI or SNRI may be substantiated on a case-by-case basis. There may also be a role for antiadrenergic agents, especially in the management of intrusive re-experiencing and hyperarousal symptoms. Some evidence for the second-generation antipsychotic agents and antiepileptic mood stabilizers is also found in the literature, and the risks and benefits of their use must be weighed carefully in each patient given the potential side effect burden. More research into safe and effective pharmacological interventions for PTSD in youth is needed.

Psychopharmacologic Interventions: Evaluation

Children and adolescents should receive a complete psychiatric evaluation before psychotropic medication is prescribed. A comprehensive evaluation is critical to developing a full understanding of problematic symptoms, underlying diagnoses, and the biopsychosocial context in which these difficulties occur to determine if medication is warranted. The best diagnostic tool for mental health related conditions is a thorough history, which typically involves an interview with parents or guardians, an interview and observation of the child or adolescent, conversations with other professionals, including medical providers and teachers, and a review of medical records. The risks and benefits of administering any specific medication to any particular patient and the rationale for its use, especially in those combating medical illness and being treated with other pharmacological agents, must be recognized and addressed. A clear understanding of the clinical picture is essential.

The patient's history must include a narrative of the major concerns, prior mental health problems or interventions, medical and surgical history, list of allergies, current medications, family psychiatric history, and the child or adolescent's developmental history and academic, social, and family functioning. Collateral sources of information are critical to a pediatric evaluation, such as teachers, tutors, and coaches. Both parents/guardians and the patient himself or herself should be interviewed. Younger children may not be able to articulate much about their inner experiences, but observations of their behavior and interactions with parents and others are highly instructive. Medical personnel involved in the management of the youngster's medical condition may also be invaluable reporters of emotional and behavioral concerns in a child or adolescent.

Rating scale/questionnaire data bolster the diagnosis and further inform the clinician regarding the most debilitating symptoms. Anxiety questionnaires that may be helpful include the Multidimensional Anxiety Scale for Child Anxiety-Related Disorders (MASC) and Screen for Anxiety Related Emotional Disorders (SCARED) (March et al. 1997; Birmaher et al. 1999). Depression questionnaires commonly used include the Children's Depression Inventory (CDI), Hamilton Depression Rating Scale (Ham-D), and Beck Depression Inventory (BDI) (Kovacs 1985; Hamilton 1960; Beck et al. 1961). For PTSD, the Child Posttraumatic Symptom Scale (CPSS) and UCLA PTSD Reaction Index are commonly used (Foa et al. 2001; Steinberg et al. 2004). Good comprehensive questionnaires soliciting symptoms in multiple domains include the Achenbach, also known as the Child Behavior Checklist (CBCL), and the Youth Self Report (YSR) (Achenbach 1991a, b). Rating scales provide quantifiable baseline data, such as frequency and intensity of symptoms. Questionnaires can also be used to measure treatment response over time.

Neurological, laboratory, and neuroimaging assessments are typically found to be normal and are generally not diagnostic. Nonetheless, baseline physical exam and laboratories including a comprehensive metabolic panel, complete blood count (CBC), thyroid panel, lead level, vitamin D level, vitamin B12 level, folic acid level, and in adolescents a pregnancy test and urine toxicology screen for drugs of abuse should be considered to rule-out possible underlying medical conditions. Biological testing should be completed before the initiation of psychopharmacotherapy to establish baseline values for potential future monitoring of the treatment. Some medications require a baseline and follow-up electrocardiogram (ECG) as well to monitor cardiac status.

Psychopharmacologic Interventions: Treatment

Medication management of psychiatric disorders is individualized and tailored to the specific needs of the patient. The most distressing or impairing symptoms should be targeted first. Clinicians are encouraged to carefully consider the target symptoms for treatment and what psychopharmacologic, psychotherapeutic, and other interventions may be necessary. Once it is decided to treat a child or adolescent with psychotropic medication, the clinician must discuss various aspects of treatment with the patient and/or their family. These points are delineated in Box 11.1 below.

Box 11.1: Treatment Discussion with Patients and Families

- Medication options to treat target symptoms and diagnoses AND non-pharmacological alternatives
- Possible risks, side effects, and benefits
- Therapeutic dosage range of medication
- Medication schedule and dose titration
- Duration of treatment to achieve an effect
- Emergency/adverse drug reaction plan
- Anticipated length of treatment

Once a medication is chosen, a full trial should be administered with adequate doses and duration of treatment. Medication management should focus on target symptoms as well as diagnoses. Successful treatment requires education of and collaboration with the family and other providers.

Clinical management of the patient being treated with psychotropic medication should monitor target symptoms and the need for any additional or different interventions, provide ongoing support to the patient and family, continue to educate the patient and family about the psychiatric condition and/or symptoms being treated, evaluate the need for school interventions and supports, and evaluate the need for any case management services.

Medication is always initiated at the lowest dose with gradual titration. Whenever possible, a single medication (monotherapy) should be used. More than one agent may occasionally need to be prescribed simultaneously (targeted combined pharmacotherapy) when monotherapy has not been efficacious or has resulted in limiting side effects, or when there are multiple target symptoms or more than one disorder is being treated. In general, it is recommended to wait a few weeks after a dose initiation or adjustment before drawing conclusions about therapeutic response and before making additional adjustments.

Special Pharmacological Considerations in Youth with Medical Conditions

SSRIs may impact platelet function, which should be considered in youth with hematologic dysfunction or with any condition or treatment that affects platelet count or action. SSRIs, SNRIs, and numerous other pharmacological agents that raise serotonin levels in the body, including certain antibiotics (e.g., linezolid), anti-migraine medications (e.g., triptans), anti-nausea medications (e.g., ondansetron), pain medications (e.g., oxycodone, tramadol), and anti-retroviral agents used to treat HIV/AIDS (e.g., ritonavir), have the potential to cause a serious acute medical problem, serotonin syndrome, alone or in combination. The symptoms of serotonin syndrome may vary in presentation and severity and may include myoclonus, hyperthermia, tachycardia, hypertension, diaphoresis, hyperreflexia, tremor, dilated pupils, diarrhea, ataxia, seizures, confusion, agitation, and loss of consciousness. Severe serotonin syndrome can be life threatening, and treatment should be pursued carefully to avoid this serious medical complication.

While fluoxetine is FDA-approved for the treatment of depression in youth and is effective for its treatment and that of the anxiety disorders, it is an agent with a long half-life and a potent inhibitor of cytochrome P450 2D6. Therefore, despite the research evidence regarding its success in treating anxiety and depressive disorders, it should be used cautiously in the medically ill population given the potential for medication interactions. Agents such as sertraline, citalopram, or escitalopram may be considered first line in youth with medical disorders given fewer medication interactions, but citalopram should be avoided in those at risk for QT prolongation, especially when a dose higher than 40 mg is likely to be necessary. Those with congestive heart failure, arrhythmias, or predisposition to hypokalemia or hypomagnesemia due to illness or medication are at higher risk of developing torsade de pointes and should be closely monitored if prescribed citalopram or some second-generation antipsychotic agents also known to cause QT prolongation (Bursch and Forgey 2013; Sakolsky and Birmaher 2012).

Propranolol should not be used in children with asthma, and it should be used cautiously in those with diabetes as it may mask signs of hypoglycemia.

Summary

Children and adolescents demonstrate variable psychological vulnerability to the impact of acute and chronic medical conditions. Furthermore, acute and chronic medical interventions may be as traumatizing for youth as the disorders they are meant to evaluate and/or treat. There are numerous cases of illness-related and iatrogenic trauma in the literature with affected children and adolescents experiencing anxiety, depressive, and trauma-related symptoms. The psychotherapies, especially cognitive-behavioral therapy (CBT), are first-line interventions in mild to moderate cases. Moderate to severe presentations often require treatment with psychopharmacological medications as well.

While medications have been shown to be effective for the management of anxiety, depressive symptoms, and posttraumatic stress, there is little direct evidence for the use of first-line agents, such as SSRIs or SNRIs, in youth coping with medical problems. The indications for their use are based primarily on research in youth with a primary psychiatric condition in the absence of medical illness.

A recent systematic review and meta-analysis examined the safety and efficacy of SSRIs and SNRIs in those younger than 18 years of age for the treatment of depressive disorders, anxiety disorders, OCD, and PTSD by examining 36 randomized, double-blind trials that met eligibility criteria with a total of 6778 participants (Locher et al. 2017). No significant conclusions could be drawn about the treatment of PTSD, as only one of the studies involved psychopharmacological intervention for this disorder. SSRIs and SNRIs were found to be more beneficial than placebo for the treatment of anxiety disorders. Response to these agents was not notably superior to placebo for depressive disorders, however. Furthermore, side effects were more common than with placebo (Locher et al. 2017). These findings are humbling, emphasize the need for more research and novel psychopharmacologic treatment strategies, and underscore the need for psychotherapeutic interventions to treat PTSD, anxiety, and depressive symptoms such as CBT.

When medications are needed for moderate to severe presentations, there is ample research data to support the use of the SSRI and SNRI medications for the anxiety disorders. Less data is available for their use in depression, with fluoxetine being a standout agent in research and meta-analyses. The empirical evidence is most scant in the area of trauma and stressor-related disorders, such as PTSD. Nonetheless, various agents have been studied and show promise, including the antidepressants, alpha-2-agonists, the alpha-1-antagonist prazosin, the beta-blocker propranolol, second-generation antipsychotics, and anticonvulsant mood stabilizers.

Psychopharmacological agents can be used safely and effectively when a thoughtful evaluation of patients is conducted to gain a comprehensive understanding of the need for intervention as well as possible risks and negative interactions. Medication should be prescribed along with other psychosocial interventions, ongoing education and support, and collaboration with all involved in the care of the child or adolescent being treated.

References

Achenbach, T. M. (1991a). *Manual for the child behavior checklist/ 4–18 and 1991 profile*. Burlington, VT: University of Vermont, Department of Psychiatry.

Achenbach, T. M. (1991b). *Manual for the youth self-report and 1991 profile*. Burlington, VT: University of Vermont, Department of Psychiatry.

Beck, A. T., Ward, C. H., Mendelson, M., Mock, J., & Erbaugh, J. (1961). An inventory for measuring depression. *Archives of General Psychiatry, 4*, 561–571.

Berard, R., Fong, R., Carpenter, D. J., Thomason, C., & Wilkinson, C. (2006). An international, multicenter, placebo-controlled trial of paroxetine in adolescents with major depressive disorder. *Journal of Child and Adolescent Psychopharmacology, 16*(1–2), 59–75.

Birmaher, B., Brent, D. A., Chiappetta, L., Bridge, J., Monga, S., & Baugher, M. (1999). Psychometric properties of the screen for child anxiety related emotional disorders (SCARED): A replication study. *Journal of the American Academy of Child and Adolescent Psychiatry, 38*(10), 1230–1236.

Birmaher, B., Axelson, D. A., Monk, K., Kalas, C., Clark, D. B., Ehmann, M., et al. (2003). Fluoxetine for the treatment of childhood anxiety disorders. *Journal of the American Academy of Child and Adolescent Psychiatry, 42*(4), 415–423.

Bridge, J. A., Iyengar, S., Salary, C. B., Barbe, R. P., Birmaher, B., Pincus, H. A., et al. (2007). Clinical response and risk for reported suicidal ideation and suicide attempts in pediatric antidepressant treatment: A meta-analysis of randomized controlled trials. *Journal of the American Medical Association, 297*(15), 1683–1696.

Brooks, R. K., & Strawn, J. R. (2014). Psychological and pharmacologic treatment of youth with posttraumatic stress disorder-an evidence-based review. *Child and*

Adolescent Psychiatric Clinics of North America, 23, 399–411.

Brosbe, M. S., Faust, J., & Gold, S. N. (2013). Complex traumatic stress in the pediatric medical setting. *Journal of Trauma & Dissociation, 14,* 97–112.

Brown, L. K., Kennard, B. D., Emslie, G. J., Mayes, T. L., Whiteley, L. B., Bethel, J., et al. (2016). Effective treatment of depressive disorders in medical clinics for adolescents and young adults living with HIV: A controlled trial. *Journal of Acquired Immune Deficiency Syndromes, 71*(1), 38–46.

Bursch, B., & Forgey, M. (2013). Psychopharmacology for medically ill adolescents. *Current Psychiatry Reports, 15*(10), 395.

Cipriani, A., Zhou, X., Del Giovane, C., Hetrick, S. E., Qin, B., Whittington, C., et al. (2016). Comparative efficacy and tolerability of antidepressants for major depressive disorder in children and adolescents: A network meta-analysis. *Lancet, 388,* 881–890.

Cohen, J. A., Mannarino, A. P., Perel, J. M., & Staron, V. (2007). A pilot randomized controlled trial of combined trauma-focused CBT and sertraline for childhood PTSD symptoms. *Journal of the American Academy of Child and Adolescent Psychiatry, 46*(7), 811–819.

Connor, D. F., Grasso, D. J., Slivinsky, M. D., Pearson, G. S., & Banga, A. (2013). An open-label study of guanfacine extended release for traumatic stress related symptoms in children and adolescents. *Journal of Child and Adolescent Psychopharmacology, 23*(4), 244–251.

Creswell, C., & Waite, P. (2016). Recent developments in the treatment of anxiety disorders in children and adolescents. *Evidence-Based Mental Health, 19*(3), 65–68.

Emslie, G. J., Wagner, K. D., Kutcher, S., Krulewicz, S., Fong, R., Carpenter, D. J., et al. (2006). Paroxetine treatment in children and adolescents with major depressive disorder: A randomized, multicenter, double-blind, placebo-controlled trial. *Journal of the American Academy of Child and Adolescent Psychiatry, 45*(6), 709–719.

Emslie, G. J., Ventura, D., Korotzer, A., Tourkodimitris, S., et al. (2009). Escitalopram in the treatment of adolescent depression: A randomized placebo-controlled multisite trial. *Journal of the American Academy of Child and Adolescent Psychiatry, 48*(7), 721–729.

Famularo, R., Kinscherff, R., & Fenton, T. (1988). Propranolol treatment for childhood posttraumatic stress disorder, acute type. A pilot study. *The American Journal of Diseases of Children, 142*(11), 1244–1247.

Foa, E. B., Johnson, K. M., Feeny, N. C., & Treadwell, K. R. H. (2001). The child PTSD symptom scale: A preliminary examination of its psychometric properties. *Journal of Clinical Child Psychology, 30*(3), 376–384.

Gibbons, R. D., Brown, C. H., Hur, K., Marcus, S. M., Bhaumik, D. K., Erkens, J. A., et al. (2007). Early evidence on the effects of regulators' suicidality warnings on SSRI prescriptions and suicide in children and adolescents. *American Journal of Psychiatry, 164*(9), 1356–1363.

Hamilton, M. (1960). A rating scale for depression. *Journal of Neurology, Neurosurgery, and Psychiatry, 23,* 56–62.

Hammad, T. A., Laughren, T., & Racoosin, J. (2006). Suicidality in pediatric patients treated with antidepressant drugs. *Archives of General Psychiatry, 63*(3), 332–339.

Harmon, R. J., & Riggs, P. D. (1996). Clonidine for posttraumatic stress disorder in preschool children. *Journal of the American Academy of Child and Adolescent Psychiatry, 35,* 1247–1249.

Horrigan, J. P., & Barnhill, L. J. (1999). Risperidone and PTSD in boys. *The Journal of Neuropsychiatry and Clinical Neurosciences, 11,* 126–127.

Ipser, J. C., Stein, D. J., Hawkridge, S., & Hoppe, L. (2010). Pharmacotherapy for anxiety disorders in children and adolescents (review). *The Cochrane Collaboration, 6,* 1–72.

Keeshin, B. R., & Strawn, J. R. (2014). Psychological and pharmacologic treatment of youth with posttraumatic stress disorder: an evidence-based review. *Child and Adolescent Psychiatric Clinics of North America, 23*(2), 399–411.

Keller, M. B., Ryan, N. D., Strober, M., Klein, R. G., Kutcher, S. P., Birmaher, B., et al. (2001). Efficacy of paroxetine in the treatment of adolescent major depression: A randomized, controlled trial. *Journal of the American Academy of Child and Adolescent Psychiatry, 40*(7), 762–772.

Kolves, K., & De Leo, D. (2016). Adolescent suicide rates between 1990 and 2009: Analysis of age group 15-19 years worldwide. *Journal of Adolescent Health, 58,* 69–77.

Kovacs, M. (1985). The children's depression inventory (CDI). *Psychopharmacology Bulletin, 21*(4), 995–998.

Locher, C., Koechlin, H., Zion, S. R., Werner, C., Pine, D. S., Kirsch, I., et al. (2017). Efficacy and safety of serotonin reuptake inhibitors, serotonin-norepinephrine reuptake inhibitors, and placebo for common psychiatric disorders among children and adolescents: A systematic review and meta-analysis. *JAMA Psychiatry, 74*(10), 1011–1020.

Looff, D., Grimley, P., Kuller, F., Martin, A., & Shonfield, L. (1995). Carbamazepine for PTSD. *Journal of the American Academy of Child and Adolescent Psychiatry, 34*(6), 703–704.

March, J. S., & Vitiello, B. (2009). Clinical messages from the treatment for adolescents with depression study (TADS). *American Journal of Psychiatry, 166*(10), 1118–1123.

March, J. S., Parker, J. D. A., Sullivan, K., Stallings, P., & Conners, C. K. (1997). The multidimensional anxiety scale for children (MASC): Factor structure, reliability, and validity. *Journal of the American Academy of Child and Adolescent Psychiatry, 36*(4), 554–565.

Meighen, K. G., Hines, L. A., & Lagges, A. M. (2007). Risperidone treatment of preschool children with thermal burns and acute stress disorder. *Journal of*

Child and Adolescent Psychopharmacology, 17(2), 223–232.

Merikangas, K. R., He, J. P., Burstein, M., Swanson, S. A., Avenevoli, S., Cui, L., et al. (2010). Lifetime prevalence of mental disorders in us adolescents: Results from the national comorbidity survey replication—Adolescent supplement (NCS-A). *Journal of the American Academy of Child and Adolescent Psychiatry, 49*, 980–989.

Nugent, N. R. (2007). *The efficacy of early propranolol administration at preventing/reducing PTSD symptoms in child trauma victims: Pilot*. Dissertation, Kent State University.

Park, E. M., & Rosenstein, D. L. (2015). Depression in adolescents and young adults with cancer. *Dialogues in Clinical Neuroscience, 17*(2), 171–180.

Perry, B. D. (1994). Neurobiological sequelae of childhood trauma: PTSD in children. In M. M. Murburg (Ed.), *Catecholamine function in posttraumatic stress disorder: Emerging concepts* (pp. 233–255). Washington, DC: American Psychiatric Press.

Piacentini, J., Bennett, S., Compton, S. N., Kendall, P. C., Birmaher, B., Albano, A. M., et al. (2014). 24- and 36-week outcomes for the child/adolescent anxiety multimodal study (CAMS). *Journal of the American Academy of Child and Adolescent Psychiatry, 53*(3), 297–310.

Robb, A. S., Cueva, J. E., Sporn, J., Yang, R., & Vanderburg, D. G. (2010). Sertraline treatment of children and adolescents with posttraumatic stress disorder: A double-blind, placebo-controlled trial. *Journal of Child and Adolescent Psychopharmacology, 20*(6), 463–471.

Rynn, M. A., Riddle, M. A., Yeung, P. P., & Kunz, N. R. (2007). Efficacy and safety of extended-release venlafaxine in the treatment of generalized anxiety disorder in children and adolescents: Two placebo-controlled trials. *American Journal of Psychiatry, 164*(2), 290–300.

Rzucidlo, S. E., & Campbell, M. (2009). Beyond the physical injuries: Child and parent coping with medical traumatic stress after pediatric trauma. *Journal of Trauma Nursing, 16*(3), 130–135.

Sakolsky, D., & Birmaher, B. (2012). Developmentally informed pharmacotherapy for child and adolescent depressive disorders. *Psychiatric Clinics of North America, 21*, 313–325.

Seedat, S., Lockhat, R., Kaminer, D., Zungu-Dirwayi, N., & Stein, D. J. (2001). An open trial of citalopram in adolescents with post-traumatic stress disorder. *International Clinical Psychopharmacology, 16*(1), 21–25.

Seedat, S., Stein, D. J., Ziervogel, C., Middleton, T., Kaminer, D., Emsley, R. A., et al. (2002). Comparison of response to a selective serotonin reuptake inhibitor in children, adolescents, and adults with posttraumatic stress disorder. *Journal of Child and Adolescent Psychopharmacology, 12*(1), 37–46.

Shatkin, J. P. (2015). *Child & adolescent mental health- a practical, all-in-one guide* (2nd ed.). New York: W.W. Norton.

Stathis, S., Martin, G., & McKenna, J. G. (2005). A preliminary case series on the use of quetiapine for posttraumatic stress disorder in juveniles within a youth detention center. *Journal of Clinical Psychopharmacology, 25*(6), 539–544.

Steinberg, A. M., Brymer, M., Decker, K., & Pynoos, R. S. (2004). The University of California at Los Angeles post-traumatic stress disorder reaction index. *Current Psychiatry Reports, 6*, 96–100.

Steiner, H., Saxena, K. S., Carrion, V., Khanzode, L. A., Silverman, M., & Chang, K. (2007). Divalproex sodium for the treatment of PTSD and conduct disordered youth: A pilot randomized controlled clinical trial. *Child Psychiatry and Human Development, 38*(3), 183–193.

Strawn, J. R., Prakash, A., Zhang, Q., Pangallo, B. A., Stroud, C. E., Cai, N., et al. (2015a). A randomized, placebo-controlled study of duloxetine for the treatment of children and adolescents with generalized anxiety disorder. *Journal of the American Academy of Child and Adolescent Psychiatry, 54*(4), 283–293.

Strawn, J. R., Welge, J. A., Wehry, A. M., Keeshin, B. R., & Rynn, M. A. (2015b). Efficacy and tolerability of antidepressants in pediatric anxiety disorders: A systematic review and meta-analysis. *Depression and Anxiety, 32*(3), 149–157.

Strawn, J. R., Mills, J. A., Sauley, B. A., & Welge, J. A. (2018). The impact of antidepressant dose and class on treatment response in pediatric anxiety disorders: A meta-analysis. *Journal of the American Academy of Child and Adolescent Psychiatry, 57*(4), 235–244.

The Research Unit on Pediatric Psychopharmacology Anxiety Study Group. (2001). Fluvoxamine for the treatment of anxiety disorders in children and adolescents. *New England Journal of Medicine, 344*(17), 1279–1285.

Uthman, O. A., & Abdulmalik, J. (2010). Comparative efficacy and acceptability of pharmacotherapeutic agents for anxiety disorders in children and adolescents: A mixed treatment comparison meta-analysis. *Current Medical Research and Opinion, 26*(1), 53–59.

Varigonda, A. L., Jakubovski, E., Taylor, M. J., Freemantle, N., Coughlin, C., & Bloch, M. H. (2015). Systematic review and meta-analysis: Early treatment responses of selective serotonin reuptake inhibitors in pediatric major depressive disorder. *Journal of the American Academy of Child and Adolescent Psychiatry, 54*(7), 557–564.

von Knorring, A. L., Olsson, G. I., Thomsen, P. H., Lemming, O. M., & Hulten, A. (2006). A randomized, double-blind, placebo-controlled study of citalopram in adolescents with major depressive disorder. *Journal of Clinical Psychopharmacology, 26*(3), 311–315.

Wagner, K. D., Ambrosini, P., Rynn, M., Wohlberg, C., Yang, R., Greenbaum, M. S., et al. (2003). Efficacy of sertraline in the treatment of children and adolescents with major depressive disorder: Two randomized controlled trials. *Journal of the American Medical Association, 290*(8), 1033–1041.

Wagner, K. D., Robb, A. S., Findling, R. L., Jin, J., Gutierrez, M. M., & Heydorn, W. E. (2004). A randomized, placebo-controlled trial of citalopram for the treatment of major depression in children and adolescents. *American Journal of Psychiatry, 161*(6), 1079–1083.

Wagner, K. D., Jonas, J., Findling, R. L., Ventura, D., & Saikali, K. (2006). A double-blind, randomized, placebo-controlled trial of escitalopram in the treatment of pediatric depression. *Journal of the American Academy of Child and Adolescent Psychiatry, 45*(3), 280–288.

Walkup, J. T., Albano, A. M., Piacentini, J., Birmaher, B., Compton, S. N., Sherrill, J. T., et al. (2008). Cognitive behavioral therapy, sertraline, or a combination in childhood anxiety. *New England Journal of Medicine, 359*(26), 2753–2766.

Xu, Y., Bai, S. J., Lan, X. H., Qin, B., Huang, T., & Xie, P. (2016). Randomized controlled trials of serotonin-norepinephrine reuptake inhibitor in treating major depressive disorder in children and adolescents: A meta-analysis of efficacy and acceptability. *Brazilian Journal of Medical and Biological Research, 49*(6), 1–8.

Zohar, J., Juven-Wetzler, A., Sonnino, R., Cwikel-Hamzany, S., Balaban, E., & Cohen, H. (2011). New insights into secondary prevention in post-traumatic stress disorder. *Dialogues in Clinical Neuroscience, 13*(3), 301–309.

Part II

Working with Specific Populations

Cognitive Behavioral Therapy in Primary Care

12

Carisa Parrish and Kathryn Van Eck

Due to the extent of individuals with co-occurring physical and behavioral problems, behavioral health integration with primary care has been recommended to improve the availability of effective services by increasing access to behavioral specialists. Most children see a primary care provider each year (Stancin and Perrin 2014), making the pediatric primary care setting a natural place to provide links and access to behavioral health services for youth. Patient-centered medical homes have become the ideal model for providing optimal care (American Academy of Family Physicians (AAFP), American Academy of Pediatrics (AAP), American College of Physicians (ACP), and American Osteopathic Association (AOA) 2007) for both physical and behavioral health. Medical homes are most effective when multidisciplinary clinical teams deliver evidence-based, scientifically informed, comprehensive approaches to diagnosis and treatment. The Joint Principles of the Patient-Centered Medical Home was amended in 2014 to emphasize the importance of integrating behavioral health to create comprehensive, whole-person care housed in the primary care setting (Working Party Group on Integrated Behavioral Healthcare et al. 2014).

The Argument for Integrated Care Models

Childhood is a critical time for the development of emotional and behavioral problems. Thus, identifying and treating these concerns quickly and effectively is vital for minimizing their long-term impact. More than half of adults diagnosed with mental health problems have been shown to display symptoms prior to the age of 14 years (Anda et al. 2007; Jones 2013; Kessler et al. 2005). In particular, the preponderance of youth with attention deficit/hyperactivity disorder (ADHD) demonstrates symptoms prior to the age of 12 years (Polanczyk et al. 2010); similarly, oppositional defiant disorder (ODD) typically emerges in childhood, although onset for conduct disorder (CD) occurs during early adolescence (Maughan et al. 2004). Thus, working with pediatricians to identify behavioral problems during childhood is critical for fostering a positive developmental trajectory for youth.

Rates of suicidal behavior increase as children move into adolescence, as does the preva-

C. Parrish (✉) · K. Van Eck
Division of Child and Adolescent Psychiatry,
Department of Psychiatry and Behavioral Sciences,
Johns Hopkins University School of Medicine,
Baltimore, MD, USA
e-mail: cparris5@jhmi.edu

lence of several additional emotional and behavioral challenges. Suicidal behavior, which is the second leading cause of death among youth, is a significant mental health problem with impact on both childhood and adolescence. About 20–24% of youth struggle with suicidal behavior (Nock et al. 2008). Although the average age of onset for substance use disorders is approximately 20 years (Jones 2013), initial substance use prior to the age of 14 years is associated with six times greater risk of developing a substance use disorder in adulthood (Substance Abuse and Mental Health Services Administration (SAMHSA 2013)). Given that 3 years on average elapses between initial use in adolescence and the presence of a substance use disorder (Wittchen et al. 2008), pediatricians have a critical window of opportunity in identifying and coordinating treatment for substance use for adolescent patients.

Mood disorders and psychotic symptoms also tend to emerge in adolescence. Females experience a three- to fourfold increase in clinical depression symptoms during middle adolescence (Lewinsohn et al. 2004). Onset of bipolar disorder is greatest during late adolescence (Kessler et al. 2005), and those at risk for psychotic disorders typically have their first experiences of psychotic symptoms during middle adolescence (Thompson et al. 2004) with diagnosis typically emerging by late adolescence (Kessler et al. 2005, 2007). Keeping youth on a stable, positive development trajectory ensures the best chance for children to move into adulthood well adjusted, with confidence and competence. With annual visits with patients across childhood, primary care affords a unique opportunity to catch and treat emerging emotional and behavioral concerns that can compromise or undermine normal development.

Despite the fact that mental health concerns are most likely to emerge during childhood and adolescence, research shows that 80% of youth who need mental health care do not receive it (Kataoka et al. 2002). For example, comprising 54% of all referral requests, disruptive behavior represents one of the most common emotional and behavioral problems for which parents seek support (Kolko et al. 2012). However, evidence suggests that less than half of children aged 4–17 years with ADHD, the most common disruptive behavior disorder, receive behavioral treatment (Weber et al. 2018), the evidence-based treatment recommended for disruptive behavior (AAP 2011). This discrepancy highlights the profound gaps that exist between our knowledge of effective treatments and patient access to them (Kolko et al. 2014).

Thus, the primary care visit provides a unique opportunity to connect youth who need it to mental health care. However, although emotional and behavioral concerns are the focus of many pediatric primary care visits, with 25% of pediatric office visits focusing on these symptoms (Rushton et al. 2002), simply referring for mental health services outside of primary care may not be enough to effectively engage youth in treatment. When mental health is offered onsite with primary care, 66% of families engaged in care compared to 5% of families who received offsite referrals (Lieberman et al. 2006). When recommended mental health services are offered within the primary care setting, 95% of children received them compared to 17% of children who had referrals for outside mental health. Similarly, the same study showed that 78% of children completed their recommended course of mental health treatment when the treatment was co-located with the primary care pediatrician, whereas 20% completed treatment when referred to outside providers (Kolko et al. 2012). These findings emphasize the importance of integrated care models that involve co-location of psychological and primary care services to ensure that pediatric patients indeed receive services that appropriately address emotional and behavioral concerns.

Models of Integrated Care

Partnership and collaboration between psychology and pediatrics has been proposed since the 1960s to address the emotional and behavioral needs of children (Stancin and Perrin 2014).

There are several models of linking behavioral health care to primary care, including co-location, collaboration, and integration (Gerrity 2016). The SAMHSA published an extensive list of various care models that are currently active (https://www.integration.samhsa.gov/integrated-care-models/behavioral-health-in-primary-care#integrated%20models%20of%20BH%20in%20PC). Models of integrated care must overcome the logistical challenges of providing CBT in primary care settings, including a compressed timeframe for assessment and intervention, high volume of patients, a wide diversity of diagnostic and behavioral presentations and concerns, multiple team and discipline demands, and lower frequency of appointments. Options can include standard (i.e., face-to-face), consultation/collaborative care, telehealth, online/computerized, and guided self-administered CBT (Twomey et al. 2015). Most of these approaches have been examined in adult rather than pediatric primary care, and when models do include children, they are predominantly designed for family medicine rather than specifically for pediatric primary care (Stancin and Perrin 2014). These results demonstrate the need for the development and evaluation of integrated models for child and adolescent primary care (see also Chap. 2, this volume).

A particularly successful model among adults has been the colocation of psychologists within primary care, which has been used and evaluated within the Veterans Affairs Health Care System. This model emphasizes the co-location of a psychologist embedded within the primary care context to promote the integration of health and mental health care. The embedded psychologist delivers traditional psychological treatments that are typically modified to mesh with the logistics and volume of primary care settings. Adaptations include shortening mental health visits (e.g., 15–30 min) or extending the time in between appointments to 2–4 weeks rather than weekly appointments (Vogel et al. 2016). Psychologists may serve in the role of consultation with an interdisciplinary care team or deliver treatment to patients directly in the primary care setting.

Findings from a recent meta-analysis of integrated care models for adult primary care in the VA and community health settings found that providing co-located mental health care with primary care had many positive outcomes for physical and mental health (Possemato et al. 2018). Patients across settings demonstrated improvements in access to care. Average wait time across studies ranged from 19 min to 21 days. Patients in practices with integrated care were significantly more likely to engage in mental health care and attend a significantly higher number of appointments. In one study, contact with a mental health provider increased by 391% when rates of mental health access were compared before and after implementation of an integrated model (Brawer et al. 2010). In another study, connecting to mental health within 2 weeks increased 54% with an integrated model as compared to 15% in an enhanced referral model (Krahn et al. 2006). Improvements in mental health included reductions in depression, anxiety, and suicidal behavior. Landis et al. (2013) focused on depressed adults and found that collocated services resulted in a large effect size in the reduction of depression symptoms ($d = 1.22$). In a longitudinal study with several follow-ups, Angantyr et al. (2015) found that both depression and anxiety decreased over time when an integrated care model was used ($d = 0.47$, $d = 0.78$, respectively). Physical health displayed improvements in at least one area across studies. Many studies also reported greater adherence to health behaviors and consistency in compliance with physician-prescribed medical regimens for patients in collocated services as compared to those who were referred to outside services. These results demonstrate the potential benefits of an integrated care model for pediatric primary care.

Stancin and Perrin (2014) detailed the range of priorities and activities that psychologists could address in pediatric primary care, including prevention, screening, and early intervention; direct interventions with emotional and behavioral problems (e.g., sleep, tantrums, fears, toileting, feeding) and diagnosed disorders (e.g., ADHD, anxiety, depression, disruptive behavior disorders); and health promotion with chronic health conditions. Care delivery could take the form of individual or group-based parent-focused interventions and brief symptom-focused interventions (Stancin and Perrin 2014).

The goal of cognitive-behavioral therapy is to target the association of thoughts, feelings, and behavior to improve functioning and reduce unwanted symptoms. Maladaptive or undesired responses to various situations can be reduced through several mechanisms, including cognitive (e.g., reappraisal, reduction of distortions) and behavioral strategies (e.g., increased exposure to feared stimuli, increased engagement with avoided activities), as well as third-wave CBT approaches of mindfulness and acceptance. These approaches can be applied to psychological disorders (e.g., anxiety, depression, ADHD) as well as physical conditions (e.g., adherence difficulties, somatic symptoms). While the ultimate treatment target is reduction of pediatric symptoms, the target for intervention could be the child, the parent, or both. Individual CBT with children and adolescents typically focuses on internalizing symptoms (e.g., anxiety, depression, adjustment). Parent-focused treatments are used to address behavioral issues of noncompliance and disruptive behavior problems using behavioral parent training (see also Chaps. 7 and 8, this volume).

Adult models of delivering individually focused CBT in primary care demonstrate that this approach can be effective. For example, results of a recent meta-analysis indicated that multiple modes of CBT were more effective than no primary care treatment or primary care treatment-as-usual for adult anxiety and depression symptoms, with evidence that CBT was more effective with anxiety than depressive symptoms (Twomey et al. 2015). A recent randomized controlled trial (RCT) in two pediatric centers suggests that these results may extend to children and adolescents as well. This RCT targeted pediatric anxiety and depression and indicated that youth receiving brief behavioral treatment had significantly higher rates of clinical improvement, greater reductions in symptoms, and better functioning compared to youth with assisted referrals to community treatment (Weersing et al. 2017). Volkenant and Hosterman (2012) evaluated an intervention in primary care for suicidal behavior, where pediatric patients who presented to primary care in crisis received a brief CBT-based intervention with the co-located psychologist. Within the 6-month trial, 16 of the 17 youth (94%) were able to reduce concerns enough to avoid psychiatric hospitalization.

Evidence from RCTs of parent-based interventions for children in primary care suggests that this approach can be effective in pediatric primary care as well. An RCT of the Incredible Years, an intervention that provides behavioral parent training, was evaluated in the pediatric primary setting with parents of toddlers with disruptive behavior problems. The results of the seven-session, parent-group intervention showed reductions in negative parenting strategies and negative parent–child interactions and increases in positive parenting behaviors compared to parents who did not receive the intervention (Perrin et al. 2014). Two small trials of Triple P: Positive Parenting Program, another parent-based, behavioral therapy intervention for children, offered promising results. The first study examined the efficacy of delivering four sessions in primary care with parents of preschool children with disruptive behavior problems; parents reported significant reductions in the intensity and frequency of their child's disruptive behavior and high levels of consumer satisfaction (Boyle et al. 2010). The second study, a community trial of Triple P, showed that attendance at the first appointment and overall service use was significantly higher for the co-located service delivery compared to the control clinics where parents were referred to outside community mental health resources (Wildman and Langkamp 2012).

Although research evaluating models of integrated pediatric primary care is nascent, these studies demonstrate that co-located pediatric services show promise of being an effective context for pediatric CBT. A meta-analysis of integrated care pilot studies for children and adolescents reported that youth had a 66% likelihood of improved outcomes when they received mental health care within an integrated model of mental health and physical health care as opposed to care from a referral outside of primary care (Asarnow et al. 2015). These results demonstrate the importance of pursuing evaluation of integrated care models for pediatric primary care and mental health care.

Future Research Needs

Finally, there is the potential for many innovations and novel intervention approaches that await discovery. The high patient volume and limited time demands on patient care require brief assessment and intervention strategies. CBT that can be delivered in modules selected and tailored to a patient's specific symptom, impairment, and health profile could facilitate maximizing face-to-face time (Chorpita et al. 2013; Weisz et al. 2011, 2012). For example, PracticeWise offers clinicians a menu of intervention modules to address a range of specific presenting problems associated with anxiety, depression, or disruptive behavior (Chorpita and Weisz 2009). These modules are intervention components selected for inclusion based on an exhaustive review of evidence-based treatment for children and adolescents (Chorpita and Daleiden 2009; Chorpita et al. 2011). Clinicians receive guidance on selection and sequencing of modules from a decision flowchart based on assessment of treatment response and adherence. Randomized controlled trials and effectiveness trials demonstrate that this intervention can lead to significant improvements in internalizing and externalizing symptoms with moderate to large effect sizes across parent and youth report of symptoms (Chorpita et al. 2013; Weisz et al. 2011). The flexibility and potential for treatment brevity with this intervention approach suggests it could be a good fit for the pediatric primary care context.

Another promising avenue may be the use of computerized, self-monitoring interventions initiated through brief patient care and sustained through preprogrammed cuing and self-engagement. These approaches could provide cost-effective strategies for behavioral change and adherence to healthy routines for pediatric patients. Use of smartphones and tablets has led to a proliferation of computer-based applications including CBT-based apps for children (e.g., SmartCAT, MobileType) and third-wave mindfulness apps (e.g., Stop, Breathe, and Think Kid; see Mani et al. 2015). Several systematic reviews have evaluated current offerings of CBT-based, smartphone options for youth with mental health concerns (Rickwood et al. 2017). Results indicated that although these tools abound, very few mobile apps have been tested in an efficacy trial, although initial evaluation of effectiveness supports the use of some mobile apps for youth. For example, pilot studies with SmartCAT, a mobile app used to supplement therapy sessions with skill development on tailored CBT strategies to manage anxiety symptoms, indicated that youth enjoyed using the app and showed modest improvements in CBT skills (Pramana et al. 2014). MobileType is designed to facilitate assessment and stepped care in the primary care context for youth with mild to moderate depression. Although depression symptoms were not significantly different, initial results of a small randomized controlled trial indicated that MobileType provided pediatricians with helpful details in the diagnostic decision-making process (Reid et al. 2013). These results demonstrate that this area of the health field is wide open for problem-solving with creative, innovative clinical and research solutions. Pursuing these lines of inquiry would significantly advance the field as would expanding the methodology typically used in this area to include control and comparison groups in study designs and the use of randomization of various components of treatment (Possemato et al. 2018; Stancin and Perrin 2014).

A major appeal for delivering CBT approaches is the ability to collaboratively set goals with patients and provide targeted strategies for improving health. CBT is a flexible approach that can be used to support psychological health symptoms (e.g., anxiety, depression) as well as physiological health conditions (e.g., adherence to medications, increased self-monitoring of physical symptoms such as headaches or stomachaches, sleep hygiene). The challenge of the primary care setting is to retain enough elements to effectively support change while ensuring adequate and sufficient support. Advances in understanding the mechanisms of behavior change has led to modular CBT treatments, as mentioned before, that may support delivery of brief forms of CBT that are well suited to primary care (Chorpita and Daleiden 2009; Chorpita et al. 2011; Weisz et al. 2012). Psychologists with expertise in evidence-based assessment and treatment can determine whether a brief course of CBT targeting a narrow goal is appropriate for primary care, versus deciding that more traditional treatment approaches are required to provide optimal intervention. In the clinical vignettes provided below, specific CBT approaches could be delivered in a primary care setting by a psychologist collaborating with the healthcare team.

Clinical Vignettes

Given the gap between research and practice in this area, we offer two vignettes to the reader as demonstration of how CBT components could be applied to pediatric health problems in the primary care setting.[1] The first vignette demonstrates how CBT concepts could address an eczema diagnosis, a health problem whose treatment requires consistent adherence to a frequent behavioral routine (e.g., applying cream to affected skin, taking medication) and inhibiting intense behavioral impulses that exacerbate the symptoms (e.g., scratching itchy, affected skin). The second vignette showcases how parent management training, the gold standard behavioral intervention for attention deficit/hyperactivity disorder (ADHD), could be delivered in the pediatric primary care setting for a child with ADHD.

Eczema Case Vignette Michael is a 6-year-old boy who was diagnosed with atopic dermatitis, or eczema, by his pediatrician when he was about a year old. His skin shows signs of habitual, frequent scratching. When his pediatrician brings up the topic of itchiness, Michael begins to scratch his arms; his mother reflexively reaches to stop him and scolds him. The doctor asks about their skin care routine and use of prescribed topical medications. Michael says he hates all the creams, and his mother sighs as she recounts her efforts to implement all the medical interventions on the recommended daily basis. She has asked before whether there is a medication that could take the place of applying thick, greasy moisturizers three to five times per day and the topical steroid cream twice a day when his skin looks inflamed. The pediatrician asks about the bleach baths that were recommended when they consulted with a pediatric dermatologist. Michael says that bathing is painful; the pediatrician sympathizes as she looks over all the scattered wounds caused by Michael's frequent scratching and considers whether a topical antimicrobial treatment is needed. Michael's mother dreads the battle of even attempting to convince him to do any of the recommended treatments. Michael's mother mentions how exhausted they are from Michael waking up scratching in the night, and how hard they try to get him to stop scratching. She does not mention her fear of using the steroid cream, despite the many attempts of the pediatrician to reassure her. The pediatrician reviews the same medical recommendations with Michael's mother and encourages them to keep trying to adhere to what the dermatologist prescribed.

Eczema is a chronic skin condition characterized by dry, itchy, rash-prone skin. Onset occurs early in childhood, with approximately 90% of affected youth diagnosed in the first 5 years of life. It is a highly prevalent condition, affecting 10–20% of children (Lyos et al. 2015). Eczema is associated with increased risk for skin infections, chronic itch/scratch behavior, and sleep disturbances. Course is typically chronic, relapsing, and requires a long-term approach to management. Typical treatment involves a consistent skin care routine of soaking baths and frequent application of moisturizers to hydrate the dry skin, intermittent, as-needed use of topical steroid creams to reduce inflammation during acute flares, and avoidance of skin irritants. Due to the chronic, relapsing nature of eczema, optimal symptom management is achieved through daily application of emollients and prescribed use of topical steroids during eczema flares. In addition, eczema frequently presents with habitual scratching, which further exacerbates skin healing. Poor or variable adherence to eczema treatment recommendations is common, as is parental steroid phobia and habitual scratching (Patel and Feldman 2017), yet pediatric providers lack training in improving adherence or decreasing habit behaviors.

As illustrated in this example, effective treatment of a chronic condition requires knowledge of medical recommendations as well as expertise in behavior change. Although there are effective treatments for eczema, which is very common skin condition, many parents and families struggle to consistently adhere to the effective recommendations. Eczema is an interesting case in support of integrating CBT approaches in primary care due to adherence as well as behavioral challenges that directly influence the expression of an underlying medical condition (Perry-Parrish 2016). Some of the adherence challenges are common to other chronic conditions (e.g., treatment fatigue, lack of effective routines to prevent forgetfulness), and some of the challenges are more unique (e.g., parental steroid phobia). CBT is a flexible treatment that can provide cognitive restructuring to reduce parental anxiety regarding the safety of a well-studied medical treatment; behavioral reinforcement to increase child compliance with parental application of medication; and behavioral modification to reduce maladaptive habits (e.g., scratching). Michael's mother appreciated the additional information regarding the safety trials that had been conducted with the prescribed topical steroid, along with the dermatologist guidance about how to monitor for the potentially feared side effects of skin thinning. Michael understood that his skin was thirsty for moisturizer whenever he felt itchy and supported the idea of increasing his moisturizer use. Use of a token economy to increase adherence to the daily skin care routines motivated Michael's cooperation with his parents applying moisturizer several times per day. After optimal compliance with medical recommendations was established, Michael's skin improved considerably, and it became easier to begin habit reversal training to reduce his scratching habit. The token economy was expanded to provide motivation for Michael to engage in repeated trials of mindfully noticing an itch sensation without scratching while parents prompted competing responses (e.g., clasping hands together, putting hands in his pocket, sitting on his hands, applying additional moisturizer). As Michael's scratching habit decreased, both Michael and his parents appeared less distressed about his skin condition, and his.

ADHD Case Vignette Lucy is an 8-year-old girl who was diagnosed with attention-deficit/hyperactivity disorder (ADHD) by her pediatrician when she was 6 years old. Her parents have been noticing signs of distractibility, excessive talking, and disorganization since kindergarten. Lucy's teachers have observed difficulties with sustained attention, lack of optimal effort, and frequently incomplete, late, or lost assignments. Deciding on a treatment course was difficult because Lucy's parents did not want to consider medication, and fitting in yet another commitment slowed them down from seeking therapy. They tried increasing how much exercise she engaged in and improving the family's diet. They frequently found themselves trying to convince Lucy of why it was so important that she try harder and expressing frustration when the lectures did not change her behavior. It was disappointing year after year when Lucy brought home progress reports that showed no improvement in her behavior. Each fall, they all felt hopeful that this year would be better, and no one took it harder than Lucy when she got repeated corrections for not paying attention, for overlooking an assignment, or interrupted the teacher. She did not understand why her classmates found her intrusive comments annoying, or why her parents became so frustrated when they repeated instructions to put her shoes on for school, to start eating breakfast, or to stop talking over her little brother. Her feelings were frequently hurt by her belief that people only noticed what she did wrong. Sometimes these hurt feelings led to outbursts of yelling, throwing things, and slamming doors. Lucy's parents felt stuck, as their responses did not seem to curb Lucy's behavior and left them feeling hopeless and ineffective. They knew that they were giving in to avoid hurting Lucy's feelings or because they were tired of working so hard to capture her attention and motivate appropriate behavior.

ADHD is a neurodevelopmental disorder with onset in early childhood. Symptoms span the domains of inattention, hyperactivity, and impulsivity, typically manifesting as a lack of self-regulation and control across situations (AAP 2011). Children diagnosed with ADHD often present with comorbid conditions, including anxiety, disruptive behavior, depression, and learning difficulties. Numerous studies indicate that behavioral therapy in the form of parent training is the most effective psychological treatment yet requires that parents agree to become trained in the delivery of behavioral modification strategies.

The pediatrician offered to introduce the family to the pediatric psychologist co-located in their clinic. The psychologist provided education to parents about ADHD symptoms and the importance of creating a positive social learning environment. The psychologist provided a list of evidence-based books about positive parenting approaches, including *The Incredible Years* (Webster-Stratton 2006), *The Kazdin Method for Parenting the Defiant Child* (Kazdin 2009), and *Taking Charge of ADHD* (Barkley 2013). After looking through each book with the psychologist, Lucy's parents decided to start with the Incredible Years, and the psychologist provided a guided tour of important parenting strategies. Their psychologist offered a follow-up book, *Raising an Emotionally Intelligent Child* (Gottman and Declaire 1998), and infused the emotion-focused coping strategies presented in this book into the parent management training tools from the Incredible Years program. In their initial consultation, parent–child time, differential attention, and praise for compliance were emphasized. In a follow-up session, they reviewed strategic ignoring for minor misbehavior and how to use a token economy to motivate and sustain compliance for more difficult and boring tasks, including daily routines and homework. With Lucy's involvement, the family selected a reward chart app that linked from Lucy's tablet to her parents' smartphones to help them track points and rewards for desired behavior. When parents continued to report occasional outbursts involving yelling and throwing things, the psychologist taught parents a time-out procedure and made plans for close follow-up as they implemented the technique at home with Lucy. Over time, Lucy's parents reported significant improvements with increased compliance for instructions, and daily routines, decreased resistance for homework, and confidence with using time-out for her infrequent outbursts. Lucy and her parents reported improved interactions and less tension at home. Parents reported feeling more effective in managing their daughter's difficulties. They reported going back through the book recommended by the psychologist to help refresh them on behavioral principles and remembering how much more difficult it was before they learned these positive parenting approaches.

Summary

As illustrated in these vignettes, CBT approaches can target changes in behavior and thoughts to improve coping with and adjustment to medical and psychological conditions and symptoms in primary care. There are common ingredients in implementation of CBT in primary care, including applying the most effective elements early in the process and tailoring those elements to symptoms of concern. Co-location of services reduces barriers to care and may enhance family receptivity to cognitive-behavioral therapy through ease of access and perceived support of the referring provider. Given the emphasis on identifying specific behavioral targets, the utility of CBT approaches in managing physical symptoms may reduce family resistance to considering a complementary psychological approach to their child's symptoms. Core ingredients include identification of objective behavioral targets, differential attention, and use of incentives, as well as education about the child's condition to provide conceptual link for the importance of improving adherence and compliance to treatment strategies. Finally, clinician consideration of skillfully introducing these elements to optimize parent buy-in may enhance motivation for change and maximize the likelihood of future session attendance.

References

American Academy of Family Physicians, American Academy of Pediatrics, American College of Physicians, American Osteopathic Association. (2007). Joint principles of the patient-centered medical home. *American Family Physician, 76*(6), 774–775.

American Academy of Pediatrics. (2011). ADHD: Clinical practice guideline for the diagnosis, evaluation, and treatment of Attention-Deficit/ Hyperactivity Disorder in children and adolescents. *Pediatrics, 128*(5), 1–18. https://doi.org/10.1542/peds.2011-2654. https://www.cdc.gov/ncbddd/adhd/guidelines.html.

Anda, R. F., Brown, D. W., Felitti, V. J., Bremner, J. D., Dube, S. R., & Giles, W. H. (2007). Adverse childhood experiences and prescribed psychotropic medications in adults. *American Journal of Preventive Medicine, 32*, 389–394. https://doi.org/10.1016/j.amepre.2007.01.005.

Angantyr, K., Rimner, A., Nordén, T., & Norlander, T. (2015). Primary care behavioral health model: Perspectives of outcome, client satisfaction, and gender. *Social Behavior and Personality: International Journal, 43*(2), 287–302. https://doi.org/10.2224/sbp.2015.43.2.287.

Asarnow, J. R., Rozenman, M., Wiblin, J., & Zeltzer, L. (2015). Integrated medical-behavioral care compared with usual primary care for child and adolescent behavioral health: A meta-analysis. *JAMA Pediatrics, 169*(10), 929–937. https://doi.org/10.1001/jamapediatrics.2015.1141.

Barkley, R. (2013). *Taking charge of ADHD: The complete authoritative guide for parents* (3rd ed.). New York, NY: Guilford Press.

Boyle, C. L., Sanders, M. R., Lutzker, J. R., Prinz, R. J., Shapiro, C., & Whitaker, D. J. (2010). An analysis of training, generalization, and maintenance effects of Primary Care Triple P for parents of preschool-aged children with disruptive behavior. *Child Psychiatry & Human Development, 41*(1), 114–131. https://doi.org/10.1007/s10578-009-0156-7.

Brawer, P. A., Martielli, R., Pye, P. L., Manwaring, J., & Tierney, A. (2010). St. Louis initiative for integrated care excellence (SLI(2)CE): Integrated-collaborative care on a large scale model. *Family, Systems, and Health, 28*(2), 175–187. https://doi.org/10.1037/a0020342.

Chorpita, B. F., & Daleiden, E. L. (2009). Mapping evidence-based treatments for children and adolescents: Application of the distillation and matching model to 615 treatments from 322 randomized trials. *Journal of Consulting and Clinical Psychology, 77*, 566–579.

Chorpita, B. F., & Weisz, J. R. (2009). *Modular approach to therapy for children with anxiety, depression, trauma, or conduct problems (MATCH–ADTC)*. Satellite Beach, FL: PracticeWise.

Chorpita, B. F., Daleiden, E. L., Ebesutani, C., Young, J., Becker, K. D., & Nakamura, B. J. (2011). Evidence-based treatments for children and adolescents: An updated review of indicators of efficacy and effectiveness. *Clinical Psychology: Science and Practice, 18*, 154–172.

Chorpita, B. F., Daleiden, E. L., Palinkas, L. A., Higa-McMillan, C. K., Aukahi Austin, A., Ward, A., et al. (2013). Long-term outcomes for the child STEPs randomized effectiveness trial: A comparison of modular and standard treatment designs with usual care. *Journal of Consulting and Clinical Psychology, 81*(6), 999–1009.

Gerrity, M. (2016). *Evolving models of behavioral health integration: Evidence update 2010–2015*. New York, NY: Milbank Memorial Fund.

Gottman, J. M., & Declaire, J. (1998). *Raising an emotionally intelligent child: The heart of parenting*. New York, NY: Simon & Schuster.

Jones, P. B. (2013). Adult mental health disorders and their age at onset. *The British Journal of Psychiatry, 202*(S), 5–10. https://doi.org/10.1192/bjp.bp.112.119164.

Kataoka, S. H., Zhang, L., & Wells, K. B. (2002). Unmet need for mental health care among U.S. children: Variation by ethnicity and insurance status. *American Journal of Psychiatry, 159*(9), 1548–1555.

Kazdin, A. (2009). *The Kazdin method for parenting the defiant child* (2nd ed.). Wilmington, MA: Mariner Books.

Kessler, R. C., Berglund, P., Demler, O., Jin, R., Merikangas, K. R., & Walters, E. E. (2005). Lifetime prevalence and age-of-onset distributions of DSM-IV disorders in the National Comorbidity Survey Replication. *Archives of General Psychiatry, 62*(6), 593–602.

Kessler, R. C., Amminger, G. P., Aguillar-Gaxiola, S., Alonso, J., Lee, S., & Ustun, T. B. (2007). Age of onset of mental disorders: A review of recent literature. *Current Opinion in Psychiatry, 20*(4), 359–364. https://doi.org/10.1097/YCO.0b013e32816ebc8c.

Kolko, D. J., Campo, J. V., Kilbourne, A. M., & Kelleher, K. (2012). Doctor-office collaborative care for pediatric behavioral problems: A preliminary clinical trial. *Archives of Pediatrics & Adolescent Medicine, 166*(3), 224–231.

Kolko, D. J., Campo, J., Kilbourne, A. M., Hart, J., Sakolsky, D., & Wisniewski, S. (2014). Collaborative care outcomes for pediatric behavioral health problems: A cluster randomized trial. *Pediatrics, 133*(4), 981–992. https://doi.org/10.1542/peds.2013-2516.

Krahn, D. D., Bartels, S. J., Coakley, E., Oslin, D. W., Chen, H., McIntyre, J., et al. (2006). PRISM-E: Comparison of integrated care and enhanced specialty referral models in depression outcomes. *Psychiatric*

Services, 57(7), 946–953. https://doi.org/10.1176/ps.2006.57.7.946.

Landis, S. E., Barrett, M., & Galvin, S. L. (2013). Effects of different models of integrated collaborative care in a family medicine residency program. *Family, Systems, and Health, 31*(3), 264–273. https://doi.org/10.1037/a0033410.

Lewinsohn, P. M., Shankman, S. A., Gau, J. M., & Klein, D. N. (2004). The prevalence and comorbidity of sub-threshold psychiatric conditions. *Psychological Medicine, 34*, 613–622.

Lieberman, A., Adalist-Estrin, A., Erinle, O., & Sloan, N. (2006). On-site mental health care: A route to improving access to mental health services in an inner-city, adolescent medicine clinic. *Child: Care, Health and Development, 32*(4), 407–413.

Lyos, J. J., Milner, J. D., & Stone, K. D. (2015). Atopic dermatitis in children: Clinical features, pathophysiology, and treatment. *Immunology and Allergy Clinics of North America, 35*(1), 161–183. https://doi.org/10.1016/j.iac.2014.09.008.

Mani, M., Kavanagh, D. J., Hides, L., & Stoyanov, S. R. (2015). Review and evaluation of mindfulness-based iphone apps. *JMIR mHealth and uHealth, 3*(3), e82.

Maughan, B., Rowe, R., Messer, J., Goodman, R., & Meltzer, H. (2004). Conduct disorder and oppositional defiant disorder in a national sample: Developmental epidemiology. *Journal of Child Psychology and Psychiatry, 45*(3), 609–621.

Nock, M. K., Borges, G., Brohmet, E. J., Cha, C. B., Kessler, R. C., & Lee, S. (2008). Suicide and suicidal behavior. *Epidemiologic Reviews, 30*, 133–154.

Patel, N., & Feldman, S. R. (2017). Adherence in atopic dermatitis. *Advanced in Experimental Medicine and Biology, 1027*, 139–159. https://doi.org/10.1007/978-3-319-64804-0_12.

Perrin, E. C., Sheldrick, R. C., McMenamy, J. M., Henson, B. S., & Carter, A. S. (2014). Improving parenting skills for families of young children in pediatric settings: A randomized clinical trial. *JAMA Pediatrics, 168*(1), 6–24. https://doi.org/10.1001/jamapediatrics.2013.2919.

Perry-Parrish, C. (2016). *Cognitive behavioral therapy in the management of eczema*. Presentation, Society for Pediatric Dermatology Annual Meeting, American Academy of Dermatology Meeting, Washington, DC.

Polanczyk, G., Laranjeira, R., Zalesk, I. M., Pinsky, I., Caetano, R., & Rohde, L. A. (2010). ADHD in a representative sample of the Brazilian population: Estimated prevalence and comparative adequacy of criteria between adolescents and adults according to the i.e. response theory. *International Journal of Methodology in Psychiatric Research, 19*, 177–184.

Possemato, K., Johnsona, E. M., Beehlera, G. P., Shepardsona, R. M., King, P., Vaire, C. L., et al. (2018). Patient outcomes associated with primary care behavioral health services: A systematic review. *General Hospital Psychiatry, 53*, 1–11.

Pramana, G., Parmanto, B., Kendall, P. C., & Silk, J. S. (2014). The SmartCAT: An m-health platform for ecological momentary intervention in child anxiety treatment. *Telemedicine Journal of Electronic Health, 20*(5), 419–427.

Reid, S. C., Kauer, S. D., Hearps, S. J., Crooke, A. H., Khor, A. S., Sanci, L. A., et al. (2013). A mobile phone application for the assessment and management of youth mental health problems in primary care: Health service outcomes from a randomized controlled trial of mobiletype. *BMC Family Practitioner, 19*, 14–84.

Rickwood, D., Soron, T. R., Aggarwal, S., Dove, E., Dogan, E., & Ashford, M. (2017). Mental health mobile apps for preadolescents and adolescents: A systematic review. *Journal of Medical Internet Research, 19*(5), e176.

Rushton, J., Bruckman, D., & Kelleher, K. (2002). Primary care referral of children with psychosocial problems. *Archives of Pediatrics & Adolescent Medicine, 156*(6), 592–598.

Stancin, T., & Perrin, E. C. (2014). Psychologists and pediatricians: Opportunities for collaboration in primary care. *American Psychologist, 69*(4), 332–343.

Substance Abuse and Mental Health Services Administration (SAMHSA). (2013). Results from the 2012 National Survey on Drug Use and Health: summary of national findings. Rockville, MD: SAMHSA.

Thompson, J. L., Pogue-Geile, M. F., & Grace, A. A. (2004). Developmental pathology, dopamine, and stress: A model for the age of onset of schizophrenia symptoms. *Schizophrenia Bulletin, 30*, 875–900.

Twomey, C., O'Reilly, G., & Byrne, M. (2015). Effectiveness of cognitive behavioral therapy for anxiety and depression in primary care: A meta-analysis. *Family Practice, 32*(1), 3–15.

Vogel, M. E., Kanzler, K. E., Aikens, J. E., & Goodie, J. L. (2016). Integration of behavioral health and primary care: Current knowledge and future directions. *Journal of Behavioral Medicine, 40*(1), 69–84. https://doi.org/10.1007/s10865-016-9798-7.

Volkenant, K., & Hosterman, S. (2012). *Integrating pediatric psychology into primary care: A pilot project*. Paper presented at the Pediatric Psychology Symposium at the Midwest Regional Conference on Pediatric Psychology, Milwaukee, WI.

Weber, L., Kamp-Becker, I., Christiansen, H., & Mingebach, T. (2018). Treatment of child externalizing behavior problems: A comprehensive review and meta-meta-analysis on effects of parent-based interventions on parental characteristics. *European Journal of Child and Adolescent Psychiatry*. https://doi.org/10.1007/s00787-018-1175-3.

Webster-Stratton, C. (2006). *The Incredible Years: A trouble-shooting guide for parents of children aged 3 to 8* (2nd ed.). Los Angeles, CA: Umbrella Press.

Weersing, V. R., Brent, D. A., Rozenman, M. S., Gonzalez, A., Jeffreys, M., Dickerson, J. F., et al. (2017). Brief behavioral therapy for pediatric anxiety and depression in primary care: A randomized clinical trial. *JAMA Psychiatry, 74*(6), 571–578.

Weisz, J. R., Chorpita, B. F., Frye, A., Ng, M. Y., Bearman, S. K., Ugueto, A. M., et al. (2011). Youth top problems: Using idiographic, consumer-guided assessment to identify treatment needs and to track change during psychotherapy. *Journal of Consulting and Clinical Psychology, 79*, 369–380.

Weisz, J. R., Chorpita, B. F., Palinkas, L. A., Schoenwald, S. K., Miranda, J., Bearman, S. K., et al. (2012). Testing standard and modular designs for psychotherapy treating depression, anxiety, and conduct problems in youth. *Archives of General Psychiatry, 69*, 274–282.

Wildman, B. G., & Langkamp, D. L. (2012). Impact of location and availability of behavioral health services for children. *Journal of Clinical Psychology in Medical Settings, 19*, 393–400. https://doi.org/10.1007/s10880-012-9324-1.

Wittchen, H. U., Behrendt, S., Höfler, M., Perkonigg, A., Lieb, R., Bühringer, G., et al. (2008). What are the high risk periods for incident substance use and transitions to abuse and dependence? Implications for early intervention and prevention. *International Journal of Methods in Psychiatric Research, 17*(Suppl. 1), S16–S29. https://doi.org/10.1002/mpr.254.

Working Party Group on Integrated Behavioral Healthcare, Baird, M., Blount, A., Brungardt, S., Dickinson, P., Dietrich, A., et al. (2014). Behavioral health addendum to the joint principles of the patient-centered medical home. *Annals of Family Medicine, 12*(2), 183–185. https://doi.org/10.1370/afm.1633.

Cognitive Behavioral Therapy in Pediatric Patients with Chronic Widespread Musculoskeletal Pain

Lauren M. Fussner and Anne M. Lynch-Jordan

Widespread musculoskeletal pain is a chronic and debilitating condition associated with declines in physical, academic, social, and emotional functioning (Palermo 2000; Kashikar-Zuck et al. 2002). Musculoskeletal pain affects up to 24% of youth (King et al. 2011; Perquin et al. 2000) and results in high rates of health care utilization and costly medical expenses (Sleed et al. 2005). Adolescent females (age 15–18 years) are most at risk for developing chronic musculoskeletal pain along with a host of other mental health conditions (Giedd et al. 2008; Zapata et al. 2006). The American College of Rheumatology criteria for chronic widespread pain include multisite joint or musculoskeletal pain (e.g., back, neck, arm, leg) every day or almost every day for at least 3 months without an organic cause (e.g., juvenile idiopathic arthritis, systemic lupus). Chronic widespread pain must be accompanied by impairment (e.g., concentration or memory problems) and significant physical symptoms (e.g., loss of appetite, nausea, headache; Wolfe et al. 2010).

The presentation of musculoskeletal pain is quite variable. While some individuals report "all over aches and pains," others describe primary localized pain (e.g., back pain) with secondary pain locations. Similarly, some youth report constant pain that fluctuates in intensity, while others report persistent severe pain. Thus, diagnosis can be a complex process that poses intervention challenges. The following case example[1] illustrates a common clinical presentation, assessment, and treatment approach for a patient with widespread musculoskeletal pain.

"Haley" is a 16-year-old female who presented to the outpatient psychology clinic at her local children's hospital reporting severe neck, back, and ankle pain. She was referred from the pediatric rheumatology clinic after an extensive diagnostic workup revealed no disease process to explain her musculoskeletal pain. Haley became visibly upset while describing her pain history:

"I started dancing at age 3 and I've been doing it ever since. Last year I hurt my ankle during rehearsal, and I've never really recovered. I was really good about doing all of my exercises to help strengthen my ankle in the beginning. I even took two weeks off, which I have never done, to try and rest it. But nothing helped. I tried to go back to dance because I love it, and that's where all my friends are, but I just couldn't keep up. I lost my solo and missed a lot of practices. I had to stop dancing completely about six months ago. Things have just gotten worse and worse since then. The

L. M. Fussner (✉)
Yale Medicine Child Study Center,
New Haven, CT, USA
e-mail: Lauren.Fussner@yale.edu

A. M. Lynch-Jordan
University of Cincinnati College of Medicine,
Cincinnati Children's Hospital Medical Center,
Cincinnati, OH, USA

[1]The case presented in this chapter represents a confabulated case example for didactic purposes. Any similarity to a specific patient is coincidental.

© Springer Nature Switzerland AG 2019
R. D. Friedberg, J. K. Paternostro (eds.), *Handbook of Cognitive Behavioral Therapy for Pediatric Medical Conditions*, Autism and Child Psychopathology Series,
https://doi.org/10.1007/978-3-030-21683-2_13

pain is spreading. It's not just my ankle but has now moved into my neck and back too. Sometimes the pain is so bad that I'm in bed all day. I haven't seen my friends in weeks, and when I do see them, my pain gets much worse after I'm done hanging out with them. My mom has taken me to lots of doctors; I've tried some medicine; nothing has helped."

Haley's story is common in children and adolescents, as musculoskeletal injury is a highly common complaint in pediatric primary care (De Inocencio 2004). While many youth recover from injury with time and proper medical care, up to 30% of youth who present to the emergency room or primary care office with musculoskeletal injury continue to have pain beyond 3 months (Holley et al. 2017), which is the benchmark criteria for chronic pain (i.e., daily or almost daily pain that has persisted beyond 3 months; Treede et al. 2015). Despite the prevalence of widespread musculoskeletal pain, its etiology is still poorly understood.

Biopsychosocial Model of Widespread Musculoskeletal Pain

Introduced by George Engel in 1977, the biopsychosocial model proposes that health is a complex interaction of biological, psychological, and social factors (Gatchel et al. 2007). This framework differed from the traditional *biomedical* approach to chronic illness, which views the mind and body as independent entities that do not interact with one another. From the biomedical perspective, symptoms must be accounted for by disease or injury, which applies to acute pain stemming from a broken bone or organic illnesses such as juvenile arthritis. However, for musculoskeletal pain *without* an identifiable cause, the biomedical model does little to explain the etiology of pain or guide appropriate intervention. As a result, physicians may have limited medical interventions to offer patients, which leave families confused and dissatisfied with medical care. The biopsychosocial model highlights multidimensional processes that reciprocally relate and interact with one another and contribute to symptoms (Gatchel et al. 2007), which readily applies to the complexities of chronic pain.

Consistent with the biopsychosocial model, the Gate Control Theory of Pain (Melzack 1996) was introduced by Melzack and Wall in 1965 to advance the biological understanding of how pain is processed in the brain. This theory highlights the critical role of the brain in processing noxious stimuli and proposes that certain chemicals (i.e., descending signals) interact with structures in the spinal cord and serve as "gates" to either increase or decrease pain signals (see Melzack 2001; Melzack and Katz 2004 for further review). Several adaptations of this theory have been made following clinical and research findings (see Mendell 2014 for discussion), yet the *multidimensional* conceptualization of pain and proposed *modulatory system* are widely accepted. This theory has set the stage for researchers and clinicians to consider how psychological symptoms (e.g., depression) and environmental factors (e.g., social support) interact with biology to influence the pain experience.

Biological Factors

Genetic factors play a pivotal role in the intergenerational transmission of risk for chronic pain. In adult chronic pain research, approximately 50% of risk for chronic pain is attributed to genetic factors (Diatchenko et al. 2013). Moreover, females are at significantly greater risk for developing chronic musculoskeletal pain compared to males, with one study reporting a threefold increase in chronic musculoskeletal pain in girls compared to boys (i.e., 34% vs. 11%; Zapata et al. 2006). These findings suggest that hormonal and genetic factors may underlie sex differences in chronic pain, although additional work is needed (see Bartley and Fillingim 2013 for discussion).

Physiological factors play an important role in the experience and maintenance of chronic pain. A significant body of work has described how the experience of pain modifies the central nervous system in a process referred to as "central sensitization," which results in hypersensitization or hyperexcitability (Meeus and Nijs 2007; Sörensen et al. 1998). The mechanisms that contribute to central sensitization are unclear, yet "wind up" has been proposed as an important process contributing to central nervous system changes (Meeus and Nijs 2007). "Wind up" occurs with prolonged activation of the nervous system (such as the experience of persistent pain) and results in increasingly greater pain intensity with even benign activities (Li et al. 1999). Thus, individuals who commonly experience pain may be more sensitive to noxious stimuli as well as typically innocuous stimuli (such as being touched; Staud and Smitherman 2002).

Psychological Factors

Psychological processes play an important role in the presentation and trajectory of chronic pain. Edwards et al. (2016) reviewed several variables that play a role in the onset, exacerbation, and/or maintenance of chronic pain in youth and adults. Distress (e.g., depression), trauma, fear, and catastrophizing (e.g., ruminating about pain-related symptoms) were described as risk factors for the development and maintenance of chronic pain, whereas social support, active coping, acceptance, and self-efficacy were described as protective factors (see Edwards et al. 2016 for further review). Poor sleep has also been found to contribute to greater pain intensity and functional disability (i.e., disrupted functioning in daily tasks and activities due to pain; Harrison et al. 2014). Greater than 70% of youth with chronic pain endorse disordered sleeping (Evans et al. 2017); thus, sleep hygiene and related healthy lifestyle behaviors (e.g., exercise, nutrition, hydration) are often included in psychological interventions for youth with chronic musculoskeletal pain (Palermo et al. 2009), in addition to methods to address the cognitive and emotional responses to chronic pain. Importantly, research suggests a multifaceted interplay between risk and resilience factors and the presentation of chronic pain (Edwards et al. 2016). Little to no research supports a causal model of psychological factors and the development of chronic pain.

Social Factors

Environmental and family factors such as conflict and social exclusion are also associated with widespread musculoskeletal pain and pain-related disability (Lewandowski et al. 2010). Youth with chronic pain have higher rates of school absenteeism (Roth-Isigkeit et al. 2005) and withdrawal from extracurricular activities (Hunfeld et al. 2001), which may contribute to poor social functioning and greater risk for bullying (Forgeron et al. 2010). Compared to healthy classmates, youth with juvenile fibromyalgia, a widespread chronic pain condition, were described by peers as more sensitive and isolated, were less well liked, and had fewer reciprocated friendships (Kashikar-Zuck et al. 2007). Youth with juvenile fibromyalgia also experience less family cohesion relative to healthy youth and youth with arthritis (Conte et al. 2003). Moreover, a significant body of literature supports the association between pain-specific parenting factors (such as solicitous responses to their child's pain and catastrophizing about their child's pain) and greater pain-related disability in youth (Claar et al. 2008). Collectively, results suggest social and environmental factors are an influential contributor to the presentation of pediatric chronic pain (see Palermo et al. 2014 for a developmental model).

> Haley's emerging chronic pain problems occurred in the context of several notable factors. Within her extended family, several family members reported a history of chronic pain including her grandmother who was diagnosed with fibromyalgia and her mother who had longstanding issues with back pain but had never been formally treated. Temperamentally, Haley was prone to anxiety, frequently worried about her grades and athletic performance, and now found herself attending to and worrying about body symptoms and each new pain complaint. Moreover, Haley's mother had begun to do the same thing, frequently assessing Haley's pain levels, her sleep quality (which was poor), and worrying aloud about the progressive nature of Haley's symptoms. As a result, family conversations often revolved around health issues. Conversely, Haley's friends started to drift away due to Haley frequently complaining of pain and declining attendance at social functions due to pain, all of which worsened Haley's mood.

Multidisciplinary Treatment

From the brief review of biological, psychological, and social correlates of chronic widespread musculoskeletal pain, it is evident that chronic pain is a complex condition and benefits from a multifaceted approach utilizing a multidisciplinary team of providers with overlapping, yet distinct areas of expertise (Palermo et al. 2013). Depending on the severity of pain and degree of impairment, youth with widespread musculoskeletal pain may initially be under the care of their primary care physician. Pains are often initially monitored or may be viewed as "growing pains." Specialized medical providers are often sought as intensity and impairment worsen and may include an orthopedist, rheumatologist, sports medicine physician, and/or pain medicine physician. The multidisciplinary treatment team may also include a psychologist, social worker, occupational therapist, and/or physical therapist. Complementary and alternative methods of pain management are sometimes pursued by families and may include a naturopath, chiropractor, and/or massage therapist, but this is based on unique family and patient preferences and may not be specifically recommended by the medical team. Importantly, collaboration between the treatment team is critical in order to reinforce the overarching goal of physical rehabilitation and resumption of normal functioning.

> Haley reported initially being evaluated by her **primary care physician** who referred her to an **orthopedist** at the local children's hospital when pain did not resolve with standard recommendations (rest, icing, over-the-counter medication). Following her orthopedic exam, decreased physical activity and **physical therapy** were recommended to address weakness and joint hypermobility in her ankle. Haley worked with her physical therapist but saw little improvement in her ankle pain and progressively expanding pain complaints, including back and neck pain. As pain symptoms intensified, Haley's sleep worsened. The family opted to engage in **massage therapy** as well. Eventually Haley's orthopedist sent her to a **pediatric rheumatologist** to further evaluate her now widespread pain, poor sleep, and physical decline. A comprehensive evaluation was completed including lab work, imaging, and extensive medical history and exam. The rheumatologist diagnosed Haley with fibromyalgia, a chronic widespread musculoskeletal pain condition, prescribed anti-inflammatory medication, and referred Haley to psychology for behavioral pain management. Haley's treatment plan emphasized a rehabilitative approach to pain management including improving coping skills, improving physical strength and endurance, making lifestyle changes to support better health and sleep, and taking medication to reduce symptom severity. Haley reported a modest understanding of this plan and relatively limited knowledge of psychological treatments for chronic pain.

Clinical practice often places initial emphasis on medical diagnosis, while also addressing comfort and functioning. Unfortunately, depending on practice and referral patterns, pain psychology may not be introduced until pain has been ongoing for several months or disability fails to improve. At larger institutions, interdisciplinary work integrating psychologists into the treatment team from the initial evaluation does occur. However, given the series of providers with whom families meet, it is understandable that some families express that no provider understands their child's pain or is able to help them. Thus, the first task of providers is to clearly explain the role of psychology and the value of adding psychological interventions to the treatment of chronic pain.

Cognitive Behavioral Therapy for Pediatric Chronic Widespread Musculoskeletal Pain

Cognitive behavioral therapy (CBT) is an empirically supported treatment approach for youth with several chronic conditions, including widespread musculoskeletal pain (Eccleston et al. 2014). Specific work has adapted CBT strategies to address the unique needs of youth with widespread musculoskeletal pain (Kashikar-Zuck et al. 2012). Findings support the effectiveness of pain-focused CBT on improving physical functioning and reducing psychological distress (Kashikar-Zuck et al. 2005; Lynch-Jordan et al. 2014). Pain-focused CBT emphasizes resumption of normal functioning and prioritizes helping youth with musculoskeletal pain gradually return to normal activities and daily routines with environmental and social support (Eccleston et al. 2014). Resuming typical activities (e.g., attending school, spending time with friends, participating in athletic practice) is often challenging for youth with chronic musculoskeletal pain, as many have attempted to return to school full time and/or resume participation in extracurricular activities and subsequently experienced an intense pain flare. This experience often leads to greater avoidance of physical activity and fear of movement, which perpetuate functional disability and chronic pain (see Crombez et al. 2012 for additional information). Thus, CBT for chronic widespread musculoskeletal pain uses a gradual approach to improve physical functioning. Given that youth with musculoskeletal pain often meet with several providers and engage in multiple treatments to achieve their functional goals, it is ideal for CBT for chronic musculoskeletal pain to be time limited (i.e., six to ten sessions) and pain-focused (rather than addressing global mental health concerns).

Treatment Components for Chronic Widespread Musculoskeletal Pain

CBT for chronic widespread musculoskeletal pain consists of several strategies designed to improve physical functioning and teach active behavioral coping. The nuances of delivering CBT for widespread pain, rather than localized pain such as headaches or abdominal pain, are highlighted here and illustrated in the case example. As with most CBT treatments, caregivers are included in several sessions to support youth in utilizing pain management strategies and engage in parenting behaviors that help promote the return to function. Key elements of CBT for pediatric widespread musculoskeletal pain include (1) assessment, (2) psychoeducation, (3) relaxation training, (4) activity pacing and behavioral activation, (5) cognitive restructuring, (6) healthy lifestyle habits, and (7) problem solving/relapse prevention (Table 13.1).

Table 13.1 Sample CBT treatment schedule for pediatric chronic widespread musculoskeletal pain

Session number	Session focus	Content
Session 1	Assessment	• Family interview (caregiver present) • Caregiver report questionnaires • Youth self-report questionnaires
Session 2	Psychoeducation	• Gate Control Theory of Pain (caregiver present) • Understanding relationship between behavior, feelings, and thoughts • Caregiver guidelines for behavioral pain management (caregiver present)
Session 3	Behavioral	• Relaxation training: • Diaphragmatic breathing, progressive muscle relaxation
Session 4	Behavioral	• Relaxation: Guided imagery, mini relaxation and/or • Mindfulness and cognitive distraction techniques
Session 5	Behavioral	• Activity pacing (caregiver present) • Behavioral activation
Session 6	Cognitive	• Identifying automatic thoughts • Challenging automatic thoughts • Calming statements
Session 7	Behavioral	• Healthy lifestyle habits: setting daily routines, sleep hygiene, graduated exercise, adequate hydration (caregiver present)
Session 8	Cognitive/behavioral	• Targeted problem solving • Maintenance of skills (caregiver present)

Assessment

As recommended by the Pediatric Initiative on Methods, Measurement, and Pain Assessment (PedIMMPACT; McGrath et al. 2008) consensus statement, assessment of chronic pain should include domains of physical functioning, pain intensity, emotional functioning, and sleep. Moreover, musculoskeletal pain is commonly associated with decreased participation in activities and fear of movement. Therefore, it can be helpful to administer brief, self-report measures specifically designed to assess these domains:

- *Functional Disability Inventory* (Walker and Greene 1991): A 15-item self-report measure assessing difficulty completing physical activities across home, school, and social settings. This measure has reliable cutoff values for minimal (0–12), moderate (13–29), and severe (30+) disability (Kashikar-Zuck et al. 2011), which can be helpful to understand the magnitude of impairment in physical functioning.
- *Tampa Scale of Kinesiophobia* (Woby et al. 2005): An 11-item self-report measure assessing fear of movement related to pain (e.g., "I'm afraid that I might hurt myself if I exercise"). This measure has two subscales assessing activity avoidance and somatic focus.
- *Fear of Pain Questionnaire-Child Report* (Simons et al. 2011): A 24-item self-report measure assessing pain-related fear (e.g., "I worry when I am in pain," "I cannot go back to school until my pain is treated"). A 23-item caregiver-proxy version also exists.
- *PROMIS Pediatric Pain Interference*: Self-report measure developed with the NIH Patient-Reported Outcomes Measurement Information System (PROMIS) initiative (Varni et al. 2010). The eight-item pain interference self-report form assesses the impact of pain on physical, psychological, and social domains (e.g., "I felt angry when I had pain," "It was hard for me to pay attention when I had pain").

Quantitative measures provide important information about symptom severity and level of functioning that cannot always be captured in the time allotted for clinical interviews. Use of both caregiver and youth report is valuable in order to understand the subjective experience of the patient while gaining caregiver information related to the context and environment in which the youth functions. Sample questions for caregivers and youth with chronic musculoskeletal pain are suggested below (Table 13.2).

> Haley and her mother participated in a clinical interview and completed assessment measures. She and her mother endorsed worsening pain-related anxiety (i.e., hypervigilance about pain symptoms, fear of re-injury), worry about being able to return to dance in a timely manner (e.g., in order to participate in her recital), and worsening pain during physical therapy exercises. Additionally, Haley endorsed fear of losing her status as an elite dancer in her company and missing out on solos that she would have otherwise received. While Haley endorsed elevated levels of generalized anxiety, pain-related disability and fear of movement appeared to be far more impairing at the initiation of treatment.

Table 13.2 Sample questions to ask youth with chronic musculoskeletal pain and their caregivers

Questions to ask caregivers of youth with chronic musculoskeletal pain
• How do you know your child is hurting? What behaviors or changes happen? (e.g., lying on the couch, retreating to bedroom, wincing, crying)
• How do you respond to your child's pain? Are there differences between caregivers in response to child's pain? (e.g., caregiver tension can occur between one caregiver engaging in a "tough love" approach and another offering support through overprotective or accommodating responses)
• What are the challenges you experience helping your child manage his/her pain? (e.g., family conflict related to pain management, witnessing a child hurting, knowing when to encourage functioning and when to allow modifications or rest)
• How have family relationships and activities been affected by pain? (e.g., sibling jealousy and/or neglect due to increased focus on the child with pain; lack of family activities such as eating dinner together or going to church; canceled vacations or plans)
Questions to ask youth with chronic musculoskeletal pain
• What have you tried to manage the pain? Do you have strategies that help? (e.g., medication, warm bath, television, or video games)
• What does your pain get in the way of or stop you from doing? (e.g., going to school, participating in extra-curricular activities, spending time with friends)
• How has pain affected your mood?
• What worries do you have about your pain or your health? (e.g., worries about etiology of pain, its duration, its impact on activities such as sports; worry about re-injury or making pain worse with movement)

Psychoeducation

Psychoeducation is the initial foundation upon which CBT skills can be built. The initial goal of intervention for musculoskeletal pain is to restore physical functioning, improve physical endurance, and enhance coping skills, with the secondary goal to reduce pain intensity. This treatment approach can be challenging for families to appreciate, given that many patients and families hold the belief that physical functioning and activity can only improve once pain intensity has reduced. This belief is accurate for the treatment of acute pain (e.g., you can't participate in soccer practice until your broken bone has healed), but a different approach is necessary when pain becomes chronic. The Gate Control Theory of Pain is a useful framework to inform patients and families about how pain is processed in the brain and why cognitive and behavioral skills can be effective for managing pain. Providing a developmentally appropriate explanation of the brain–body connection to patients of all ages provides a justification for making functional changes prior to pain reduction and must be emphasized repeatedly throughout treatment to both the youth and the caregiver. Below is a sample clinician script describing the Gate Control Theory of Pain to Haley.

> Now we're going to start with a science lesson about how your body feels pain using a theory called the Gate Control Theory. This explanation can help you understand why the coping skills we'll discuss can be so helpful for managing pain.
>
> Many years ago, we used to think that the way we felt pain was quite simple. We thought that there were specific nerves in our body that picked up the pain signal and carried it straight to a pain center in our brain, kind of like an electrical wire. Once our brain received this pain signal, we would know we were hurt.
>
> We now know that the way our body feels pain is a lot more complicated. It involves our central nervous system—our brain and spinal cord—and our peripheral nervous system—all the nerves throughout our body. According to the Gate Control Theory of pain, pain messages flow along the nerves up to the spinal cord. However, before the pain message reaches the brain, it passes through what we refer to as "pain gates." Obviously, you don't actually have gates in your body, but nerves and brain chemicals that work like gates. These gates can make the pain message either stronger (so the pain would hurt more) or weaker (and the pain would hurt less).
>
> Now we're going to talk about certain things that help close pain gates and decrease the pain signal. One way the pain signal can be made weaker or even blocked is by medication. This may be why your physician initially prescribed medication. Scientists have also found other areas in your brain that are connected to pain gates. These include the center for your thoughts and the center for your feelings. For example, let's say you were watching a really funny TV show or were spending time with your best friend and having a really good time. For many people, these activities partially close their pain gates and make pain feel a bit better. The reason this happens is that positive mood (how we may feel when we're watching a funny show) and enjoyable activities (spending time with our friend) distract our brain from the pain signal and partially close pain gates. Importantly, positive mood and fun activities don't make pain go away, but they affect how many pain signals our brain receives and therefore the intensity of the pain we feel.
>
> Our thoughts and our feelings can also open pain gates and increase the pain signal our brain receives. While distraction and being in a positive mood can help close pain gates, attention to pain (or thinking a lot about pain) and being in a negative mood can open pain gates. This is because thinking about pain "primes" the brain to feel more pain. The same can be true for when we're having a bad day or when we feel frustrated with our siblings. These thoughts and feelings open the pain gates and increase the pain signal.
>
> Finally, the tension in our body can also serve to open or close pain gates. The relaxation response in our body causes many physical things to happen—heart rate slows,

breathing slows, muscles become less tight and tense, and the pain gates close. Thus, learning deep relaxation, including how to relax muscles, can help close pain gates and interrupt the pain and tension cycle.

Throughout treatment, we're going to discuss specific strategies that can be useful in closing pain gates. Knowing a bit more about how our body experiences pain can help you understand why these strategies may help you manage pain.

Throughout treatment, clinicians should continue to discuss how behaviors, thoughts, and feelings can affect the position of the pain gate and emphasize that youth will learn specific cognitive and behavioral strategies to help close their pain gate as well as reduce muscle tension and proactively address overexertion to prevent pain flares.

Caregiver Guidelines Parenting a child with chronic musculoskeletal pain is challenging, and caregivers may initially react in a protective manner while diagnostic workup is being completed for fear of making symptoms worse. Once significant medical conditions and/or injuries have been ruled out (or medically addressed), caregivers may need to be prompted to shift their expectations and encourage their child to function despite pain and fatigue. It is helpful to review caregiver guidelines to help caregivers support their child in active coping strategies. The following guidelines were discussed with Haley and her mother.

Guideline 1: Encourage your child to manage his/her physical symptoms independently The goal of guideline 1 is to promote independent self-management of pain symptoms and reduce over-reliance on caregivers for coping strategies.

> Haley informed her psychologist that she often texts her mother from school when she experiences pain. The psychologist encouraged mother to help Haley problem solve how to manage pain while remaining at school by utilizing the skills she learns throughout treatment. As Haley learned new strategies to manage pain, she kept a list of them in her planner that she could reference at school, prior to calling home.

Guideline 2: Eliminate status checks. Do not ask about pain Caregivers often show their love and support by giving their children attention and asking questions about their symptoms. Once pain persists, this approach can become a habit and the center of family conversations; however, attention to pain can inadvertently open pain gates. Thus, avoidance of pain talk is the best method to *decrease* attention to pain symptoms and help close pain gates.

> Haley and her mother endorsed that Haley's mother frequently asked how she is feeling, despite her mother being able to visibly see when pain is higher by Haley limping. Additionally, Haley mentioned that frequent questions about her health made her focus on her lack of progress and how pain seemed to be the defining feature of her life.

Guideline 3: Praise your child for actively coping and using the new skills they are learning Positively reinforcing a behavior increases the likelihood of that behavior being repeated. Thus, caregivers are instructed to *decrease* attention to pain symptoms and behaviors (Guideline 2) and *increase* attention to active coping efforts (Guideline 3). Active coping refers to behaviors that either physiologically relax the body or actively distract the child and help close pain gates. Avoidance of passive coping techniques, such as rest, sleep, or lying down, is important as these unintentionally contribute to deconditioning, poor endurance, sleep disruption, and ongoing physical impairment. The use of electronics for distraction is often a source of contention between caregivers and youth. While effective for distraction, electronics should not be the sole coping strategy because they cannot be utilized across multiple settings (e.g., school, dance practice).

> With support from psychology providers, Haley's parents developed a reinforcement plan in which Haley earned time on her phone when she engaged in relaxation strategies rather than napping to cope with pain flares after school.

Guideline 4: Help your child maintain normal activity/routines The goal of maintaining functioning and resuming normal routines is to ultimately change the brain's experience of chronic pain. Protective, avoidance behaviors such as rest and withdrawal from activities are counterproductive and can unintentionally reinforce attention to pain and delay recovery. Thus, caregivers are instructed to help their child maintain normal activity and routines even in the presence of pain.

> Haley and her family were encouraged to resume family pizza night on Mondays, light chores, and game night on Thursdays (all of which they had stopped when Haley's pain persisted and worsened). While some activities needed to be modified to help Haley be successful, modifications are preferential to avoidance.

Relaxation Training

A wealth of literature supports the use of relaxation training to significantly reduce pain (Palermo et al. 2010). Patients with widespread musculoskeletal pain may particularly benefit from learning a variety of relaxation strategies as a method to ease muscle tension, reduce physiological arousal, and promote physical comfort (particularly in settings where certain positions flare their musculoskeletal pains). Progressive muscle relaxation (PMR) is particularly helpful in this regard, although caution should be used for patients with joint problems or hypermobility since some PMR stretches might unintentionally worsen an unstable joint. Thus, it is important for clinicians to ask the patient about problematic body areas prior to practicing relaxation strategies in order to offer methods of adapting exercises for painful areas (i.e., engage in an autogenic progressive muscle relaxation rather than the more traditional muscle tightening and releasing for a particular area).

> Haley reported experiencing intense ankle pain prior to practicing PMR. Therefore, her psychologist modified PMR instructions to simply observe any tension she was experiencing in her ankle and notice what her ankle felt like if tension was released. This modification worked well for Haley and she was able to participate fully in the remainder of PMR practice. Additionally, a practice plan was developed, comparable to her home exercise program in physical therapy. Haley chose to practice PMR at bedtime to ease the aches of the day and help obtain a comfortable sleep position. She also decided to use PMR after her physical therapy session as a method to recover from the pain flare that typically occurred following completion of physical therapy exercises.

Activity Pacing

Activity pacing and behavioral activation are highly relevant strategies for overcoming activity avoidance in patients with widespread chronic pain. For adults with chronic pain, there is strong evidence to suggest activity avoidance and/or overexertion are significantly correlated with disability and poor outcomes, although results for activity pacing are less clear and may be dependent on the outcome variable, its measurement, and/or how pacing was utilized (i.e., reactively versus proactively; Andrews et al. 2012; Karsdorp and Vlaeyen 2009; McCracken and Samuel 2007). Similar to adults with chronic pain, youth have often gone from moderate or high levels of physical activity (i.e., playing sports, dancing) to sedentary behavior. As a result, muscle weakness and poor endurance compound to create pain flares for even mild levels of activity. Thus, the first goal of pacing is exposure to increased physical activity in a graduated manner.

Activity pacing emphasizes remaining active despite pain but with breaks to proactively avoid pain flares. Short, frequent breaks are often more effective than being active for longer periods of time followed by extended recovery. Importantly, youth may be resistant to adopting this approach for a variety of reasons including inconvenience, fear of looking different than their peers, or fear of adults (coaches, caregivers, teachers) being upset with them for taking breaks. Thus, the psychologist must first develop a behavioral plan for activity pacing, then identify and problem solve obstacles for implementation (Table 13.3).

> Upon initiating treatment, Haley was inactive and worried about creating pain flares with move-

ment. Thus, activity pacing goals were to (1) increase Haley's overall activity level and (2) pace physically demanding activities. As described earlier, Haley's psychologist encouraged active coping and restricted daily naps and resting in bed. To comply with her physician's request to resume aerobic exercise, Haley agreed to a graded exercise plan and she chose to use the family's elliptical machine to do so. Based on previous attempts at exercise, Haley reported that working out on the elliptical machine for more than 10 minutes resulted in increased fatigue and achiness. Thus, the following pacing plan was developed:

In addition to identifying a specific exercise Haley could complete during active minutes (i.e., using the elliptical machine), the psychologist and Haley brainstormed what she could do during her break. Haley agreed to hydrate with water, engage in a few targeted physical therapy stretches, and take slow, deep breaths. Following her break, she would resume exercise on the elliptical machine, repeating the sequence for a total of three rounds. Haley chose to exercise every 2–3 days to give her body a chance to recover between activity.

As described above, it is critical to assess baseline levels of activity prior to developing an activity pacing plan. Given that Haley reported exercising for more than 10 min resulted in increased fatigue and pain, the psychologist encouraged Haley to take brief breaks following no more than 5 min of activity. Alternating activity with rest may help youth gradually develop endurance while decreasing the likelihood of a pain flare due to overexertion. In addition to collaboratively developing an activity pacing plan, several strategies are recommended to increase compliance with activity pacing. First, write the behavioral plan down and thoroughly describe the type of activity to be completed, the duration of activity and rest breaks, and specific behaviors and coping skills to engage in during rest breaks. Second, problem solve with youth and caregivers to identify and address potential barriers to implementing the pacing plan. Some youth benefit from scheduling a specific time to engage in physical activity, using phone alarms to track activity duration and rest breaks, and receiving positive reinforcement following implementation of activity pacing. Activity pacing can be applied to several distinct activities including family outings, social events, being in school all day, and participating in gym class. Clinicians should help families prioritize activity goals when collaboratively developing an activity pacing plan.

Cognitive Restructuring for Fear of Movement

Dysfunctional beliefs and cognitive biases play a critical role in affect and behavior change (Beck 2008). Pain has historically been recognized as a warning signal for danger (Price 1988). As such, attentional models propose that pain "interrupts, distracts, and demands attention" (Eccleston and Crombez 1999: 357). For acute pain or injury, this appraisal and response is necessary. However, when pain becomes chronic, the belief that "pain signals danger" becomes dysfunctional and can actually promote activity avoidance and contradict rehabilitation goals. Fear of pain, such as worrying whether pain will ever go away, and fear of movement, such as believing that movement is physically dangerous, are common among individuals with chronic pain (Leeuw et al. 2007; Roelofs et al. 2007). These beliefs are linked to greater activity withdrawal (Crombez et al. 2012), emotional distress, and

Table 13.3 Haley's pacing plan

Week	Goal	Schedule	Total active minutes	Total time
Week 1	~15 active minutes 2–3/week	5:00 exercise/3:00 break for three rounds	15	24
Week 2	~20 active minutes 2–3/week	7:00 exercise/3:00 break for three rounds	21	30
Week 3	~25 active minutes 2–3/week	9:00 exercise/3:00 break for three rounds	27	36
Week 4	~30 active minutes 2–3/week	11:00 exercise/3:00 break for three rounds	33	42

functional impairment (Severeijns et al. 2001; Stroud et al. 2000; see Crombez et al. 2012 for discussion of Fear Avoidance Model). Therefore, cognitive restructuring is an essential component of CBT for individuals with widespread musculoskeletal pain. Cognitive restructuring helps patients generate more positive, realistic, and functional thinking styles (Mills et al. 2008). The goal for patients with chronic musculoskeletal pain is to identify and challenge dysfunctional beliefs about pain and movement and ultimately generate more helpful, calming beliefs.

> For Haley, her fear of being active was the result of a strong belief that pain would never improve and that she would reinjure herself if she engaged in physical activity. Additionally, Haley took an extreme, all-or-nothing approach to coping skills, reporting them to be ineffective if they did not markedly improve her symptoms. These attitudes affected her overall motivation to engage in physical therapy as well as behavioral coping strategies, and led to inconsistent use of coping skills in the beginning of the treatment. In response, Haley's psychologist helped her reconceptualize the purpose of coping skills to include emotional calming not pain reduction, the need for a variety of tools, and that efficacy of skills was associated with practice. When Haley identified that a coping technique was not working well, problem solving was employed to modify the technique or the situation rather than abandon the technique. For example, Haley disliked taking breaks on the elliptical machine because it disrupted her exercise rhythm; thus, breaks were re-conceptualized as decreasing effort on the elliptical machine to low-intensity movement to prevent her muscles from getting cold and tight. Her psychologist also gradually integrated cognitive strategies (identifying and challenging automatic thoughts) into each session while continuing to introduce behavioral strategies. This approach allowed Haley to use her experience with behavioral strategies, such as activity pacing, to help modify cognitive beliefs (e.g., "I did not get injured when I started back on the elliptical. I was sore after using the elliptical, but the next day my joints felt better").

As evidenced in the above description, it is critical to integrate cognitive strategies throughout treatment, even if formal instruction on cognitive restructuring occurs later after teaching other pain coping skills.

Healthy Lifestyle Habits

Proper sleep and nutrition are vital to maintaining health, emotional well-being, and recovery from illness or pain (Hagan et al. 2017). Sleep problems including frequent night-time awakenings and extreme tiredness are common in adolescents with chronic musculoskeletal pain (Harrison et al. 2014). As a result, youth may utilize electronics for distraction or feel the need to sleep during the day, ultimately perpetuating unhealthy sleep habits. Moreover, individuals with chronic widespread musculoskeletal pain commonly report headaches, dizziness, and fatigue, symptoms which may be improved with proper hydration and nutrition. Thus, youth with chronic musculoskeletal pain often benefit from psychoeducation and behavioral plans to promote healthy sleeping and eating habits. [Refer Chaps. 17 and 18 for a more thorough review of behavioral plans to promote healthy nutrition and sleep.]

> Upon initiating treatment, Haley's sleep was poor. She frequently took long naps after school and would not fall asleep until approximately 1 a.m. As mentioned above, Haley's parents implemented a reinforcement plan in which Haley earned time on her phone when she engaged in relaxation strategies rather than napping to cope with pain flares after school. To further support healthy sleeping habits, Haley was advised to use her bed only for sleeping at night (not for resting, watching TV, or playing on her phone). If she needed a break during the day, Haley was instructed to do so in a common area of the home such as the living room or kitchen. Additionally, Haley agreed to initiate a sleep routine including a warm bath and calming activities (e.g., drawing, reading) before bed with the goal of being ready to sleep by 10:30 p.m. Finally, Haley's family decided to make a group lifestyle change whereby phones from all family members were left to charge in the kitchen at night, thus reducing the temptation to use electronics as a bedtime coping distraction.

Problem Solving for School Coping

One common challenge youth with chronic musculoskeletal pain experience is attending school full time, as they feel more confident in their ability cope with pain symptoms at home rather than at school. Developing school-based coping plans and identifying modifications to support comfort and functioning can be helpful. Psychologists are in the best position to develop accommodation plans including identifying activities during the school day that are most painful for the patient (i.e., walking between classes quickly; physical education class, carrying a heavy back pain), recommending accommodations that may be helpful (i.e., extra time between classes; ability to substitute low-intensity exercise for high-intensity exercise in physical education class), and formulating plans to putting accommodations into place (i.e., developing a plan to leave class 5 min early to avoid rushing between classes). Modifications should be presented as tools to improve school attendance and physical comfort.

> Haley identified that walking between classes quickly and being at school for an entire day worsened pain and fatigue. The psychologist and Haley generated a few helpful changes to improve these issues including being allowed to arrive a few minutes late to each class without receiving a tardy and having a 10-minute mid-morning and mid-afternoon break in a quiet area (guidance office) to practice her relaxation strategies. Haley's psychologist wrote a letter supporting these modifications, which Haley, her mother, and the school guidance counselor reviewed together. Haley reported that having a formal, written plan made her feel more comfortable using the accommodations and gave the school specific information about what she needed. Additionally, Haley liked having routine relaxation breaks built into her daily schedule so that she did not have to determine if/when she needed the accommodations and did not have to repeatedly approach teachers to request help. Because Haley's plan was written and specific, teachers were more likely to follow Haley's school coping plan.

The need for and types of modifications are unique to each patient. Common modifications for youth with chronic musculoskeletal pain are presented in Box 13.1.

The sample modifications support the adolescent in achieving the overarching goal of reducing school avoidance and attendance issues, and promoting active coping in the school environment. The acceptance of behavioral coping plans and requirement of a formal accommodation plan (e.g., 504 Plan) vary widely between school districts. However, certain accommodations such as homebound instruction or an attendance waiver are not consistent with a rehabilitative, functional approach to managing chronic pain.

Box 13.1 Common Modifications for Youth with Chronic Musculoskeletal Pain

- Extra time between classes (leaving class early or arriving to class a few minutes late)
- Use of the elevator as needed
- Ability to stand and stretch (either in the classroom or via more frequent bathroom breaks)
- Access to a top locker
- Ability to have a second set of books to leave at home to reduce backpack load
- Ability to leave heavy textbooks in the classroom rather than carry them to a locker
- Modified physical education class (ability to take breaks, substitute low-impact activity for high-impact activity)
- Ability to practice relaxation exercises in a quiet location

---

Relapse Prevention

The conclusion of CBT for youth with chronic musculoskeletal pain involves skill consolidation and development of maintenance plans to support independent self-management of pain while preparing the patient for inevitable pain flares and challenges implementing coping skills. To support effective coping, youth often benefit from planned maintenance sessions at times of the year that are more problematic (e.g., returning to school after an extended break, prior to exam week) or following a designated period of time (e.g., 1 month after concluding weekly treatment). For youth with additional mental health needs, psychologists need to either re-focus treatment or refer the patient to another mental health provider who can continue to address other problematic symptoms. Reviewing patient-reported assessment outcomes can be a useful tool to help families recognize when treatment has been effective (i.e., functional impairment has reduced) even in the absence of pain reduction. Finally, some youth continue to struggle with generalizing or implementing coping skills and require periodic assistance in refining behavioral coping plans to address novel challenges.

Conclusion

Chronic musculoskeletal pain is diverse in presentation and associated with functional impairment and disability. Treatment of chronic musculoskeletal pain often requires a multidisciplinary approach to intervention with the overarching goal to resume normal functioning and gradually return to daily activities with environmental and social support. Providers working with youth with chronic musculoskeletal pain should continually integrate psychoeducation with behavioral and cognitive strategies. The long-term medical and emotional outcomes of youth who complete CBT for chronic musculoskeletal pain are yet unknown. However, the immediate benefits of CBT are notable and hopefully provide youth with effective self-management techniques and increased coping efficacy to manage a complex pain condition.

References

Andrews, N. E., Strong, J., & Meredith, P. J. (2012). Activity pacing, avoidance, endurance, and associations with patient functioning in chronic pain: A systematic review and meta-analysis. *Archives of Physical Medicine and Rehabilitation, 93*(11), 2109–2121.

Bartley, E. J., & Fillingim, R. B. (2013). Sex differences in pain: A brief review of clinical and experimental findings. *British Journal of Anaesthesia, 111*(1), 52–58.

Beck, A. T. (2008). The evolution of the cognitive model of depression and its neurobiological correlates. *American Journal of Psychiatry, 165*(8), 969–977.

Claar, R. L., Simons, L. E., & Logan, D. E. (2008). Parental response to children's pain: The moderating impact of children's emotional distress on symptoms and disability. *Pain, 138*(1), 172–179.

Conte, P. M., Walco, G. A., & Kimura, Y. (2003). Temperament and stress response in children with juvenile primary fibromyalgia syndrome. *Arthritis and Rheumatism, 48*(10), 2923–2930.

Crombez, G., Eccleston, C., Van Damme, S., Vlaeyen, J. W., & Karoly, P. (2012). Fear-avoidance model of chronic pain: The next generation. *The Clinical Journal of Pain, 28*(6), 475–483.

De Inocencio, J. (2004). Epidemiology of musculoskeletal pain in primary care. *Archives of Disease in Childhood, 89*(5), 431–434.

Diatchenko, L., Fillingim, R. B., Smith, S. B., & Maixner, W. (2013). The phenotypic and genetic signatures of common musculoskeletal pain conditions. *Nature Reviews Rheumatology, 9*(6), 340.

Eccleston, C., & Crombez, G. (1999). Pain demands attention: A cognitive–affective model of the interruptive function of pain. *Psychological Bulletin, 125*(3), 356.

Eccleston, C., Palermo, T. M., de C Williams, A. C., Holley, A. L., Morley, S., Fisher, E., et al. (2014). Psychological therapies for the management of chronic and recurrent pain in children and adolescents. *The Cochrane Database of Systematic Reviews*, (5), CD003968.

Edwards, R. R., Dworkin, R. H., Sullivan, M. D., Turk, D. C., & Wasan, A. D. (2016). The role of psychosocial processes in the development and maintenance of chronic pain. *The Journal of Pain, 17*(9), T70–T92.

Engel, G. L. (1977). The need for a new medical model: A challenge for biomedicine. *Science, 196*(4286), 129–136.

Evans, S., Djilas, V., Seidman, L. C., Zeltzer, L. K., & Tsao, J. C. (2017). Sleep quality, affect, pain, and disability in children with chronic pain: Is affect a mediator or moderator? *The Journal of Pain, 18*(9), 1087–1095.

Forgeron, P. A., King, S., Stinson, J. N., McGrath, P. J., MacDonald, A. J., & Chambers, C. T. (2010). Social functioning and peer relationships in children and adolescents with chronic pain: A systematic review. *Pain Research and Management, 15*(1), 27–41.

Gatchel, R. J., Peng, Y. B., Peters, M. L., Fuchs, P. N., & Turk, D. C. (2007). The biopsychosocial approach to chronic pain: Scientific advances and future directions. *Psychological Bulletin, 133*(4), 581.

Giedd, J. N., Keshavan, M., & Paus, T. (2008). Why do many psychiatric disorders emerge during adolescence? *Nature Reviews Neuroscience, 9*(12), 947.

Hagan, J. F., Shaw, J. S., & Duncan, P. M. (2017). *Bright futures: Guidelines for health supervision of infants, children, and adolescents* (4th ed.). Elk Grove Village: American Academy of Pediatrics.

Harrison, L., Wilson, S., & Munafò, M. R. (2014). Exploring the associations between sleep problems and chronic musculoskeletal pain in adolescents: A prospective cohort study. *Pain Research and Management, 19*(5), e139–e145.

Holley, A. L., Wilson, A. C., & Palermo, T. M. (2017). Predictors of the transition from acute to persistent musculoskeletal pain in children and adolescents: A prospective study. *Pain, 158*(5), 794.

Hunfeld, J. A., Perquin, C. W., Duivenvoorden, H. J., Hazebroek-Kampschreur, A. A., Passchier, J., van Suijlekom-Smit, L. W., et al. (2001). Chronic pain and its impact on quality of life in adolescents and their families. *Journal of Pediatric Psychology, 26*(3), 145–153.

Karsdorp, P. A., & Vlaeyen, J. W. (2009). Active avoidance but not activity pacing is associated with disability in fibromyalgia. *Pain®, 147*(1–3), 29–35.

Kashikar-Zuck, S., Vaught, M. H., Goldschneider, K. R., Graham, T. B., & Miller, J. C. (2002). Depression, coping, and functional disability in juvenile primary fibromyalgia syndrome. *The Journal of Pain, 3*(5), 412–419.

Kashikar-Zuck, S., Swain, N. F., Jones, B. A., & Graham, T. B. (2005). Efficacy of cognitive-behavioral intervention for juvenile primary fibromyalgia syndrome. *The Journal of Rheumatology, 32*(8), 1594–1602.

Kashikar-Zuck, S., Lynch, A. M., Graham, T. B., Swain, N. F., Mullen, S. M., & Noll, R. B. (2007). Social functioning and peer relationships of adolescents with juvenile fibromyalgia syndrome. *Arthritis Care & Research, 57*(3), 474–480.

Kashikar-Zuck, S., Flowers, S. R., Claar, R. L., Guite, J. W., Logan, D. E., Lynch-Jordan, A. M., et al. (2011). Clinical utility and validity of the Functional Disability Inventory among a multicenter sample of youth with chronic pain. *Pain®, 152*(7), 1600–1607.

Kashikar-Zuck, S., Ting, T. V., Arnold, L. M., Bean, J., Powers, S. W., Graham, T. B., et al. (2012). Cognitive behavioral therapy for the treatment of juvenile fibromyalgia: A multisite, single-blind, randomized, controlled clinical trial. *Arthritis and Rheumatism, 64*(1), 297–305.

King, S., Chambers, C. T., Huguet, A., MacNevin, R. C., McGrath, P. J., Parker, L., et al. (2011). The epidemiology of chronic pain in children and adolescents revisited: A systematic review. *Pain, 152*(12), 2729–2738.

Leeuw, M., Goossens, M. E., Linton, S. J., Crombez, G., Boersma, K., & Vlaeyen, J. W. (2007). The fear-avoidance model of musculoskeletal pain: Current state of scientific evidence. *Journal of Behavioral Medicine, 30*(1), 77–94.

Lewandowski, A. S., Palermo, T. M., Stinson, J., Handley, S., & Chambers, C. T. (2010). Systematic review of family functioning in families of children and adolescents with chronic pain. *The Journal of Pain, 11*(11), 1027–1038.

Li, J., Simone, D. A., & Larson, A. A. (1999). Windup leads to characteristics of central sensitization. *Pain, 79*(1), 75–82.

Lynch-Jordan, A. M., Sil, S., Peugh, J., Cunningham, N., Kashikar-Zuck, S., & Goldschneider, K. R. (2014). Differential changes in functional disability and pain intensity over the course of psychological treatment for children with chronic pain. *Pain®, 155*(10), 1955–1961.

McCracken, L. M., & Samuel, V. M. (2007). The role of avoidance, pacing, and other activity patterns in chronic pain. *Pain, 130*(1–2), 119–125.

McGrath, P. J., Walco, G. A., Turk, D. C., Dworkin, R. H., Brown, M. T., Davidson, K., et al. (2008). Core outcome domains and measures for pediatric acute and chronic/recurrent pain clinical trials: PedIMMPACT recommendations. *The Journal of Pain, 9*(9), 771–783.

Meeus, M., & Nijs, J. (2007). Central sensitization: A biopsychosocial explanation for chronic widespread pain in patients with fibromyalgia and chronic fatigue syndrome. *Clinical Rheumatology, 26*(4), 465–473.

Melzack, R. (1996, June). Gate control theory: On the evolution of pain concepts. In *Pain forum* (Vol. 5, No. 2, pp. 128–138). Elsevier.

Melzack, R. (2001). Pain and the neuromatrix in the brain. *Journal of Dental Education, 65*(12), 1378–1382.

Melzack, R., & Katz, J. (2004). The gate control theory: Reaching for the brain. *Pain: Psychological Perspectives*, 13–34.

Melzack, R., & Wall, P. D. (1965). Pain mechanisms: A new theory. *Science, 150*(3699), 971–979.

Mendell, L. M. (2014). Constructing and deconstructing the gate theory of pain. *Pain®, 155*(2), 210–216.

Mills, H., Reiss, N., & Dombeck, M. (2008). Self-efficacy and the perception of control in stress reduction. *Mental Help*.

Palermo, T. M. (2000). Impact of recurrent and chronic pain on child and family daily functioning: A critical review of the literature. *Journal of Developmental and Behavioral Pediatrics, 21*(1), 58–69.

Palermo, T. M., Wilson, A. C., Peters, M., Lewandowski, A., & Somhegyi, H. (2009). Randomized controlled trial of an Internet-delivered family cognitive–behavioral therapy intervention for children and adolescents with chronic pain. *Pain, 146*(1–2), 205–213.

Palermo, T. M., Eccleston, C., Lewandowski, A. S., Williams, A. C. D. C., & Morley, S. (2010). Randomized controlled trials of psychological therapies for management of chronic pain in children and adolescents: An updated meta-analytic review. *Pain®, 148*(3), 387–397.

Palermo, T., Eccleston, C., Goldschneider, K., McGinn, K. L., Sethna, N., Schechter, N., & Turner, H. (2013). Assessment and management of children with chronic pain: A position statement from the American Pain Society. Chicago, IL: American Pain Society.

Palermo, T. M., Valrie, C. R., & Karlson, C. W. (2014). Family and parent influences on pediatric chronic pain: A developmental perspective. *American Psychologist, 69*(2), 142.

Perquin, C. W., Hazebroek-Kampschreur, A. A., Hunfeld, J. A., Bohnen, A. M., van Suijlekom-Smit, L. W., Passchier, J., et al. (2000). Pain in children and adolescents: A common experience. *Pain, 87*(1), 51–58.

Price, D. D. (1988). Classical and current theories of pain mechanisms. In D. D. Price (Ed.), *Psychological and neural mechanisms of pain* (pp. 212–231). New York: Raven Press.

Roelofs, J., Sluiter, J. K., Frings-Dresen, M. H., Goossens, M., Thibault, P., Boersma, K., et al. (2007). Fear of movement and (re) injury in chronic musculoskeletal pain: Evidence for an invariant two-factor model of the Tampa Scale for Kinesiophobia across pain diagnoses and Dutch, Swedish, and Canadian samples. *Pain, 131*(1–2), 181–190.

Roth-Isigkeit, A., Thyen, U., Stöven, H., Schwarzenberger, J., & Schmucker, P. (2005). Pain among children and adolescents: Restrictions in daily living and triggering factors. *Pediatrics, 115*(2), e152–e162.

Severeijns, R., Vlaeyen, J. W., van den Hout, M. A., & Weber, W. E. (2001). Pain catastrophizing predicts pain intensity, disability, and psychological distress independent of the level of physical impairment. *The Clinical Journal of Pain, 17*(2), 165–172.

Simons, L. E., Sieberg, C. B., Carpino, E., Logan, D., & Berde, C. (2011). The Fear of Pain Questionnaire (FOPQ): Assessment of pain-related fear among children and adolescents with chronic pain. *The Journal of Pain, 12*(6), 677–686.

Sleed, M., Eccleston, C., Beecham, J., Knapp, M., & Jordan, A. (2005). The economic impact of chronic pain in adolescence: Methodological considerations and a preliminary costs-of-illness study. *Pain, 119*(1–3), 183–190.

Sörensen, J., Graven-Nielsen, T., Henriksson, K. G., Bengtsson, M., & Arendt-Nielsen, L. (1998). Hyperexcitability in fibromyalgia. *The Journal of Rheumatology, 25*(1), 152–155.

Staud, R., & Smitherman, M. L. (2002). Peripheral and central sensitization in fibromyalgia: Pathogenetic role. *Current Pain and Headache Reports, 6*(4), 259–266.

Stroud, M. W., Thorn, B. E., Jensen, M. P., & Boothby, J. L. (2000). The relation between pain beliefs, negative thoughts, and psychosocial functioning in chronic pain patients. *Pain®, 84*(2–3), 347–352.

Treede, R. D., Rief, W., Barke, A., Aziz, Q., Bennett, M. I., Benoliel, R., et al. (2015). A classification of chronic pain for ICD-11. *Pain, 156*(6), 1003.

Varni, J. W., Stucky, B. D., Thissen, D., DeWitt, E. M., Irwin, D. E., Lai, J. S., et al. (2010). PROMIS Pediatric Pain Interference Scale: An item response theory analysis of the pediatric pain item bank. *The Journal of Pain, 11*(11), 1109–1119.

Walker, L. S., & Greene, J. W. (1991). The functional disability inventory: Measuring a neglected dimension of child health status. *Journal of Pediatric Psychology, 16*(1), 39–58.

Woby, S. R., Roach, N. K., Urmston, M., & Watson, P. J. (2005). Psychometric properties of the TSK-11: A shortened version of the Tampa Scale for Kinesiophobia. *Pain, 117*(1–2), 137–144.

Wolfe, F., Clauw, D. J., Fitzcharles, M. A., Goldenberg, D. L., Katz, R. S., Mease, P., et al. (2010). The American College of Rheumatology preliminary diagnostic criteria for fibromyalgia and measurement of symptom severity. *Arthritis Care & Research, 62*(5), 600–610.

Zapata, A. L., Moraes, A. J. P., Leone, C., Doria-Filho, U., & Silva, C. A. A. (2006). Pain and musculoskeletal pain syndromes in adolescents. *Journal of Adolescent Health, 38*(6), 769–771.

Cognitive Behavioral Therapy for Functional Abdominal Pain Disorders

Kari Baber and Kelly A. O'Neil Rodriguez

Introduction

Functional Abdominal Pain Disorders

Functional abdominal pain disorders (FAPDs) are a subcategory within the broader classification of functional gastrointestinal disorders (FGIDs). Functional gastrointestinal disorders (FGIDs) include symptoms of the gastrointestinal tract (e.g., abdominal pain, nausea, vomiting, bowel symptoms) and are among the most common functional disorders in pediatrics. FGIDs, including FAPDs, are described by symptom-based diagnostic criteria; these are commonly referred to as the "Rome criteria," named after the nonprofit organization (The Rome Foundation) that supports and organizes international groups of experts to develop consensus- and research-based guidelines for FGID diagnosis and treatment. The current Rome criteria (Rome IV; Hyams et al. 2016) describe three categories of FGIDs affecting children and adolescents: functional abdominal pain disorders (FAPDs: functional dyspepsia, irritable bowel syndrome, abdominal migraine, functional abdominal pain—not otherwise specified), functional nausea and vomiting disorders (cyclic vomiting syndrome, functional nausea and functional vomiting, rumination syndrome, aerophagia), and functional defecation disorders (functional constipation, nonretentive fecal incontinence). Recent large, community-based studies of FGID epidemiology describe that more than 20% of youth experience symptoms consistent with Rome IV FGID criteria. The most common FGIDs included the functional abdominal pain disorders, endorsed by 8–17% of the sample, and functional constipation, endorsed by 10–14% (Robin et al. 2018; Saps et al. 2018).

Similar to other types of pediatric chronic illness and chronic pain disorders in particular (e.g., Lewandowski et al. 2010), functional abdominal pain disorders can have a profound impact on child and family functioning. In cross-sectional studies, pediatric FGIDs are associated with decreased health-related quality of life (Robin et al. 2018; Varni et al. 2015), increased school absences and parental missed work (Robin et al. 2018), and high health care utilization (Varni et al. 2015). In a recent qualitative study, families of children with functional abdominal pain described high levels of uncertainty and caregiving stress (Brodwall et al. 2018). In longi-

K. Baber (✉) · K. A. O'Neil Rodriguez
Department of Child and Adolescent Psychiatry and Behavioral Sciences, The Children's Hospital of Philadelphia, Philadelphia, PA, USA

Department of Pediatrics/Division of Gastroenterology, Hepatology and Nutrition, The Children's Hospital of Philadelphia, Philadelphia, PA, USA
e-mail: baberk@email.chop.edu; rodrigueka@email.chop.edu

tudinal studies, pediatric FAPDs are associated with higher current and lifetime risk of anxiety disorders, higher lifetime risk of depressive disorders (Shelby et al. 2013), and higher incidence of FGID symptoms in adulthood (Horst et al. 2014).

Cognitive Behavior Therapy for Functional Gastrointestinal Symptoms

The first studies of cognitive behavioral interventions for pediatric patients with functional gastrointestinal symptoms were published nearly three decades ago (Finney et al. 1989; Sanders et al. 1989), when the nomenclature "recurrent abdominal pain" was used to describe chronic abdominal pain without an organic etiology. Since that time, cognitive behavior therapy (CBT) interventions have demonstrated positive effects in reducing pain and improving daily functioning for youth with functional gastrointestinal symptoms (Brent et al. 2008; Rutten et al. 2015). As a result, treatment guidelines for nearly all pediatric FGIDs now include behavioral and cognitive behavioral therapies (Hyams et al. 2016). This is especially true for the functional abdominal pain disorders (FAPDs), which have been the most widely studied and are the focus of this chapter.

Recent investigations of CBT for FAPDs have described positive treatment effects including decreased pain (Bonnert et al. 2017; Lalouni et al. 2016, 2017; Van der Veek et al. 2013; Zucker et al. 2017), improved gastrointestinal symptoms (Bonnert et al. 2017; Lalouni et al. 2016, 2017; Van der Veek et al. 2013), decreased medication use (Bonnert et al. 2017), fewer school absences (Bonnert et al. 2017; Lalouni et al. 2016, 2017) and caregiver work absences (Lalouni et al. 2017), decreased pain-related functional impairment (van der Veek et al. 2013; Zucker et al. 2017), and improved quality of life (Bonnert et al. 2017; Lalouni et al. 2016, 2017; Wassom et al. 2013). Additionally, recent investigations have supplemented traditional outcome measures (pain, symptoms, disability, quality of life) with process variables that may contribute to treatment outcomes and can be specifically targeted in CBT for pediatric FAPDs. Specifically, CBT has demonstrated positive treatment effects in reducing maladaptive pain behaviors (e.g., avoidance; Bonnert et al. 2017; Lalouni et al. 2017) and passive coping (Wassom et al. 2013) and in promoting increased use of distraction (Levy et al. 2010) and decreased caregiver monitoring and overprotective responses to pain (Lalouni et al. 2016; Levy et al. 2010). Recent developments including technology-supported interventions (GutStrong CD-ROM and workbook; Wassom et al. 2013), web-based interventions (Bonnert et al. 2017; Lalouni et al. 2017; Nieto et al. 2015), and hybrid interventions including both in-person and web-based sessions (ADAPT; Cunningham et al. 2018; Zucker et al. 2017) have further advanced the literature by assessing feasibility and acceptability of service delivery models with the potential to more broadly disseminate evidence-based treatment for pediatric FAPDs.

Biopsychosocial Conceptualization of Pediatric Functional Abdominal Pain Disorders

Biopsychosocial conceptualization of pediatric FAPDs reflects the understanding that biological, psychological, and environmental factors reciprocally interact to contribute to the clinical presentation, including gastrointestinal symptom severity and related impairment in daily functioning, health-related quality of life, and health care use (Drossman 2016; Van Oudenhove et al. 2016). Research in the field of neurogastroenterology suggests that physiological and psychosocial factors interact at the level of neural and hormonal pathways between the central nervous system (brain, spinal cord) and the enteric nervous system in the gut via the autonomic nervous system (ANS) and hypothalamic-pituitary-adrenal (HPA) axis. This "brain–gut axis" is bidirectional; gut physiology can influence mood and behavior, and in turn, cognitions and emotions affect perception of sensation, motility, and so forth in the gut. The evidence base for the role of the brain–gut axis in FGIDs is so compelling that these conditions are now considered "disorders of gut-brain interaction" (Drossman 2016: 1268). There is also evidence that the gut microbiome plays a role in symptoms of FGIDs and therefore should be included in the gut-brain model (Kennedy et al. 2014).

Biological factors involved in the gut-brain dysfunction of FGIDs may include physiological factors such as altered sensation, motility, immune function, food and diet, and gut microbiome (Drossman 2016). In FAPDs, visceral hypersensitivity is thought to play an important physiological role and is a target of directed pharmacological treatment in pediatric FGIDs (Rosen et al. 2014). Visceral hypersensitivity describes a decreased threshold for pain or discomfort and is increasingly understood to be related to psychological processes influencing perception of normal activity of the gut as painful (Van Oudenhove et al. 2016). The biopsychosocial conceptualization of FAPDs includes the potential role of visceral hypersensitivity and of symptoms or treatments associated with comorbid acute or chronic health problems.

Psychological factors to consider in evaluation and conceptualization of pediatric FAPDs include psychiatric comorbidities, coping skills, and symptom-related cognitions and beliefs. Psychological factors with demonstrated relationships to functional gastrointestinal symptoms in pediatric and adult populations include anxiety (Campo et al. 2004; Cunningham et al. 2015), depression (Campo et al. 2004; Pinto-Sanchez et al. 2015; Yacob et al. 2013), catastrophizing (Hunt et al. 2009; Langer et al. 2009; van Tilburg et al. 2013, 2015), and GI symptom-specific anxiety (Wilpart et al. 2017). Consistent with understanding of the brain–gut axis as bidirectional, these psychological factors may contribute to, exacerbate, and maintain functional gastrointestinal symptoms through altered perception or interpretation, ANS and stress hormone system response (HPA axis; Van Oudenhove et al. 2016), or changes in health-related behaviors. Likewise, gastrointestinal symptoms may also contribute to disturbances in mood and anxiety through disease-related distress and impairments in daily functioning (e.g., school absenteeism, limited participation in social or enjoyed activities).

Environmental or contextual factors to include in evaluation and conceptualization of youth with FAPDs include trauma history, chronic and acute stressors for the child and/or family, social support, and caregiver modeling and responses regarding GI symptoms. Environmental factors with links to functional GI symptoms in pediatric and adult populations include early adverse life events and history of trauma (Bradford et al. 2012; Sherman et al. 2015), perceived social support (Lackner et al. 2010), negative social interactions (Lackner et al. 2013), parental pain modeling (Stone and Walker 2017), and maladaptive (e.g., solicitous, protective, critical) parental responses to symptom reports (Claar et al. 2008; DuPen et al. 2016; Levy et al. 2004; Walker et al. 2006). Parental responses to symptom reports warrant particular attention in the clinician's evaluation and conceptualization of FAPDs: parents' cognitions about their children's symptoms may mediate treatment response (Levy et al. 2014), and caregiver responses to pain can be targeted in cognitive-behavioral therapy (e.g., Levy et al. 2010).

Finally, the biopsychosocial conceptualization as applied to youth with FAPDs must include developmental considerations, particularly in regard to psychological and social aspects of the framework (Palermo et al. 2014). For example, among younger children or those with limited autonomy and independence, caregiver responses to pain behaviors may have greater influence on coping and impairment than those for older youth. For children and adolescents with high levels of autonomy over daily routines, sleep dysregulation associated with physical symptoms may contribute to significant sleep schedule shifts, with associated impact on daily activities.

Case Example of Biopsychosocial Conceptualization for Pediatric FAPD

Tiana[1] is a 14-year-old biracial female referred by her gastroenterologist for psychological evaluation and intervention related to chronic GI symptoms of abdominal pain, bloating, and diarrhea. Tiana was diagnosed with lactose intolerance by a positive lactose breath test. However, her symptoms have persisted following elimination of lactose in her diet, leading the gastroenterologist to identify visceral hypersensitivity as another potential physiological factor in her presentation and diagnose Irritable Bowel Syndrome-Diarrhea Predominant. Tiana's GI symptoms have contributed to frequent school absences. Tiana's mother also shared with the gastroenterologist that the guidance counselor has expressed concerns about Tiana's adjustment to high school.

The psychological evaluation revealed that Tiana was experiencing subclinical depressive symptoms and GI symptom-specific anxiety. Tiana reported worrying both about experiencing future symptoms and about potentially embarrassing social aspects of her GI symptoms (e.g., "My stomach feels off. I'll probably have to go 10 times today and it would be better to stay home," and "My friends will start to notice how much I go to the bathroom and laugh."). This GI symptom-specific anxiety appeared to be contributing to Tiana's frequent school absences.

During the psychological evaluation, the family also described Tiana's recent transition to a new school as difficult due to challenges in making new friends. Tiana indicated that she had experienced relational aggression from a peer at her new school. Although the relational aggression had not been directly related to her GI symptoms to date, Tiana worried about the possibility that her symptoms or bathroom trips could become a target of the peer's aggression. Tiana frequently texted her mother at work in the morning to report GI symptoms of abdominal pain and diarrhea and then requested to stay home from school, which her mother accommodated due to concerns about sending Tiana to school "sick." Tiana's mother also noted that, as a single, working parent experiencing chronic financial strain, she had difficulty leaving work to take Tiana to school for a partial day if she had missed the bus in the morning due to symptoms. Tiana's mother described limited extended family or other social support available locally to help with transportation and childcare.

The psychologist working with Tiana and her mother shared the impression that, from a biopsychosocial perspective, biological (lactose intolerance, visceral hypersensitivity), psychological (depressive symptoms, GI symptom-specific anxiety), and environmental factors (peer victimization, school transition, caregiver protective responding, financial strain, limited social support) were reciprocally interacting to contribute to Tiana's symptoms and related impairment in her daily functioning, including school absenteeism (Fig. 14.1).

CBT Interventions in Treatment of Pediatric FAPDs

Most studies of CBT for FAPDs describe multicomponent protocols that include intervention strategies for both patients and caregivers. At this point, the "active ingredients" of these CBT protocols have not been isolated, and these protocols have not been disseminated for clinical use. However, the principles and strategies described in treatment studies are familiar to many clinicians with foundational CBT skills. In this section, we describe the practice of CBT for FAPDs as informed by the existing treatment literature, including recent work in the treatment of youth with chronic pain and other somatic symptoms. Based on a biopsychosocial conceptualization of FAPDs, CBT typically includes elements of psychoeducation, caregiver support and training, relaxation training, cognitive restructuring, graded engagement/exposure, and support for lifestyle changes (See also Chaps. 7 and 8 in this volume).

---

[1]This case example was confabulated and does not contain any patient-identifying information.

Fig. 14.1 Case conceptualization for "Tiana," an adolescent female with lactose intolerance and irritable bowel syndrome (IBS)

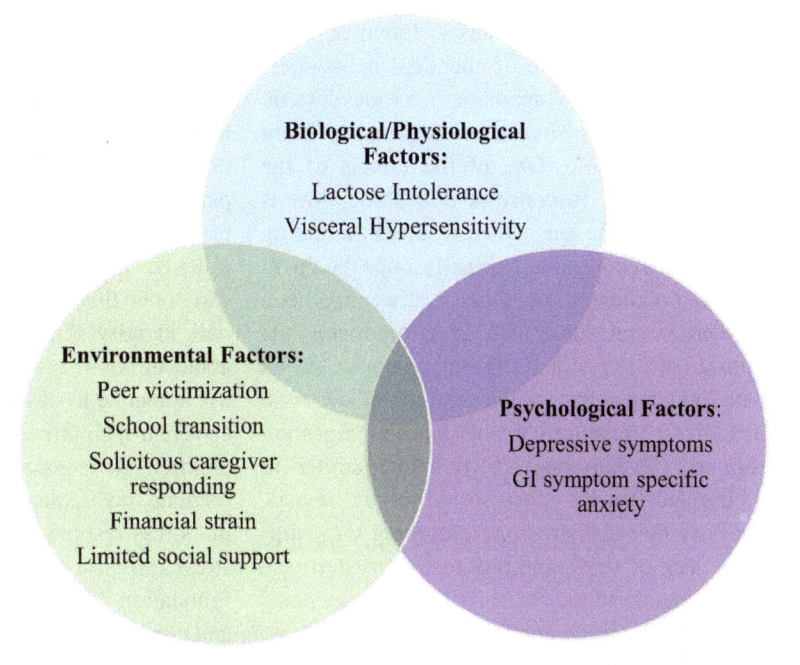

Biological/Physiological Factors:
Lactose Intolerance
Visceral Hypersensitivity

Environmental Factors:
Peer victimization
School transition
Solicitous caregiver responding
Financial strain
Limited social support

Psychological Factors:
Depressive symptoms
GI symptom specific anxiety

Psychoeducation

As in other applications of CBT, psychoeducation is a foundational intervention in the treatment of youth with gastrointestinal symptoms (Brent et al. 2008). Nearly all CBT treatment studies for FAPDs in the past decade describe a psychoeducational component (Bonnert et al. 2017; Cunningham et al. 2018; Lalouni et al. 2016; Levy et al. 2010; Nieto et al. 2015; Van der Veek et al. 2013; Wassom et al. 2013; Zucker et al. 2017). Psychoeducation is grounded in the biopsychosocial model and explicitly includes information about how biological and physiological factors including the gut–brain axis, the body's stress response system, and pain processing contribute to the gastrointestinal symptom experience.

It has been recommended that psychoeducation about the biological and physiological aspects of the child's symptoms begin in the first visit, as this establishes the behavioral health provider's knowledge and interest in helping the child and family understand and manage the bothersome gastrointestinal symptoms that are the basis of the referral (Reed-Knight et al. 2017). Failure to include biological processes in the biopsychosocial conceptualization and in psychoeducation may inadvertently reinforce a dualistic mindset in which the psychological and social aspects of the illness are viewed as distinct from the biological or "medical" aspect. For youth and families seeking services within medical clinics or integrated care clinics, such an oversight may have a negative impact on treatment acceptability and completion.

Education for youths and families about the gut–brain axis should promote the understanding that digestive system functioning is regulated by the enteric nervous system. Simply, the enteric nervous system and the central nervous system communicate back and forth, with the gut both sending information to and receiving information from the brain. Gut messages to the brain include some signals that reach our awareness—for example, pain and signals about hunger, fullness, or the need to have a bowel movement. Visceral hypersensitivity contributes to an amplified pain experience that can be further exacerbated by the stress response.

The brain's communication to the gut is complex; among the most important brain signals for youth with gastrointestinal symptoms to understand are those related to the body's stress response. The brain responds to threat or stress by initiating a cascade of chemical messengers that activate the sympathetic nervous system, producing what is often referred to as the "fight or flight" response. One of the effects of the "fight or flight" response is that blood flow is diverted from the gut, which results in a halting or slowing of digestion. Normally, once the threat has been addressed, the body's parasympathetic nervous system kicks into gear, producing the relaxation, or "rest and digest," response. As its name indicates, one of the features of the "rest and digest" response is that normal digestion resumes. It is important for youth and families to understand that the stress response can be activated by physical stressors (including GI symptoms, lack of sleep, and physical over-exertion), psychological stressors (including worry or anxiety), and environmental/social stressors (e.g., exposure to unsafe environments). Stressors are conceptualized as any circumstances that result in a perceived imbalance between situational demands and one's ability to cope (Lazarus and Folkman 1984); there is no absolute list of "stressful" and "non-stressful" life events or experiences that will trigger the body's stress response system. Youth and caregivers are educated that treatment may include keeping a pain or symptom diary to identify stressors that may contribute to the gastrointestinal symptom experience.

The stress response can also be discussed as a facilitator of pain signaling within the central nervous system. Melzack and Wall's pioneering conceptualization of the gate control theory of pain (1965) provides a helpful metaphor that can be referenced throughout treatment (See also Chap. 13 this volume). Simply, this theory describes how neurons in the spinal cord act as "gates" controlling the flow of information from the peripheral nervous system to the central nervous system. These gates open and close depending on a variety of factors, including how much "traffic" is headed toward the brain and whether any physiological, cognitive, or psychological processes are serving to shut down or open up the gates. Vigilance and attention to pain also can serve to "open the gates."

Following initial psychoeducation about the stress response and its implications, it is important to highlight that humans can learn voluntary, behavioral, and cognitive strategies to modulate or override body responses that are typically happening automatically. It can be helpful to illustrate this concept by considering automatic, reflexive activities like blinking. Most humans can notice that they are blinking. Similarly, most will identify that they do not normally think about or control their blinking. However, if you ask someone to have a staring contest, he or she can control blinking for periods of time. Similarly, children and teens can use voluntary strategies to regulate involuntary processes associated with the stress response. Education about the body's stress response and pain processing provides the foundation for introducing relaxation training and coping skills including active distraction and problem-solving in response to pain or other bothersome GI symptoms.

Explicit psychoeducation about the cognitive behavioral model helps pediatric patients develop a biopsychosocial conceptualization of their illness. As in other applications, initial psychoeducation may include a straightforward teaching example about how thoughts, feelings, and actions interact. It also is helpful to use an example relevant to the patient's gastrointestinal symptoms to illustrate the cognitive behavioral case conceptualization. Because they are seeking treatment for pain and bowel symptoms, it is often quite easy for young people to describe situations in which their symptoms have caused distress or disruption of activities. Commonly elicited automatic thoughts may include expectations of worsening symptoms or impairment. Common behavioral responses may include avoidance or other maladaptive coping patterns (e.g., rest, social isolation). Affective responses may include a range of negative emotions. It is helpful to include individuals' physical symptoms in the cognitive behavioral conceptualization to demonstrate the exacerbating impact of cognitive and affective reactions and maladaptive behavioral responses. Some authors describe conceptualizing gastrointestinal symptoms as an addition to the traditional triadic CBT model

(Ballou and Keefer 2017), or symptoms may be included alongside "feelings" or emotional/affective response. In the latter approach, it is useful to distinguish "body feelings" from "mood feelings" to promote insight about the connection between emotional states and physiologic responses. Psychoeducation about the cognitive behavioral model provides the context for CBT interventions including cognitive restructuring and graded engagement or exposure.

Throughout the process of psychoeducation, it is appropriate to validate children's and caregivers' desire for symptom alleviation. By the time the child with gastrointestinal symptoms has completed medical evaluation and received a FAPD diagnosis, he or she may have been experiencing symptoms for months or even years. Pain and bowel symptoms are uncomfortable and can be profoundly disruptive of daily functioning. Social stigma around "bathroom issues" is common. Many youth and families describe receiving stigmatizing messages about the nature of FAPD symptoms, along the lines of "it's all in your head." Parents of children with chronic digestive symptoms may worry about the underlying cause of these symptoms, particularly if there is a family history of bowel disease. It is consistent with the biopsychosocial model for GI symptoms to be discussed openly, along with associated worries. Indeed, when discussion of the individual's GI symptoms is avoided, the child and caregivers may lose trust in the behavioral health provider's intervention. It is possible, and quite helpful, to validate the distress caused by these symptoms without reinforcing the associated impairment.

Caregiver Support and Training

Parents and other caregivers are integral participants in CBT for FAPDs, and nearly all recent studies of CBT for pediatric FAPD have included a component of caregiver education (Bonnert et al. 2017; Cunningham et al. 2018; Lalouni et al. 2016; Levy et al. 2010; Nieto et al. 2015; Van der Veek et al. 2013; Zucker et al. 2017). Although the mechanisms are not yet comprehensively understood (Palermo et al. 2014; Van der Veek et al. 2011), it is widely accepted that parents and other caregivers, and their interactions with their children, can have a significant impact on children's pain experience. Social learning theory has had a lasting impact on the treatment of chronic pediatric pain, including FAPDs. As applied to coping with chronic pediatric pain, the social learning theory posits that caregiver modeling of maladaptive pain behavior (e.g., withdrawal from usual activities) and solicitous responses to child pain behavior (e.g., reducing demands, limiting usual activities) reinforce and therefore increase the frequency of maladaptive pain behaviors and associated functional impairment (see Levy et al. 2007). Additionally, the concept of "miscarried helping" (Anderson and Coyne 1991) can be applied to understand dynamic parent–child interactions that may co-occur with social learning processes in the setting of chronic illness management (Harris et al. 2008). In the context of chronic pain, miscarried helping describes an evolving process in which caregivers' initial involvement in symptom management may reduce child autonomy and independence. As demands of chronic illness management increase and are renegotiated within the parent–child relationship, conflict arises and compromises illness management. In clinical practice with youth with FAPDs, "miscarried helping" in the form of parental accommodation or reduced expectations for functioning can complicate treatment as youth are encouraged to use active coping strategies and participate in graded engagement and exposure activities.

Psychoeducation and caregiver training supports caregivers in understanding how their responses (and those of other influential individuals in the child's life) can unintentionally model and shape pain responses that are contradictory to adaptive management of chronic pain and other symptoms. Caregivers of younger children may benefit from modeling and in-session practice of encouraging alternate activities (active distraction) in response to pain reports. Caregiver training also may expand upon the CBT strategies that children are learning. Caregivers are often involved in relaxation training and are viewed as essential collaborators in coaching the use of distraction and other active coping strategies during symptom episodes that occur between visits. Additionally, the cognitive behavioral model can be used to identify and address the impact of caregivers' catastrophizing predictions on overprotective behaviors that may unintentionally reinforce the child's maladaptive coping responses or activity limitations.

Relaxation Training

Relaxation training is a common component of CBT for pediatric FAPDs, having been included in most published treatment trials to date (Cunningham et al. 2018; Levy et al. 2010; Nieto et al. 2015; van der Veek et al. 2013; Wassom et al. 2013). Relaxation strategies are used to downregulate the body's sympathetic response to stress. Additionally, learning behavioral strategies to regulate the body's autonomic response, associated symptoms, worry, and other stressors promotes mastery and builds confidence. Relaxation training typically includes diaphragmatic breathing, progressive muscle relaxation, and guided imagery; specific description and evidence base for each will be described in greater detail below. Of note, recently published treatment guides for pediatric chronic pain and somatic symptoms include helpful scripts and educational handouts describing each of these relaxation strategies (Palermo 2012; Williams and Zahka 2017).

In general, relaxation training can include any combination of face-to-face instruction and practice with handouts, worksheets, or online videos. Parents are often included in teaching and initial practice of relaxation strategies so that they can effectively coach home practice. Alternatively, the patient and clinician can practice together, and the patient can demonstrate the use of the technique to his or her parent at the end of the session. Home practice of relaxation strategies is essential. As in other forms of CBT, home practice is initially recommended to include daily practice at a time when the patient is not experiencing disruptive gastrointestinal symptoms. Once the child can demonstrate relaxation skills "on demand," he or she is encouraged to begin using these skills when symptoms begin or when he or she becomes aware of feeling "stressed" or having gastrointestinal symptoms. Practice of relaxation skills in session, particularly when the child describes experiencing physical symptoms or emotional distress, allows real-time review of their effectiveness.

Diaphragmatic breathing Diaphragmatic breathing is included in all of the recent CBT treatment studies that specifically describe relaxation components techniques (e.g., Cunningham et al. 2018; Levy et al. 2010; Nieto et al. 2015; van der Veek et al. 2013; Wassom et al. 2013). Diaphragmatic breathing is typically taught with the child placing one hand on his or her chest and the other on his or her lower abdomen. First, the child is encouraged to breathe normally with attention to the movement of his or her hands. The clinician can then model, with hands on his or her own chest and lower abdomen, the difference between "normal breathing" and "diaphragmatic breathing" (or "belly breathing"). Next, the child is encouraged to inhale deeply through the nose with focused attention on expanding the lower abdomen. Younger children can be encouraged to imagine they are filling a balloon in the belly with air. Once the deep inhale is complete, the child is encouraged to exhale slowly. Some children prefer to exhale through their mouths; others, and particularly those who are self-conscious about being observed using relaxation strategies, prefer to exhale through their noses. We are not aware of compelling evidence to support or recommend against either form of exhalation. Inhalation through the nose is typically recommended: inhalation through the mouth can promote excessive air swallowing (aerophagia) that can cause additional gastrointestinal discomfort or symptoms (belching).

Progressive muscle relaxation Like diaphragmatic breathing, progressive muscle relaxation

(PMR) is included in all of the recent CBT treatment trials that specifically describe training in relaxation techniques (Cunningham et al. 2018; Levy et al. 2010; Nieto et al. 2015; van der Veek et al. 2013; Wassom et al. 2013). Progressive muscle relaxation was first developed by physician Edmund Jacobson in the 1930s and describes sequential tension and release of different muscle groups with focus on the sensation of muscle release or relaxation. The technique has a long history of use in behavioral medicine; Carlson and Hoyle provided an early review (1993). Progressive muscle relaxation scripts are readily available, including those adapted for young children. Because youth with FAPDs often experience visceral hypersensitivity and associated anxiety about gastrointestinal symptoms, some may describe increased distress when prompted to tense and release abdominal muscles. For this reason, clinicians may choose to allow the patient to refrain from using the abdominal muscles during PMR for relaxation (and may also choose to use "engagement of abdominal muscles during PMR" as a graded exposure task, as described below).

Guided imagery Compared to diaphragmatic breathing and progressive muscle relaxation, guided imagery has been included in relatively fewer multicomponent CBT treatment studies (Cunningham et al. 2018; Levy et al. 2010; Van der Veek et al. 2013; Wassom et al. 2013). However, it is unique among these relaxation strategies in having been evaluated as a stand-alone treatment for FAPDs (Van Tilburg et al. 2009). Guided imagery is closely related to clinical hypnosis, which is considered a viable "first-line" treatment for chronic pain (Jensen et al. 2014). A recent review of randomized controlled trials of guided imagery and hypnotherapy interventions for pediatric FAPD described positive treatment effects in the form of decreased abdominal pain (Rutten et al. 2013).

In clinical practice for the treatment of pediatric FAPDs, guided imagery can be used to facilitate general relaxation or more specifically to promote symptom-reduction. In the former case, guided imagery involves helping the child develop and elaborate upon imagery of a situation in which the child feels comfortable and relaxed. This can be based on an actual memory or an imaginary scenario. When using guided imagery to promote symptom alleviation, the child is encouraged to develop an image that represents their symptom experience (e.g., pain may be described as a small burning ball over the belly button). Working collaboratively, an image that attenuates the symptom experience is developed (e.g., a light breeze that initially causes the flames to flicker but then continues to the point that the flames are extinguished). The extent to which the child can elaborate on the sights, sounds, smells, and any other associated sensory features may promote a more vivid and engaging imagery exercise. Once the image and accompanying narrative have been sufficiently elaborated, the child can be encouraged to write, draw, or record elements of the narrative to assist with later rehearsal. Commercially available guided imagery exercises or personalized recordings can also be introduced.

Biofeedback In practice, some clinicians routinely use biofeedback-assisted relaxation training for youth and adults with FAPDs. However, the evidence base for biofeedback to decrease pain and symptoms in youth with FAPDs is limited: existing studies tend to be characterized by small sample sizes and variability in biofeedback protocols. Nearly two decades ago, Humphreys and Gevirtz (2000) described promising results of skin temperature biofeedback as an adjunct to fiber supplementation in youth with functional abdominal pain. More recently, Sowder et al. (2010) described positive effects of a six-session course of biofeedback aimed at increasing heart rate variability among youth with functional abdominal pain, while Schurman and her colleagues (2010) described positive treatment effects of a biofeedback-assisted relaxation training program including muscle tension, respiration rate, skin temperature, and electrodermal response feedback among youth with functional dyspepsia. Therefore, while clinical practice may reasonably include biofeedback-assisted relaxation training, future research is needed. In particular, well-controlled studies examining the role of psychological processes (e.g., mastery, perceived control) in mediating treatment effects may further support the use of biofeedback to target gastrointestinal symptoms (Tsao and Zeltzer 2005).

Cognitive Restructuring

As in other CBT applications, cognitive restructuring begins with education and practice in identifying automatic thoughts and distinguishing these from feelings. Common automatic thought patterns related to GI symptoms include catastrophizing predictions about symptom severity or impact on activities. These can be elicited through the use of a symptom diary that includes the elements of a traditional CBT thought record (Appendix). Using collaborative empiricism, the clinician and young person (with or without the caregiver) explore the accuracy and helpfulness of these automatic thought patterns. Even when individuals maintain steadfast expectations that symptoms will worsen, they can often identify that these expectations produce negative emotions and result in unhelpful behavioral responses (e.g., staying home instead of going out with friends). This process can facilitate openness to developing coping statements or employing problem-solving to establish a coping plan. Cognitive restructuring for youth with FAPDs can help them develop more accurate and helpful thought patterns, including those that reinforce continued engagement in meaningful activities, thereby promoting distraction and opportunities for enjoyment and other positive emotional experiences. Cognitive restructuring work can also be modeled for parents of youth with FGIDs, who may benefit from developing more adaptive beliefs about their children's symptoms and coping capacities (DuPen et al. 2016).

Graded Engagement and Exposure

Many youth with FAPDs describe cycles of daily impairment that begin with gastrointestinal symptoms and associated worry or catastrophizing and result in activity avoidance. Activity avoidance may initially decrease anxiety, negatively reinforcing the avoidance behavior. However, avoidance behavior fosters increased anxiety over time, as the young person misses opportunities to discover that symptoms improve or resolve or that they are able to cope effectively with symptoms. This cycle is consistent with the fear-avoidance model of chronic pain (Vlaeyen and Linton 2000). A rehabilitative approach to chronic pain prioritizes improved daily functioning, as opposed to pain relief, as a primary treatment goal in pediatric chronic pain, including pain associated with FAPDs.

Graded engagement describes a combination of compatible elements of exposure and behavioral activation (Weersing et al. 2008, 2012). This technique was initially described as part of a brief behavioral intervention for the treatment of anxiety and depression in primary care but has also been applied with individuals presenting with combined internalizing emotional symptoms and somatic symptoms (Weersing et al. 2012). While not always termed "graded engagement," interventions with the goal of intentionally increasing participation in enjoyable activities that have been restricted due to pain are a component in most of the recent treatment trials for CBT for FAPDs (Cunningham et al. 2018; Van der Veek et al. 2013; Wassom et al. 2013).

Applied to the treatment of pediatric FAPDs, graded engagement begins with identifying activities of daily living that are being avoided or otherwise limited due to bothersome gastrointestinal symptoms. When school attendance has been affected by FAPD symptoms, graded engagement may include incrementally increasing the amount of time spent in school each week. When enjoyable activities have been limited or avoided, a gradual return to these activities may become a treatment goal. Understanding the interests of the individual and his or her caregivers is essential; pursuit of activity engagement despite pain or other bothersome symptoms requires a high level of motivation and requires that the goal for increased functioning supersedes the goal for immediate pain relief (Crombez et al. 2012). Graded engagement is implemented in CBT for FAPDs to promote developmentally appropriate role functioning (e.g., school attendance, completion of household chores), decrease social isolation, promote positive mood, and provide evidence to modify maladaptive thinking patterns about pain and functioning.

As youth with FAPDs prepare to re-engage in activities that have been limited or avoided due to gastrointestinal symptoms, they are encouraged to use behavioral and cognitive strategies (relaxation, distraction, cognitive coping statements) to cope with physical symptoms or affective responses that might undermine their progress (Coakley and Wihak 2017). Caregivers are encouraged to coach their children in using these strategies and to celebrate successes. When pragmatic problems like lack of awareness of bathroom locations are identified, teaching families to use a formal problem-solving approach can be helpful to promote adherence to graded engagement assignments.

There is also a growing body of evidence that graded exposure to GI symptoms, by symptom provocation, may benefit youth with FAPDs (Bonnert et al. 2017; Lalouni et al. 2016, 2017). This work is modeled from the treatment of adults with IBS (Craske et al. 2011; Ljotsson et al. 2014). For youth with FAPDs, graded exposure may extend graded engagement. For example, many youth who describe being bothered by bowel symptoms in the early morning may resort to school-based accommodations for late arrivals. While this may represent improvement from a previous level of impairment, the late arrival program may also have unintended negative consequences for the student. For example, late arrival may negatively impact the ability to complete an elective course, may supplant a study period, or may have negative social consequences. Graded exposure may include tasks like purposefully eating foods that provoke symptoms, going to school or sports practice with increasingly bothersome symptoms, and refraining from other symptom-avoidance behaviors (e.g., staying home from school or activities when anticipating stress or symptoms) in order to promote further activity engagement.

Collaboration with the medical treatment team is particularly important when applying graded engagement and exposure to youth with FAPDs. In general, collaboration between the behavioral health clinician and the treating medical team reinforces the biopsychosocial conceptualization and treatment model (Reed-Knight et al. 2017). Specific to graded engagement and exposure, such collaboration can be essential to effective treatment. For example, efforts to increase school attendance are less likely to be successful when the medical team is supporting homebound education. Efforts to decrease avoidance of specific foods may be contraindicated for youth for whom avoidance of dietary triggers is part of their medical management.

Addressing Sleep Problems

Sleep problems are common in youth with chronic pain, including those with FAPDs, and may impact both symptoms and functioning (Schurman et al. 2012; Valrie et al. 2013). Clinically, some youth describe that sleep is disrupted by pain or bowel symptoms; others describe longstanding sleep difficulties or interference by anxiety. Therefore, biopsychosocially oriented treatment for FAPDs may include promoting adequate sleep hygiene and offering behavioral strategies to support improved sleep routines. In particular, addressing sleep problems early in treatment may serve to increase treatment acceptability and build positive momentum for change. If sleep problems persist despite improvement in sleep hygiene, referral to a sleep specialist or pulmonologist for a sleep study may be indicated in consultation with the child's medical treatment team.

Treatment of Psychiatric and Medical Comorbidities

As with other chronic medical conditions, youth with FAPDs often present with comorbid psychiatric illness. Anxiety disorders are a particular common comorbidity; one recent study of 100 patients with functional abdominal pain reported that greater than 50% of the sample reported clinically significant anxiety (Cunningham et al. 2015). Some of the CBT strategies for pediatric FAPDs target worry about gastrointestinal symptoms and their impact. However, it is important to distinguish that CBT for FAPDs is not a substitute for evidence-based treatment of a clinically significant anxiety disorder. In fact, within the pediatric pain literature, there is preliminary evidence that the presence of clinically significant anxiety symptoms attenuates response to CBT for chronic pain (Cunningham et al. 2016). Future research is needed to identify whether youth with FAPDs who do not respond to CBT may be characterized by higher rates of anxiety disorder than those who demonstrate positive treatment effects. In practice, youth with clinically significant anxiety disorders, depression, or other mood disorders may be treated with CBT for FAPD symptoms but should also be referred for treatment of the comorbid psychiatric condition. Collaboration with the child's medical treatment team may further inform decision making about psychiatric referral, as central neuromodulators commonly prescribed by psychiatrists are increasingly being used in the treatment of chronic gastrointestinal symptoms and FGIDs (Drossman et al. 2018).

Thorough assessment of potential psychiatric comorbidities is recommended, as these conditions may impact response to treatment and prognosis for recovery. For example, undiagnosed or untreated psychiatric conditions including attention-deficit/hyperactivity disorder and learning disabilities may contribute to school-related stressors that consequently impact functional gastrointestinal symptoms. Youth presenting with FAPDs exhibit a range of behavioral responses that can include restricting oral intake or making other dietary modifications in order to avoid provoking symptoms. When concerns for disordered eating arise, referral for appropriately specialized evaluation and treatment is clearly indicated. Finally, individuals with FGIDs are more likely than the general population to report a history of trauma (Bradford et al. 2012; Sherman et al. 2015). If, in the course of CBT for FAPD symptoms, it becomes evident that a child or teen has experienced or is experiencing ongoing trauma, referral to specialized care is indicated.

Case Example of CBT for Pediatric FAPD

Treatment for Tiana[2] began with psychoeducation regarding the brain-gut connection, the stress response system, and pain processing. The clinician also reviewed the biopsychosocial approach to treatment of IBS. Following psychoeducation and discussion of the biopsychosocial treatment approach, Tiana continued to have questions about the nature of interdisciplinary treatment for IBS. This is common among patients referred for psychological intervention by their medical providers and warrants specific discussion with the patient.

> Tiana: "So, from now on will I see you instead of Dr. Sloan?"
> Clinician: "That's a great question. You will definitely keep seeing your gastroenterologist along with working with me for CBT. Remember when we talked about the biopsychosocial approach? It will be important to keep working with Dr. Sloan to find the right medical treatment for your visceral hypersensitivity, one of the biological factors in your IBS. We'll also talk about strategies for staying consistent with your lactose-free diet. However, our work together will focus on the other pieces of the biopsychosocial approach- what's going on in your thoughts and emotions, and in the rest of your life and the world around you that affect your IBS symptoms, and make it difficult for you to do the things you want and need to do."

Next, the clinician introduced diaphragmatic breathing, progressive muscle relaxation, and guided imagery. Tiana was encouraged to practice

---

[2]This case example was confabulated and does not contain any patient-identifying information.

one of these skills daily when GI symptoms were not present and then begin to use them to manage her GI symptoms and stress.

> Clinician: "When do you think a good time to practice your relaxation skills will be?"
> Tiana: "I think I'll do it at night, when I'm trying to go to sleep. Maybe they would also help when my stomach hurts in the morning."
> Clinician: "Excellent plan, Tiana. Bedtime, when your stomach tends to be okay and you're pretty relaxed, is a great time to practice. I like the idea about using one of these strategies in the morning too. We've talked about how the stress response system affects what goes on in your gut. It sounds like your "fight or flight" response often goes off in the morning just thinking about your new school and the girls who have been unkind, and this can make your abdominal pain worse. If you use one of your relaxation skills in the morning and activate your "rest and digest" response, you might find that you can close the gate on pain a bit."

Tiana and the clinician reviewed the cognitive behavioral model and the role of thoughts in influencing emotions and behaviors. Tiana was able to identify the types of maladaptive cognitions she tends to experience (e.g., catastrophizing), and the pair practiced questioning and modifying a negative thought with a coping model example from the clinician. Then, it was time to challenge some of Tiana's GI symptom-related cognitions.

> Clinician: "Tiana, you mentioned that the thought that pops into your head often in the morning when your stomach feels off is 'I'll probably have to go 10 times today and it would be better to stay home.' Let's ask some of our evidence-gathering questions about this thought. For example, do you know for sure this will happen? What has happened before?"
> Tiana: "Well, you know that I definitely have had diarrhea at school before and have had to go to the bathroom a bunch of times. But, no, I don't know for sure this will happen. It's true that yesterday I only went one or twice. It's maybe like half the time that it is that bad."
> Clinician: "And if it's a bad day, what's the worst thing that could happen?"
> Tiana: "Well the worst thing is leaving class again and again to go. I always feel like people are noticing, but I guess that's maybe not true because no one has ever said anything. So obviously I survive it, I just would really rather not go through it."
> Clinician: "I think you caught yourself 'mind-reading' about your classmates noticing your bathroom trips- you're really getting the hang of this! So now that we've gathered the evidence, what do you think would make a good alternative response in the morning when you notice that your stomach is off and that thought pops into your head?"
> Tiana: "I guess I can remind myself, it doesn't always happen. There's a 50% chance things will be fine today with my stomach. And even if I do have diarrhea, it's terrible, but it's not the end of the world. I can handle it because I have before."

Once Tiana was regularly and comfortably using relaxation skills and cognitive restructuring to help manage GI symptoms and related anxiety, treatment focused on graded engagement in daily and pleasant activities that Tiana was avoiding due to GI symptom-specific anxiety and depressive symptoms. Tiana's hierarchy included attending school on days she had IBS symptoms (first partial days and then full), spending time with new friends from school, and eating at restaurants (avoided due to concerns about accidentally eating something with lactose and having GI symptoms).

> Clinician: "Tiana, you're working so hard and you're ready to take your life back from IBS! Looking at our list of activities and places IBS has kept you from, and probably choosing something lower on the list, what seems like a good first challenge to take on?"
> Tiana: "I want to be able to go out to eat with my mom this week for her birthday. So maybe I should do that one first?"
> Clinician: "I know how close you are with your mom, so going out for a birthday dinner seems like a great way to not let IBS get in the way of doing things that are important to you. Let's make a plan for how to have a successful dinner out! What are some of the coping strategies that you think might be most helpful to you before and during the dinner?"
> Tiana: "I think I will go through the progressive muscle relaxation before I leave for the restaurant. That is really working well in the morning for school. And I can remind myself 'What's the worst that can happen? I can handle it even if I accidentally eat lactose and have diarrhea. It's not like that hasn't happened before.'"
> Clinician: "Tiana, I think you've come up with a solid plan. You've noticed that progressive muscle relaxation works well for you to prepare for other situations and so it's a great strategy to use before leaving for the restaurant. And at this point you've identified some go-to alternative responses that fit for a lot of situations you have previously been

avoiding due to IBS. I wonder if there is something you might plan to try if, despite your preparation beforehand, you still find yourself getting anxious about IBS symptoms during the meal?"

Tiana: "Maybe the diaphragmatic breathing? Since it's fast and easy to do anywhere?"

Clinician: "That's definitely a good option for when you need something fast and easy to activate your "rest and digest" response. When your mom joins us today, is there any way in which we should ask her to support you before or during the dinner? Or some way you'd like to celebrate your effort with her afterwards, after your successful dinner out?"

Tiana: "She actually does the muscle relaxation with me sometimes when I play it without my headphones, so maybe we could both do it. And afterwards, I mostly just want to watch our favorite TV show together. We have a lot of episodes to catch up on since she's been so busy with work."

Clinician: "I bet your mom would be happy to support and celebrate you in those ways. Let's bring her in."

Throughout treatment, Tiana's mother received psychoeducation about IBS and the cognitive behavioral model and was encouraged to reinforce Tiana's use of coping skills and approach of previously avoided activities. The clinician also consulted one of the clinic's social workers to assist Tiana's mother with issues of financial strain, transportation, and social support for herself as a single parent. The clinician connected with the school guidance counselor to facilitate in-school support for Tiana regarding the relational aggression she experienced from the peer at school. Together, Tiana and her mother were able to get Tiana back to regular school attendance despite her IBS symptoms. Once she started attending school regularly, Tiana developed some new friendships and started to enjoy her new school more. By the end of treatment, Tiana's mood had improved, as well as her GI symptom-specific anxiety. She continued to experience abdominal pain, bloating, and diarrhea, although on a less frequent basis and with minimal impairment in her daily functioning.

Conclusion

Functional abdominal pain disorders (FAPDs; functional abdominal pain, irritable bowel syndrome, and functional dyspepsia) are common in children and teens and can result in high levels of health service utilization, impaired daily functioning, emotional distress, and reduced quality of life. An evolving intervention research literature demonstrates that youth and families who participate in multicomponent CBT interventions experience benefits ranging from symptom alleviation to improved coping and improved daily functioning. Informed by a biopsychosocial conceptualization, clinicians can apply many familiar CBT skills to treat youth with FAPDs and their families.

Appendix: Symptom Diary

Please use this chart to help your care team learn about your pain/other symptoms.

Keep track of this information for 2 weeks and then return this diary to your care provider.

Date/time	Situation	Body feelings/symptoms	Emotions	Thoughts	Coping	Other notes
	What was I doing when symptoms started? Include any food/drink, physical activity.	Rate Intensity: Pain (0 = no pain to 10 = worst possible pain) Bowel Symptoms (Bristol Stool Scale 1–7) Other:	What mood am I in? How do I feel?	What do I think is happening? What am I expecting next?	What did I try? What happened?	
.						
.						
.						

References

Anderson, B. J., & Coyne, J. C. (1991). "Miscarried helping" in the families of children and adolescents with chronic diseases. In J. H. Johnson & S. B. Johnson (Eds.), *Advances in child health psychology* (pp. 167–177). Gainesville: University of Florida Press.

Ballou, S., & Keefer, L. (2017). Psychological interventions for irritable bowel syndrome and inflammatory bowel diseases. *Clinical and Translational Gastroenterology, 8*, e214. https://doi.org/10.1038/ctg.2016.69.

Bonnert, M., Olen, O., Lalouni, M., Benninga, M. A., Engelbrektsson, J., Hedman, E., et al. (2017). Internet-delivered cognitive behavioral therapy for adolescents with irritable bowel syndrome (IBS): A randomized controlled trial. *American Journal of Gastroenterology, 112*, 152–162.

Bradford, K., Shih, W., Videlock, E., Presson, A. P., Naliboff, B. D., Mayer, E. A., et al. (2012). Association between early adverse life events and irritable bowel syndrome. *Clinical Gastroenterology and Hepatology, 10*(4), 385–390.

Brent, M., Lobato, D., & LeLeiko, N. (2008). Psychological treatments for pediatric functional gastrointestinal disorders. *Journal of Pediatric Gastroenterology and Nutrition, 48*, 13–21.

Brodwall, A., Glavin, K., & Lagerløv, P. (2018). Parents' experience when their child has chronic abdominal pain: A qualitative study in Norway. *BMJ Open*. https://doi.org/10.1136/bmjopen-2017-021066.

Campo, J. V., Bridge, J., Ehmann, M., Altman, S., Lucas, A., Birmaher, B., et al. (2004). Recurrent abdominal pain, anxiety, and depression in primary care. *Pediatrics, 113*(4), 817–824. https://doi.org/10.1542/peds.113.4.817.

Carlson, C. R., & Hoyle, R. H. (1993). Efficacy of abbreviated progressive muscle relaxation training: A quantitative review of behavioral medicine research. *Journal of Consulting and Clinical Psychology, 61*(6), 1059–1067.

Claar, R. L., Simons, L. E., & Logan, D. E. (2008). Parental response to children's pain: The moderating impact of children's emotional distress on symptoms and disability. *Pain, 138*, 172–179.

Coakley, R., & Wihak, T. (2017). Evidence-based psychological interventions for the management of pediatric chronic pain: New directions in research and clinical practice. *Children*. https://doi.org/10.3390/children4020009.

Craske, M. G., Wolitzky-Taylor, K. B., Labus, J., Wu, S., Frese, M., Mayer, E. A., et al. (2011). A cognitive-behavioral treatment for irritable bowel syndrome using interoceptive exposure to visceral sensations. *Behavior Research and Therapy, 49*, 413–421.

Crombez, G., Eccleston, C., van Damme, S., Vlaeyen, J. W. S., & Karoly, P. (2012). Fear-avoidance model of chronic pain: The next generation. *Clinical Journal of Pain, 28*, 475–483.

Cunningham, N. R., Cohen, M. B., Farrell, M. K., Mezoff, A. G., Lynch-Jordan, A., & Kashikar-Zuck, S. (2015). Concordant parent child reports of anxiety predict impairment in youth with functional abdominal pain. *Journal of Pediatric Gastroenterology and Nutrition, 60*(3), 312–317.

Cunningham, N. R., Jagpal, A., Tran, S. T., Kashikar-Zuck, S., Goldschneider, K. R., Coghill, R. C., et al. (2016). Anxiety adversely impacts response to cognitive behavioral therapy in children with chronic pain. *Journal of Pediatrics, 171*, 227–233.

Cunningham, N. R., Nelson, S., Jagpal, A., Moorman, E., Farrell, M., Pentiuk, S., et al. (2018). Development of the Aim to Decrease Anxiety and Pain Treatment for pediatric functional abdominal pain disorders. *Journal of Pediatric Gastroenterology and Nutrition, 66*, 16–20.

Drossman, D. A. (2016). Functional gastrointestinal disorders: History, pathophysiology, clinical features, and Rome IV. *Gastroenterology, 150*, 1262–1279.

Drossman, D. A., Tack, J., Ford, A. C., Szigethy, E., Tornblom, H., & van Oudenhove, L. (2018). Neuromodulators for functional gastrointestinal disorders (disorders of gut-brain interaction): A Rome Foundation working team report. *Gastroenterology, 154*, 1140–1171.

DuPen, M. M., van Tilburg, M. A. L., Langer, S. L., Murphy, T. B., Romano, J. M., & Levy, R. (2016). Parental protectiveness mediates the association between parent-perceived child self-efficacy and health outcomes in pediatric functional abdominal pain disorder. *Children*. https://doi.org/10.3390/children3030015.

Finney, J. W., Lemanek, K. L., Cataldo, M. F., Katz, H. P., & Fuqua, R. W. (1989). Pediatric psychology in primary health care: Brief targeted therapy for recurrent abdominal pain. *Behavior Therapy, 20*, 283–291.

Harris, M. A., Antal, H., Oelbaum, R., Buckloh, L. M., White, N. H., & Wysocki, T. (2008). Good intentions gone awry: Assessing parental "miscarried helping" in diabetes. *Families, Systems and Health, 26*(4), 393–403.

Horst, S., Shelby, G., Anderson, J., Acra, S., Polk, B., Saville, B. R., et al. (2014). Predicting persistence of functional abdominal pain from childhood into young adulthood. *Clinical Gastroenterology and Hepatology, 12*(12), 2026–2032.

Humphreys, P. A., & Gevirtz, R. N. (2000). Treatment of recurrent abdominal pain: Components analysis of four treatment protocols. *Journal of Pediatric Gastroenterology and Nutrition, 31*(1), 47–51.

Hunt, M. G., Milonova, M., & Moshier, S. (2009). Catastrophizing the consequences of gastrointestinal symptoms in irritable bowel syndrome. *Journal of Cognitive Psychotherapy, 23*, 160–173.

Hyams, J. S., Di Lorenzo, C., Saps, M., Shulman, R. J., Staiano, A., & van Tilburg, M. (2016). Childhood functional gastrointestinal disorders: Child/adolescent. *Gastroenterology, 150*(6), 1456–1468.

Jensen, M. P., Day, M. A., & Miro, J. (2014). Neuromodulatory treatments for chronic pain: Efficacy and mechanisms. *Nature Reviews Neurology, 10*(3), 167–178.

Kennedy, P. J., Cryan, J. F., Dinan, T. G., & Clarke, G. (2014). Irritable bowel syndrome: A microbiome-gut-brain axis disorder? *World Journal of Gastroenterology, 20*(39), 14105–14125.

Lackner, J. M., Brasel, A. M., Quigley, B. M., Keefer, L., Krasner, S. S., Powell, C., et al. (2010). The ties that bind: Perceived social support, stress, and IBS in severely affected patients. *Neurogastroenterology & Motility, 22*(8), 893–900.

Lackner, J. M., Gudleski, G. D., Firth, R., Keefer, L. A., Brenner, D. M., Guy, K., et al. (2013). Negative aspects of close relationships are more strongly associated than supportive personal relationships with illness burden of irritable bowel syndrome. *Journal of Psychosomatic Research, 74*(6), 493–500.

Lalouni, M., Olen, O., Bonnert, M., Hedman, E., Serlachius, E., & Ljotsson, B. (2016). Exposure-based cognitive behavior therapy for children with abdominal pain: A pilot trial. *PLoS One*. https://doi.org/10.1371/journal.pone.0164647.

Lalouni, M., Ljótsson, B., Bonnert, M., Hedman-Lagerlöf, E., Högström, J., Serlachius, E., et al. (2017). Internet-delivered cognitive behavioral therapy for children with pain-related functional gastrointestinal disorders: Feasibility study. *JMIR Mental Health, 4*(3), 1–21.

Langer, S. L., Romano, J. M., Levy, R. L., Walker, L. S., & Whitehead, W. E. (2009). Catastrophizing and parental response to child symptom complaints. *Children's Health Care, 38*(3), 169–184.

Lazarus, R. S., & Folkman, S. (1984). *Stress, appraisal and coping*. New York: Springer Publishing Company.

Levy, R. L., Whitehead, W. E., Walker, L. S., Von Korff, M., Feld, A. D., Garner, M., et al. (2004). Increased somatic complaints and health-care utilization in children: Effects of parent IBS status and parent response to gastrointestinal symptoms. *American Journal of Gastroenterology, 99*, 2442–2451.

Levy, R. L., Langer, S. L., & Whitehead, W. E. (2007). Social learning contributions to the etiology and treatment of functional abdominal pain and inflammatory bowel disease in children and adults. *World Journal of Gastroenterology, 13*(17), 2397–2403.

Levy, R. L., Langer, S. L., Walker, L. S., Romano, J. M., Christie, D. L., Youssef, N., et al. (2010). Cognitive-behavioral therapy for children with functional abdominal pain and their parents decreases pain and other symptoms. *The American Journal of Gastroenterology, 105*(4), 946–956.

Levy, R. L., Langer, S. L., Romano, J. M., Labus, J., Walker, L. S., Murphy, T. B., et al. (2014). Cognitive mediators of treatment outcomes in pediatric functional abdominal pain. *Clinical Journal of Pain, 30*(12), 1033–1043.

Lewandowski, A. S., Palermo, T. M., Stinson, J., Handley, S., & Chambers, C. T. (2010). Systematic review of family functioning in families of children and adolescents with chronic pain. *The Journal of Pain, 11*(11), 1027–1038.

Ljotsson, B., Hesser, H., Andersson, E., Lackner, J. M., El Alaoui, S., Falk, L., et al. (2014). Provoking symptoms to relieve symptoms: A randomized controlled dismantling study of exposure therapy in irritable bowel syndrome. *Behavior Research and Therapy, 55*, 27–39.

Melzack, R., & Wall, P. D. (1965). Pain mechanisms: A new theory. *Science, 150*, 971–979.

Nieto, R., Hernandez, E., Boixados, M., Huguet, A., Beneitez, I., & McGrath, P. (2015). Testing the feasibility of DARWeb: An online intervention for children with functional abdominal pain and their parents. *Clinical Journal of Pain, 31*, 493–503.

Palermo, T. M. (2012). *Cognitive-behavioral therapy for chronic pain in children and adolescents*. New York: Oxford University Press.

Palermo, T. M., Valrie, C. R., & Karlson, C. W. (2014). Family and parent influences on pediatric chronic pain: A developmental perspective. *American Psychologist, 69*(2), 142–152.

Pinto-Sanchez, M. I., Ford, A. C., Avila, C. A., Verdu, E. F., Collins, S. M., Morgan, D., et al. (2015). Anxiety and depression increase in a stepwise manner in parallel with multiple FGIDs and symptom severity and frequency. *The American Journal of Gastroenterology, 110*, 1038–1048.

Reed-Knight, B., Maddux, M., Deacy, A. D., Lamparyck, K., Stone, A. L., & Mackner, L. (2017). Brain-gut interactions and maintenance factors in pediatric gastroenterological disorders: Recommendations for clinical care. *Clinical Practice in Pediatric Psychology, 5*(1), 93–105.

Robin, S. G., Keller, C., Zwiener, R., Hyman, P. E., Nurko, S., Saps, M., et al. (2018). Prevalence of pediatric functional gastrointestinal disorders utilizing the Rome IV criteria. *The Journal of Pediatrics, 195*, 134–139.

Rosen, J. M., Cocjin, J. T., Schurman, J. V., Colombo, J. M., & Friesen, C. A. (2014). Visceral hypersensitivity and electromechanical dysfunction as therapeutic targets in pediatric functional dyspepsia. *World Journal of Gastrointestinal Pharmacology and Therapeutics, 5*(3), 122–138.

Rutten, J. T. M., Reitsma, J. B., Vlieger, A. M., & Benninga, M. A. (2013). Gut-directed hypnotherapy for functional abdominal pain or irritable bowel syndrome in children: A systematic review. *Archives of Disease in Childhood, 98*, 252–257.

Rutten, J. T. M., Korterink, J. J., Venmans, L. M. A. J., Benninga, M. A., & Tabbers, M. (2015). Nonpharmacologic treatment of functional abdominal pain disorders: A systematic review. *Pediatrics, 135*(3), 522–535.

Sanders, M. W., Rebgetz, M., Morrison, M., Bor, W., Gordon, A., Dadds, M., et al. (1989). Cognitive-behavioral treatment of recurrent nonspecific abdominal pain in children: An analysis of generalization, maintenance, and side effects. *Journal of Consulting and Clinical Psychology, 57*(2), 294–300.

Saps, M., Velasco-Benitez, C. A., Langshaw, A. H., Ramirez-Hernandez, C. (2018). Prevalence of functional gastrointestinal disorders in children and adolescents: Comparison between Rome III and Rome IV criteria. *Journal of Pediatrics, 199*, 212–216.

Schurman, J. V., Wu, Y. P., Grayson, P., & Friesen, C. A. (2010). A pilot study to assess the efficacy of biofeedback-assisted relaxation training as an adjunct treatment for pediatric functional dyspepsia associated with duodenal eosinophilia. *Journal of Pediatric Psychology, 35*(8), 837–847.

Schurman, J. V., Friesen, C. A., Dai, H., Danda, C. E., Hyman, P. E., & Cocjin, J. T. (2012). Sleep problems and functional disability in children with functional gastrointestinal disorders: An examination of the potential mediating effects of physical and emotional symptoms. *BMC Gastroenterology.* https://doi.org/10.1186/1471-230X-12-142.

Shelby, G. D., Shirkey, K. S., Sherman, A. L., Beck, J. E., Haman, K., Shears, A. R., et al. (2013). Functional abdominal pain in childhood and long-term vulnerability to anxiety disorders. *Pediatrics, 132*(3), 475–482.

Sherman, A. L., Morris, M. C., Bruehl, S., Westbrook, T. D., & Walker, L. S. (2015). Heightened temporal summation of pain in patients with functional gastrointestinal disorders and history of trauma. *Annals of Behavioral Medicine, 49*(6), 785–792.

Sowder, E., Gevirtz, R., Shapiro, W., & Ebert, C. (2010). Restoration of vagal tone: A possible mechanism for functional abdominal pain. *Applied Psychophysiology and Biofeedback, 35*(3), 199–206.

Stone, A. L., & Walker, L. S. (2017). Adolescents' observations of parent pain behaviors: Preliminary measure validation and test of social learning theory in pediatric chronic pain. *Journal of Pediatric Psychology, 42*, 65–74.

Tsao, J. C. I., & Zeltzer, L. K. (2005). Complementary and alternative medicine approaches for pediatric pain: A review of the state-of-the-science. *eCAM, 2*(2), 149–159.

Valrie, C. R., Bromberg, M. H., Palermo, T., & Schanberg, L. E. (2013). A systematic review of sleep in pediatric pain populations. *Journal of Developmental and Behavioral Pediatrics, 34*(2), 120–128.

Van der Veek, S. M. C., Derkx, B. H. F., De Haan, E., Benninga, M. A., Plak, R. D., & Boer, F. (2011). Do parents maintain or exacerbate pediatric functional abdominal pain? A systematic review and meta-analysis. *Journal of Health Psychology, 17*(2), 258–272.

Van der Veek, S. M. C., Derkx, B. H. F., Benninga, M. A., Boer, F., & De Haan, E. (2013). Cognitive behavior therapy for pediatric functional abdominal pain: A randomized controlled trial. *Pediatrics, 132*(5), e1163–e1172.

Van Oudenhove, L., Levy, R. L., Crowell, M. D., Drossman, D. A., Halpert, A. D., Keefer, L., et al. (2016). Biopsychosocial aspects of functional gastrointestinal disorders: How central and environmental processes contribute to the development and expression of functional gastrointestinal disorders. *Gastroenterology, 150*, 1355–1367.

Van Tilburg, M. A. L., Chitkara, D. K., Palsson, O. S., Turner, M., Blois-Martin, N., Ulshen, M., et al. (2009). Audio-recorded guided imagery treatment reduces functional abdominal pain in children: A pilot study. *Pediatrics, 124*, e890–e897.

Van Tilburg, M. A. L., Palsson, O. S., & Whitehead, W. E. (2013). Which psychological factors exacerbate irritable bowel syndrome? Development of a comprehensive model. *Journal of Psychosomatic Research, 74*(6), 486–492.

Van Tilburg, M. A. L., Claar, R., Romano, J. M., Langer, S. L., Walker, L. S., Whitehead, W. E., et al. (2015). The role of coping with symptoms in depression and disability: Comparison between inflammatory bowel disease and abdominal pain. *Journal of Pediatric Gastroenterology and Nutrition, 61*(4), 431–436.

Varni, J. W., Bendo, C. B., Nurko, S., Shulman, R. J., Self, M. M., Franciosi, J. P., et al. (2015). Health-related quality of life in pediatric patients with functional and organic gastrointestinal diseases. *The Journal of Pediatrics, 166*, 85–90.

Vlaeyen, J. W. S., & Linton, S. J. (2000). Fear-avoidance and its consequences in chronic musculoskeletal pain: A state of the art. *Pain, 85*, 317–332.

Walker, L. S., Williams, S. E., Smith, C. A., Garber, J., Slyke, D. A., & Lipani, T. A. (2006). Parental attention versus distraction: Impact on symptom complaints by children with and without chronic functional abdominal pain. *Pain, 122*, 43–52.

Wassom, M. C., Schurman, J. V., Friesen, C. A., & Rapoff, M. A. (2013). A pilot study of "Gutstrong" for adolescents with functional gastrointestinal disorders. *Clinical Practice in Pediatric Psychology, 1*(3), 201–213.

Weersing, V. R., Gonzalez, A., Campo, J. V., & Lucas, A. N. (2008). Brief behavioral therapy for pediatric anxiety and depression: Piloting an integrated treatment approach. *Cognitive and Behavioral Practice, 15*, 126–139.

Weersing, V. R., Rozenman, M. S., Maher-Bridge, M., & Campo, J. V. (2012). Anxiety, depression and somatic distress: Developing a transdiagnostic internalizing toolbox for pediatric practice. *Cognitive Behavioral Practice, 19*(1), 68–82.

Williams, S. E., & Zahka, N. E. (2017). *Treating somatic symptoms in children and adolescents.* New York: Guilford Press.

Wilpart, K., Tornblom, H., Svedlund, J., Tack, J. F., Simren, M., & Van Oudenhove, L. (2017). Coping skills are associated with gastrointestinal symptom severity and somatization in patients with irritable bowel syndrome. *Clinical Gastroenterology and Hepatology, 15*, 1565–1571.

Yacob, D., Di Lorenzo, C., Bridge, J. A., Rosenstein, P. F., Onorato, M., Bravender, T., et al. (2013). Prevalence of pain-predominant functional gastrointestinal disorders and somatic symptoms in patients with anxiety or depressive disorders. *The Journal of Pediatrics, 163*, 767–770.

Zucker, N., Mauro, C., Craske, M., Wagner, H. R., Datta, N., Hopkins, H., et al. (2017). Acceptance-based interoceptive exposure for young children with functional abdominal pain. *Behaviour Research and Therapy, 97*, 200–212.

Cognitive Behavioral Therapy for Enuresis

15

Edward R. Christophersen
and Christina M. Low Kapalu

The formal definition for nocturnal enuresis (NE), according to the DSM 5 (American Psychiatric Association 2013) includes: (a) repeated voiding of urine into bed or clothes (whether voluntary or intentional); (b) the behavior is clinically significant as manifested by either a frequency of twice a week for at least 3 consecutive months or the presence of clinically significant stress or impairment in a social, academic (occupational) or other important area of functioning; (c) the chronological age is at least 5 years (or equivalent developmental level); and (d) the behavior is not due exclusively to the direct physiological effects of a substance (e.g., laxatives) or a general medical condition except through a mechanism involving constipation.

The two specific types of enuresis are nocturnal only, diurnal only, or a combination of nocturnal and diurnal. Primary enuresis refers to a patient who has never stopped wetting. Secondary enuresis refers to a patient who was continent for some time, then started wetting. The vast majority of the research on the treatment of enuresis involves the use of cognitive behavioral strategies to address NE and DE. As such, this chapter will first cover the assessment and treatment of NE and then cover what is known about the treatment of DE.

Prevalence

Primary nocturnal enuresis or NE refers to children who have never been dry at night for any length of time whereas the term "secondary nocturnal enuresis" refers to children who have been dry for a period of time, with the prevalence quite dependent upon the length of time they were dry (AACAP 2009). NE is generally a self-limiting condition with a spontaneous cure rate of 12–15% a year, that is, each year approximately 15% of children with NE will stop the wetting without any intervention (Christophersen and Friman 2010). It is estimated that 10% of school-age children have NE (Shepard et al. 2017). There is evidence that prevalence rates decline steadily with age, with 20% prevalence in 5-year-old children and 1–2% prevalence in late adolescence (Shepard et al. 2017).

Joinson et al. (2016) examined the association between psychological factors and NE. They reported that there is evidence for a link, but the

E. R. Christophersen (✉)
Children's Mercy Hospital—Kansas,
Overland Park, KS, USA

Children's Mercy Hospital—Kansas City,
Kansas City, MO, USA
e-mail: echrist@cmh.edu

C. M. Low Kapalu
Children's Mercy Hospital—Kansas City,
Kansas City, MO, USA

University of Missouri Kansas City School of Medicine, Kansas City, MO, USA
e-mail: Cmlow@cmh.edu

direction of this association is unclear (do psychological problems result in a higher risk for NE or does having NE result in a higher risk for psychological problem). A positive family history of NE has frequently been noted. In families with no history of NE, only 15% of their children had NE, whereas in families in which one parent had a history of bed-wetting, 43–44% of their children were enuretic, and in families in which both parents had a history of bed-wetting, 77% of their children had enuresis (Christophersen and VanScoyoc 2013).

Cultural Issues

The incidence of nocturnal enuresis in children does not appear to differ between the United States (Cohen 1975), United Kingdom (Richman et al. 1982), Sweden (Hjalmas 1998), and Ireland (Devlin and O'Cathain 1990). Unlike a number of different problem areas experienced by children, the literature on enuresis includes outcome studies from many different countries. Although there have been occasional references to the way contemporary culture tolerates enuresis (Moffatt 1997), an extensive literature review revealed no published articles that specifically addressed the manner in which different cultures do tolerate enuresis. Byrd et al. (1996) did collect cross-sectional data on 10,960 children in the United States, aged 5 through 17. They reported no significant differences based upon race, poverty, or maternal education.

Course and Prognosis

Enuresis, a relatively benign condition and one that resolves over time in virtually every case, can impose social and psychological burdens on afflicted children and their families. Of concern are the psychological outcomes that can result from how the enuretic child is treated by important others, most notably by family members, teachers, and peers. If the social response to a child's NE is punishing in any way, then the children are in effect being punished for a behavior they cannot control. Examples of punishment from parents include reduced privileges, nagging and threatening, corporal punishment, and the promise of unattainable rewards (e.g., the child is promised a bicycle if bed-wetting stops; Christophersen and Friman 2010).

Most empirical research shows that enuretic children as a group exhibit a slight elevation in other psychological problems, but that only a small minority are significantly impaired (e.g., Friman et al. 1998). Therefore, the prognosis for the child with enuresis appears to be quite good with two caveats: (1) all forms of punishment should be prevented or eliminated, and (2) timely and effective treatment should be made available. Improvement is usually reflected in gradual reductions in the volume and frequency of accidents (Christophersen and Friman 2010).

Nocturnal Enuresis

Assessment

Medical Assessment The Clinical Practice Guidelines of the American Academy of Child and Adolescent Psychiatry (AACAP 2009) recommend a thorough physical examination prior to any intervention attempts. A history of constipation, encopresis, or palpable stool impaction suggests mechanical pressure on the bladder which should be addressed prior to focusing on the NE. Routine laboratory tests need only include urinalysis and possibly urine culture; more invasive tests are pursued only with specific indications. In the event that possible medical issues have not already been ruled out, referral to an appropriate professional is highly recommended (Christophersen and Friman 2010).

The Role of Constipation in Enuresis Shepard et al. (2017) estimated that up to "one-third of youth with nocturnal enuresis experience comorbid constipation, and another small subset experience diurnal urinary dysfunction. Incontinence during the night may have physiological causes, including reduced production of the hormone vasopressin, reduced functional bladder capacity, and possible maturational delays (Shepard et al. 2017: 768)". McGrath et al. (2007) reported that parents were poor at identifying constipation in their children compared to experienced clinicians. This may be due, at least in part, to the fact that after children have finished toilet training, bowel and bladder functioning become much more private and parents do not necessarily have access to the child's "products of elimination" and parents are also poorer at identifying constipation because of their own bowel habits and the lack of awareness of optimal stool frequency and consistency. For just that reason, we will sometimes elect to recommend that parents offer their child a tangible reward for not flushing the toilet so that the parents can see, with their own eyes, what the child has passed. At the very least, these studies support including the child's bowel history as a part of the assessment of a child with NE.

Psychological/Behavioral Assessment For the child referred by their primary-care physician, the majority of patients can be screened behaviorally with commonly available global screen measures, completed by a parent and a teacher, along with obtaining a good family history. Examples of such measures include, but are not limited to: Achenbach Child Behavior Checklist (CBCL; Achenbach 1991), the Behavioral Assessment System for Children (BASC-3; Reynolds and Kamphaus 2008); or the Conners Comprehensive Behavior Rating Scales (CBRS; Conners 2008). Absent other significant issues, there should be no initial need for an extensive psychological evaluation (Friman et al. 1998). Although children with NE may not screen positively for clinical emotional problems, the clinician may want to evaluate any impact the NE has had on the child's self-confidence or self-concept (Joinson et al. 2016). Some children with enuresis may avoid developmentally appropriate activities such as sleepovers and nights spent with grandparents out of fear of having their wetting discovered. Periodic review of emotional functioning as well as emotional support and encouragement may prove to be important components for securing adherence to prescribed treatments (Christophersen and VanScoyoc 2013).

Neveus et al. (2010) reported on the results of the International Children's Continence Society consensus statements on Monosymptomatic Enuresis. They concluded that due to the lack of rigorous research using random assignment to alternative treatments, the evidence is weak. They stated that no expensive examinations were a substitute for a well-conducted history. They recommend that parents keep a daily record of their child's symptoms that suggest that they were holding their urine including pressing their heel into their perineum, interrupted micturition, a weak stream, and the need to use abdominal pressure in order to pass urine. Questions about bowel habits should also be posed and, if constipation is reported, it must be treated first. They further reported that the physical examination of a child with NE is usually normal. With regard to treatment, they stated that "alarm therapy should be considered in every child with NE but especially in those with well-motivated parents (p. 142)."

Behavioral Interventions

The Clinical Practice Guidelines of the American Academy of Child and Adolescent Psychiatry (AACAP), in their review of the published literature on the treatment of nocturnal enuresis (2009), stated that:

> Conditioning, using a modern, portable, battery-operated alarm along with a written contract (with the child), thorough instruction, frequent monitoring, overlearning, and intermittent reinforcement before discontinuation, makes this behavioral treatment highly effective as the first line of treatment with cooperative, motivated families. (p. 1542)

Bell-and-Pad or Urine-Alarm Training

Mowrer and Mowrer (1938) published the first paper that offered the "bell-and-pad" or "urine-alarm" behavioral strategy for dealing with NE

(Christophersen and VanScoyoc 2013). The bed-wetting alarm was a rather simple device that when the child wet the bed, it completed a circuit that turned on a bell or buzzer. Mellon and McGrath (2000) reviewed the literature on enuresis and reported that there have been over 70 published research studies on the urine-alarm. There have been many more published since 2000. They concluded that: "for successful treatment of NE, the urine-alarm must be present. We need no longer debate whether the urine-alarm is effective in altering the course of NE. (p. 198)."

Apos et al. (2018) reported on a retrospective clinical audit of 2861 cases treated with practitioner-assisted bell-and-pad alarm over 7 different Australian clinical practices. The overall success rate of the bell-and-pad strategy was 76%, irrespective of the child's age. The mean treatment time to achieve dryness was 62.1 ± 30.8 days with a relapse rate of 23%. They reported that concurrent bowel dysfunction was associated with a slightly lower success rate (74%) and concurrent lower urinary tract symptoms were associated with a lower success rate (73%) and greater relapse rate (1.75 times more like to relapse). Children with secondary enuresis had significantly higher success than those with primary enuresis (82% vs. 74%).

Unlike the various medications for NE, the urine-alarm is actually a protocol, with multiple steps that caregivers need to be educated about. Although tempting, they cannot just be handed a urine-alarm, as has been done in multiple studies comparing the urine-alarm with medication, and expect the caregiver to be able to correctly implement the urine-alarm. On average, studies that have appropriately educated the family on the uses of the alarm have shown that the urine-alarm treatment initially eliminates enuresis in approximately 75% of children, with treatment duration ranging from a mean of 5–12 weeks (Doleys et al. 1977). Relapse rates are generally high, in about 46% of cases, but reinstatement of the procedures usually results in a complete cure (Taylor and Turner 1975). The urine-alarm treatment has also been shown to be superior to no treatment, short-term psychotherapy, and imipramine (Ramakrishnan 2008) and is considered a cost-effective treatment with enduring results (Mikkelsen 2001).

There are two major types of urine alarms:

1. The original bell-and-pad alarm consisted of two metallic pads (e.g., aluminum foil), that are placed on the child's bed, separated by a sheet of paper like a newspaper, that senses the presence of urine and sends an electronic signal either through a wire or wirelessly to a device that can be adjusted to sound an alarm (with the type and volume of the alarm chosen by the caregiver), vibrate a device on the child's bed, or both. The advantage of the bell-and-pad strategy is that some children do not want anything attached to their clothing. The disadvantage is that false alarms are more likely with the bell-and-pad, by, for example, the child moving off of the pad while they are sleeping or just turning over in their sleep.
2. A small sensor that is either placed in the crotch of the child's underwear with Velcro or its equivalent, near the opening of the urinary meatus (the opening though which the child passes urine) or special underwear that actually has the sensor woven into them. The advantage of the small, worn sensor is a reduction in false alarms. The sensor activates either an alarm that is attached to the child's bedclothes or a wireless type can activate an alarm placed either near the child or caregiver's bed. There are even units available now that include two devices such that one can be placed next to the child and one can be placed next to the caregiver. The disadvantage is that some children do not want to wear a sensor of either type while they are sleeping.

In the experience of the present authors, regardless of whether the parents choose a wired alarm or a wireless alarm, many children with NE are not awakened by the alarm. So, the wired alarm will usually need an extension that will allow the alarm to be placed next to the parent's bed. Wireless alarms are advertised to work up to 75 ft from the sensor to the alarm which is usually adequate except in homes where the child's bedroom is a significant distance from the parent's bedroom.

In numerous studies that have compared the bed-wetting alarm with an alternative, typically a medication, there is little or no discussion of the procedures followed when introducing the bed-wetting alarm to the child and the parents. In fact, it is not unusual for researchers to simply recommend that the parents purchase and use a bed-wetting alarm. Alternatively, when evaluating a medication, researchers typically either provide the medication or they make sure that the cost of the medication will be covered by the parent's health insurance. Christophersen and Friman (2010) list the empirically supported components that have been used in conjunction with a urine-alarm such as reward systems, overlearning (described below), and retention-control training. The use of urine alarms, as well as behavioral strategies requires a commitment from the child and parent in order to be successful. Clinicians may ask families to obtain a urine-alarm and bring it in to their next appointment so they can practice setting it up correctly. Families should be informed that the elimination of night wetting may take a month or two, or more, and will require both parent and child to get up in the night. They should also know that use of the urine-alarm needs to be continued for at least 2 weeks after the child has stopped wetting. In the event of a relapse, it is recommended that the family reinstate the urine-alarm protocol.

In larger clinical settings, there are enuresis clinics available, either through pediatric practices or through a children's hospital, staffed with individuals experienced in the treatment of NE, both physicians and allied health providers. It is best to check by phone, when calling for the initial appointment, to ascertain what kind of support services are available. While a urine-alarm is a device, the protocol for implementation of the device typically requires more than the simple purchase and installation of the alarm which, in turn, requires the services of an experienced practitioner who can take the time necessary to introduce the family to the proper implementation of the urine-alarm.

Dry-Bed Training

The concept of "Dry-Bed Training" was introduced to the literature in by Azrin and Foxx (1974) as an improvement over the use of just the urine-alarm. Dry-bed training combined a number of behavioral procedures with the use of a urine-alarm, including cleanliness training, positive practice, nighttime awakening, retention-control training, and positive reinforcement (See Table 15.1; Azrin and Foxx 1974). Reported success with dry-bed training approached 85%, with relapse rates reported between 7 and 29% (Azrin and Foxx 1974). As with urine-alarm treatment, relapsed children were cured when the training procedures were reinstated although Azrin and colleagues did not provide data on the length of reinstatement time required. One little quoted fact is that Azrin and Foxx (1974) used professional therapists with extensive experience implementing the Dry-Bed Training protocol, not the parents (Azrin, personal communication,, circa 1975) which is quite different from the instructing parents, during an office visit, on how to implement the protocol and is likely to yield better outcomes. The present authors have taken the position that there are enough data in the

Table 15.1 Treatment components of dry-bed training

Treatment component	Definition
Cleanliness training	Child is encouraged to change their own wet bedclothes and bedding
Positive practice	Parents are instructed to encourage the child to practice getting up and going to the bathroom multiple times after each enuretic episode
Nighttime awakening	When the urine-alarm sounds, the parents are told to gently awaken their child, finish urinating in the toilet, and change their bedclothes and wet bedding
Retention-control training Positive reinforcement	Child is rewarded, when they have the urge to urinate, to lay on their bed and focus on the sensations from their bladder as long as they can
Overlearning	Child is encouraged to consume extra liquids prior to bedtime to facilitate learning how it feels to have a full bladder

literature to support the use of overlearning and dry-bed training over just the bed-wetting alarm (c.f., Glazener et al. 2009; Mellon and McGrath 2000) to justify the combination of the urine-alarm, dry-bed training, and overlearning.

Overlearning

Overlearning refers to a procedure in which a child, after he or she is dry at night from using a bed-wetting alarm, is encouraged to drink extra liquids prior to bedtime until the child attains 14 additional consecutive dry nights (Houts 1996). Drinking extra fluids should make it more difficult for the child to avoid bed-wetting; thereby, training them attain a higher criterion. Forty-eight children achieved initial arrest of enuresis, and only one had relapsed at 1-year follow-up. These results, using 1-h group training sessions, supported the efficacy of the overlearning and retention-control training procedures, in addition to using the bell-and-pad. Overlearning usually results in a relapse of wetting, but in the majority of cases, that lasts only a week or so (Moffatt 1997).

Medical Treatments

Although, for a time, the medication "imipramine" was used and recommended for the treatment of NE, the Physician's Desk Reference (PDR Staff 2011) stated that it should only be used as contemporary adjunctive therapy for children with enuresis 6 years of age and older. Like any other powerful pharmacological agent, imipramine has potentially serious side effects and should be reserved for cases where more conventional therapies are not practical or effective. A recent Cochrane Database (2016) report on the use of tricyclic and related drugs for NE, concluded that tricyclics are effective at reducing the number of wet nights during treatment, but do not have a sustained effect after treatment stops, with most children relapsing. In contrast, there was evidence that alarm therapy has better short- and long-term outcomes.

Currently, the most popular medication for NE is some formulation of desmopressin or DDAVP. Moffatt (1997) reported that, for studies that had not preselected for DDAVP response, the best estimate for dryness was only approximately 25%. The relapse rate, when reported, also was high. Only 5.7% of the test subjects remained dry after withdrawal of the drug. Moffatt et al. (1993) reported an average of only 24% of the subjects achieved short-term dryness. In three studies reporting on long-term dryness, only 5.7% maintained dryness after stopping DDAVP. The authors concluded that, on the basis of current knowledge, DDAVP is inferior to conditioning alarms (i.e., urine alarms) as a primary therapy. As Moffatt (1997) concluded, DDAVP and tricyclic antidepressants are a second line of management when the alarm has failed or is impractical. For children who are known responders to medication, it can be used as needed for special occasions, such as sleepovers and camps. Thompson and Rey (1995) arrived at essentially the same conclusions about desmopressin, based upon their review of 61 published articles, which indicated an average of only 25% of patients becoming dry after the use of desmopressin. More recently, desmopressin has been available in a form that melts on the child's tongue with preliminary reports of outcomes superior to the original DDAVP (Robson et al. 2007). Much of the literature on desmopressin has been a little misleading in that it reports how many of the research participants were dry at night while still taking the medication, referring to such a practice as long-term follow-up. At the very least, each such study should include the fact that the participant continues to take the medication during follow-up assessment. Since the medication is expensive, even if the cost is covered by health insurance, this is not a minor issue. There have not been any published studies that the present authors are aware of that had participants continue with a urine-alarm for a year or two after the onset of treatment which would likely result in better long-term outcomes.

A review of the relevant literature suggests including DDAVP with alarm-based treatment has the potential to boost the already high success obtained by the alarm to 100% (Mellon and McGrath 2000). That optimistic perspective, however, shifted toward pessimism due to the discovery of potentially fatal side effects resulting from DDAVP. As recently as 2015, the FDA has repeated their caution regarding the potential for serious side effects. Further, as one of the known side effects of DDAVP is constipation, and constipation is a known condition preceding NE, the prescribing physician should routinely monitor the child for constipation.

Kasaeeyan et al. (2015) reported on randomly assigning 120 children with NE to either a urine vibrating alarm group or a DDAVP group. They reported that "the long term response rate in the vibratory alarm group was more than in the desmopressin group and it seems that vibratory alarm device may be a choice for the first-line treatment in primary nocturnal enuresis (p. 37)." At 12-month follow-up, 73% of the patients in the urine-alarm group were no longer exhibiting NE compared to 47% in the DDAVP group. Unfortunately, the manuscript does not reveal whether the long-term response to DDAVP was after the medication was discontinued or while the patients were still on the medication. The authors also used the DDAVP nasal spray which is no longer approved for use with children in the United States.

The urine-alarm can be combined with medication as a second line of treatment for NE. Kamperis et al. (2008) conducted a retrospective analysis on data from 423 children treated at clinics with a urine-alarm. Children were treated with a urine-alarm alone before the addition of desmopressin which was added after 6 weeks with patients who did not exhibit an adequate response to the urine-alarm or after 2 weeks for patients experiencing multiple enuretic episodes per night or showing no indication of improvement. A total of 290 children (74%), out of 315, became dry. A total of 108 children (26%) were treated with a combination of a urine-alarm and desmopressin, with 80 becoming dry at night. The authors concluded that children needing the addition of desmopressin have a higher nocturnal urine production on wet nights but do not seem to differ in terms of bladder reservoir function characteristics.

Case Example: Nocturnal Enuresis

History Fred, a 10-year-old boy, was living at home with his natural parents and two younger sisters, ages 6 and 8, with whom he got along well, with the exception of some teasing because of his bed-wetting. He was in the fifth grade and did well in school both behaviorally and academically. He presented at an Outpatient Behavioral Pediatric and Family Services Clinic with complaints of chronic bed-wetting. His medical, psychiatric, educational, and developmental histories were unremarkable. His parents were both professionals and worked full-time jobs outside the home. Both parents were college educated.

The clinical history indicated that beyond the current concern, there were no other behavioral complaints. Fred had been daytime trained since the age of 3 and had yet to have an accident-free night. His social life was somewhat constrained because he had had urinary accidents on sleepovers and at camp. He had worn a pull-up to bed up until age 8 when he requested to be allowed to go to bed in pajamas.

The referring psychologist requested a physical examination to be conducted by his primary-care doctor, which ruled out medical causes of the nocturnal enuresis. A family history revealed that his mother had been nocturnally incontinent until the age of 9, and an uncle on his father's side had been nocturnally incontinent until the age of 11. A developmental screening was negative for delays and a psychological screening was negative for significant behavioral and emotional problems. As indicated, however, there was mounting evidence of social problems stemming from his chronic incontinence. Specifically, he refused to attend camp and denied requests from friends to spend the night. He also discontinued the practice of inviting friends to spend the night at his house. An assessment of parental attitudes toward enuresis indicated tolerance on the part of both parents, although it was somewhat more limited in the father than in the mother. Both parents and child were highly motivated to seek treatment.

Assessment The assessment of Fred's accidents indicated that they occurred once or twice a night. His parents intermittently woke him to visit the bathroom, and if an accident had already occurred, they changed his bedding and required that he change his pajamas. He never changed his bedding or pajamas on his own without prompting from parents, and his mother routinely changed his bedding during the day. He provided no assistance with the laundry of his wet pajamas and bedding. No consequences were applied for accidents, and because he had not yet had a dry night, parental response for success was moot. During the assessment period, Fred assented to measurement of his daytime urine output and use of a common household measuring cup for six urinations showed an average of 4 oz, which was quite small for a child his age. He urinated an average of 8–10 times a day.

Case Conceptualization Fred's urinary accidents met the diagnostic criteria from the DSM-IV for Primary Monosymptomatic Nocturnal Enuresis. As is typical of most cases of enuresis, it appeared to be inherited, with potential genetic lines of transmission on both sides of the family. The case was not complicated by extraneous psychosocial factors, nor was it yet complicated by comorbid behavioral problems. But there was evidence of a gradually shrinking social life, and Fred rarely slept away from his home. There was also clear evidence of reduced functional bladder capacity and overly frequent daytime urinations. The average volume for a continent child his age should be between 10 and 14 oz, and his was around 4 oz. Additionally, 4–6 urinations a day should be sufficient for a 10-year-old boy.

Treatment Consistent with the description of treatment for enuresis in this paper, the primary component of treatment selected for Fred was the urine-alarm—one that attached to his pajamas. As discussed previously, the effectiveness of treatment increases as additional components are added to a treatment plan. These are best selected collaboratively by therapist, child, and parents, as was done in this case. Fred and his parents selected the following additional components:

1. A motivational system involving the dot-to-dot program, wherein Fred would earn a cherished videogame when his drawing was complete.
2. Responsibility training requiring Fred to bring stained bed clothing and pajamas to the basement laundry room and to remake his own bed after an accident.
3. A 2-week period of overlearning during which Fred drank extra fluids before bed and during the day on weekends.
4. Dry Kegel exercises conducted several times during the day and at least one start/stop exercise conducted while urinating each day.
5. Retention Control Training on the weekends.
6. A self-monitoring system involving Fred recording wet and dry nights on a calendar supplied by the therapist.
7. A weekly parent monitoring system involving sizing urine stains on either Saturday or Sunday night.
8. A visualization exercise requiring Fred to imagine waking up in a dry bed in the morning.
9. Tablet-based DDAVP to be supplied as needed whenever Fred spent the night away from home.

Outcome Fred's therapist monitored progress by interviewing the parents and Fred himself, inspecting Fred's self-monitoring calendar, and reviewing progress on the dot-to-dot drawing and variations in the urine spot measurement. During a 2-week pretreatment baseline, Fred wet the bed nightly and the urine spots were very large because of the overlearning component of the treatment that was imposed during baseline. In the first week following treatment, Fred's frequency of accidents sank to five nights a week and continued to fall for five continuous weeks, at which point accidents ceased altogether. At that point, the major components of the program were phased out. In the 6 months following, Fred had two accidents, both of which involved small amounts of urine. At the 1-year follow-up, Fred had not had an accident for at least 6 months.

Shared with permission from Christophersen and Friman (2010).

Conclusions

NE can be successfully managed using a urine-alarm, achieving good initial results and long-term complete dryness, without the need for expensive pharmacologic interventions. Cutting et al. (2007) published 2-year outcome data on a supportive program that made management less arduous for the child and their family. The few outcome studies that have reported long-term follow-up after discontinuation of medications to reduce nighttime wetting typically report that less than one-third of the participants remained dry at night. The most recent advance in medication for NE has been the formulation of desmopressin that melts in the child's mouth which, when the dose is gradually titrated down, results in the best medication outcome data with the least negative side effects, as long as the child is cautioned to avoid drinking many fluids after the evening meal. In general, "Random Controlled Trial results support the use of desmopressin in addition to urine-alarm training for short-term improvement of nightly bed-wetting, but also suggest the lack of long-term symptom remission" (Shepard et al. 2017, see p. 771).

Diurnal Enuresis (Day Wetting)

The vast majority of cases of enuresis are nocturnal and, correspondingly, most of the literature on enuresis is devoted to the nocturnal type. Nonetheless, enuresis cases that involve a diurnal component are a notable concern, especially in late preschool and early elementary school. Although the pertinent literature is small, it strongly suggests that diurnal enuresis is a justifiable cause of concern for afflicted children, their caretakers, and teachers. Along with the risk of secondary psychological problems, there are public health concerns associated with daytime wetting. For example, the increase in the prevalence of infectious disease (e.g., hepatitis, infectious diarrhea) seen in daycare settings and preschools over the past few decades has been partially attributed to the spread of bacteria through child incontinence (Christophersen and Friman 2010).

In a survey of more than 3000 7-year-old students7 years old, Hjalmas (1998) reported that day wetting of any kind occurred in 6% of students. Over 70% of the children who wet during the day also had increased urgency. Combined daytime and nighttime incontinence was reported by 17% of the children, whereas 22% were wet only during the day and 61% wet only at night. None of the students had a previously indicated organic cause for their incontinence. Savaser et al. (2018), in a study of 2750 primary school students between the ages of 11 and 14 years of age in Istanbul, reported an incidence of diurnal enuresis (DE) of only 0.9%, supporting their statement that the incidence of diurnal enuresis decreases with age.

Medical Assessment

The vast majority of referrals for day wetting, from the primary-care physician, will already have had reasonable medical conditions already ruled out. If a patient presents who has not seen a physician first, then referral for a physical is indicated (Christophersen and Friman 2010). The AACAP (2009) recommends a physical examination including enlarged adenoids or tonsils, bladder distention, fecal impaction, genital abnormalities, spinal cord anomalies, and neurologic signs noted. Routine lab tests need only include urinalysis and possible urine culture (Hobson 2009). Unfortunately, studies have shown that as few as 38% of children with enuresis had seen any physician about their symptoms (Foxman et al. 1986). There does seem to be general agreement in the literature regarding etiology (AACAP 2009).

Behavioral Assessment

Most patients with DE can be adequately screened for behavioral and emotional problems through the use of a thorough interview and behavior rating scales. The AACAP (2009) recommends separate interviews of the child and their caregiver, to explore every aspect of urinary incontinence. Since a history of punishment is common in day wetters (perhaps not physical punishment but the loss of privileges), parents are strongly discouraged from providing any forms of punishment for wetting and are provided with psychoeducation so that they understand that the day wetting is out of the child's control.

Behavioral Treatment

The AACAP (2009) recommends, as the first line of treatment for day wetting, the use of a battery-operated bed-wetting alarm along with a written contract, thorough instruction, frequent monitoring, overlearning, and intermittent reinforcement before discontinuation of the alarm. Despite this recommendation, few medical providers are aware of this intervention or recommend it to families (Christophersen 2005). The majority of medication studies on bed-wetting alarms treat the alarm almost like a medication in that the researchers recommend that the family purchase a bed-wetting alarm and follow the instructions that come with the alarm. But the use of a bed-wetting alarm is actually a protocol, typically including discussion, a written contract between the parent and the child and providing thorough, hands on, instruction on how to use the bed-wetting alarm. There are two often-quoted studies supporting the use of a bed-wetting alarm for day wetting. Friman and Vollmer (1995) reported, with long-term objective follow-up data using a reversal design, the successful use of a bed-wetting alarm. Halliday et al. (1987) with random assignment to one of the two groups: alarm sounding contingent upon wetting and random alarm sounding that was not contingent upon wetting also reported the efficacy of this intervention. Two-thirds of the children in the contingent alarm condition responded by becoming daytime continent. The non-contingent alarm produced just as good a response and was recommended for routine use in children with day wetting. They reported that 23% of those who responded to treatment relapsed up to 2 years after completion of the trial. Although Christophersen and Friman (2010) recommend reinstitution of the alarm for any relapse, just as physicians recommend reinstitution of medication in the event of a relapse, none was reported. Another contrast with medication studies is that the medication is typically continued for months or years until the child is dry, whereas the alarm studies typically are only implemented for a few weeks, at most months. Neither of the alarm studies reported any negative side effects so often reported in the literature on medication management of day wetting, making this intervention both effective and low risk.

Medical Treatment

The two medications that are currently recommended, in the event that the bed-wetting alarm has not reduced or stopped the day wetting, or the family is not willing or able to implement the alarm procedure, are imipramine and DDAVP. Meadow and Berg (1982), in a controlled trial of imipramine in DE, reported that no evidence emerged to support that imipramine was superior to placebo in the treatment of DE.

Case Vignette: Diurnal Enuresis

History Sam, a 6-year-old boy, lived at home with his natural parents and older brother, Tom, age 12. He was in the first grade. His teacher had no complaints about his academic progress, but she was concerned about emerging socially withdrawn behavior and a pattern of diurnal incontinence that she felt was at least partially responsible for the withdrawal. He presented at an Outpatient Behavioral Pediatric and Family Services Clinic for treatment of the daytime wetting problems. His medical, psychiatric, educational, and developmental histories were unremarkable. His father was a plumber and his mother held a part-time job as a sales clerk. Both parents had high-school educations. The clinical history indicated that with the exception of the incontinence and the emerging social problems, there were no other behavioral complaints. He had been toilet trained successfully at the age of 3 but began having urinary accidents when he entered kindergarten. He was continent at night. His parents managed his wetting accidents using absorptive undergarments (pull-ups), but following the advice of friends, they had made a small number of attempts to address the wetting with reward systems, scheduling, and removal of the absorptive undergarments. The results of their efforts were unfortunately unsuccessful and resulted in two accidents at school that were detected by his teacher and his peers. Subsequently, he returned to wearing the absorptive undergarments which he was using at the time of the referral.

The referring psychologist requested a physical examination to be conducted by his primary-care physician, which ruled out medical causes of the diurnal wetting. A family history revealed that an uncle on his mother's side had been a bedwetter though the parents could not recollect daytime wetting problems in their own histories nor in the histories of other close relatives. A developmental screening was negative for delays, and a psychological screening was negative for significant behavioral and emotional problems. However, the screening did indicate psychometric evidence of the social withdrawal noted by his teacher. In addition to avoiding others on the playground, he refused to attend camp and expressed little interest in having friends visit him at his home. He was also reluctant to visit friends at their homes, and at the time of the referral, the parents and the boy could not identify any classmate or neighbor as a close friend. An assessment of parental attitudes toward the wetting indicated tolerance on the mother's part and intolerance on the father's part. The father believed that Sam was inattentive and mildly lazy about his toileting responsibilities. His mother believed that he simply couldn't help it. Both the mother and Sam were highly motivated to pursue treatment, but the father did not participate in any clinic visits. The mother reported that the father was supportive but unable to find the time to come to the clinic.

Assessment Assessment of Sam's urinary patterns indicated that he was completely continent at night. Because he wore a pull-up, the frequency of his accidents during the day was impossible to determine on school days, but he came home wet at least 4 days a week. To estimate accident frequency during the assessment period, he did not wear pull-ups on the weekends, and the frequency across 4 weekend days was 1.25 accidents a day. Parental response to the accidents varied depending on the parent. The mother tended to note neutrally that he had had an accident, guide him to the bathroom, encourage him to attempt to urinate, and then change his clothing. His father was more firm and sometimes more critical, and supplied much less assistance. He would merely note that his boy had an accident, comment critically, and tell him to go change his clothes. The mother also assessed his urinary output using a glass measurement container on three occasions, and the result indicated an average of approximately 3.5 oz per measure. She also estimated that he urinated an average of seven to nine times a day when he was not in his pull-up.

Case Conceptualization Sam's urinary accidents met criteria from the DSM-IV for Primary Diurnal Enuresis. It also fit criteria for a secondary classification because he had had a period of complete continence lasting longer than 6 months. There was modest evidence supporting its being an inherited condition. There was also evidence that the chronic accidents were producing an increasingly growing detrimental effect on Sam's social life, largely because he had had accidents at school, and peers and teachers had detected them. There was also evidence of substantially reduced functional bladder capacity and overly frequent daytime urinations. There was no evidence that the onset of the accidents was occasioned by a trauma or chronic encounter with serious distressful events. These facts supported the view that it was an idiopathic ("garden variety") case of diurnal enuresis.

Treatment The core component for treatment for Sam's incontinence while at home was the vibrating urine-alarm. But, because of the potential for enhanced detection at school by classmates, it was not used there. Because of the elevated motivation of Sam and his mother, multiple components were assembled to create a treatment package. These included the following:

1. A motivational system involving the dot-to-dot program mentioned earlier. The ultimate reward he selected was a basketball.
2. A toileting schedule was implemented both at home and at school. At school, he was directed to use the toilet between two classes in the morning and two classes in the afternoon.
3. A toileting pass program was implemented at school which allowed him to leave class whenever he felt the urge to urinate, at which point he would surrender his pass. For each unused pass, he was provided one sticker, and the accumulation of five stickers allowed him to withdraw one small reward from a classroom reward bag.
4. The use of pull-ups was discontinued at school.
5. Wet Kegel exercises were conducted two to three times a week at home.
6. Retention Control Training was conducted on the weekends.
7. A self-monitoring system with which Sam recorded accident-free days on a specially constructed chart at home was implemented.
8. A modification of the father's typical response to accidents was requested and, according to the mother, actually realized. The father was simply asked to provide a neutral response to accidents and avoid any form of criticism.
9. Although Sam was too young to assist with laundry, he was required to bring his own soiled clothing to the laundry basket whenever he had an accident.

Outcome Sam's therapist monitored his progress through telephone contacts with the mother and periodic clinic visits. He would either inquire about or actually inspect the self-monitoring calendar and the dot-to-dot drawing. During a 2-week baseline, Sam was wet almost every day and slightly more frequently on the weekends. Immediately following the implementation of treatment, accidents at school stopped but continued periodically on the weekends. By week 4, he was completely accident-free, at which point the use of the alarm was discontinued. When he completed his dot-to-dot program and earned his reward, the system was discontinued as was the calendar-based monitoring system. At week 7, all major components of the program were discontinued. At the 6-month follow-up, Sam had not had an accident for at least 4 months.

Shared with permission from Christophersen and Friman (2010).

Training and Supervision for the Evaluation and Treatment of Enuresis

Because the vast majority of psychologists have little or no experience in the evaluation and treatment of enuresis, APA Ethical Guidelines discourage beginning to evaluate and treat a new condition without actual supervised clinical experience. The practitioner who desires to add the evaluation and treatment of enuresis to the services that they offer in their clinic would do well to arrange for supervision by an experienced practitioner, either from a nearby APA approved training program or from a local practitioner who was trained to routinely treat enuresis. This is recommended *in addition to* attendance of clinical trainings or workshops and additional readings.

Discussion

Few problems addressed by the pediatric psychologist are as prevalent as enuresis and few problems have the high success rate of an inexpensive treatment as the urine-alarm does. Granted, implementing a urine-alarm is not as easy as giving a child a pill to swallow, but there are literally no negative physiological side effects of using a urine-alarm which must be contrasted with the potentially serious side effects of the few medications that have demonstrable effectiveness in the treatment of enuresis, as long as the child continues to take the medication for months and, in many cases, years, at significant expense either to the family or to the family's insurance provider. In cases where the urine-alarm is not practical, medication is a second line of treatment with moderate efficacy as long as the medication is given daily. The recent addition of the desmopressin melt has resulted in similar treatment effects with less reported negative side effects (as long as the parents refrain, as instructed, from allowing their child to drink many fluids after the evening meal).

The outcome literature on the treatment of enuresis is significantly limited by the lack of random controlled studies that assign participants to either the urine-alarm or a medication trial. While there are numerous studies with large sample sizes that have evaluated the urine-alarm and medication, random assignment between the urine-alarm and medication are lacking. In the studies that have compared the urine-alarm to medication, the medication arm of the study typically gets a lot of attention in the sense of titrating the dosage of the medication and carefully tracking potential negative side effects. However, few physicians have the training and experience to comprehensively approach the implementation of the urine-alarm (Tables 15.2, 15.3, 15.4, 15.5, and 15.6).

Table 15.2 Enuresis intake form

Parents

1. What word does your child use for urinating? _____
2. Has your child ever been potty trained? _____

	Age started	Age accomplished
Bladder trained? _____	_____	_____
Bowel trained? _____	_____	_____

3. What potty-training method did you use? _____
4. Was there ever a time when your child did not wet the bed? Yes _____ No _____
5. If so, when did bed-wetting begin? _____
6. When did you decide that it was a problem? _____
    Your spouse? _____
    Your child? _____
7. What about bed-wetting makes it a problem for you? _____
    For your spouse? _____
    For your child? _____
8. Does your child wet the bed every night? _____
    If not, how often? _____ -
9. Has your child ever gone for 2 months without wetting the bed? _____
    How long? _____
    How often? _____
10. What methods have you used in the past to stop the bed-wetting? _____ _____
11. Are you still using any of these methods? _____
12. What is your child's responsibility when he/she wets the bed? _____
13. Does your child ever wet his/her pants during the day? _____
    How much? Small _____ Medium _____ Large _____
14. Does your child ever dribble in his/her pants during the day? _____
15. Does your child ever complain of burning when he/she urinates? _____
16. Does your child have to go more frequently than you think is normal? _____
17. Does your child complain that it doesn't feel like he/she has completely emptied his/her bladder when finished? _____
18. When your child has to urinate, can he/she wait a while or does he/she have to go right then or have an accident? _____
19. Have you ever noticed any irritation around the end of his penis/her meatus? _____
20. Has your child ever had a work-up for a urinary tract infection or any other urinary problem? When? _____
21. By whom? _____
22. Where? _____
23. Results? _____
24. Is your child a sound sleeper? _____
25. When your child stays overnight with relatives or a friend, does he/she wet the bed? _____
26. What do you believe causes bed-wetting? _____
27. Has your child ever had problems with constipation? Yes _____ No? _____
28. Has your child ever had a problem with soiling?
29. To your knowledge, did anyone in either the biological mother's or father's family wet the bed?
    If so, who? _____

(continued)

Table 15.2 (continued)

	Child
1.	Tell me why you're here? _____
2.	Do you want to stop wetting the bed? _____
3.	Does wetting the bed cause you any problems? _____
4.	What do Mom and Dad say/do when you wet the bed? _____
5.	Have you ever gone without wetting the bed? _____
6.	When you wet the bed, what do you do about it? _____
7.	What do you like to do with your Mom? _____ With your Dad? _____

Christophersen, E.R. (1994). Pediatric Compliance: A Guide for the Primary-Care Physician. New York: Plenum. Reprinted with permission

Table 15.3 Practical tips for successful use of an enuresis alarm

- Inform parents that successful training takes time; suggest a 3-month commitment. Contract with the parent and child for a 3-month trial
- Recommend an appointment schedule of every 3 weeks until further notice
- Inform parents that their involvement is necessary (including assistance in the middle of the night) as their child may not arouse on their own initially
- Provide a diary to complete before the first visit and during treatment. Record number of wet nights, how many episodes per night, estimated size of wetness on the sheet
- Suggest that the parent place the actual alarm component of the urine-alarm near their bed since many children will not arouse on their own to the alarm
- Emphasize to parent and child that arousal is key and should be rewarded. Emphasize and reward arousal
- Evaluate improvement by decreases in number of wet nights, decreases in frequency per night, and decreases in size of wetness on sheets. Use a decreased frequency of wet nights, a decreased number of episodes per night, and a decreased size of wet spot as signs of improvement
- Initial goal should be 14 consecutive dry nights with no bed-wetting. Continue until the child achieves 14 consecutive dry nights (no alarm sound for even a spot of urine)
- Once initial goal has been reached, implement overlearning as follows: intake of fluid before bedtime, increasing in 2-oz increments until 17 oz is reached. Increase only after each addition is mastered (defined as two additional weeks with bed-wetting). After initial goal is achieved, use overlearning, that is, either 16 oz of fluid before bed or gradual 2-oz increments, increasing as each step is mastered, until 16 oz is reached
- End overlearning when child is dry for 14 consecutive nights after 16 oz of fluid at bedtime. Continue overlearning until the child achieves 14 consecutive dry nights
- End urine-alarm and extra drinking when overlearning goal has been reached. When overlearning is completed, stop the alarm and extra drinking
- Inform family that relapses are normal and the same treatment protocol can be used again successfully. Relapses can be retreated successfully in the same manner, in many cases

From: Christophersen, E.R. & Vanscoyoc, S.M. Diagnosis and management of nocturnal enuresis. In: E.R. Christophersen and S.M. Vanscoyoc (2013). Treatments that work with children: Empirically supported strategies for managing childhood problems. Second Edition. Washington, D.C.: American Psychological Association. 129–142
Reprinted with permission

Table 15.4 Dry-bed training procedures

I.	Recording: Use calendar progress chart to record dry or wet for each night
(A)	Parent praises child if dry
(B)	Parent encourages child to keep working if wet
II.	At bedtime
(A)	Child feels sheets and comments on their dryness
(B)	Child describes what he will do if he has the urge to urinate
(C)	Child describes current need to urinate and does so
(D)	Parent expresses confidence in child and reviews progress
(E)	Alarm is placed on bed or on child
(F)	Alarm is connected and turned "on"
(G)	Child goes to sleep
III.	Nightly awakening
(A)	Awaken child once during the night
1.	Use minimal prompt in awakening, but be sure the child is awake
2.	Child feels sheets and comments on dryness
3.	Parent praises child for dry sheets
4.	Child goes to bathroom, urinates as much as possible, returns to bed
5.	Child feels sheets again
6.	Child states what he will do if he feels urge to urinate
7.	Parent expresses confidence to child
8.	Keep alarm on bed if it has not sounded before awakening
9.	If alarm has sounded more than 30 min before scheduled awakening, awaken at schedule time
10.	If alarm has sounded less than 30 min before scheduled awakening, awaken at the scheduled time
(B)	Adjust time of nightly awakening
1.	On first night, awaken child 5 h before his or her usual time of awakening
2.	After child has six consecutive dry nights, awaken him or her 1 h earlier the next night. Continue to move the awakening time 1 h earlier after each six dry nights until the awakening time is 8 h before the usual time of awakening
3.	When dry for 14 nights at 8-h awakening, discontinue awakening and discontinue alarm
IV.	When alarm sounds
(A)	Awaken child and give mild reprimand for wetting
(B)	Child feels sheets and comments on wetness
(C)	Child walks to bathroom and finishes wetting
(D)	Child takes quick bath
(E)	Child changes into dry clothes
(F)	Child removes wet sheets and places them in laundry
(G)	Child remakes bed with dry sheets
(H)	Child feels bed sheets and comments on dryness
(I)	Do not reconnect alarm
(J)	Child returns to sleep
V.	During day
(A)	Child and parents describe progress to relevant friends or family members
(B)	Parents repeatedly express confidence in child and praise him or her
(C)	Parent calls therapist at set times to report progress

Reproduced from Azrin, N. H., Sneed, T. J., & Foxx, R. M. (1974) with permission

Table 15.5 Some alarm devices for the treatment of primary enuresis

Device	Manufacturer	Cost
Wet-Stop	Palco Labs	$65.00
	Santa Cruz, CA	
	800-346-4488	
Nytone Enuretic Alarm	Nytone Medical Products	53.50
	Salt Lake City, UT	
	801-973-4090	
Potty Pager	Ideas for Living	49.95
	Boulder, CO	
	800-497-6573	
Nite Train'r	Koregon Enterprises	69.00
	Beaverton, OR	
	800-544-4240	
Sleep Dry	Star Child Labs	45.00
	Aptos, CA	
	800-346-7283	

Reprinted (and updated) from Christophersen and Friman (2010) with written permission

Table 15.6 Positive practice for toileting accidents

After they have been toilet trained, some children occasionally have periods of frequent wetting or soiling. The children should first be examined by a physician to rule out physical conditions, such as urinary tract infections, that may be causing the accidents

When you find your child with wet or soiled pants, use the following guidelines:

1. Show verbal disapproval for the wetting or soiling
   (a) Tell your child why you are displeased, saying something like, "You wet your pants"
   (b) Express your disapproval of the accident by saying something like, "You shouldn't wet your pants. You should use the toilet"
2. Have your child do positive practice of self-toileting
   (a) Tell your child what you are doing and why by saying something like, "Bobby wet his pants. Bobby has to practice going to the bathroom"
   (b) Guide your child quickly to the toilet or potty chair
   (c) Guide your child to quickly lower his/her pants and sit on the toilet/potty
   (d) After sitting 1 or 2 s (do not allow urination), guide your child to quickly raise his/her pants
   (e) Guide your child back to the area where you discovered the accident for a total of five positive practices from where your child had the accident. Then, guide your child to practice from five other parts of the house (for example, from the front door, from the back door, from the kitchen) to the bathroom or potty chair
   (f) If your child refuses to do the positive practice trials, or if he/she has a temper tantrum, direct him to time-out. After he/she completes the time-out, begin the positive practice from where you left off
3. Make your child responsible for cleaning up
   (a) If there is urine on the floor, guide your child to get a cloth and wipe up the spot
   (b) With a minimum of guidance, require your child to remove his/her soiled pants
   (c) Guide your child to put his/her soiled clothing in an appropriate place
   (d) If your child has had a bowel movement, guide him/her to clean himself/herself up or to take a quick partial bath
   (e) Guide your child to put on clean clothes
4. After the accident has been corrected, do not continue to talk about it. Your child should start with a clean slate
5. Remember to praise and hug your child when he/she eliminates in the toilet/potty chair

Source: Adapted from Azrin, N.H. and Foxx, R.M. (1976). *Toilet training in less than a day*. New York: Pocket Books

References

Achenbach. (1991). *Manual for the child behavior checklist: 4-18 and 1991 profile*. Burlington: University of Vermont, Department of Psychiatry.

American Academy of Child and Adolescent Psychiatry. (2009). Practice parameters for the assessment and treatment of children and adolescents with enuresis. *Journal of the American Academy of Child and Adolescent Psychiatry, 43*, 1540–1550.

American Psychiatric Association. (2013). *Diagnostic and statistical manual of mental disorders* (5th ed.). Arlington: American Psychiatric Publishing.

Apos, E., Schuster, S., Reese, J., Whitaker, S., Murphy, K., Golder, J., et al. (2018). Enuresis management in children: Retrospective clinical audit of 2861 cases treated with practitioner-assisted bell-and-pad alarm. *The Journal of Pediatrics, 193*, 211–216.

Azrin, N. H., & Foxx, R. M. (1974). *Toilet training in less than a day*. New York: Simon and Schuster.

Azrin, N. H., Sneed, T. J., & Foxx, R. M. (1974). Dry-bed training: Rapid elimination of childhood enuresis. *Behaviour Research and Therapy, 12*, 147–156.

Byrd, R. S., Weitzman, M., Lanphear, N. E., & Auinger, P. (1996). Bed-wetting in US children: Epidemiology and related behavior problems. *Pediatrics, 98*, 414–419.

Caldwell, P. H., Sureshkumar, P., & Wong, W. C. (2016). Tricyclic and related drugs for nocturnal enuresis in children. *Cochrane Database Systematic Review*, (1), CD002117.

Christophersen, E. R. (2005). Is evidence-based treatment sufficient to manage nighttime wetting problems (Enuresis)? Yes and No. *Archives of Pediatric & Adolescent Medicine, 159*, 1182–1183.

Christophersen, E. R., & Friman, P. C. (2010). Elimination disorders in children and adolescents: Enuresis and encopresis. In D. Weddding (Ed.), *Advances in psychotherapy: Evidence-based practice series*. Goettingen: Hogrefe & Huber.

Christophersen, E. R., & VanScoyoc, S. M. (2013). Diagnosis and management of nocturnal enuresis. In E. R. Christophersen & S. M. VanScoyoc (Eds.), *Treatments that work with children: Empirically supported strategies for managing childhood problems* (2nd ed.). Washington, DC: APA.

Cohen, M. W. (1975). Enuresis. *Pediatric Clinics of North America, 22*, 545–560.

Conners, C. K. (2008). *Conners comprehensive behavior rating scales*. New York: Multi-Health Systems.

Cutting, D. A., Paallant, J. F., & Cutting, F. M. (2007). Nocturnal enuresis: Application of evidence-based medicine in community practice. *Journal of Paediatrics and Child Health, 43*, 167–172.

Devlin, J. B., & O'Cathain, C. (1990). Predicting treatment outcome in nocturnal enuresis. *Archives of Disease in Children, 65*, 1158–1161.

Doleys, D. M., Ciminero, A. R., Tollison, J. W., Williams, W., & Wells, K. C. (1977). Dry-bed training and retention control training: A comparison. *Behavior Therapy, 8*, 54–548.

Foxman, B., Burciaga-Valde, Z. R., & Book, R. H. (1986). Childhood enuresis: Prevalence, perceived impact and prescribed treatments. *Pediatrics, 77*, 482–486.

Friman, P. C., & Vollmer, D. (1995). Successful use of the nocturnal urine alarm for diurnal enuresis. *Journal of Applied Behavior Analysis, 28*, 89–90.

Friman, P. C., Handwerk, M. L., Swearer, S. M., McGinnis, C., & Warzak, W. J. (1998). Do children with primary nocturnal enuresis have clinically significant behavior problems? *Archives of Pediatrics and Adolescent Medicine, 152*, 537–539.

Glazener, C. M. A., Evans, J. H. C., & Peto, R. E. (2009). *Alarm interventions for nocturnal enuresis in children*. Chichester: Wiley, Cochrane Incontinence Group.

Halliday, S., Meadow, S. R., & Berg, A. I. (1987). Successful management of daytime enuresis using alarm procedures: A randomly controlled trial. *Archives of Disease in Childhood, 62*, 132–137.

Hjalmas, K. (1998). Functional daytime incontinence: Definitions and epidemiology. *Scandinavian Journal of Urology and Nephrology, 141*, 39–44.

Hobson, W. L. (2009). Evaluation and management of enuresis. *New England Journal of Medicine, 360*, 1429–1436.

Houts, A. C. (1996). Behavioral treatment of enuresis. *Clinical Psychologist, 49*, 5–6.

Joinson, C., Sullivan, S., von Gontard, A., & Heron, J. (2016). Early childhood psychological factors and risk for bedwetting at school age in a UK cohort. *European Journal of Child and Adolescent Psychiatry, 25*, 519–528.

Kamperis, K., Hagstroem, S., Rittig, S., & Djurhuus, J. C. (2008). Combination of the enuresis alarm and desmopressin: Second line treatment for nocturnal enuresis. *Journal of Urology, 179*, 1128–1131.

Kasaeeyan, A. A., Nakhjavany, N. H., Aliramaji, A., & Shafi, H. (2015). Comparison of long-term efficacy between vibratory alarm and desmopressin in treatment of Primary Nocturnal Enuresis. *Caspian Journal of Applied Sciences Research, 4*, 37–41.

McGrath, K. H., Caldwell, P. H. Y., & Jones, M. P. (2007). The frequency of constipation in children with nocturnal enuresis: A comparison with parental reporting. *Journal of Paediatrics and Child Health, 44*, 19–27.

Meadow, R., & Berg, I. (1982). Controlled trial of imipramine in diurnal enuresis. *Archives of Disease in Childhood, 57*, 714–716.

Mellon, M. W., & McGrath, M. L. (2000). Empirically supported treatments in pediatric psychology: Nocturnal enuresis. *Journal of Pediatric Psychology, 25*(4), 193–214.

Mikkelsen, E. J. (2001). Enuresis and encopresis: Ten years of progress. *Journal of the American Academy of Child and Adolescent Psychiatry, 40*, 1146–1158.

Moffatt, M. E. (1997). Nocturnal enuresis: A review of the efficacy of treatments and practical advice for clinicians. *Journal of Developmental and Behavioral Pediatrics, 18*, 49–56.

Moffatt, M. E., Harlos, S., Kirshen, A. J., & Burd, L. (1993). Desmopressin acetate and nocturnal enuresis: How much do we know? *Pediatrics, 92*, 420–425.

Mowrer, O. H., & Mowrer, W. M. (1938). Enuresis—A method for its study and treatment. *American Journal of Orthopsychiatry, 8*, 436–459.

Neveus, T., Eggert, P., Evans, J., Macedo, A., Rittig, S., Tekgul, S., et al. (2010). Evaluation of and treatment for monosymptomatic enuresis: A standardization document from the International Children's Continence Society. *The Journal of Urology, 183*(2), 441–447.

PDR Staff. (2011). *Physicians' desk reference*. PDR Network.

Ramakrishnan, K. (2008). Evaluation and treatment of enuresis. *American Family Physician, 78*, 489–496.

Reynolds, C. R., & Kamphaus, R. W. (2008). *Behavior assessment system for children: Manual*. Circle Pines: American Guidance.

Richman, N., Stevenson, J. E., & Graham, P. J. (1982). Prevalence of behavior problems in 3-year-old children: An epidemiological study in a London borough. *Journal of Child Psychology and Psychiatry, 16*, 277–287.

Robson, W. L. M., Leung, A. K. C., & Norgaard, J. P. (2007). The comparative safety of oral versus intranasal desmopressin for the treatment of children with nocturnal enuresis. *The Journal of Urology, 178*(1), 24–30.

Savaser, S., Beji, N. K., Aslan, E., & Gozen, D. (2018). The prevalence of diurnal urinary incontinence and enuresis and Quality of Life: Sample of school. *Urology Journal, 15*, 173–179.

Shepard, J. A., Poler, J. E., & Grabman, J. H. (2017). Evidence-based psychosocial treatments for pediatric elimination disorders. *Journal of Clinical Child & Adolescent Psychology, 46*, 767–797.

Taylor, P. D., & Turner, R. K. (1975). A clinical trial of continuous intermittent and overlearning "bell and pad" treatments for nocturnal enuresis. *Behaviour Research and Therapy, 3*, 281–293.

Thompson, S., & Rey, J. M. (1995). Functional enuresis: Is desmopressin the answer? *Journal of the American Academy of Child & Adolescent Psychiatry, 34*, 266–271.

Cognitive Behavioral Therapy for Encopresis

Christina M. Low Kapalu and Edward R. Christophersen

Dylan is a 5-year-old boy who was seen by his pediatrician for his 5-year well-child visit. At this visit, his mother reported that he recently began to "poop in his pants" when at school. She stated that 3 months ago, he began to refuse to use the toilet when asked and began to have accidents in his underwear. As a result of frequent accidents, he was put back into pull ups so that his parents could help keep him and the furniture clean. Dylan reportedly denied having an accident even though others could smell it and would not get cleaned up. Refusal to clean up after a soil caused a lot of distress for Dylan and his parents. His parents stated that they cannot understand why he is "doing this all of a sudden." During the visit, Dylan was observed to sit on his heels and rock back and forth at times.[1]

Encopresis, also known as fecal incontinence, is one of the two main elimination disorders. This condition occurs when a child passes stool into inappropriate locations such as onto the floor or, more frequently, into their underwear. This condition is known as a biobehavioral or biopsychobehavioral (Cox et al. 1998) condition, meaning that complex biological and psychosocial/behavioral factors interact to influence presentation and consequently treatment (Culbert and Banez 2007). For the purposes of this chapter, the Diagnostic and Statistical Manual, Fifth Edition (DSM-5; American Psychiatric Association 2013) diagnostic criteria will be utilized to define encopresis.

Fecal soiling must occur at least once a month for at least 3 months, in a child who has the chronological age, or developmental equivalent, of 4 years in order to qualify for a diagnosis of encopresis (American Psychiatric Association 2013). Soiling cannot be the direct result of a substance, medication (e.g., laxative overuse), or another medical condition (e.g., neurogenic bowel, Hirschprung's Disease). The exception to this rule is constipation, as most children with encopresis present with constipation at some point in the course of this condition. Some distinguish encopresis (previous period of fecal continence) from delayed bowel training (never bowel trained); however, this distinction is not consistently utilized in the literature.

There are two specifiers for encopresis: with constipation and overflow incontinence or with-

---

[1] All cases, including names, are fictional.

C. M. Low Kapalu (✉)
Children's Mercy Hospital—Kansas City, Kansas City, MO, USA

University of Missouri Kansas City School of Medicine, Kansas City, MO, USA
e-mail: Cmlow@cmh.edu

E. R. Christophersen
Children's Mercy Hospital—Kansas, Overland Park, KS, USA

Children's Mercy Hospital—Kansas City, Kansas City, MO, USA
e-mail: echrist@cmh.edu

out constipation and overflow incontinence. It is estimated that between 85 and 95% of children with encopresis have a current or past history of constipation that contributes to soiling (Levine 1975; Molnar et al. 1983; Loening-Baucke 2007). Soiling is thought to occur for different reasons for these two subtypes. In children with constipation and overflow incontinence, also known as retentive fecal incontinence, soiling is thought to result from chronic constipation, fecal impaction, and/or stool retention in the rectum. The frequency of soiling is often related to the degree and chronicity of constipation as well as the resultant physiological deconditioning of the colon and rectum. Fecal soiling for a child with constipation is thought to be an involuntary process in which softer stools "leak" around large, hard masses of stool in the rectum (Christophersen and Friman 2010). This "seepage" or soiling is the result of an involuntary reflex and is often not detected by the child. Thus, parental frustration related to the child not cleaning up following an accident can be tempered by providing education about the involuntary nature of soiling.

In children with encopresis without constipation and overflow incontinence or nonretentive fecal incontinence, stools are soft, easy to pass, and occur at a regular frequency. Soiling in this type of encopresis is intermittent and there are no signs of fecal retention such as retentive posturing or reported withholding (Hyams et al. 2016). In children without constipation, soiling is often less frequent and may be related to behavioral difficulties such as oppositional and/or defiant behavior (American Psychiatric Association 2013).

Prevalence and Etiology of Encopresis

Encopresis occurs in between 1 and 4% of 5-year-old children and between 1 and 2% of 11–12-year-old children (American Psychiatric Association 2013; Van der Wal et al. 2005). Males are more likely to have encopresis than females (van der Wal et al. 2005). Encopresis and enuresis are commonly co-occurring (Hansakunachai et al. 2005; Unal and Pehlivantürk 2003).

Most children with encopresis do not present with clinically significant emotional disturbance or psychiatric comorbidities (Friman et al. 1988; Cox et al. 2002); however, there are a small subset of children with encopresis who present with significant behavioral complexity and encopresis symptoms may be more treatment resistant in this group (Cox et al. 2002; Friman et al. 2006). Higher prevalence rates of encopresis are found in youth with anxiety/depression (Cox et al. 2002), attention deficit hyperactivity disorder (Mellon et al. 2013), developmental disabilities (von Wendt et al. 1990), obesity (Fishman et al. 2004), and children from lower socioeconomic backgrounds (van der Wal et al. 2005).

Better clinical outcomes of medical treatment of encopresis are found for older children (over age 5 years), females, those with nonretentive encopresis, and those with a collaborative child and family relationship (Mohammed and Mekael 2012).

Constipation

Constipation is defined as infrequent, hard, or difficult to pass stools. Prevalence of constipation in children varies widely based upon the study; however, a systematic review suggested an average prevalence rate of about approximately 14% (Mugie et al. 2011). Constipation may be accompanied by abdominal pain and/or distension, lethargy, vomiting, foul smelling flatulence, decreased appetite, and urinary incontinence. For most children, constipation is functional (Pashankar 2005). This means that there is no identifiable biological cause for constipation. Functional constipation is also known as chronic idiopathic constipation. The Rome Foundation publishes guidelines for the assessment and treatment of functional gastrointestinal disorder (FGIDs) including functional constipation in children (Hyams et al. 2016). Functional abdominal pain is fully discussed in Chap. 14 of this volume. Diagnosis is made through review of history and physical examination by a medical provider.

Functional constipation occurs in between 4 and 36% of children (Van der Wal et al. 2005; de Araújo Sant and Calçado 1999; Yong and Beattie

1998). Constipation in youth can be the result of a number of factors including slow motility, dietary inadequacies, stool retention, and medication side effects. Constipation can occur across the life span and commonly begins in childhood after a major life change such as toilet training, starting school, or painful bowel movements (Danda and Hyman 2014). Constipation is thought to persist into adulthood for up to 25% of children with functional constipation (Bongers et al. 2010). Evaluating stool withholding is important as this behavior can contribute to the onset and maintenance of constipation.

Functional constipation often first occurs around the time of toilet training (Culbert and Banez 2007; Danda and Hyman 2014) and there are no sex differences (van den Berg et al. 2006) in the prevalence of constipation. However, there are higher rates of fecal incontinence in boys when compared to girls. Functional constipation occurs in all age groups/social classes.

> Betsy is a 6-year-old girl who recently started soiling after a period of about 2 years of fecal continence. At the last visit, Betsy was having a bowel movement in the toilet every 3–4 days. Her mother stated that stools are large (about the diameter of a pop can), hard (cracked log shaped stools), and are difficult for Betsy to pass. Betsy sometimes has blood tinged stools. When she sits on the toilet, Betsy appears to be pushing, sometimes becoming red in the face from straining. A review of recent history suggests that Betsy's difficulties with soiling began about 1 month after she started kindergarten. Prior to starting school, Betsy was having bowel movements about every other day and they were soft formed and easy to pass.[1]

Assessment of Encopresis

Interdisciplinary Evaluation

Interdisciplinary evaluation includes simultaneous evaluation of a patient by two or more treating providers. This method of evaluation and treatment is less common, perhaps due to the more time consuming and resource heavy nature, but is well suited to addressing the biopsychosocial nature of encopresis. Simultaneous evaluation, as opposed to serial evaluation, is often preferred by families as it allows for coordination of medical and psychological care and prevents redundant history gathering. Although there is significant overlap in the interventions recommended by medical and psychological providers, each type of assessment will be addressed separately below.

Medical Assessment (Table 16.1)

Routine medical assessment of encopresis will involve collection of a full medical history, obtaining family medical history, and conducting a physical examination. If any warning signs, discussed below, are uncovered, further evaluation may be necessary. Providers will obtain a description of the onset, duration, and frequency of associated symptoms as well as the size, consistency, and frequency of bowel movements and soils in order to determine the most appropriate bowel management plan.

The Bristol Stool Scale (Lewis and Heaton 1997), a visual representation of stool firmness, is frequently utilized during an initial evaluation. Physical examination may include abdominal palpation, and looking for any warning signals of organic causes for constipation including abnormal anal appearance or location or the presence of a sacral dimple. The diagnostic consensus paper on the treatment of functional constipation in infants and children suggests that a full medical examination, blood work, and X-rays are not needed to evaluate uncomplicated constipation and encopresis in the absence of warning symp-

Table 16.1 Goals of medical evaluation

- Gather stooling history and determine whether warning signals are present
- Determine the current stool burden and assess for need of clean out
- Assess previous medical interventions for constipation and encopresis
- Determine which medical intervention is most appropriate for presentation and patient specifics
- Refer for further medical evaluation should warning signals be present

toms (Tabbers et al. 2014) such as delayed passage of meconium, failure to thrive, family history of Hirschprung's disease, anorectal malformation, or sacral dimple (Hyams et al. 2016). If warning signals are present, additional testing may be warranted to rule out biological causes for constipation (Tabbers et al. 2014).

Psychological/Behavioral Assessment

Psychological or behavioral evaluation of children presenting with encopresis begins in much the same fashion as it does for medical evaluation of this condition. The mental health professional will likely conduct a diagnostic interview with the child and parent. Information collected may include demographic information, medical history, family history, and emotional/behavioral information in order to obtain a better understanding of any contextual factors that contribute to encopresis. A full toilet training history will also be obtained. Valuable information will include toilet training history, past and present stooling patterns, developmental history, and an evaluation of toileting-related behaviors. Mental health providers will evaluate if any behavior excesses (e.g., disruptive behavior, aggression) or skills deficits (e.g., inability to recognize the signal to defecate) contribute to ongoing toileting difficulties.

Formal psychodiagnostic or neuropsychological evaluation procedures are not required for the treatment of encopresis. However, brief behavioral screening is often conducted at the outset and periodically throughout treatment to monitor behavioral comorbidities that can contribute to toileting problems. Screening measures may include broadband (e.g., Behavioral Assessment System for Children (BASC), Reynolds et al. 2015; Child Behavior Checklist (CBCL); Achenbach and Ruffle 2000) and narrowband (e.g., Parental Opinions of Pediatric Constipation Questionnaire (POOP-C), Silverman et al. 2015; Virginia Encopresis-Constipation Apperception Test, Cox et al. 2003) measures as clinically indicated. Further, evaluation of common comorbidities such as attention deficit hyperactivity disorder (ADHD) and enuresis by history will be conducted so as to inform comprehensive treatment planning and connection of the family with resources to address psychosocial con-

> **Box 16.1 Goals of Psychological Assessment**
> - Obtain toilet training and stooling history
> - Evaluate, by history, cognitive, behavioral, and contextual factors that may play a role in the development and maintenance of encopresis
> - Gain understanding of parent and child knowledge about constipation and encopresis
> - Assess current toileting-related skills
> - Screen for psychological or behavioral comorbidities that may impact treatment
> - Determine readiness for intervention

tributors. Behavioral reevaluation throughout the treatment, particularly during times of treatment plateau, is recommended (Christophersen and Friman 2010).

When considering contextual variables, it is important to evaluate family dynamics and parental responses to soiling as well as child self-esteem. Parent stress related to toileting difficulties has been documented (Macias et al. 2006) and should be considered when treatment planning. Similarly, encopresis, particularly chronic fecal soiling, is thought to negatively impact self-esteem (Landman et al. 1986) and quality of life (Bongers et al. 2010), which can then lead to low self-efficacy, or the belief that one can successfully create change. Tertiary evaluation of other contributing factors such as limited diet, restricted fluid intake, poor bodily awareness, difficulties with transitions, and behavioral rigidity may also be helpful.

Comorbidities As up to 25% of children with encopresis have clinically significant symptoms of ADHD, brief screening for ADHD symptoms may also be helpful in treatment planning and referrals (for evaluation and behavioral treatment) if symptoms interfere with the treatment of encopresis (Johnston and Wright 1993). The existing literature does not support that the presence of fecal soiling in isolation is an indicator of sexual abuse in children (Mellon et al. 2006).

Treatment of Encopresis Overview

Biopsychosocial treatment of encopresis is recognized clinically as the gold standard treatment for this condition. A combined medical and psychological/behavioral treatment plan is used to increase appropriate toileting behaviors (e.g., defecating in the toilet, cleaning up after soils) and decrease inappropriate toileting behaviors (e.g., hiding soiled undergarments or stool withholding). Combined treatment is especially relevant for children who have been treated via medical intervention only for a duration of time and have not progressed. Cognitive behavioral treatment of encopresis should be initiated simultaneous with or subsequent to medical management of constipation. The general treatment guidelines offered apply to both retentive and nonretentive encopresis; however, there is less research regarding the efficacy of treatment for the latter. Specific treatment examples for both retentive and nonretentive encopresis will be provided at the end of this chapter.

Broadly, treatment of encopresis involves provision of education to children and families about the condition and management of symptoms, medical management of constipation, and cognitive and behavioral strategies that can be used to increase appropriate toileting behavior and subsequently decrease incompatible behaviors. Treatment progresses in phases including the initial bowel clean out, medical and behavioral maintenance, and relapse prevention. Bowel output tracking is often conducted as a part of treatment in order to inform bowel management programs.

Medical Treatment

Box 16.2 Goals of Medical Treatment

- Evaluate for fecal impaction and recommend bowel clean out as necessary
- Create bowel management regimen designed to produce frequent, soft, and easy-to-pass stools
- Maintain soft stools for a prolonged period of time
- Taper medications
- Educate regarding how to respond to recurrence of constipation in the future

Bowel cleanout As the vast majority of children with encopresis present with constipation, addressing chronic constipation is the first step of treatment. Medical treatment often begins with bowel clean out for colonic disimpaction (Tabbers et al. 2014) or the removal of large or hard masses in the colon. This step is meant to "prepare" the colon for retraining, reduce overflow soiling, and encourage normal stooling patterns (e.g., frequent, soft, and easy-to-pass stools). Bowel clean outs can be achieved by using high doses of oral laxatives for short periods of time (usually 2–3 days) or rectal therapies (e.g., enemas or suppositories).

Maintenance medications Once fecal disimpaction is achieved, maintenance laxative medications are prescribed with the goal of promoting regularly occurring, soft, and easy-to-pass bowel movements. Additionally, medications are used to avoid future impaction that could hinder progress toward resolution of encopresis. For children with a fear of defecation, prolonged periods of soft and easy-to-pass stools are necessary to "decondition" the fear of stooling and resultant stool withholding.

Providers have a range of oral laxative medications to choose from including stimulant laxatives, stool softeners, or a combination of these.

The choice of medication used and how it should be administered will depend on a number of factors. Evaluation of barriers to medication adherence is vital to treatment success. Below please find an illustrative therapeutic dialogue addressing barriers to medication adherence.

> Provider: To help your child have soft bowel movements, I would like to recommend that Suzy take a medicine every day.
> Parent: I'm not sure she can.
> Provider: Tell me more about your concerns with medication.
> Parent: Well, she can't swallow pills and she often fights me when I try to give her liquid medications she doesn't like the taste of.
> Provider: Do you think she would drink 8 ounces of juice with a medication that can be dissolved in it?
> Parent: Yeah, I think she might take that if I call it her "sugar medicine."
> Provider: What might you do if she refuses to take it?
> Parent: I'm not sure how I could convince her.
> Provider: Perhaps you could consider offering her a small reward for finishing the beverage with medication in it. It will also be helpful to ignore any refusal behaviors such as pushing the drink away or saying, "I'm not going to drink this" in order to avoid accidentally reinforcing these behaviors.

Rectal therapies, such as suppositories or enemas, are sometimes used, although less frequently, in combination with oral laxatives for bowel management.

During the establishment of a bowel management program, a family may be asked to complete bowel output tracking logs for several days or weeks in order to learn more about when, where (e.g., soil vs. in the toilet) and how often a child stools as well as the firmness of stools. If the child is very young, the parents may complete this measure, but for older children and teens, the responsibility may be shared. The Bristol Stool Scale (Lewis and Heaton 1997) is often used to describe the consistency of stools in a more subjective manner. Review of bowel tracking data can be useful for adjusting medication doses and timing, planning scheduled toilet sits, identifying patterns related to toileting, and tracking progress over time (Fig. 16.1).

As mentioned previously, additional medical testing is often not required for the treatment of uncomplicated encopresis. However, for a small group of children who present with warning symptoms or whose constipation and soiling have not improved despite combined and ongoing treatment, referral to a specialist such as a gastroenterologist is recommended.

Adjunctive nutritional goals Standard nutritional recommendations to address constipation include increasing fluid consumption, limiting dairy consumption due to constipating effects, and increasing dietary fiber. It should be noted however that fluid and dietary recommendations are not currently recommended by the North American Society for Pediatric Gastroenterology, Hepatology, and Nutrition (NASPGHAN) Evaluation and Treatment Guidelines for constipation (2014) as there is insufficient evidence to suggest that these interventions are efficacious in the treatment of constipation. Due to the low risk and potential for even small positive effects, these interventions are commonly recommended clinically.

Psychological/Psychosocial Interventions

> **Box 16.3 Goals of Psychological/Psychosocial Interventions**
> - Provide education about condition and treatment
> - Address any parental punishment of soiling
> - Teach new/appropriate toileting skills and behaviors
> - Create an individualized treatment plan to address specific contributing and maintaining factors
> - Utilize operant conditioning procedures/behavior modification strategies to increase appropriate behaviors and decrease inappropriate toileting behaviors
> - Increase self-efficacy and motivation to change
> - Relapse prevention and more education

Education/Cognitive intervention Psychological treatment of encopresis

POOP CHART

Date	Time of Poop	Accident	Poop in Toilet	How Much Poop?	Poop Type (Bristol)	Go on my own	Notes
7/18/2018	7:00am		x	1/4 cup	5	No	During toilet sit
	7:15am	X		1 tbsp	6	No	Playing videogames
	6:00pm	X		smear	6	No	Outside playing
7/19/2018	8:00am		X	1 cup	5	Yes	
7/20/2018	8:30am		X	1 cup	6	No	Went during a sit
7/21/2018	8:00am	X		1 tsp	6	No	
	8:15am		x	1 cup	6	No	Finished during sit

Fig. 16.1 Sample bowel tracking log

begins and ends with education. Children and families are taught about the causes, characteristics, and effects of constipation and encopresis at the outset of treatment. This knowledge provides the family with the foundation needed to proceed with combined medical–behavioral treatment of encopresis and helps to reduce both parent and child distress related to this chronic and often distressing condition. This initial education process is often referred to as "demystification" of the soiling process.

Families are told about the biology of constipation, using diagrams and pictures as necessary. They are shown how chronic constipation impacts the functioning of the colon by stretching the rectum which leads to decreased sensation and functioning over time. They are also taught about the cycle of constipation and stool withholding whereby withheld stool dries out, hardens, and becomes compacted, therefore potentiating constipation. Education regarding the involuntary nature of fecal soiling and overflow incontinence is described as a physiologically mediated process that is outside of the child's control and often awareness. Use of developmentally appropriate language and visuals to explain these concepts to youth is recommended. The importance of ongoing medical management of constipation, the primary cause of encopresis, is stressed in order to prevent early termination of treatment and eventual relapse. Families are informed of the commitment required of them over the next months or even years in order to overcome this condition. They are reassured that encopresis is common, despite the fact it is not talked about, and is very treatable.

Providers must take care to address parental and child concerns that encopresis is indicative of serious psychosocial problems or that the condition is lifelong. Providing education is a critical component of treatment as it is helpful for reducing parental frustration related to encopresis, and thereby helps to decrease negative interactions between parents and the child. Further, youth shame and embarrassment related to soiling are often abated when they receive additional information about encopresis.

Then, the process of stool withholding is explained to children and families. This process is described as a reasonable or rational response to past painful defecation. Children who have had painful stooling experiences due to large caliber or hard stools, attempt to avoid subsequent painful experiences by withholding stool instead of passing it into the toilet or a pull up. Eventually, the body does its job and passes the stool; however, because it was withheld, it is even firmer and possibly larger than it was before. The cycle of stool withholding and treatment is described. Treatment for this fear of defecation and stool withholding is explained including the need for these children to have a great number of soft and easy-to-pass bowel movements that are not accompanied by pain, conflict, or punishment in order to decondition their fear of stooling. Parents are encouraged to be patient and consistent throughout the treatment process.

Finally, but perhaps most importantly, providers must stress the importance of avoidance of punishment, in all forms, for soiling. Families are informed that while frustration regarding soiling is absolutely normal, punishment, shaming, or blaming the child may actually make the problem worse. Many parents express remorse for previously punishing their child for soiling and children may become angry with their parents for punishing them for behaviors they now learn were likely out of their control. Psychologists take great care to normalize parent and child concerns and validate their feelings regarding this often stressful condition.

Behavioral intervention When constipation is adequately managed, behavioral intervention can proceed. Behavior modification for the treatment of encopresis has long been studied and has been proven to have efficacy (Freeman et al. 2014). The specific causal factors or treatment components associated with behavior change related to soiling are less clear however. Limited research is available to suggest which components of behavioral treatments are needed to produce positive outcomes.

Behavioral modification, or behavioral intervention, has several goals: Increase appropriate toileting behaviors, decrease inappropriate toileting behaviors, and increase skills needed to stool effectively. Providers assess these areas at the outset of treatment and create an individualized treatment plan, paying particular attention to address barriers to treatment progress such as interfering behaviors, limited motivation, or family conflict (Table 16.2).

It is also important to consider the child's developmental level and current skills when creating a toileting plan. It may be that they do not know how to evacuate stool effectively because they have been withholding for so long that they do not engage their pelvic floor muscles correctly. As a result, they need to be "taught" to push effectively and respond right away when they notice a change in their body that indicates they need to stool.

Operant conditioning procedures are often utilized to achieve behavioral toileting goals. At the core of these procedures is the notion that a behavior can be strengthened by reinforcement and weakened by a punishment. In behavioral toilet training, reinforcement in the form of token economies, sticker charts, or other reward systems is often utilized to incentivize appropriate

Table 16.2 Behavioral targets

Behaviors to increase	Behaviors to decrease
Sitting on the toilet when asked	Refusing to sit on the toilet
Sitting on the toilet for a duration of time	Getting up quickly
Increasing awareness of and response to the urge to stool	Delayed defecation
Effective "pushing" when sitting on the toilet	Stool withholding or paradoxical contraction
Recognizing a soil and getting cleaned up	Continuing to play and refusing clean up
Taking medications	Refusing medications

toileting behaviors, taking into consideration the child's likes and dislikes. Rewards are provided contingently. This means that they are given when a child demonstrates a behavior you want to see but not otherwise. Toileting skills are broken down into component skills (e.g., pulling down one's pants or sitting on the toilet) and taught in a sequential fashion, starting with the most basic and progressing to more advanced skills. Reinforcement is given along the way. Parents are encouraged to use reinforcement as the primary intervention for toilet training and punishment is often discouraged or limited. Mild consequences such as being asked to clean up after a soil are permissible but should not be paired with lecturing, nagging, or shaming. Punitive consequences are actively discouraged as they are ineffective or counterproductive (Christophersen and Friman 2010). A strong foundation in behavioral theory is often required for the treatment of more challenging toileting cases.

Behavioral plans are tailored to the youth and families' needs and powerful rewards are selected based on the child's interests. The first target of a reward system will depend on the barriers to toileting uncovered during the initial assessment. For example, a treatment target for a child who is compliant with sits but is having difficulty eliminating successfully might be to practice appropriate defecation dynamics in order to eliminate. A child who is noncompliant with sitting on the toilet might initially work on following directions and receiving rewards for compliance. Creation of short- and long-term goals is recommended. Creating behavioral momentum is often vital to the success of a reward plan as a child who feels unable to reach goals is unlikely to persevere in completing difficult tasks. In this vain, it is important to consider offering rewards or incentives for compliance with bowel management plans rather than just successful elimination, at least initially, in order to encourage child "buy in" to the toileting program. Many parents will report having tried and failed toilet training using reward systems. Table 16.3 lists the top reasons for the failure of reward systems. Nonjudgmental inquiry about the specifics of unsuccessful behav-

Table 16.3 Top reasons for the failure of reward systems

Reasons for failure	Example	Solution
Goals were unachievable or too difficult	Child has never been bowel trained and does not sit on the toilet. Rewards offered only for stooling in the toilet	Offer a reward for sitting on the toilet
Prerequisite skills absent	Reward offered for independent toileting but the child cannot get on and off the toilet by themselves	Teach child to get on and off of the toilet using a step stool first
Rewards were not desired by the child	Sticker chart used as a reward for a 12-year-old boy	Consider offering access to electronics for short intervals when goals are met
Rewards were not offered consistently	Rewards for elimination in the toilet offered when parent remembers	Put the rewards in the bathroom in a jar so that they are given immediately following elimination
Rewards are not "powerful" enough	Plan includes electronics time as a reward for doing toilet sits but child has unlimited access to tablet on weekends	All tablet time must be earned for toileting behaviors (e.g., sits, clean up, elimination) and offered contingently
Delayed rewards	Child selects a special toy as their breakthrough reward for eliminating in the toilet for the first time but the parents have not purchased it yet	Purchase breakthrough reward and place in a location that the child can see but does not have access to
Rewards accompanied by punitive consequences	Child earns a small prize for stooling in toilet but it is then taken away because they soil the next day	Offer rewards contingently and do not punish for accidents. Talk about the next opportunity to earn a prize

ior plans can help the practitioner to identify areas for improvement.

Behavioral treatment for encopresis typically progresses in the following fashion.

Treatment begins by encouraging frequent but short-duration toilet sits three or more times per day. Toilet sits are often encouraged 0–30 min following a meal to take advantage of the gastrocolic reflex or the body's natural increase in gut functioning following a meal. Families are encouraged to have their child elevate their feet on a step stool or other device when sitting on the toilet in order to aid in effective elimination, mimicking a squatting position (Sakakibara et al. 2010; Sikirov 2003). While there is not conclusive evidence to suggest that this intervention is helpful for all individuals with constipation, the intervention is relatively inexpensive, poses low risk to patients, and is acceptable to most families, making it an appropriate adjunctive component to treatment.

For reluctant or nervous children, the treating provider may request that children be allowed to complete pleasurable activities such as looking at their favorite book, playing with a toy, or blowing bubbles when sitting on the toilet. This serves to decrease anxiousness about sitting or elimination and may increase compliance with a direction for a previously non-preferred task such as sitting on the toilet. Further, allowing the child to relax on the toilet will help to reduce any additional tension, which could make stooling more difficult. Similarly, although there is not any empirical support to suggest that having boys sit to urinate can be effective in treating elimination disorders, the authors have anecdotally observed that children are more likely to "hit the mark" (e.g., eliminate in the toilet) if they spend greater time in contact with it.

Behavioral treatment of elimination disorders will include the use of operant conditioning procedures to shape behavior as well as behavioral parent training. Reinforcement of desired behaviors will be strongly encouraged and appropriate reward systems created during clinic visits. Revision of behavioral toileting goals will occur as the child meets treatment goals, increasing the difficulty of toileting tasks incrementally and

> **Box 16.4 Behavioral Treatment Steps**
> - Step 1: Teach toilet sitting behavior
> - Step 2: Establish a reward system for appropriate toileting behaviors
> - Step 3: Teach children and families how to respond to soils
> - Step 4: Encourage effective pushing
> - Step 5: Maintain toileting supports for at least several months after soiling has discontinued

building upon newly established foundational skills. Further, parents should be provided with training in behavioral management of interfering behaviors such as noncompliance, disruptive behaviors, or aggression as these factors often warrant intervention prior to the implementation of toileting recommendations. Education on the power of attending to behaviors, especially those that are incompatible with appropriate toileting, will need to be discussed. Parents are coached on the delivery of directions related to toileting in order to diffuse power struggles between child and parent. Further, negative interaction styles that may have developed as a result of prolonged stress and conflict related to toileting difficulties, may need to be addressed before progressing with toileting treatment. The logic follows that if interactions with the child's parents are not reinforcing for the child, they will not be motivated to increase appropriate toileting behaviors. Parents are also encouraged to manage their own stress related to their child's toileting difficulties and get support from friends and family members as needed.

Targeted toilet sit routines can be created based on review of bowel tracking data, optimizing the likelihood for the child to defecate in the toilet if established bowel habits have been identified. Finally, as medical treatment of constipation is integral to treatment success, behavioral strategies may need to be employed to maintain medication adherence.

Another important aspect of treatment of encopresis is how to respond to soils. Both children and their parents have established behavioral routines regarding soiling, whether they know it or not. Children may hide their underwear or clothing, deny soiling, refuse to clean up, or "lie" about soiling-related difficulties. Parents may use an accusatory tone when talking about soils, ask questions when they already know the answer (e.g., "did you have an accident?"), and provide back-handed compliments. Bringing these response styles out into the open allows for all relevant parties to engage in cognitive reframing of the problem as well as engage in behavior change. Rewards can be implemented for remaining soil free for a period of time or being honest about and responding to a soil, using a pants check procedure. During this procedure, a parent can ask a child if they have soiled and reward and praise honesty once they verified the child's response. Other children are rewarded for telling an adult when they have soiled so that they can get cleaned up more quickly, thereby promoting healthy hygiene habits, and avoid hiding soiled clothing.

The key to setting realistic and achievable goals is to create treatment goals that are just beyond the child's current capabilities. When they achieve these goals, they feel a sense of self-efficacy, or the ability to succeed in a given task, which fosters internal motivation to tackle more difficult toileting tasks. Behavioral interventions are often based on trial and error and will require an ongoing feedback loop to determine how to adjust plans to meet the child and family's needs. Providing guidance about potential times for greater difficulties, will normalize this experience and often goes a long way to promote perseverance in treatment.

As children begin to develop prerequisite toileting behaviors such as sitting on the toilet after meals and stopping a preferred task to go to the bathroom, they can progress to learning how to recognize and respond appropriately to the urge to stool. Many children with encopresis have engaged in stool withholding for extended periods of time, which has made them less aware of the signals sent to their brain telling them that they need to defecate. Teaching them to respond to signals immediately, rather than waiting, will help to establish habits consistent with fecal continence.

If a child presents with fear of toileting or toilet refusal, strategies such as graduated exposure, use of adaptive coping skills, and reinforced practice can be taught to help children learn to conquer these fears and move toward more appropriate toileting behaviors. It should be noted however, that cognitive behavioral strategies are most appropriate for youth who do not have significant language or intellectual impairment as they require higher order thinking skills and the ability to think about one's own thinking.

Anecdotally, it is known that children with encopresis struggle with self-esteem, particularly older children and those in which soiling has persisted for longer periods of time. The literature on self-esteem in children with encopresis is mixed however, with some studies finding reduced levels of self-esteem in children who soil compared to children who are soil free (Landman et al. 1986; Owens-Stively 1987); and others finding no differences in self-esteem for children with and without soiling (Cox et al. 2002; Joinson et al. 2006). Differences in samples, and perhaps duration of disorder, may partially explain mixed findings. Many individuals report hiding soils to avoid getting in trouble, to limit the social impact of soiling, and to reduce being teased by peers. Long-term exposure to these stressors can lead to low self-esteem and/or mood symptoms. It is then not uncommon to see children and adolescents with this condition demonstrate avoidance of toileting, denial of soiling or problems related to soiling, and learned helplessness as clinically observed outcomes of prolonged soiling. Assessing for bullying and other social impacts of soiling that can also negatively impact self-esteem is recommended.

A critical component of any behavioral intervention is preemptive assessment of barriers to treatment or adherence to treatment plan. Conducting this type of evaluation at the outset of treatment may improve provider ability to give anticipatory guidance, increase the likelihood of adherence with treatment plans, and decrease dropout rate. Barriers may be educational (e.g., soiling is involuntary), medication related (e.g., inadequate treatment of constipation), behavioral (e.g., noncompliance with toilet sit requests), skills deficits (e.g., ineffective pushing while trying to pass a bowel movement), structural (e.g., limited access to running water or adequate toilet facilities), or motivational (e.g., child does not appear to care if they are soiled).

Review of the Treatment Literature for Encopresis

The treatment literature supporting the efficacy of various treatments for pediatric encopresis has had a slow progression over the past 30–40 years, necessitating discussion of both relatively distant and more recent studies. In looking at the literature, relatively few studies have included adequate control groups or randomization, making generalization of results challenging. Further, differential definitions of treatment success, failure to separate retentive and nonretentive subtypes, and vague packages of behavioral interventions make identification of the critical elements of treatment difficult. To our knowledge, only three systematic reviews (McGrath et al. 2000; Brooks et al. 2000; Shepard et al. 2017) and two meta-analyses (Brazzelli et al. 2011; Freeman et al. 2014) on the efficacy of encopresis interventions exist.

McGrath et al. (2000) suggested that medical intervention plus positive reinforcement with increased dietary fiber, medical intervention plus positive reinforcement, but without increased dietary fiber recommendations, medical intervention with biofeedback for paradoxical contraction, and an intervention that included a package of medical, behavioral strategies, and biofeedback were probably efficacious. Brooks and colleagues (2000) reported that combined medical and behavioral treatment as well as behavioral treatment in isolation to be equally effective in the treatment of pediatric encopresis. They concluded that there was no evidence to suggest benefit related to adding biofeedback to medical-behavioral treatment. More recently, Brazzelli et al. (2011) completed a Cochran Review of treatments for encopresis and concluded that behavioral intervention paired with laxative therapy may improve bowel continence in children with functional fecal incontinence with constipation. They concluded that biofeedback training was not efficacious in treating encopresis.

Freeman et al. (2014) completed a systematic review and meta-analysis examining behavioral interventions for fecal incontinence and constipation. They concluded that behavioral intervention was more effective at reducing soiling than treatment as usual or medication only treatments. Finally, and most recently, a review of the evidence base for the treatment of encopresis was conducted using the Task Force on the Promotion and Dissemination of Psychological Procedures guidelines. Authors of this review identified only seven encopresis intervention studies occurring in the past 15 years (Shepard et al. 2017). There were no treatments that were identified as well-established treatments and only two probably efficacious interventions-biofeedback training and enhanced toilet training.

It should be noted that the literature on efficacious treatments of encopresis is variable, limited, and sometimes conflicting. Further randomized controlled trials, with clearly defined and outlined treatment protocols, and separation of encopresis subtypes (retentive vs. nonretentive) are needed.

Enhanced Toilet Training

Enhanced Toilet Training (ETT; Cox et al. 1996) was first established in 1996 as a bundled behavioral intervention which included standard elements of care including education, behavioral modification strategies, and skills practice, training in, and of modeling of appropriate defecation dynamics. This intervention is deemed as probably efficacious as research supporting its efficacy has only been completed by one research group and replication is needed.

ETT is unique in that it is the only intervention that clearly delineates the process of teaching the mechanics of defecation. Children who have encopresis often demonstrate what is called "paradoxical contraction" whereby they constrict the external anal sphincter (EAS) instead of relaxing it while sitting on the toilet. This contraction makes stooling more difficult and can account for the parent observation that their child appears to be pushing when sitting on the toilet (e.g., face turning red and straining) but they are not able to pass stool into the toilet.

Enhanced toilet training, created by Cox et al. (1996), teaches children about paradoxical constriction of the (EAS) and provides therapist lead training and modeling of appropriate defecation dynamics (e.g., relaxing one's legs and bottom, sitting up straight, and pushing down with one's lower abdomen while exhaling). These skills are practiced multiple times daily during toilet sits to help children develop better stooling habits. ETT has been studied in various forms, since its inception, with good support for each iteration of this intervention. In the initial study, researchers compared laxative therapy only, laxative therapy plus ETT, and laxative therapy plus ETT and anal sphincter biofeedback. ETT and biofeedback were superior to laxative therapy in reducing the frequency of soiling.

In a subsequent study conducted in 2002, ETT was compared to intensive medical therapy (IMT) only, IMT plus and ETT, and IMT plus ETT plus external anal sphincter electromyographic biofeedback (BF) in a randomized control trial. ETT was found to be somewhat more effective in the treatment of pediatric encopresis than intensive medical therapy or biofeedback therapy alone (Borowitz et al. 2002). Children in the ETT group required less laxative medication and fewer treatment visits when compared to children in the medication treatment only group. Additionally, ETT resulted in "statistically significant decreases in the daily frequency of soiling for the greatest number of children" when comparing treatment groups. In a subsequent randomized controlled trial, researchers found decreased soiling postintervention and at 1-year follow-up for children who received online delivery of ETT compared to treatment as usual controls (Ritterband et al. 2013).

Maintenance of Treatment Gains

A critical component of the treatment of encopresis is relapse prevention. Constipation is often cyclical, making it important to educate parents about the importance of monitoring for and aggressively treating recurrence of constipation. Signs of increasing constipation may include less frequent or reduced stool output, harder stools, difficulty "emptying" when stooling, the reemergence of soiling, or urinary incontinence. Managing constipation quickly has the potential to prevent the reoccurrence of soiling. Further, families should be educated about how to address the reemergence of soiling, which often involves returning to bowel management basics including laxative medication use, frequent toilet sits, and cleanout as necessary. Although there is no evidence to suggest this, anecdotally we know that children are more likely to experience a reoccurrence of constipation and/or soiling following a transition or major life stressor, during or after illness, and during or after travel. Parents and children are encouraged to proactively manage any relapses in order to reduce the amount of time it takes to return to toileting baseline.

Interdisciplinary Treatment of Encopresis with Constipation and Overflow Incontinence/ Retentive Encopresis

As mentioned previously, co-management of encopresis is recommended for the treatment of refractory or long-standing presentations. The success of this treatment hinges upon integrated treatment targets across all providers, with medical providers offering medical and pharmaceutical expertise and the behavioral health provider offering their expertise in behavior and learning. The child and their family are also integral team members as they provide expertise regarding the patient, routines, and contextual variables that must be considered when creating an achievable treatment plan. Care coordination between team members and the primary care provider is also recommended.

Table 16.4 Psychobiological considerations

Domain	Contributors	Treatment goal	Interventions
Biological	• Constipation • Result of taking Iron?	• Create soft stools	• Rule out other medical comorbidities that could explain symptoms • Bowel clean out • Maintenance laxative therapies • Increase fluid intake • Increase dietary fiber
Psychological/behavioral	• Noncompliance with toileting behaviors (e.g., sitting on the toilet)	• Follow parent directions related to toileting	• Develop a toileting routine to build compliance • Reinforce compliance • Respond appropriately to refusal • Implement reward system that is motivating for the child • Adjust goals as child achieves success
Psychological/behavioral	• Stool withholding	• Respond appropriately to urge to defecate	• Keep stools consistently soft for at least several months • Establish sitting program • Reward stool evacuation
Psychological/behavioral	• Medication nonadherence	• Get child to take oral laxatives	• Determine why child won't take medication • Offer alternative formats of medication • Reward compliance with taking medications • Create a routine for medication taking • Encourage parent supervision during medication administration
Social	• Parent and child frustration	• Decrease conflict around soiling	• Provide education about encopresis and treatment • Do away with punishment for soiling • Increase positive parent-child interactions • Encourage use of reinforcement strategies
Social	• Bullying → learned helplessness	• Increase self-efficacy	• Explain that soiling is not the child's fault and is involuntary • Help Bobby achieve small successes to build motivation • Help parents to advocate for their child regarding bullying • Reward all child attempts to manage encopresis

The case below illustrates the interplay between medical and behavioral factors in pediatric encopresis (Table 16.4).

Bobby is an 8-year-old boy with attention deficit hyperactivity disorder who began to soil 3 months ago. He was previously fully toilet trained and has never had problems with soiling in the past. Bobby was prescribed iron supplements by his pediatrician approximately 4 months ago due to low ferritin levels and began to experience constipation as a result. Review of history suggested that he stools about once per week in the toilet and stools are large caliber, hard, and painful to pass. Bobby admitted that he doesn't like to defecate and often tries to "hold poop in" when he feels the urge to go. Soils are liquid to pasty and occur in his underwear. A physician examining Bobby noted that he likely had fecal impaction after reviewing symptoms and palpating his abdomen.

Bobby's parents were very frustrated that Bobby soils as he "should know better at his age." Bobby reportedly hid his soiled underwear in his room to avoid consequences, resulting in smelly discoveries by his parents, who responded by taking away Bobby's electronics privileges. Bobby became increasingly defiant over the last several months, refusing to sit on the toilet, denying the occurrence of soils, and not getting cleaned up when he has an accident. Bobby reported being bullied by other children about soiling and stated "this will never get better."

Bobby's pediatrician prescribed fiber gummies and 1 cap of MiraLAX® every day for maintenance. Bobby's parents stated that Bobby takes fiber gummies regularly but only takes MiraLAX® 1–2 times a week because he often refuses to drink beverages with MiraLAX® dissolved into it.[1]

Bobby's pediatrician referred him to the Gastroenterology division of a local children's hospital, where he was seen in an interdisciplinary toileting clinic staffed by a gastroenterologist and psychologist. They conducted the initial evaluation and treatment proceeded as follows.

Given symptoms and physical exam findings, the gastroenterologist recommended an initial bowel clean out for Bobby. He was instructed to take 6–8 doses of MiraLAX® per day (one cap every 2 h or so) over a period of 2–3 days with the goal of producing many liquid stools. Bobby was then prescribed maintenance laxative medications to take daily. Medications were adjusted until Bobby was stooling regularly (perhaps daily or every other day) and stools were soft formed and easy to pass. Bobby was reluctant to take MiraLAX®, so his family and the provider discussed how to best increase medication adherence. Bobby stated that he does not like the taste or texture of MiraLAX®. The gastroenterologist suggested that the medication be mixed into another clear liquid that Bobby prefers (e.g., a sports' drink) and that the medication is stirred for at least 2 min in order to dissolve all granules. With these interventions, Bobby no longer refuses maintenance medications and takes them at least 6/7 days per week. Increasing dietary fiber and fluid intake was recommended. Limiting, but not eliminating, dairy was recommended.

Bobby and his family were asked to complete a bowel tracking log for 1–2 weeks following bowel cleanout to help titrate medications appropriately. Bobby and his family were provided with education about encopresis and its treatment. This education included mention of the brain-gut connection, the cycle of constipation and stool withholding, and the involuntary nature of soiling. The psychologist recommended that any punishment for soiling be discontinued immediately and instilled hope that this problem will get better with treatment. The importance of consistent bowel management for several months or even a year was discussed to prevent early termination of the bowel management plan.

> **Box 16.5 Treatment Plan for Bobby**
> - Bowel clean out using oral laxatives
> - Addition of daily maintenance medications
> - Psychoeduction about encopresis
> - Addition of scheduled toilet sits daily
> - Creation of a reward system
> - Assessment of barriers and collaborative problem solving
> - Relapse prevention

Review of the bowel tracking log suggested that Bobby soils most often when at school and typically had a bowel movement in the toilet as soon as he got home from school each day. Based on this information, it was theorized that Bobby likely had the urge to stool at school each day and he did not want to or delayed stooling, resulting in a soil. He stooled in the toilet once he got home because he was more comfortable in this setting. The providers recommended that Bobby complete a 5-min toilet sit 20–30 min after each meal, including one after breakfast but before going to school. Additionally, a letter was written to Bobby's school to request that he complete one toilet sit at school after lunch and be allowed an "anytime bathroom pass" due to unpredictable bowel activity. This letter was provided to the family so that they could give it to Bobby's educational team. As Bobby was somewhat resistant to sitting on the toilet when prompted by his parents, he was initially offered rewards (e.g., 5 min of electronics time after each sit) for following the direction to sit on the toilet and not evacuation. As he became more compliant with sitting, he was offered a reward for sitting on and stooling in the toilet. After he reached that goal, he was offered a reward for remaining soil free for a period of time. Prior to creation of the reward system, the psychologist asked Bobby about what items or activities were most motivating to him and worked with his family to identify rewards for meeting toileting goals.

After several weeks of stooling regularly in the toilet, Bobby reported increased awareness of the urge to defecate and began to go to the restroom on his own. Soiling gradually decreased in frequency over the next several weeks. When soiling occurred, his parents used a nonjudgmental tone to tell him to get cleaned up and no punishment was given out for soiling. Bobby was less resistant to clean up once he knew that he was not going to get into trouble. Bobby's family followed up with the providers 2 months after their initial visit, at which time he was having daily soft stools and was no longer soiling. His family asked about discontinuing laxative medications at 2-month follow-up. They were encouraged to begin to taper medications slowly after another several soil-free months in order to allow Bobby's colon to continue to return to normal structure and function. Warning signs of increasing constipation were discussed and the family was encouraged to proactively treat constipation should it occur.[1]

Treatment of Encopresis Without Constipation and Overflow Incontinence or Nonretentive Encopresis

As mentioned previously, nonretentive encopresis or encopresis without constipation, is uncommon, occurring in between 5 and 15% of cases (Levine 1975; Molnar et al. 1983; Loening-Baucke 2007). Less is known about the treatment of this relatively rare condition as limited research has been conducted in this area. To the author's knowledge, there is only one set of treatment guidelines for the treatment of nonretentive encopresis. The American Family Physician Treatment Guidelines for Primary Nonretentive Encopresis and Stool Toileting Refusal are very similar to those used to manage retentive encopresis. Similar behavioral interventions to encourage appropriate defecation are recommended but ongoing medical intervention (e.g., laxatives) is not recommended unless otherwise indicated. The authors of these guidelines suggest medical assessment of these children is grossly normal and does not reveal active or past constipation (Kuhn et al. 1999). They also describe subgroups of children who present with fecal soiling, which include those who were not toilet trained by a developmentally appropriate age, those who had toileting-related fears, those with a stronger behavioral component to toileting difficulties (e.g., refusal to complete activities related to toileting), and those with medical causes of stooling difficulties (Kuhn et al. 1999). The authors of a 2007 review article suggested that approximately 30–40% of children with nonretentive functional encopresis have never been toilet trained (Bongers et al. 2007).

Medical Assessment

Medical evaluation of a child with nonretentive encopresis begins with the medical provider collecting a comprehensive toileting history including information about toilet training and past and current stooling habits. A physical examination can also be conducted to rule out potential biological causes for soiling and evaluate for warning symptoms mentioned previously. Children with nonretentive encopresis will present with normal stooling patterns, historically soft stools, and infrequent soiling (when compared to children with retentive encopresis). Children with nonretentive encopresis are often referred to mental and behavioral health providers for assistance with behavior management and skills development.

Box 16.6 Treatment Goals for Nonretentive Encopresis

- Decrease toileting refusal and increase compliance with toileting directives
- Teach and practice appropriate defecation dynamics
- Decrease disruptive and/or interfering behaviors
- Decrease any fears of the toilet or stooling
- Increase stooling in the toilet

Psychological Assessment

In addition to comprehensive history taking, mental health providers will want to identify behavioral or contextual factors that contributed to the genesis or maintenance of encopresis. Assessment of toileting skills as well as interfering behaviors will be important when treatment planning for children with nonretentive encopresis. Factors such as significant aggression, noncompliance, disruptive behavior, or lack of parental understanding of behavioral modification will need to be addressed as a part of treatment. The prevalence of such behavioral difficulties in children with nonretentive encopresis is unknown and findings vary by study, suggesting that this group of children is heterogeneous in its behavioral presentation.

Box 16.7 Treatment Plan for Nonretentive Encopresis

- Provide education about encopresis and treatment
- Teach prerequisite toileting skills
- Work on overall compliance with parental instructions, thereby decreasing disruptive behaviors
- Implement scheduled toilet sits without pressure to defecate
- Help the child to form positive associations with sitting on the toilet or stooling
- Encourage parent use of behavioral modification strategies
- Use gradual exposure or shaping procedures to address any toileting fears or phobias

Psychological/Behavioral Treatment

Treatment of nonretentive encopresis mirrors the treatment of retentive encopresis; however, with a greater focus on behavioral challenges that prevented toilet training may be required. Bongers et al. (2007), suggested treatment components including education, toilet training, bowel tracking, and use of reward systems based on their clinical experiences and limited data available.

Case Example

Gwen is a 6-year-old girl who had never been bowel trained. She was fully urine trained by 3 years of age. Review of history suggested that Gwen stooled daily or every other day and stools were soft formed. During physical examination, she did not have hard palpable stool or fecal impaction. Although she wore underwear during the day, she requested pull ups to stool in each evening. When she put the pull ups on, she stooled in them while hiding in a closet in her room. When she had finished, she went to the bathroom to get cleaned up and requested parent help as needed. Gwen's parents had tried withholding pull ups from Gwen in the past, but she would not stool without them, going several days without defecating. As a result, her parents continued to offer pull ups to her. When she presented for treatment, her parents stated that they were unable to get her to sit on the toilet in the evenings when they knew she had to stool. If they asked her to sit on the toilet to defecate, she said, "no" and began to cry. Gwen sat on the toilet for 10–15 s to urinate without distress. Gwen's parents reported a history of "forcing her" to sit on the toilet during toilet training, which resulted in lots of tears and no defecation. Gwen was referred by her primary care provider to a psychologist for behavioral toilet training.

The psychologist began treatment by conducting an evaluation of previous experiences related to toileting. They provided Gwen and her family with education about encopresis and outlined treatment components. Gwen's parents were encouraged to monitor for constipation in the future. The psychologist identified the things that Gwen was most interested in and was motivated to earn. The psychologist used this information to create a reward system to incentivize sitting on the toilet. Gwen's parents were encouraged to ask Gwen to sit on the toilet two times each evening as this is when she was most likely to stool. Gwen earned a sticker each time she sat on the toilet for 30 s. A timer was used to show Gwen when her time had elapsed. Gwen's parents were instructed not to talk about stooling in the toilet when Gwen does her sits, instead simply asking her to sit on the toilet to earn her sticker. When Gwen earned six stickers, she picked a small grab bag prize from a bag. Gwen was made aware of the fact that she could earn three bonus stickers if she passed any stool into the toilet. Gwen was encouraged to take toys or books with her to the bathroom to keep toilet sits positive and decrease any anxiety she had about sitting on the toilet.

Gwen's parents were given information about how to avoid power struggles if Gwen refused toileting directives. After explaining the reward system to Gwen, she was asked if she would like to earn her first sticker by doing a toilet sit in the office restroom. She replied, "yes" and her parents walk her to the bathroom. She completed the sit and was excited to return to the psychologist's office to tell them of her success and earn her first sticker. Gwen's parents were asked to repeat this procedure for the next week and return to clinic the following week. When rewarded toilet sits were instituted at home, her parents were told to allow Gwen to continue to have access to pull ups to stool in. They were kept in the bathroom so that she had to enter the bathroom when she needed to defecate.

Gwen's parents provided an update to the psychologist after 5 days, stating that Gwen was sitting on the toilet without protest and was excited to earn her rewards. She stooled in the toilet on the fifth day because she really wanted to earn a small toy from her prize bag. Her parents provided her with lots of praise and even called Gwen's grandparents to share her success. Over the next few days, Gwen stooled in the toilet during scheduled sits and continued to earn rewards. Gwen continued to stool in the toilet for the next week; however, on treatment day 13, she repeatedly asked for a pull up to stool in and did not stool for the next 2 days. Her parents were encouraged to ignore this behavior, continue with scheduled toilet sits, and add in a laxative, as guided by their pediatrician. Additionally, they were asked to add new and novel prizes to her prize bag to increase Gwen's motivation to continue. Parents were cautioned not to return to allowing Gwen to stool in pull ups or provide negative feedback about Gwen's refusal to toilet as this could cause a setback. Gwen eventually returned to stooling in the toilet and did not ask for pull ups again. Prizes for stooling were faded overtime as Gwen became fully continent of stool.[1]

Treatment Complicating Factors

Should symptoms of encopresis persist despite medical and behavioral intervention, reevaluation may be necessary. Several factors can complicate the treatment and warrant intervention. Medical reevaluation may be needed for refractory constipation, paying attention to any warning signals present, or the need for additional or alternative medications. Prior to making medication changes, it is important to assess medication adherence, aiming for a goal of at least 80% of all medications taken regularly. If adherence is poor, determining the cause for this will be important for treatment planning. For example, if children do not take their medications consistently because they cannot swallow pills, they can be referred to a psychologist for pill swallowing training or switched to a different formulation. For children whose progress has stalled despite well-managed constipation and no evidence of stool withholding, reevaluation of psychological comorbidities is necessary. Comorbidities such as ADHD and anxiety are particularly common in children with encopresis and can hinder toileting progress for a subgroup of children. Referral for individual therapy to address these comorbidities is recommended in these cases.

Training and Supervision for the Evaluation and Treatment of Encopresis

Specialized training and supervised experience in the treatment of elimination disorders is highly recommended for the provider unfamiliar with assessment and treatment of this condition.

Conclusion

Elimination disorders are considered biobehavioral conditions, best managed with combined medical and behavioral treatment. The most common cause of fecal soiling is constipation, which is observed in the vast majority of children with encopresis. Initial medical evaluation may suggest that bowel clean out is necessary prior to the use of oral laxatives to keep stools soft and easy to pass. Once constipation is well managed, behavioral interventions aimed at increasing adaptive toileting skills and decreasing interfering behaviors can commence. Operant conditioning principles are used to incentivize, and therefore increase the likelihood of helpful toileting behaviors such as sitting on the toilet and cleaning up after a soil. Relapse prevention strategies are key to the continued success of children with encopresis. Future research is needed to determine the causal mechanisms of improvement of symptoms of encopresis and critical components of treatment. Finally, behavioral categorization of the different presentations of encopresis (e.g., stooling withholding, behavioral toilet refuser, child who soils due to delayed stooling) may be helpful for informing treatment recommendations.

References

Achenbach, T. M., & Ruffle, T. M. (2000). The Child Behavior Checklist and related forms for assessing behavioral/emotional problems and competencies. *Pediatrics in Review, 21*(8), 265–271.

American Psychiatric Association. (2013). *Diagnostic and statistical manual of mental disorders* (5th ed.). Arlington: American Psychiatric Publishing.

Bongers, M. E., Tabbers, M. M., & Benninga, M. A. (2007). Functional nonretentive fecal incontinence in children. *Journal of Pediatric Gastroenterology and Nutrition, 44*(1), 5–13.

Bongers, M. E., van Wijk, M. P., Reitsma, J. B., & Benninga, M. A. (2010). Long-term prognosis for childhood constipation: Clinical outcomes in adulthood. *Pediatrics, 126*(1), e156-e162.

Borowitz, S. M., Cox, D. J., Sutphen, J. L., & Kovatchev, B. (2002). Treatment of childhood encopresis: A randomized trial comparing three treatment protocols. *Journal of Pediatric Gastroenterology and Nutrition, 34*(4), 378–384.

Brazzelli, M., Griffiths, P. V., Cody, J. D., & Tappin, D. (2011). Behavioural and cognitive interventions with or without other treatments for the management of faecal incontinence in children. *Cochrane Database of Systematic Reviews, (12)*.

Brooks, R. C., Copen, R. M., Cox, D. J., Morris, J., Borowitz, S., & Sutphen, J. (2000). Review of the treatment literature for encopresis, functional constipation, and stool-toileting refusal. *Annals of Behavioral Medicine, 22*(3), 260–267.

Christophersen, E. R., & Friman, P. C. (2010). Elimination disorders in children and adolescents: Enuresis and encopresis. In E. Wedding (Ed.), *Advances in psychotherapy: Evidence-based practice series*. Goettingen: Hogrefe & Huber.

Cox, D. J., Sutphen, J., Ling, W., Quillian, W., & Borowitz, S. (1996). Additive benefits of laxative, toilet training, and biofeedback therapies in the treatment of pediatric encopresis. *Journal of Pediatric Psychology, 21*(5), 659–670.

Cox, D. J., Sutphen, J., Borowitz, S., Kovatchev, B., & Ling, W. (1998). Contribution of behavior therapy and biofeedback to laxative therapy in the treatment of pediatric encopresis. *Annals of Behavioral Medicine, 20*(2), 70–76.

Cox, D. J., Morris, J. B., Jr., Borowitz, S. M., & Sutphen, J. L. (2002). Psychological differences between children with and without chronic encopresis. *Journal of Pediatric Psychology, 27*(7), 585–591.

Cox, D. J., Ritterband, L. M., Quillian, W., Kovatchev, B., Morris, J., Sutphen, J., et al. (2003). Assessment of behavioral mechanisms maintaining encopresis: Virginia encopresis-constipation apperception test. *Journal of Pediatric Psychology, 28*(6), 375–382.

Culbert, T. P., & Banez, G. A. (2007). Integrative approaches to childhood constipation and encopresis. *Pediatric Clinics of North America, 54*(6), 927–947.

Danda, C. E., & Hyman, P. E. (2014). Management of functional constipation in children. In C. Martin & T. Dovey (Eds.), *Pediatric gastrointestinal disorders: A psychosocial perspective* (pp. 137–150). London: Radcliffe Publishing Ltd.

de Araújo Sant, A. M. G., & Calçado, A. C. (1999). Constipation in school-aged children at public schools in Rio de Janeiro, Brazil. *Journal of Pediatric Gastroenterology and Nutrition, 29*(2), 190–193.

Fishman, L., Lenders, C., Fortunato, C., Noonan, C., & Nurko, S. (2004). Increased prevalence of constipation and fecal soiling in a population of obese children. *The Journal of Pediatrics, 145*(2), 253–254.

Freeman, K. A., Riley, A., Duke, D. C., & Fu, R. (2014). Systematic review and meta-analysis of behavioral interventions for fecal incontinence with constipation. *Journal of Pediatric Psychology, 39*(8), 887–902.

Friman, P. C., Mathews, J. R., Finney, J. W., Christophersen, E. R., & Leibowitz, J. M. (1988). Do encopretic children have clinically significant behavior problems? *Pediatrics, 82*, 407–409.

Friman, P. C., Hofstadter, K. L., & Jones, K. M. (2006). A biobehavioral approach to the treatment of functional encopresis in children. *Journal of Early and Intensive Behavior Intervention, 3*(3), 263.

Hansakunachai, T., Ruangdaraganon, N., Udomsubpayakul, U., Sombuntham, T., & Kotchabhakdi, N. (2005). Epidemiology of enuresis among school-age children in Thailand. *Journal of Developmental & Behavioral Pediatrics, 26*(5), 356–360.

Hyams, J. S., Di Lorenzo, C., Saps, M., Shulman, R. J., Staiano, A., & van Tilburg, M. (2016). Childhood functional gastrointestinal disorders: Child/adolescent. *Gastroenterology, 150*(6), 1456–1468.

Johnston, B. D., & Wright, J. A. (1993). Attentional dysfunction in children with encopresis. *Journal of Developmental & Behavioral Pediatrics, 14*(6), 381–385.

Joinson, C., Heron, J., Butler, U., von Gontard, A., & Avon Longitudinal Study of Parents and Children Study Team. (2006). Psychological differences between children with and without soiling problems. *Pediatrics, 117*(5), 1575–1584.

Kuhn, B. R., Marcus, B. A., & Pitner, S. L. (1999). Treatment guidelines for primary nonretentive encopresis and stool toileting refusal. *American Family Physician, 59*(8), 2171–2178.

Landman, G. B., Rappaport, L., Fenton, T., & Levine, M. D. (1986). Locus of control and self-esteem in children with encopresis. *Journal of Developmental and Behavioral Pediatrics, 7*(2), 111–113.

Levine, M. D. (1975). Children with encopresis: A descriptive analysis. *Pediatrics, 56*(3), 412–416.

Lewis, S. J., & Heaton, K. W. (1997). Stool form scale as a useful guide to intestinal transit time. *Scandinavian Journal of Gastroenterology, 32*(9), 920–924.

Loening-Baucke, V. (2007). Prevalence rates for constipation and faecal and urinary incontinence. *Archives of Disease in Childhood, 92*(6), 486–489.

Macias, M. M., Roberts, K. M., Saylor, C. F., & Fussell, J. J. (2006). Toileting concerns, parenting stress, and behavior problems in children with special health care needs. *Clinical Pediatrics, 45*(5), 415–422.

McGrath, M. L., Mellon, M. W., & Murphy, L. (2000). Empirically supported treatments in pediatric psychology: Constipation and encopresis. *Journal of Pediatric Psychology, 25*(4), 225–254.

Mellon, M. W., Whiteside, S. P., & Friedrich, W. N. (2006). The relevance of fecal soiling as an indicator of child sexual abuse: A preliminary analysis. *Journal of Developmental & Behavioral Pediatrics, 27*(1), 25–32.

Mellon, M. W., Natchev, B. E., Katusic, S. K., Colligan, R. C., Weaver, A. L., Voigt, R. G., & Barbaresi, W. J. (2013). Incidence of enuresis and encopresis among children with attention-deficit/hyperactivity disorder in a population-based birth cohort. *Academic pediatrics, 13*(4), 322–327.

Mohammed, A. A., & Mekael, F. M. (2012). Encopresis in children. *Saudi Medical Journal, 33*(6), 648–653.

Molnar, D., Taitz, L. S., Urwin, O. M., & Wales, J. K. (1983). Anorectal manometry results in defecation disorders. *Archives of Disease in Childhood, 58*(4), 257–261.

Mugie, S. M., Benninga, M. A., & Di Lorenzo, C. (2011). Epidemiology of constipation in children and adults: A systematic review. *Best Practice & Research Clinical Gastroenterology, 25*(1), 3–18.

Owens-Stively, J. A. (1987). Self-esteem and compliance in encopretic children. *Child Psychiatry and Human Development, 18*(1), 13–21.

Pashankar, D. S. (2005). Childhood constipation: Evaluation and management. *Clinics in Colon and Rectal Surgery, 18*, 120–129.

Reynolds, C. R., Kamphaus, R. W., & Vannest, K. J. (2015). *BASC3: Behavior assessment system for children*. PsychCorp.

Ritterband, L. M., Thorndike, F. P., Lord, H. R., Borowitz, S. M., Walker, L. S., Ingersoll, K. S., et al. (2013). An RCT of an internet intervention for pediatric encopresis with one-year follow-up. *Clinical Practice in Pediatric Psychology, 1*(1), 68.

Sakakibara, R., Tsunoyama, K., Hosoi, H., Takahashi, O., Sugiyama, M., Kishi, M., et al. (2010). Influence of body position on defecation in humans. *LUTS: Lower Urinary Tract Symptoms, 2*(1), 16–21.

Shepard, J. A., Poler, J. E., Jr., & Grabman, J. H. (2017). Evidence-based psychosocial treatments for pediatric elimination disorders. *Journal of Clinical Child & Adolescent Psychology, 46*(6), 767–797.

Sikirov, D. (2003). Comparison of straining during defecation in three positions: Results and implications for human health. *Digestive Diseases and Sciences, 48*(7), 1201–1205.

Silverman, A. H., Berlin, K. S., Di Lorenzo, C., Nurko, S., Kamody, R. C., Ponnambalam, A., et al. (2015). Measuring health-related quality of life with the parental opinions of pediatric constipation questionnaire. *Journal of Pediatric Psychology, 40*(8), 814–824.

Tabbers, M. M., DiLorenzo, C., Berger, M. Y., Faure, C., Langendam, M. W., Nurko, S., et al. (2014). Evaluation and treatment of functional constipation in infants and children: Evidence-based recommendations from ESPGHAN and NASPGHAN. *Journal of Pediatric Gastroenterology and Nutrition, 58*(2), 258–274.

Unal, F., & Pehlivantürk, B. (2003). Comorbid psychiatric disorders in 201 cases of encopresis. *The Turkish Journal of Pediatrics, 46*(4), 350–353.

Van der Wal, M. F., Benninga, M. A., & Hirasing, R. A. (2005). The prevalence of encopresis in a multicultural population. *Journal of Pediatric Gastroenterology and Nutrition, 40*(3), 345–348.

Van Den Berg, M. M., Benninga, M. A., & Di Lorenzo, C. (2006). Epidemiology of childhood constipation: a systematic review. *The American Journal of Gastroenterology, 101*(10), 2401.

Von Wendt, L., Similä, S., Niskanen, P., & Järvelin, M. R. (1990). Development of bowel and bladder control in the mentally retarded. *Developmental Medicine & Child Neurology, 32*(6), 515–518.

Yong, D., & Beattie, R. M. (1998). Normal bowel habit and prevalence of constipation in primary-school children. *Ambulatory Child Health, 4*, 277–277.

Cognitive-Behavioral Therapy for Chronic Headache Disorders in Children and Adolescents

17

Karen Kaczynski

Introduction

Almost everyone has experienced a headache at least once in their life. Minor disruptions to our daily routines, such as a poor night's sleep, too much or too little caffeine, dehydration, hunger, or a particularly stressful interaction at school or work can cause a headache. In most cases, headaches are irritants that resolve with some Ibuprofen, a glass of water, and rest. In other cases, such as migraines, headaches are more debilitating and disruptive to daily life. However, by identifying and avoiding triggers and taking prescribed medication when needed, these headaches can often be managed. When children and adolescents complain of headaches, our common experience with headaches combines with a tendency to question whether childhood complaints are legitimate or have another purpose, like getting out of a math test. Indeed, any school nurse will tell you that students often show up in her office complaining of headaches on test days. Further complicating the picture is the fact that headaches are largely subjective, relying on the report of the person experiencing the pain rather than objective evidence, as would be available with a fever or strep throat.

For these reasons, children and adolescents with chronic headaches and associated disability often have their symptoms minimized, questioned, or even dismissed by their family, teachers, and doctors. It is important to consider this context when working with children and adolescents with chronic headaches. Some initial effort may be needed to validate the symptoms and build trust, particularly with psychosocial interventions which patients may already be resistant to due to their perception that psychological treatment implies a psychological cause. However, as with other chronic pain conditions, once patients and families buy-in to the value of psychosocial interventions, there is much potential for improvement. A combination of education about chronic pain, problem-solving around school and other functional difficulties, and cognitive-behavioral techniques such as reframing and relaxation skills can go a long way towards helping children and adolescents with chronic headache manage their symptoms better and lead fuller lives. This chapter will provide an overview of the most common primary headache disorders in children and adolescents, a biopsychosocial explanation of chronic headache and associated disability, a brief review of medical interventions, and a more detailed explanation of psychological treatment of chronic

K. Kaczynski (✉)
Pediatric Headache Program, Division of Pain Medicine, Department of Anesthesia, Perioperative, and Pain Medicine, Boston Children's Hospital and Harvard Medical School, Waltham, MA, USA
e-mail: karen.kaczynki@childrens.harvard.edu

pediatric headache with reference to case examples.

Headache Prevalence

Headaches are one of the most common complaints in children and adolescents. Approximately 60% of children and adolescents worldwide experience headaches of varying degrees of intensity (Abu-Arafeh et al. 2010). Headaches account for a large proportion of pediatric primary care or emergency room visits. While patients and parents often fear catastrophic causes (e.g., brain tumors), the vast majority of pediatric headaches are due to a primary headache disorder such as migraine or a relatively benign acute process such as a viral illness (Blume 2012).

Chronic pain affects one in four children and adolescents, and headache is the most common chronic pain complaint in pediatrics (Perquin et al. 2000). Chronic headache is defined as ≥ 15 headache days per month (Blume 2012). Almost 20% of children in the US experience frequent or severe headaches, and the rate increases substantially from childhood (13%) to early adolescence (22%) to late adolescence (27%) (Lateef et al. 2009). Girls are more likely to experience headaches than boys (Abu-Arafeh et al. 2010), and girls' headaches tend to be more intense, persistent, and disabling than boys' headaches (Isensee et al. 2016).

Similarly, migraine is a common disorder, affecting almost one in ten youth (Abu-Arafeh et al. 2010). Although there is no gender difference in the prevalence of migraine in childhood (Eidlitz-Markus and Zeharia 2017), adolescent girls are approximately 1.5 times more likely to experience migraines than boys (Buse et al. 2013; Eidlitz-Markus and Zeharia 2017). Headache accounts for 1 in 50 pediatric emergency room visits in the USA (Kedia et al. 2014), and migraine is one of the leading causes of nonfatal disability worldwide (Vos et al. 2012). Thus, headaches are a common disorder that cause significant distress and disability in a large number of children and adolescents.

Headache Types

When discussing headache treatment, it is helpful to understand the different types of headache that may present in children and adolescents. While there are similarities in the psychosocial correlates and cognitive-behavioral management of headache across subtypes, it is important to understand the differences in underlying pathophysiology and presentation in order to target treatment most effectively. Therefore, a brief description of the most common primary headache disorders in pediatrics is presented here. Chronic post-concussive headache is also described, due to the prevalence of sports-related concussion in children and adolescents. Less common headache types, such as occipital or trigeminal neuralgia and cluster headaches, are not included in the interest of space. Interested readers are directed to Blume (2012) for more information.

Tension-Type Headache

Tension-type headache (TTH) is typically bilateral pain lasting several minutes to several days that is described as pressing or squeezing in quality. Pain intensity is rated as mild to moderate. The headache may be associated with some light or sound sensitivity, but nausea and vomiting are not typical during TTH episodes. Routine physical activity does not intensify the pain.

TTH is extremely common, and almost everyone will experience TTH at least once in their lifetime. Therefore, to avoid over-diagnosis of headache disorders, the *International Classification of Headache Disorders, third edition* (ICHD-3; International Headache Society 2018), distinguishes between the following subtypes of TTH:

- Infrequent episodic TTH
  - <1 headache episode per month on average
- Frequent episodic TTH
  - At least ten episodes occurring on 1–14 days per month
- Chronic TTH
  - ≥ 15 episodes per month

Although infrequent episodic TTH is relatively easy to manage with basic lifestyle changes (e.g., rest, hydration, nutrition) and over-the-counter medications (e.g., NSAIDS, Tylenol), frequent episodic and chronic TTH are more challenging to address and may require specialized medical attention. It is these more frequent subtypes of TTH that are the focus of the following discussion.

Despite the descriptive name, the physiological cause of tension-type headache is not known. However, tenderness and tension in the muscles around the skull and at the neck, shoulders, and upper back are common. These peripheral pain mechanisms contribute to episodic TTH, while chronic TTH likely involves both peripheral and central pain processes.

Migraine

Migraine is typically unilateral, although it may be bilateral in children. The pain is frontal and/or temporal and is pulsating or throbbing in quality. Pain intensity is moderate to severe. Migraine episodes last 2–72 h and may be associated with nausea, vomiting, and sensitivity to light and/or sound. Pain is aggravated by routine physical activity. Migraine with aura involves the gradual development of visual and/or sensory and/or speech symptoms that occur prior to the onset of the pain. These may include loss of vision or blurry vision, seeing spots or squiggly lines, numbness or tingling in one side of the face or in the arms or legs, or word finding difficulties. Aura symptoms last up to 1 h and resolve completely when the headache episode is over. Chronic migraine is diagnosed when either migraine or TTH occurs on 15 or more days per month, with eight of the headache episodes meeting criteria for migraine with or without aura.

Migraine involves severe pain and associated symptoms that often interfere in daily functioning. It may be necessary to stop regular activity and rest or sleep in a dark room during a migraine episode. Prescription medications, such as triptans (e.g., Sumatriptan, Rizatriptan) or antiemetics (e.g., Ondansetron), may be required.

Migraine is a neurobiological disorder, although the underlying pathophysiology is not fully understood. While migraine was previously thought to involve changes in vasodilation and vasoconstriction, it has become clearer recently that the central nervous system plays a role due to the sensitization of pain pathways. Regional cerebral blood flow imaging studies suggest that changes in blood flow in the brain stem are also involved. Neurotransmitters, the chemical messengers in the brain, also appear to be disrupted during migraine episodes. For example, serotonin, a neurotransmitter which regulates pain, is decreased. Cortical spreading depression, which involves the gradual inhibition of the cerebral cortex, has been identified in migraine with aura. The trigeminovascular system has been identified as the primary brain circuit involved in migraine.

New Daily Persistent Headache

A chronic headache that develops on a specific day, that occurs all day, every day since onset, and that lasts for 3 months or longer is diagnosed as new daily persistent headache (NDPH). It is notable that the patient or family often distinctly remembers the exact date and even sometimes the time when the headache started. Pain may increase or decrease over time, but it is always present. The symptoms of NDPH may be similar to TTH, migraine, or a combination. Often, there is no previous history of headache.

NDPH is often triggered by a viral illness, although it may also be triggered by a psychosocial stressor, or, in some cases, may develop spontaneously with no clear trigger or precipitant (Li and Rozen 2002; Mack 2004). There is limited research on NDPH and the cause is not known. However, hypermobility of the joints in the neck may increase the likelihood of developing NDPH (Tyagi 2012). It has also been suggested that NDPH is due to chronic inflammation in the central nervous system, particularly in cases that are triggered by infection.

As many as one in 1000 people develop NDPH, and the disorder is more common in women than in men, similar to other headache disorders (Castillo et al. 1999). NDPH often resolves on its own after several months with no additional treatment required. However, a subset of patients with NDPH experience headaches that persist for months or years and that do not improve with aggressive treatment efforts. The lack of clear knowledge about the underlying cause of this disorder, prolonged course, and poor response to treatment makes this an incredibly challenging diagnosis for patients, families, and treatment providers.

Post-concussive Headache

The American Academy of Neurology defines concussion as "a clinical syndrome of biomechanically induced alteration of brain function, typically affecting memory and orientation, which may involve loss of consciousness" (Giza et al. 2013). Twenty percent of American high school students have experienced a concussion in their lifetime, and the rate of concussion is higher in boys, older adolescents, and those who play contact sports (Veliz et al. 2017). Headache that develops within 7 days of a concussion is considered a post-concussive headache. The headache may involve symptoms of TTH and/or migraine. Therefore, the close temporal relation between the head injury and the development of the headache is key to diagnosis. Headache may be the only symptom or may be associated with other post-concussive symptoms, such as fatigue, dizziness, nausea, and difficulties with concentration and memory. A post-concussive headache that lasts for 3 months or less is considered acute, while a headache that persists for longer than 3 months is considered chronic. As many as 14% of school-age children develop chronic post-concussive symptoms following a concussion (Barlow et al. 2010). Symptoms may develop following a single, relatively minor head trauma, or may not develop until several head injuries have occurred. Children and adolescents may be more susceptible to concussion, and may take longer to recover, than adults (Gómez and Hergenroeder 2013). Post-concussive symptoms, including headache, may be due to mild brain injury, inflammation, or alternations in brain functioning.

The Impact of Headache

Primary headache disorders can be severe and disabling, impacting a child's functioning and quality of life substantially (Hershey 2010). Frequent headaches may affect every aspect of a child or adolescent's life, including mood, school, sports, and peer and family relationships. A child may be unable to participate in daily activities due to their pain and associated symptoms. Furthermore, headaches are often made worse by both physical and mental activity, and therefore a child or adolescent may avoid daily activities, including school and sports, to prevent their headaches from getting worse. Increased stress due to missed activities may serve to maintain the headache pain, ultimately resulting in greater difficulty functioning. An inability to perform daily activities due to pain and/or other somatic symptoms is called "functional disability."

Mood

Chronic headaches are frequently associated with symptoms of anxiety and depression, such as worry, increased tension, sleep disruption, and irritability. While most youth with chronic headache do not qualify for a comorbid anxiety or depressive disorder (Slater et al. 2012), the vast majority experience elevated symptoms of anxiety and depression (Pakalnis et al. 2007; Rousseau-Salvador et al. 2014). Anxiety and depression symptoms may have been present prior to the onset of headaches and may play a role in the development and persistence of the child's chronic headaches. Anxiety and depression symptoms may also develop in response to chronic, unremitting pain and functional disability. Often, a vicious cycle develops with headaches making anxiety and depression symptoms worse, and anxiety and depression symptoms making the headaches worse. The combination of chronic headache and associated anxiety and depression symptoms can make daily functioning extremely difficult.

Sleep

Sleep problems are quite common in youth, occurring in 37% of children and 20% of adolescents (Mindell and Owens 2015). However, sleep problems are three times more common in children and adolescents with frequent headache than in the general population (Luntamo et al. 2012). In fact, there appears to be a bidirectional relationship between sleep disturbance and headache in children and adolescents. That is, poorer sleep results in more frequent and severe headaches (Houle et al. 2012) and frequent headaches also interfere in sleep quality (Heyer et al. 2014). Symptoms of anxiety and depression may also intensify sleep difficulties in children and adolescents with chronic headache (Rabner et al. 2017).

School

Children and adolescents with chronic headaches often struggle in school. In fact, youth with chronic headaches report more difficulties with school than children with other chronic illnesses, including cancer (Powers et al. 2003). The cognitive demands of being in school may intensify headaches, making school attendance especially challenging. Indeed, school absences are common in youth with chronic headache, especially migraines (Laurell et al. 2005; Rousseau-Salvador et al. 2014). Furthermore, headache-related emergency room visits increase in September and January (Kedia et al. 2014), suggesting that stress related to the return to school after vacation triggers headache pain. Even when children are able to attend school, headaches may affect their ability to retain information and complete tests and assignments, resulting in declines in performance. Stress related to frequent absences, make-up work, and declining performance may aggravate headaches further, resulting in an escalating cycle of pain and school-related disability. School is the primary domain for the development of cognitive, social, and community-related skills, and thus school impairment related to chronic headaches may have pervasive negative effects on child and adolescent development (Eccleston et al. 2004; Powers et al. 2006).

Sports and Other Extracurricular Activities

Children and adolescents with chronic headache are often unable to participate in regular sports and other extracurricular activities. They may not be willing or able to play sports due to their headaches and the possibility that physical activity may intensify their pain. They may also need to prioritize doctor's appointments and completing missed schoolwork in the afternoons, when they would otherwise be participating in sports. Often, when students are frequently absent from school, they are not allowed to participate in sports and other school-based extracurricular activities. While it is reasonable to prioritize school and medical treatments, there is also a cost to limiting regular afterschool activities in children and adolescents with chronic headaches. Sports and other extracurricular activities often provide children and adolescents with valuable physical conditioning, stress reduction, and opportunities for unstructured peer interactions. These benefits may help with pain management and may motivate youth to continue daily activities.

Family Functioning

The impact of chronic headaches often extends beyond the individual child, and family functioning is frequently disrupted (Palermo and Chambers 2005). Family stress may increase due to the daily demands of caring for a child with a chronic illness, including the need to stay home with a child who is absent from school, to schedule and attend multiple doctor's visits, and to coordinate a complex treatment plan. Family conflict may increase when a child and his or her parents respond to the child's headaches in different ways. For example, the child may have a difficult time performing daily activities while managing their pain and other associated somatic symptoms and may prefer to limit activity. In contrast, the parents may try to encourage continued adaptive functioning despite pain and other somatic symptoms. Such a conflict may cause children to perceive their parents as less supportive of their needs, potentially leading to increased headache pain. Alternatively, some parents may inadvertently reinforce their child's persistent pain and disability by relieving them of responsibilities and demands. Although well-meaning, parents' overly solicitous responses to their child's headaches (e.g., focusing excessive attention on pain, providing special privileges, allowing the child to stay home from school) may lead to greater pain and disability in the long run (Claar et al. 2008; Kaczynski et al. 2009; Welkom et al. 2013). Thus, parenting a child with chronic headaches requires a delicate balance between supporting the child emotionally while also encouraging daily functioning despite pain, and this process often puts undue strain on family relationships.

Peer Relationships

Children and adolescents with chronic headaches often struggle with peer relationships. They may miss out on regular peer interactions due to absences from school and extracurricular activities. Friendships may become strained, or it may be difficult to form friendships in the first place, due to the lack of regular peer contact. Comorbid anxiety or depression symptoms may also make it difficult for children and adolescents with chronic headache to interact with their peers in socially acceptable ways and develop healthy peer relationships. Indeed, children with chronic pain tend to have fewer reciprocal friendships and to be more socially isolated than healthy children (Forgeron et al. 2010). Peer victimization, including traditional and cyber-bullying, is common in traditional school settings and may trigger headaches in children and adolescents with a pain vulnerability (Herge et al. 2016; Kowalski and Limber 2013). While rates of bullying are similar in children with chronic pain and healthy children, recent research suggests that children with chronic pain are more distressed by the experience of being bullied (Fales et al. 2018). Thus, bullying may contribute to increased pain, emotional distress, and school avoidance in children and adolescents with chronic headaches.

Biopsychosocial Formulation of Pediatric Chronic Headache

Pediatric chronic primary headache disorders are complex and multifactorial. The biopsychosocial model is a theoretical framework that explains the complex interplay of biological, psychological, and social factors that contribute to the development and persistence of chronic headaches (Andrasik et al. 2011). While the specific factors involved may differ in different individual cases, a combination of multiple triggering and maintenance factors is almost always involved when headaches become chronic.

Biological factors may include a predisposition to develop chronic headaches due to a positive family history of headache and other chronic pain conditions. This biological vulnerability may increase the child's risk for developing chronic headaches if other factors are present. Biological factors may also precipitate the development of chronic headaches. For example, viral illnesses and head injuries are often identified as the initial trigger for a child's headaches. Additional biological factors, such as allergies and hormonal changes related to the onset of puberty, may also play a role in chronic headaches.

Psychological factors include comorbid symptoms of anxiety and/or depression, which may exacerbate headache pain. Headaches may also represent a somatic expression of underlying anxiety or depression symptoms in some cases. Youth with chronic pain may internalize or underreport emotional distress due to a desire to present themselves more positively (Logan et al. 2008), potentially increasing the likelihood that distress is expressed somatically. Children and adolescents with chronic pain conditions tend to be high academic achievers with perfectionistic tendencies (Randall et al. 2018; Wojtowicz and Banez 2015), and the stress of meeting their high expectations for themselves while managing headaches and functional difficulties may also contribute to the persistence of their pain. It is also possible that a child has an undiagnosed or untreated learning or attention deficit disorder that is not being adequately addressed in school, resulting in excessive cognitive strain which intensifies headaches. Additional psychosocial stressors, such as family and peer conflict which are common in adolescence, may also contribute to the development and maintenance of chronic headaches. Lastly, the strategies a child uses to cope with their pain, emotional distress, and daily stressors may determine whether they are able to push through their pain and continue regular daily activities, or become stuck in the cycle of chronic pain and disability. Unfortunately, there is a tendency for children and adolescents with chronic headaches to engage in passive coping strategies, such as rest and reduction of activities, which perpetuate the cycle of chronic pain, activity avoidance, distress, and disability (Wager et al. 2014; Wojtowicz and Banez 2015).

Social factors may also contribute to chronic headaches in children and adolescents, and these primarily involve interactions with family, peers, and teachers. Parents who are either overly solicitous or overly dismissive of their child's pain complaints may unintentionally contribute to the persistence of pain and functional disability. There may be inconsistency or disagreement between two parents in the same family about how to respond to the child's headaches, which can be quite confusing and stressful for the child. Siblings may become jealous of their brother or sister with chronic headaches because of the increased parental attention and relief from household responsibilities he or she receives, resulting in increased sibling conflict. Peers and teachers may question the severity of the child's symptoms and the need to miss multiple days of school. Increased conflict or stress in any of the child's important relationships may result in increased pain and may also contribute to functional disability as the child attempts to avoid distressing social interactions.

Case Example 1: Maya A[1]

Maya is a 15-year-old Arab American girl who developed chronic daily headaches following a minor head injury when she was 10. She was evaluated in a multidisciplinary pediatric headache program and diagnosed with new daily persistent headache. She has seen several neurologists and has tried multiple medications and alternative interventions (e.g., acupuncture, Botox), with limited improvement. Maya tends to be a perfectionist, and she is having a very difficult time completing her schoolwork because she cannot maintain her usual high standards due to her headaches. She attended an academically rigorous private school but was asked to leave due to excessive school absences and inability to complete assignments. She transferred to the local public high school, but continues to have issues with attendance and completion of assignments. She has struggled in her relationships with peers because her friends do not understand her headaches and become frustrated with her when cancels plans due to a headache. She has been unable to participate in extracurricular activities and her parents limit peer activities outside of school so her opportunities to make friends are limited. Her parents immigrated to the USA from the Middle East as young adults and have high expectations for Maya's academic performance but limited understanding of the challenging social dynamics in American schools. Maya and her parents continue to search for a clear diagnosis and a medical treatment that will resolve her pain.

Multidisciplinary Treatment of Chronic Pediatric Headache

In most children and adolescents, headaches are infrequent and time-limited, and they can easily be addressed with over-the-counter medications and lifestyle changes at home or in the primary care setting if needed. However, when headaches become more frequent, chronic, and disruptive to daily functioning, multidisciplinary treatment is often required to address the pain as well as the combination of factors that maintain the pain and disability (Soee et al. 2013). Treatment for children and adolescents with chronic headache and associated disability often involves a combination of medication, psychological, complementary, and lifestyle interventions. Each type of intervention will be reviewed below, with a more detailed description of psychological treatment of chronic pediatric headache.

Medication

Medications for chronic headache include both acute and preventive medications. Acute medications are taken at the time of a headache episode to reduce the intensity or duration of the pain. Preventive medications are taken daily and are intended to reduce the frequency or intensity of headache episodes overall. Preventive treatment should be considered if a child or adolescent has one or more headache episodes per week (Blume 2012). For frequent headaches, a combination of daily preventive medications and acute medications to be taken during headache episodes is often recommended. The choice of medications depends on the child's age, comorbidities, and the side effect profile.

Acute Pain Medications
Analgesics are acute medications that are used to reduce pain. These include acetaminophen and nonsteroidal anti-inflammatory drugs (e.g., ibuprofen, naproxen). Analgesics can be very effective at reducing acute pain due to episodic TTH or migraine, as long as they are taken early in the headache episode. Side effects are minimal and include gastrointestinal distress with long-term use. Unfortunately, these medications are not usually effective when headaches are frequent or daily. In addition, prolonged daily use can result in medication overuse headache (MOH), which can complicate diagnosis and treatment. MOH may develop when analgesic medication is taken on 15 or more days per month for 3 months or longer, which can exacerbate an underlying headache disorder. MOH is similar to the headache that may develop with caffeine withdrawal and requires discontinuation of the frequently used medication and possibly steroid treatment to overcome the withdrawal symptoms.

Rescue Medications for Migraine
Abortive medications are intended to interrupt a migraine episode. They can be quite effective and include triptans (e.g., Sumatriptan, Zolmitriptan, Rizatriptan) and dihydroergotamine (DHE). They must be taken at the earliest sign that a migraine is coming on in order to be effective. Therefore, these medications are often prescribed only for patients with migraine with aura because the aura provides the warning signal that a migraine is coming on and allows the patient to take the medication early enough for it to be effective. Triptans often cause drowsiness, which is an added benefit because sleep can help with migraine recovery. Additional possible side effects include muscle tension, tingling, dizziness, hot flashes, and nausea.

Medications for Associated Symptoms of Headache
Adjunct medications can be used to address other symptoms that are associated with the headache. For example, antiemetics (e.g., ondansetron, reglan) are often used to treat headache-related nausea. Sleep is often disrupted due to chronic headaches, and antihistamines (e.g., cyproheptadine, hydroxyzine) can provide pain reduction while also promoting restorative sleep. Dietary supplements such as magnesium, riboflavin, and butterbur are often also recommended to reduce the frequency and/or intensity of chronic headaches.

Preventive or Prophylactic Medications

When headaches occur once a week or more, a daily preventive medication may be recommended to reduce the frequency or intensity of headache episodes. There are several types of medication that may be used for headache prevention, including antihistamines (e.g., cyproheptadine), tricyclic antidepressants (e.g., amitriptyline, nortriptyline), anticonvulsants (e.g., topiramate, zonisamide, gabapentin), beta blockers (e.g., propranolol), and calcium channel blockers (e.g., verapamil). These medications must be taken daily to be effective and can take up to 1 month to provide symptom reduction. Cyproheptadine is the first-line drug of choice in prepubertal children, whereas a trial of amitriptyline or topiramate is often recommended first in adolescents. The specific medication prescribed depends on the child's age, comorbidities, and side effects that may be either beneficial or problematic. For example, amitriptyline can cause drowsiness, which may be helpful for sleep difficulties but disruptive to school functioning. Common side effects that may occur with daily headache medications include mental clouding, sedation, and changes in mood. Side effects are minimal if the medications are started at low doses that are gradually increased and they often wear off within a few days.

While medications may be somewhat helpful in some patients, they are usually not a complete solution for chronic headaches. Limited research has been conducted to evaluate the efficacy of headache medications in children and adolescents, and results are mixed (Lewis et al. 2007; Winner et al. 2005). Results of a recent multi-site, randomized, double-blind, placebo-controlled study comparing amitriptyline, topiramate, and placebo in adolescents with chronic migraine (Powers et al. 2017) showed that, while amitriptyline and topiramate both reduced the frequency of migraine episodes in about 50% of the participants, there was no difference on any outcome measures between the active treatment groups and the placebo group. Furthermore, the active medications caused more adverse side effects than the placebo. So, while medications may reduce the frequency of headache episodes in some patients, the effect may be no better than a placebo, and the benefit must be weighed against the risk of adverse effects.

Psychological Treatment for Headache

Psychosocial factors often play a central role in the development and maintenance of chronic headaches in children and adolescents. Therefore, psychological interventions are an important component of effective multidisciplinary treatment for chronic headaches. Evidence-based psychological treatments for headache include relaxation training, cognitive-behavioral therapy (CBT), and biofeedback (Sieberg et al. 2012). These interventions may be used separately or in combination, depending on the age and preferences of the patient, headache characteristics, and associated psychosocial factors. With exception of temperature biofeedback, which has been found to be particularly effective at preventing migraine episodes (Penzien and Taylor 2014), these psychological interventions are appropriate for any primary headache diagnosis.

Relaxation Training

Relaxation training involves teaching the patient skills that reduce stress and tension. These strategies alter pain-related physiological changes and decrease general nervous system hyperarousal. Relaxation skills can be used during headache episodes or to manage psychosocial stressors that may trigger headaches. As with any new skill, these strategies are most effective when practiced regularly. The most common relaxation skills are diaphragmatic breathing, progressive muscle relaxation (PMR), and visual imagery. Diaphragmatic breathing (i.e., belly breathing) involves slow, regular, deep breathing using the diaphragm to fully expand the lungs. This type of breathing is incompatible with stress and promotes calm and relaxation. PMR involves progressively tensing and releasing various muscle groups while engaging in diaphragmatic breathing. Chronic tension in the muscles in the face, neck, and scalp may contribute to chronic TTH, and PMR allows for increased awareness and conscious control of muscle tension and release. Visual imagery involves the conscious and deliberate mental creation of a relaxing experience as if it were actually happening (e.g., lying on the beach), including all the sounds, sights, smells, tastes, and feelings involved in the experience. Calm, focused awareness of a relaxing internal experience promotes deep relaxation. Visual imagery may also be used to directly alter or reduce pain. For example, the patient may be coached to imagine what the pain looks like and then use a mental process to alter it or reduce its impact. A therapist can guide the patient through a visual imagery practice in session and record a relaxation script for home practice. There are also several apps available that provide visual imagery scripts (e.g., Calm, Headspace, Insight Timer).

Cognitive-Behavioral Therapy

Cognitive-behavioral therapy (CBT) for chronic headaches involves cognitive interventions to address negative thought patterns related to pain and stress and behavioral strategies to improve active coping and promote adaptive functioning (Law et al. 2017). Psychoeducation about chronic pain in general and headache in particular is an important cognitive component that can help the child or adolescent and his or her family shift their thinking away from a desire for a clear diagnosis and immediate treatment response towards a more realistic understanding of the biopsychosocial model of chronic pain and the need for a more functional approach. There are several excellent books for parents of children with chronic pain which can be very helpful in educating parents, including:

- Conquering Your Child's Chronic Pain: A Pediatrician's Guide for Reclaiming a Normal Childhood by Christina Blackett Schlank and Lonnie Zeltzer
- When Your Child Hurts: Effective Strategies to Increase Comfort, Reduce Stress, and Break the Cycle of Chronic Pain by Rachael Coakley

For children, a helpful reference with good hands-on explanations and exercises is:

- Be the Boss of Your Pain: Self-Care for Kids by Rebecca Kajander and Timothy Culbert

Parents often have negative beliefs or fears about the headaches (e.g., "Is it a brain tumor?") that may increase attention to pain and intensify stress, resulting in increased pain perception and activity avoidance. It is important to identify and challenge these negative thoughts, replacing irrational fears with more realistic information (e.g., Brain tumors are exceedingly rare in children and adolescents and frequently involve neurological changes that are not typical in primary headache disorders; Wilne et al. 2006). Cognitive modification can also be used to help the child or adolescent reappraise psychosocial stressors that may trigger headaches, such as school or peer stressors. Reducing negative thought patterns can decrease stress and promote effective problem-solving.

Clinical Example[1]

Therapist: It's pretty common for kids with chronic headaches to become frustrated and have some negative thoughts about their headaches, like, "why me?" or "this isn't fair." What thoughts do you have about your headaches?
Maya: I don't really think about my headaches. I just know that the doctors can't figure out what's wrong with me.
Therapist: That sounds like a thought to me! What makes you think that the doctors can't figure out what's wrong?
Maya: Well, they've done a lot of tests and they haven't found anything. There must be something else going on that they haven't found yet. Because it's not normal to have headaches that don't ever go away at my age. I don't know anyone else who has this problem.
Therapist: Chronic pain is actually more common than you think, even in kids. About 1 out of 4 teenagers experience chronic pain, and headaches are the most common type of chronic pain.
Maya: Really?
Therapist: Yep! But since chronic pain is invisible, you can't see it and you can't tell who has it. Just

---

[1]Fictional dialogue based on interactions with many adolescent patients with chronic headache.

like not everyone at school knows about your chronic headaches, there are most likely other kids at school with chronic pain that you don't know about.
Maya: I guess that's possible. But I still think there's something wrong that the doctors haven't figured out.
Therapist: Well, what evidence do you have that makes you think that?
Maya: They've done a lot of different tests, like blood tests and MRIs and stuff, and they haven't been able to figure out why I have these headaches.
Therapist: It's actually good news that they haven't found anything that explains your headaches, because anything that they would find would be pretty serious and scary. Sometimes in medicine, we have to rule out the bad stuff first, and fortunately we have been about to do that for you.
Maya: But it still really hurts.
Therapist: I know. And the pain is real. It just isn't caused by an underlying injury or condition. Chronic pain itself is the issue. And there is no specific test for chronic pain. It's diagnosed by talking with the patient, doing a physical exam, and ruling out any other possible causes for the pain.
Maya: So I guess I just have chronic pain. Does that mean it will never go away?
Therapist: No, the "chronic" in chronic pain just means your pain has lasted 3 months or more. It doesn't mean it will never go away. And the good news is that we have really great ways to treat chronic pain, including cognitive-behavioral therapy, like we are doing right now. You are doing the right things to help yourself feel better and get back to the things you enjoy in life.
Maya: Well, I guess that makes me feel better.
Therapist: Good!

Behavioral strategies for chronic headache include coping strategies to use during headache episodes to reduce pain intensity. The relaxation skills described above (i.e., diaphragmatic breathing, progressive muscle relaxation, visual imagery) can be used to reduce stress and muscle tension and decrease the focus of attention on pain. Training in these skills provides the child or adolescent with greater self-efficacy as they learn to manage their headaches on their own, without relying on medical interventions. It is also helpful to develop a list of the patient's preferred activities (e.g., listening to music, doing artwork, going for a walk, talking with a friend, playing with pets). Any activity that the child or adolescent intrinsically enjoys can be used as a relaxation or distraction strategy during headache episodes.

The goal is to develop an active strategy to cope with the headaches while continuing to function, rather than relying on rest and activity avoidance.

It is also helpful to evaluate the antecedents and consequences of headaches, particularly when headaches are episodic. Treatment can then be targeted to address any specific antecedents or triggers that are identified. For example, headaches may develop or intensify on Sunday evenings in some children, suggesting that anticipatory anxiety about school triggers headache episodes. Addressing school stress by providing appropriate school support may reduce the frequency of school-related headaches. The consequences of a child's headaches may also contribute to persistent pain and associated disability. For example, if the child experiences a reward during headache episodes, such as being allowed to stay home from school, headaches will be reinforced and may become more frequent. It is important to teach active coping and continuation of regular activities during headache episodes to minimize inadvertent reinforcement of passive coping and disability.

Clinical Example[2]

Therapist: One way to decrease the frequency of your headaches is to figure out if there are any specific triggers. Is there anything that you've noticed triggers or brings on a headache? Or that causes your headache to get worse?
Maya: My headache always gets worse when I have to do a lot or reading or writing, like in History.
Therapist: What about reading and writing for History class makes your headache worse?
Maya: I think because it's hard and I have to think a lot to do it. It's too much of a strain on my brain.
Therapist: So the cognitive effort involved in doing your schoolwork for History makes your pain worse.
Maya: Yes. So I can't get any of my History homework done. I just keep putting it off and it piles up.
Therapist: That must be stressful.
Maya: It is!
Therapist: The strain of doing your History homework makes your pain worse, so you avoid it. But then it piles up and gets more overwhelming

---
[2]Fictional dialogue based on interactions with many adolescent patients with chronic headache.

and stressful. I bet that makes your headache even worse when you think about how much work you have to do in History!
Maya: Yes! But I don't know what to do about it because I just can't get any work done because my pain is too bad.
Therapist: It sounds like stress and cognitive strain triggers your pain. It is normal to try to avoid the things that cause us pain. Avoiding doing your History schoolwork reduces your pain in the short term. But in the long term, this is not a good solution.
Maya: I know, because it just makes me more stressed and makes my pain even worse.
Therapist: That's right! Let's work on breaking this cycle. One thing we could do is communicate with your History teacher and guidance counselor about this problem and see if there are any accommodations that would help you. Maybe they would be willing to reduce the amount of make-up work you have to do or give you some deadline extensions. Would that be ok?
Maya: Yes, I think that would help!

Chronic headaches can affect the whole family, and parental involvement is a key component of CBT for chronic pediatric headache disorders (Sieberg and Manganella 2015). Parents should be educated about their child's headaches, including the difference between acute and chronic pain and the importance of focusing on coping and adaptive functioning rather than symptom resolution. It is helpful to inform parents about the various coping skills their child may be learning in therapy so that the parents can encourage their child to practice the skills regularly and use them during headache episodes. Family interactions that contribute to the child's headaches should also be addressed in treatment. These may include family conflict which may increase the child's stress, excessive parental attention to the child's pain, and parental responses to the child's headaches that unintentionally reward passive, avoidant responses to headaches.

Clinical Example[3]

Therapist (to parent): When your child has a headache, how do you usually respond?

---

[3]Fictional dialogue based on interactions with parents of children with chronic headache.

Parent: I tell her to stay home from school and rest. I feel bad leaving her at home alone while I go to work, but I don't have a choice. I usually text her or call her every couple of hours to ask how she's feeling and get her to rate her pain.
Therapist: Does that help?
Paerent: Not really. Her pain just seems to stay the same and then it's harder for her to go back to school. But I don't know what else to do.
Therapist: As a parent, it's natural to try to comfort your child when they aren't feeling well. But even though staying home from school and resting works for acute pain, like pain related to an illness, it's not very effective for chronic pain. And it can just make other issues worse, like school stress that may intensify the pain.
Parent: I can see that. But how can I make her go to school when her pain is an 8/10?
Therapist: First of all, it's not very helpful to keep asking her to rate her pain. That just puts more focus on the pain intensity and makes it more difficult to cope with it. I would recommend not asking her to rate her pain so often. If there is a significant change in her pain, she will let you know.
Parent: OK, I can try that.
Therapist: Good. Next, remember that the treatment for chronic pain is learning coping strategies and returning to regular activities, like school. It's easier said than done, but if you stick with it, it will help.
Parent: That's what the doctor told us, but it's hard to believe.
Therapist: I know. But there is a lot of good research that says that it works. Plus, you've tried letting her stay home and rest and that hasn't worked. Your child has been working on learning relaxation skills to help her manage her headaches. Let's support her in being an active coper by encouraging her to use those strategies at school rather than staying home. Can we give that a try?
Parent: Ok.

School issues often go hand in hand with chronic headaches, as children and adolescents may be absent from school or have difficulty completing assignments due to their headaches. School stress and difficulties with school-related functioning may, in turn, trigger increased headaches. Therefore, school collaboration is often necessary to address school-related stressors that perpetuate the headaches and to promote a return to functioning. School personnel may have misconceptions about the child or adolescent's headaches and frequent absences, and it can be very helpful to clarify the child's diagnosis and treatment plan with relevant school personnel, such as the school nurse or guidance counselor. School accommodations may be necessary to support the student's functioning in school while they manage their headaches. This can be done either informally or through a formal section 504 plan. Accommodations should be individualized to each student's needs, and may include a reduced workload, extended deadlines, excused absences, partial schedules, and additional academic supports such as class notes or tutoring. Acknowledgement on the part of school personnel that the child or adolescent is coping with a real illness and that they qualify for accommodations often goes a long way towards reducing school-related stress and improving school functioning.

CBT has been found to be very effective at reducing pain and improving functioning in children and adolescents with chronic headache (Ng et al. 2017; Palermo et al. 2010; Trautmann et al. 2006). CBT is also effective at addressing comorbid symptoms that frequently co-occur with headaches in children and adolescents, such as anxiety and depressive symptoms (Rith-Najarian et al. 2019). Furthermore, since CBT involves learning new skills, the benefits are maintained at long-term follow-up (Ng et al. 2017; Kröner-Herwig 2011), unlike medications which stop working when the child stops taking them. Combining CBT with a preventive medication provides a greater reduction in headache days and overall disability than preventive medication and headache education alone (Powers et al. 2013).

Biofeedback

Biofeedback involves using technology to get information about the body and using that information to improve functioning. A scale is an example of biofeedback with which most people are familiar. The number on the scale provides a person's weight, and based on that number the person can alter their diet or activity level to increase or decrease their weight. In the case of chronic headaches, biofeedback is used to assess different aspects of the physiological stress response which may be activated due to pain or stress, such as muscle tension, heart rate, breathing rate, and blood pressure. These physiological responses can intensify pain when activated, so reducing them helps decrease pain and increase subjective feelings of control.

During treatment with biofeedback, noninvasive sensors are used to assess various aspects of the physiological stress response. This information is read into a computer program that allows the patient to see how their body is functioning in the moment. Relaxation strategies can then be practiced with immediate feedback about how the body is responding. Graphs, pictures, and sounds are used to show changes in physiological responses during relaxation training. EMG biofeedback to reduce muscle tension in the forehead, neck, and upper back has been found to be particularly helpful for TTH (Grazzi et al. 2001), but is also beneficial for migraine prevention. Thermal biofeedback, which involves using relaxation and imagery to increase hand temperature, has been found to be effective for reducing migraine frequency (Scharff et al. 2002). Biofeedback can improve buy-in and effectiveness of relaxation strategies, as there is clear feedback that the strategies are resulting in the desired reduction in physiological arousal. Biofeedback was found to be an effective treatment for reducing the frequency of headaches in a pediatric headache clinic (Blume et al. 2012). Results of a recent meta-analysis of randomized-controlled trials showed that biofeedback can reduce the frequency, duration, and intensity of migraine episodes in children and adolescents, although more research is needed to confirm these findings (Stubberud et al. 2016).

Lifestyle and Other Complementary Interventions

Lifestyle factors can be very important to address in children and adolescents with chronic headache. It is essential that they maintain a healthy diet with excellent hydration. A consistent sleep schedule is also crucial to headache management. Regular physical activity is also an important component of headache treatment. Daily habits that promote health and well-being can be discussed in medical visits and targeted in CBT. When patients are severely deconditioned and disabled, physical therapy may be necessary to guide physical rehabilitation. Additional complementary interventions that can be helpful for headache management include aromatherapy (e.g., lavender, jasmine, peppermint), acupressure (pressure points between the eyes at just above the bridge of the nose and on the webbing between the thumb and pointer finger), and acupuncture.

Case Example 2: Sarah L[4]

Sarah is a 14-year-old girl with a history of chronic migraine without aura and anxiety. She uses mostly avoidant coping strategies to manage her headaches and anxiety, and therefore has missed a significant amount of school. She is temperamentally inhibited and worries about pleasing other people. She has very high standards for herself and will only engage in an activity if she can perform very well; otherwise, she will opt out. She struggles to keep up in school because she often misses school when she has a severe headache, and she has difficulty concentrating and paying attention in school when she is able to attend. Her mother is a homemaker who will do anything to help Sarah feel better; she often allows her to stay home from school to rest and buys her gifts, such as books and games, to help her cope with her pain. Her father works long hours to support the family and is rarely home or available. There is an older sister with chronic joint pain who also struggles with school. Sarah has several friends, but she is not able to see them often, and she feels "out of the loop" with them. They rarely contact her to make plans anymore because she usually doesn't feel well enough to join them, and when she is feeling better she doesn't feel comfortable contacting them because she is worried they will question her headaches.

[4]Identifying information has been changed to protect patient identity.

Following a multidisciplinary headache evaluation, CBT was initiated to treat Sarah's chronic headaches, anxiety, and disability. She and her mom were educated about the difference between an acute headache and a chronic headache disorder, the biopsychosocial model of chronic pain, and the process of pain rehabilitation. Sarah's rigid, perfectionistic beliefs about herself were challenged and modified. She gradually learned to think about her health and her performance in a more flexible way. She was taught relaxation strategies and did thermal and EMG biofeedback to increase her ability to actively cope with her headaches. The role of school stress in perpetuating her headaches was identified, and a 504 plan was established to provide flexibility and support in the school setting. With time, she and her mom became aware of the escalating cycle of headache pain, school absences, school stress, and increased pain, and were willing to work hard to interrupt the cycle. Sarah was taught to use the behavioral and cognitive skills she learned in treatment to manage her pain and anxiety in order to attend school more regularly. Her school stress gradually decreased with more consistent attendance. Structured guidance, role plays, and reinforcement were also used to help her re-engage in peer relationships. Fortunately, her friends were supportive of her efforts to reconnect and welcomed her back into their lives. She was more motivated to remain in school because of her improved peer relationships. Last, mom was educated about the impact of her reactions to Sarah's headaches and was given alternative responses that allowed her to feel nurturing while also supporting Sarah's active coping and adaptive functioning. Sarah's headaches became much less frequent and her functioning improved substantially through treatment.

Brief Conclusion

Chronic headache, including migraine and tension-type headache, is extremely common in children and adolescents and can have a negative impact on emotional adjustment and daily functioning. The biopsychosocial model describes the combination of biological, psychological, and social factors that are involved in the development and maintenance of chronic headaches. Chronic headache and associated functional disability often require a multidisciplinary treatment approach, including both medication and psychological treatment. Medications can be helpful for treating headache episodes or preventing headaches in some patients. Psychological interventions such as relaxation training, cognitive-behavioral therapy, and biofeedback are also effective at reducing headache intensity and frequency and improving functioning. The cognitive and behavioral strategies learned in psychological treatment are excellent life skills that can be used to manage headaches and other psychosocial stressors that the child or adolescent may encounter during their lives.

References

Abu-Arafeh, I., Razak, S., Sivaraman, B., & Graham, C. (2010). Prevalence of headache and migraine in children and adolescents: A systematic review of population-based studies. *Developmental Medicine & Child Neurology, 52*(12), 1088–1097. https://doi.org/10.1111/j.1469-8749.2010.03793.x.

Andrasik, F., Buse, D. C., & Lettich, A. (2011). Assessment of headaches. In D. C. Turk, R. Melzack, D. C. Turk, & R. Melzack (Eds.), *Handbook of pain assessment* (pp. 354–375). New York: Guilford Press.

Barlow, K. M., Crawford, S., Stevenson, A., Sandhu, S. S., Belanger, F., & Dewey, D. (2010). Epidemiology of postconcussion syndrome in pediatric mild traumatic brain injury. *Pediatrics, 126*(2), e374–e381. https://doi.org/10.1542/peds.2009-0925.

Blume, H. K. (2012). Pediatric headache: A review. *Pediatrics in Review, 33*(12), 562–576.

Blume, H. K., Brockman, L. N., & Breuner, C. C. (2012). Biofeedback therapy for pediatric headache: Factors associated with response. *Headache: The Journal of Head and Face Pain, 52*(9), 1377–1386. https://doi.org/10.1111/j.1526-4610.2012.02215.x.

Buse, D. C., Loder, E. W., Gorman, J. A., Stewart, W. F., Reed, M. L., Fanning, K. M., et al. (2013). Sex differences in the prevalence, symptoms, and associated features of migraine, probable migraine and other severe headache: Results of the American Migraine Prevalence and Prevention (AMPP) study. *Headache: The Journal of Head and Face Pain, 53*(8), 1278–1299. https://doi.org/10.1111/head.12150.

Castillo, J., Muñoz, P., Guitera, V., & Pascual, J. (1999). Kaplan Award 1998. Epidemiology of chronic daily headache in the general population. *Headache, 39*, 190–196.

Claar, R. L., Simons, L. E., & Logan, D. E. (2008). Parental response to children's pain: The moderating impact of children's emotional distress on symptoms and disability. *Pain, 138*(1), 172–179.

Eccleston, C., Crombez, G., Scotford, A., Clinch, J., & Connell, H. (2004). Adolescent chronic pain: Patterns and predictors of emotional distress in adolescents with chronic pain and their parents. *Pain, 108*(3), 221–229.

Eidlitz-Markus, T., & Zeharia, A. (2017). Symptoms and clinical parameters of pediatric and adolescent migraine, by gender—A retrospective cohort study. *The Journal of Headache and Pain, 18*, 80.

Fales, J. L., Rice, S., Aaron, R. V., & Palermo, T. M. (2018). Traditional and cyber-victimization among adolescents with and without chronic pain. *Health Psychology, 37*(3), 291–300. https://doi.org/10.1037/hea0000569.

Forgeron, P. A., King, S., Stinson, J. N., McGrath, P. J., MacDonald, A. J., & Chambers, C. T. (2010). Social functioning and peer relationships in children and adolescents with chronic pain: A systematic review. *Pain Research & Management, 15*, 27–41. https://doi.org/10.1155/2010/820407.

Giza, C. C., Kutcher, J. S., Ashwal, S., et al. (2013). Summary of evidence-based guideline update: Evaluation and management of concussion in sports: Report of the Guideline Development Subcommittee of the American Academy of Neurology. *Neurology, 80*, 2250–2257.

Gómez, J. E., & Hergenroeder, A. C. (2013). New guidelines for management of concussion in sport: Special concern for youth. *Journal of Adolescent Health, 53*(3), 311–313. https://doi.org/10.1016/j.jadohealth.2013.06.018.

Grazzi, L., Andrasik, F., D'Amico, D., Leone, M., Moschiano, F., & Bussone, G. (2001). Electromyographic biofeedback-assisted relaxation training in juvenile episodic tension-type headache: Clinical outcome at three-year follow-up. *Cephalalgia, 21*(8), 798–803. https://doi.org/10.1046/j.1468-2982.2001.218193.x.

Herge, W. M., La Greca, A. M., & Chan, S. F. (2016). Adolescent peer victimization and physical health problems. *Journal of Pediatric Psychology, 41*, 15–27. https://doi.org/10.1093/jpepsy/jsv050.

Hershey, A. D. (2010). Current approaches to the diagnosis and management of paediatric migraine. *The Lancet Neurology, 9*, 190–204.

Heyer, G. L., Rose, S. C., Merison, K., Perkins, S. Q., & Lee, J. E. M. (2014). Specific headache factors predict sleep disturbances among youth with migraine. *Pediatric Neurology, 51*(4), 489–493.

Houle, T. T., Butschek, R. A., Turner, D. P., Smitherman, T. A., Rains, J. C., & Penzien, D. B. (2012). Stress and sleep duration predict headache severity in chronic headache sufferers. *Pain®, 153*(12), 2432–2440.

International Headache Society. (2018). Headache Classification Committee of the International Headache Society (IHS). The International Classification of Headache Disorders. *Cephalalgia, 38*(1), 1–211.

Isensee, C., Fernandez Castelao, C., & Kröner-Herwig, B. (2016). Developmental trajectories of paediatric headache—Sex-specific analyses and predictors. *The Journal of Headache and Pain, 17*, 32.

Kaczynski, K. J., Claar, R. L., & Logan, D. E. (2009). Testing gender as a moderator of associations between psychosocial variables and functional disability in children and adolescents with chronic pain. *Journal of Pediatric Psychology, 34*(7), 738–748.

Kedia, S., Ginde, A. A., Grubenhoff, J. A., Kempe, A., Hershey, A. D., & Powers, S. W. (2014). Monthly variation of United States pediatric headache emergency department visits. *Cephalalgia, 34*(6), 473–478. https://doi.org/10.1177/0333102413515346.

Kowalski, R. M., & Limber, S. P. (2013). Psychological, physical, and academic correlates of cyberbullying and traditional bullying. *Journal of Adolescent Health, 53*(1 Suppl), S13–S20. https://doi.org/10.1016/j.jadohealth.2012.09.018.

Kröner-Herwig, B. (2011). Psychological treatments for pediatric headache. *Expert Review of Neurotherapeutics, 11*(3), 403–410. https://doi.org/10.1586/ern.11.10.

Lateef, T. M., Merikangas, K. R., He, J., Kalaydjian, A., Khoromi, S., Knight, E., et al. (2009). Headache in a national sample of American children: Prevalence and comorbidity. *Journal of Child Neurology, 24*(5), 536–543.

Laurell, K., Larsson, B., & Eeg-Olofsson, O. (2005). Headache in schoolchildren: Association with other pain, family history and psychosocial factors. *Pain, 119*(1), 150–158.

Law, E. F., Beals-Erickson, S. E., Fisher, E., Lang, E. A., & Palermo, T. M. (2017). Components of effective cognitive-behavioral therapy for pediatric headache: A mixed methods approach. *Clinical Practice in Pediatric Psychology, 5*(4), 376–391. https://doi.org/10.1037/cpp0000216.

Lewis, D. W., Winner, P., Hershey, A. D., & Wasiewski, W. W. (2007). Efficacy of zolmitriptan nasal spray in adolescent migraine. *Pediatrics, 120*(2), 390–396. https://doi.org/10.1542/peds.2007-0085.

Li, D., & Rozen, T. D. (2002, February). The clinical characteristics of new daily persistent headache. *Cephalalgia, 22*(1), 66–69.

Logan, D. E., Claar, R. L., & Scharff, L. (2008). Social desirability response bias and self-report of psychological distress in pediatric chronic pain patients. *Pain, 136*(3), 366–372. https://doi.org/10.1016/j.pain.2007.07.015.

Luntamo, T., Sourander, A., Rihko, M., Aromaa, M., Helenius, H., Koskelainen, M., et al. (2012). Psychosocial determinants of headache, abdominal pain, and sleep problems in a community sample of Finnish adolescents. *European Child & Adolescent Psychiatry, 21*(6), 301–313.

Mack, K. J. (2004, August). What incites new daily persistent headache in children? *Pediatr Neurol, 31*(2), 122–125.

Mindell, J. A., & Owens, J. A. (2015). *A clinical guide to pediatric sleep: Diagnosis and management of sleep problems*. Philadelphia: Lippincott Williams & Wilkins.

Ng, Q. X., Venkatanarayanan, N., & Kumar, L. (2017). A systematic review and meta-analysis of the efficacy of cognitive behavioral therapy for the management of pediatric migraine. *Headache: The Journal of Head and Face Pain, 57*(3), 349–362. https://doi.org/10.1111/head.13016.

Pakalnis, A., Butz, C., Splaingard, D., Kring, D., & Fong, J. (2007). Emotional problems and prevalence of medication overuse in pediatric chronic daily headache. *Journal of Child Neurology, 22*(12), 1356–1359. https://doi.org/10.1177/0883073807307090.

Palermo, T. M., & Chambers, C. T. (2005). Parent and family factors in pediatric chronic pain and disability: An integrative approach. *Pain, 119*(1), 1–4.

Palermo, T. M., Eccleston, C., Lewandowski, A. S., Williams, A. C., & Morley, S. (2010). Randomized controlled trials of psychological therapies for management of chronic pain in children and adolescents: An updated meta-analytic review. *Pain, 148*(3), 387–397. https://doi.org/10.1016/j.pain.2009.10.004.

Penzien, D. B., & Taylor, F. R. (2014). Behavioral and other nonpharmacologic treatments for headache. *Headache: The Journal of Head and Face Pain, 54*(5), 955–956. https://doi.org/10.1111/head.12369.

Perquin, C. W., Hazebroek-Kampschreur, A. A., Hunfeld, J. A., Bohnen, A. M., van Suijlekom-Smit, L. W., Passchier, J., et al. (2000). Pain in children and adolescents: A common experience. *Pain, 87*(1), 51–58.

Powers, S. W., Patton, S. R., Hommel, K. A., & Hershey, A. D. (2003). Quality of life in childhood migraines: Clinical impact and comparison to other chronic illnesses. *Pediatrics, 112*(1), e1–e5.

Powers, S. W., Gilman, D. K., & Hershey, A. D. (2006). Headache and psychological functioning in children and adolescents. *Headache, 46*(9), 1404–1415.

Powers, S. W., Kashikar-Zuck, S. M., Allen, J. R., LeCates, S. L., Slater, S. K., Zafar, M., et al. (2013). Cognitive behavioral therapy plus amitriptyline for chronic migraine in children and adolescents: A randomized clinical trial. *JAMA, 310*(24), 2622–2630. https://doi.org/10.1001/jama.2013.282533.

Powers, S. W., Coffey, C. S., Chamberlin, L. A., Ecklund, D. J., Klingner, E. A., Yankey, J. W., et al. (2017). Trial of amitriptyline, topiramate, and placebo for pediatric migraine. *New England Journal of Medicine, 376*, 115–124. https://doi.org/10.1056/NEJMoa1610384.

Rabner, J., Kaczynski, K., Simons, L., & Lebel, A. (2017). Pediatric headache and sleep disturbance: A comparison of diagnostic groups. *Headache: The Journal of Head and Face Pain, 58*(2), 217–228.

Randall, E. T., Smith, K. R., Kronman, C. A., Conroy, C., Smith, A. M., & Simons, L. E. (2018). Feeling the pressure to be perfect: Effect on pain-related distress and dysfunction in youth with chronic pain. *The Journal of Pain, 19*(4), 418–429. https://doi.org/10.1016/j.jpain.2017.11.012.

Rith-Najarian, L. R., Mesri, B., Park, A. L., Sun, M., Chavira, D. A., & Chorpita, B. F. (2019). Durability of cognitive behavioral therapy effects for youth and adolescents with anxiety, depression, or traumatic stress: A meta-analysis on long-term follow-ups. *Behavior Therapy, 50*(1), 225–240. https://doi.org/10.1016/j.beth.2018.05.006.

Rousseau-Salvador, C., Amouroux, R., Annequin, D., Salvador, A., Tourniaire, B., & Rusinek, S. (2014). Anxiety, depression and school absenteeism in youth with chronic or episodic headache. *Pain Research & Management, 19*(5), 235–240. https://doi.org/10.1155/2014/541618.

Scharff, L., Marcus, D. A., & Masek, B. J. (2002). A controlled study of minimal-contact thermal biofeedback treatment in children with migraine. *Journal of Pediatric Psychology, 27*(2), 109–119. https://doi.org/10.1093/jpepsy/27.2.109.

Sieberg, C. B., & Manganella, J. (2015). Family beliefs and interventions in pediatric pain management. *Child and Adolescent Psychiatric Clinics of North America, 24*(3), 631–645. https://doi.org/10.1016/j.chc.2015.02.006.

Sieberg, C. B., Huguet, A., von Baeyer, C. L., & Seshia, S. S. (2012). Psychological interventions for headache in children and adolescents. *The Canadian Journal of Neurological Sciences, 39*(1), 26–34. https://doi.org/10.1017/S0317167100012646.

Slater, S. K., Kashikar-Zuck, S. M., Allen, J. R., LeCates, S. L., Kabbouche, M. A., O'Brien, H. L., et al. (2012). Psychiatric comorbidity in pediatric chronic daily headache. *Cephalalgia, 32*(15), 1116–1122. https://doi.org/10.1177/0333102412460776.

Soee, A. L., Skov, L., Skovgaard, L. T., & Thomsen, L. L. (2013). Headache in children: Effectiveness of multidisciplinary treatment in a tertiary paediatric headache clinic. *Cephalalgia, 33*(15), 1218–1228. https://doi.org/10.1177/0333102413490349.

Stubberud, A., Varkey, E., McCrory, D. C., Pedersen, S. A., & Linde, M. (2016). Biofeedback as prophylaxis for pediatric migraine: A meta-analysis. *Pediatrics, 138*(2), 1–13. https://doi.org/10.1542/peds.2016-0675.

Trautmann, E., Lackschewitz, H., & Kröner-Herwig, B. (2006). Psychological treatment of recurrent headache in children and adolescents—A meta-analysis. *Cephalalgia, 26*(12), 1411–1426. https://doi.org/10.1111/j.1468-2982.2006.01226.x.

Tyagi, A. (2012). New daily persistent headache. *Annals of Indian Academy of Neurology, 15*(Suppl. 1), S62–S65. https://doi.org/10.4103/0972-2327.100011.

Veliz, P., McCabe, S. E., Eckner, J. T., & Schulenberg, J. E. (2017). Prevalence of concussion among US adolescents and correlated factors. *Journal of the American Medical Association, 318*(12), 1180–1182.

Vos, T., Flaxman, A. D., Naghavi, M., Lozano, R., Michaud, C., Ezzati, M., et al. (2012). Years lived with disability (YLDs) for 1160 sequelae of 289 diseases and injuries 1990–2010: A systematic analysis for the Global Burden of Disease Study 2010. *The Lancet, 380*(9859), 2163–2196. https://doi.org/10.1016/S0140-6736(12)61729-2.

Wager, J., Zernikow, B., Darlington, A., Vocks, S., & Hechler, T. (2014). Identifying subgroups of paediatric chronic pain patients: A cluster-analytic approach. *European Journal of Pain, 18*(9), 1352–1362. https://doi.org/10.1002/j.1532-2149.2014.497.x.

Welkom, J. S., Hwang, W. T., & Guite, J. W. (2013). Adolescent pain catastrophizing mediates the relationship between protective parental responses to pain and disability over time. *Journal of Pediatric Psychology, 38*(5), 541–550.

Wilne, S. H., Ferris, R. C., Nathwani, A., & Kennedy, C. R. (2006). The presenting features of brain tumours: A review of 200 cases. *Archives of Disease in Childhood, 91*(6), 502–506.

Winner, P., Pearlman, E. M., Linder, S. L., Jordan, D. M., Fisher, A. C., & Hulihan, J. (2005). Topiramate for migraine prevention in children: A randomized, double-blind, placebo-controlled trial. *Headache: The Journal of Head and Face Pain, 45*(10), 1304–1312. https://doi.org/10.1111/j.1526-4610.2005.00262.x.

Wojtowicz, A. A., & Banez, G. A. (2015). Adolescents with chronic pain and associated functional disability: A descriptive analysis. *Journal of Child Health Care, 19*(4), 478–484. https://doi.org/10.1177/1367493514523157.

Cognitive Behavioral Treatment for Pediatric Sleep Difficulties

18

Karla K. Fehr, Danielle Chambers, and Jennifer Ramasami

Introduction

Approximately 20–40% of children and adolescents experience difficulties with sleep that impact the daily functioning of the child and the child's family (Bruni et al. 2004; Meltzer et al. 2014). While it is known that sleep is an essential biological process, the purpose of sleep is widely debated. Sleep may be a time for the nervous system to rest (Zepelin and Rechtschaffen 1974), a time for the body to repair and restore energy lost during wakefulness (Vanderkerckhove and Cluydts 2010), and/or a time for synaptic plasticity and brain development to occur (Frank and Cantera 2014). Each of these theories highlights the importance of obtaining sufficient sleep.

Boerner et al. (2015) surveyed 46 sleep experts and concluded that being knowledgeable about healthy sleep habits is a core competency required for practitioners who treat children and adolescents with sleep difficulties. For example, providers addressing children's sleep should be knowledgeable about appropriate amounts of sleep and common sleep difficulties at each developmental phase. Infants (age 0–12 months) should obtain 12–17 h of sleep per day (National Sleep Foundation 2015). Common sleep problems during this age include difficulties initiating and maintaining sleep independently and returning to sleep following night wakings (Meltzer and Crabtree 2015). Children from age 1 to 2 years should receive 11–14 h of sleep daily, and children ages 3–5 should receive 10–13 h of sleep in a 24-h period (National Sleep Foundation 2015). During this early childhood stage, frequency of napping decreases with only 25% of children napping at age 5 (Meltzer and Crabtree 2015). Increased desire for independence and increasingly complex cognitive abilities contribute to increases in nighttime fears, night wakings, and bedtime resistance in preschool-aged children (Byars and Simon 2016; Owens 2001; Sadeh et al. 2009). It is recommended that school-age children (age 6–13 years) obtain 9–11 h of sleep per night (National Sleep Foundation 2015). Circadian rhythm preferences begin to emerge at this age. Children who are "night owls" are less likely to get a sufficient amount of sleep due to the combination of staying up late and waking up early for school (Minges and Redeker 2016). Cognitive abilities also continue to develop, contributing to increased nighttime fears and difficulty initiating sleep (Meltzer and Crabtree 2015). Last, adolescents should obtain 8–10 h of sleep per night (National Sleep Foundation 2015).

All cases in this chapter are confabulated.

K. K. Fehr (✉) · D. Chambers · J. Ramasami
Department of Psychology, Southern Illinois University, Carbondale, IL, USA
e-mail: Kfehr@siu.edu

Insufficient sleep is the most common problem in this age group with most adolescents averaging 7.5 h of sleep per night (Moore 2012; National Sleep Foundation 2004). Providers addressing children's sleep should also be knowledgeable about circadian rhythms, cultural influences on sleep, homeostatic processes, and sleep–wake regulation (Boerner et al. 2015). For additional description of healthy sleep habits and sleep processes, see Meltzer and Crabtree (2015) or Mindell and Owens (2015).

Research has shown that sleep difficulties are related to a plethora of negative outcomes. Such effects can be seen as early as infancy with sleep difficulties related to delays in learning to crawl and walk (Scher 2005). Sleep difficulties have been associated with higher rates of behavior problems in children and adolescents (e.g., Bélanger et al. 2018; Gruber et al. 2012). Insufficient sleep is also related to emotion regulation and internalizing difficulties such as irritability and depression (e.g., Meltzer and Mindell 2014). Studies have shown that adolescents express less positive affect and more negative affect after getting 2–6 h of sleep rather than the recommended 8 h of sleep (Kahn et al. 2014; Talbot et al. 2010). Sleep difficulties are also associated with academic difficulties, lower school attendance, impaired memory, and decreased executive functioning (e.g., Astill et al. 2012; Gruber et al. 2012). Further, sleep difficulties can have a negative impact on one's health. Studies have shown that insufficient sleep increases the risk for hypertension, diabetes, obesity, and decreased overall immune system functioning (Bhushan et al. 2014; Lange and Born 2011).

Sleep problems are persistent through childhood and adolescence and typically do not resolve with age, making treatment for such difficulties essential (Kataria et al. 1987). Although research has shown that medication is the most common treatment for pediatric sleep difficulties (Goodday et al. 2014), there are no medications approved by the Food and Drug Administration for treating sleep difficulties in children (Owens et al. 2003; Stojanovski et al. 2007). However, substantial empirical support has been found for a variety of behavioral and cognitive-behavioral strategies, which will be discussed further in this chapter.

Biopsychosocial Conceptualization of Treatment

James is a 4-year-old boy who recently started preschool, which is the first time he received caregiving outside the home. Since starting school, he has been resistant to going to bed. In particular, he argues with each step of the bedtime routine to delay bedtime. When he is finally in bed, he continues to come out of his room to make requests such as another drink, a snack, another story, or to be tucked in until one of his parents lie down with him while he falls asleep. He also wakes multiple times per night and eventually falls asleep by getting in bed with his parents. Due to difficulties falling asleep and multiple night wakings, he is getting significantly less sleep than usual. His parents wonder if there is anything they can do to help him but don't want to give him medication and don't mention it to his pediatrician. They hope this is a phase that he will outgrow.

In order to receive treatment, a child must be identified as having abnormal or problematic sleep habits. It has been estimated that 12–15% of children have unidentified sleep difficulties (National Institute of Health 2001). Research on parent knowledge about healthy sleep habits has found that parents respond correctly to approximately 30–45% of questions (Schreck and Richdale 2011; Owens and Jones 2011; Owens et al. 2011), suggesting that there may be gaps in parents' knowledge about what healthy sleep habits are in childhood. Higher knowledge about childhood sleep corresponds with positive sleep habits (Owens et al. 2011). Mindell and Owens (2010) proposed that napping, persistent daytime sleepiness, and behavioral signs of sleepiness reported by parents or teachers could indicate sleep difficulties in school-aged children. Declines in school or work performance, use of alertness-promoting agents, increased risk-taking behaviors, and sleeping in on the weekends (i.e., shift in weekday to weekend sleep duration) may be symptoms of problematic sleep in adolescents (see Mindell and Owens 2015).

Even when parents recognize that their child has difficulties with sleep, there still may be barriers to seeking treatment. In some cases, parents may endorse symptoms of sleep difficulties, but they may not feel that their child has a sleep problem. In a sample of children with intellectual disabilities, approximately 63% of parents endorsed symptoms of sleep difficulties but only 27% endorsed that their child had a sleep problem (Robinson and Richdale 2004). Other parents may identify concerns with their child's sleep, but that may not translate to seeking treatment. In a national study of parents, 62% of parents who endorsed that their child had difficulties with their sleep had not spoken with anyone about their concerns (Fehr 2015). Further, very few parents were aware of behavioral or cognitive-behavioral treatment options to improve childhood sleep (Fehr 2015). Thus, additional assessment and education may be needed to assist parents with identifying when their child's sleep could benefit from intervention and the empirically supported treatment options.

Formal sleep assessment may be needed to determine the nature of the sleep difficulty and rule out medical sleep disorders (see Mindell and Owens 2015, for further information). Sleep assessments as part of behavioral or cognitive-behavioral treatment often include sleep diaries, in which parents monitor children's daily sleep habits. Sleep diaries can be particularly helpful to determine sleep patterns as well as monitor treatment progress. In addition, a variety of questionnaires have been validated to assess self- and parent-report of sleep habits and daytime sleepiness (see Lewandowski et al. 2011, for review).

A variety of factors can contribute to sleep difficulties in youth, including behavioral factors and biological processes. Regardless of the cause, the first-line treatments for difficulties with sleep initiation and maintenance are primarily behavioral in nature. These sleep difficulties, including behavioral insomnia of childhood and delayed sleep–wake phase disorder, are the focus of this chapter. Other sleep disorders, including those with a primarily biological cause, can also benefit from behavioral and/or cognitive-behavioral intervention to optimize the medical treatment and/or improve functional outcomes. Although not the primary focus of this chapter, behavioral and cognitive-behavioral treatment components for parasomnias, obstructive sleep apnea, and narcolepsy are briefly reviewed below. It is important to note that even in cases of sleep disorders with medical etiology, behavioral sleep difficulties commonly co-occur. Further, clinicians working with families with behavioral sleep difficulties must be aware of the symptoms of these disorders to ensure that appropriate referrals are made when medical sleep disorders must be ruled out (see Meltzer and Crabtree 2015, for further information on these disorders as well as restless-legs syndrome, periodic limb movement disorder, and sleep-related rhythmic movement disorder).

Behavioral Insomnia of Childhood

Behavioral insomnia of childhood (BIC) is the most common sleep problem children experience and involves difficulties with bedtime compliance, sleep initiation, and sleep maintenance (American Academy of Sleep Medicine 2014). The two main factors that impact a child's ability to initiate sleep are sleep-onset associations and parental limit setting. Difficulties with sleep initiation and maintenance can be caused by either of these independently or in combination.

Sleep-Onset Associations Sleep-onset associations are formed by pairing environmental cues with sleep initiation. The more consistent the pairings, the stronger the associations will be. Sleep-onset associations can be helpful with sleep initiation. For example, a child with a strong sleep-onset association may get drowsy when placed in bed. Sleep-onset associations can interfere with falling asleep if the paired stimuli are not present. For instance, if a child is used to sleeping on the couch, being rocked to sleep, or lying down with a parent, they would likely have difficulty falling asleep if placed in their bed. Negative sleep-onset associations are important to consider if a child is having difficulty with frequent and/or prolonged night wakings. Sleep-onset associations require that the same environment be present during night wakings as at bedtime in order to initiate sleep. Thus, they can impact a child's ability to fall asleep after night wakings, including those that occur naturally with each sleep cycle (e.g., Mindell and Owens 2015). Similarly, if a child's sleep environment is variable, it may be more difficult for him or her to initiate sleep as a strong environmental cue has likely not been developed. Sleep-onset associations include all the cues present at sleep onset. In addition to the physical sleeping environment, this includes having a special blanket or stuffed animal and whether music or other sounds are playing. It is important for parents to be thoughtful about these cues. They can be helpful in cases where the physical environment cannot be kept consistent (e.g., offering the same blanket when traveling) or during night wakings (e.g., choosing a fan or white noise machine that runs throughout the night over music that plays only until the child falls asleep).

Limit Setting The limit setting subtype of BIC involves situations where there are inadequate or inconsistent parental limits that result in the child resisting going to bed, which can subsequently impede the child's ability to fall asleep at the appropriate time to obtain sufficient total sleep time. Bedtime resistance is the most common sleep problem in school-aged children (Blader et al. 1997) and can involve attempts to stall at bedtime, "curtain calls" (i.e., coming out of the room after being put to bed to make additional requests such as a drink or to be tucked in again), or bedtime refusal (for further information, see Mindell and Owens 2015). In addition to avoiding bedtime, these behaviors are often aimed at gaining parental attention. However, this should be considered as there could be other explanations for the child avoiding bedtime (e.g., hunger, anxiety) that may need to be addressed. It is also possible that the child is not tired yet due to a delayed circadian rhythm (e.g., Meltzer and Crabtree 2015), especially if the bedtime resistance is habitual or if there is an early bedtime that does not align with age-appropriate expectations for sleep duration.

Parents may have difficulties setting or enforcing limits at bedtime and/or during night wakings for a variety of reasons. Environmental factors, such as when a child shares a room, can also play a role in parents' responses to bedtime resistance (see Mindell and Owens 2015, for review of additional factors that may impact parent limit setting at bedtime). It can be distressing for the child when a parent attempts to set limits and requires the child be independent at night. Furthermore, parents report a high degree of stress when having to manage their child's crying and protests at bedtime (e.g., Adams and Rickert 1989). Nighttime fears and separation anxiety are common in young children, and this can be a challenge for parents to manage at bedtime. Understanding and addressing the reasons for parent limit setting difficulties is often an important treatment component.

Although in James' case it is possible that his sleep difficulties could be transient and related to adjustment to formal schooling, a number of behaviors put him at risk for continued bedtime difficulties. Once these behavioral patterns are established, they typically do not resolve spontaneously. In regard to sleep-onset associations, James appears to be developing a sleep-onset association with parental presence as he is only able to fall asleep when they lay down with him or when he gets in bed with them. Further, moving to his parents' bed in the middle of the night likely decreases the association he has with his own bed. In regards to parent limit setting, it appears that his parents are struggling to set limits at bedtime due to difficulties seeing him upset and worry that if they don't lay down with him he will receive even less sleep. The assessment further indicates that both parents have returned to work full time this year after having at least one of them at home with James and that they are experiencing some guilt regarding not being available to spend as much time with him during the day.

Delayed Sleep–Wake Phase Disorder

Chloe (age 16) presents for treatment of "insomnia." She reports that she regularly is unable to fall asleep until 2 am. She participates in sports and must wake at 6 am for practice before school, though she often oversleeps and is late. She reports that she is so tired that she takes a 2-h nap after school before starting her homework, which she often does not complete until midnight or 1 am. On the weekends, she also stays up until approximately 2 am watching movies. However, she is able to fall asleep quickly at that time and can feel rested the next day after sleeping in until noon or later.

Delayed sleep–wake phase disorder occurs when the circadian rhythm is shifted such that children receive an age-appropriate amount of sleep but at a time later than when they or their caregivers desire (American Academy of Sleep Medicine 2014). Youth with delayed sleep–wake phase disorder typically fall asleep between 2 and 6 am (Mindell and Owens 2015). A delayed schedule may occur inadvertently when sleep onset is regularly delayed, such as when bedtime resistance is common or when homework or other scheduling issues result in a later bedtime. Children with a delayed sleep phase may present with complaints about difficulties with sleep initiation as they may struggle if they attempt to go to bed prior to the time their body is naturally falling asleep. Thus, a comprehensive evaluation of current sleep habits is important for differential diagnosis. Biological processes, including a later circadian rhythm shift, occur naturally in early adolescent development and with the onset of puberty, which may also contribute to a shifted schedule in adolescence (for review, see Owens et al. 2014). Insufficient sleep may occur secondarily when youth are required to wake relatively early for school or other responsibilities.

Parasomnias

Parasomnias are a set of episodic sleep disorders that occur while asleep or during the transition from sleep to partial wakefulness (Sadeh 2005). These include sleepwalking, confusional arousals (characterized by acting in an odd, confused manner when waking up or after waking up), and night terrors (i.e., episodes during which an individual may scream, kick, and experience intense fear while asleep, usually during the slow-wave sleep period), among others. Prevalence rates differ depending on the type of parasomnia. For example, the prevalence rate for occasional sleep walking in children aged 1.5–13 years is approximately 29%, while the prevalence rate for night terrors is around 56% (Petit et al. 2015). Parasomnias that occur on a regular basis appear in approximately 2–6% of the population (Klackenberg 1987; Goodwin et al. 2004). If parasomnias occur infrequently (1–2 times per month), treatment is usually not needed as the occurrence of these disturbances typically decreases over time and likely resolves spontaneously in 1–2 years (Kotagal 2009; Sadeh 2005). Therefore, parental psychoeducation about parasomnias and discussing ways to ensure child safety during episodes may be sufficient. In addition, obtaining adequate sleep is important for children who experience parasomnias, given that insufficient sleep can be a trigger for parasomnias (Kotagal 2009). Thus, improving sleep hygiene and implementing other behavioral techniques that increase sleep duration may prevent or decrease parasomnias, particularly when difficulties with sleep initiation or maintenance are also present (Kotagal 2009; Stores 2009). Scheduled naps may also be considered in younger children to increase the amount of sleep received. If parasomnias begin to negatively impact the child's safety or family functioning, additional behavioral strategies, such as scheduled awakenings (discussed later in this chapter), may be helpful in reducing the occurrence of childhood parasomnias (Sadeh 2005).

Obstructive Sleep Apnea

Obstructive sleep apnea (OSA) is characterized by disordered breathing due to partial upper airway obstructions and/or complete obstructions at irregular intervals during sleep (Epstein et al. 2009). These obstructions of airway passages disrupt breathing and regular sleep patterns. Pediatric OSA affects approximately 2% of children (Marcus et al. 2012). Without treatment for OSA, children commonly suffer from excessive daytime sleepiness, inattention, and hyperactivity (Marcus et al. 2012), possibly due to the impact of regular sleep disruptions and/or reduced intake of oxygen (Bucks et al. 2017). Typically, tonsillectomy and adenoidectomy are the first line of medical treatment for children (Friedman et al. 2009). In a review of the level of effectiveness for these treatments, tonsillectomy and adenoidectomy were found to successfully treat approximately 82.9% of pediatric patients (Brietzke and Gallagher 2006). However, approximately 17% of these children still suffered from pediatric OSA even after these procedures. Another primary treatment for pediatric OSA is continuous positive airway pressure (CPAP). CPAP involves administering low levels of pressure to the respiratory cycle through devices (i.e., face or nasal mask) that provide a continuous stream of compressed air to keep the airways open throughout the night (Alison et al. 2008). When used for treatment of pediatric OSA, it is highly effective (Marcus et al. 2006). However, adherence to CPAP therapy has proven challenging for many children with OSA. Common problems for children include irritation from wearing the CPAP face mask for long periods of time or feeling discomfort due to the constant pressure of air (Sadeh 2005). Further, certain psychosocial factors can also negatively impact youth's level of adherence, such as conditioned anxiety resulting from negative experiences with CPAP equipment, unstable family structure, and lack of CPAP knowledge in youth (Koontz et al. 2003; Prashad et al. 2013). These issues may then impact compliance and adherence rates (Marcus et al. 2006). On average, children's use of CPAP ranges from 3 to 5.3 h each night (Difeo et al. 2012; Marcus et al. 2006). Furthermore, research indicates that only about half of children with OSA immediately adhere to using CPAP; those who do not immediately comply with CPAP use may take anywhere from 9 to 295 days from its introduction to accept CPAP (O'Donnell et al. 2006).

Many behavioral interventions can be implemented to increase adherence rates of CPAP in children and adolescents. These include differential positive reinforcement for adherence approximations, gradual exposure to the mask and/or air pressure, and counter conditioning by systematically pairing an enjoyable, distracting activity, and praise with potentially distressing CPAP equipment (Koontz et al. 2003). Koontz et al. (2003) found that the use of these behavioral interventions for CPAP adherence resulted in significant increases in the tolerance of the CPAP equipment as well as increases in documented hours of usage compared to children who did not receive behavioral intervention. Preliminary evidence for the use of these behavioral interventions with preschool children has also been found (Slifer et al. 2007). Behavioral interventions may be critical to implement in order to effectively increase adherence of CPAP, and ultimately daytime functioning, in children with pediatric OSA.

Narcolepsy

Narcolepsy is a chronic neurological disorder characterized by excessive daytime sleepiness and additional symptoms that may include abrupt loss of muscle tone (cataplexy), sleep paralysis, hypnogogic hallucinations (i.e., sensory events that occur during transition from wakefulness to sleep), and irregular sleep at night (Guilleminault and Pelayo 1998). In children, this most often initially presents as daytime sleepiness (Meltzer and Mindell 2009). Children with narcolepsy have higher rates of behavior and educational problems as well as more depressive symptoms compared to same-aged peers; it has been posited that excessive daytime sleepiness in this population is likely the cause of these difficulties (Stores et al. 2006).

Lifelong treatment for narcolepsy is likely necessary for those with this diagnosis (Guilleminault and Pelayo 2000). Medical treatment includes the use of stimulant medications to reduce daytime sleepiness and sleep episodes (Guilleminault and Pelayo 2000; Meltzer and Mindell 2009). Behavioral interventions are frequently incorporated into treatment to improve functioning such as implementation and maintenance of regular sleep–wake schedules and scheduled daytime naps (Guilleminault and Pelayo 2000; Meltzer and Mindell 2009). Scheduled naps that are approximately 15–20 min in length aid in maintaining alertness throughout the day (Guilleminault and Pelayo 2000). These approaches are used in an effort to reduce the symptoms of narcolepsy and optimize functioning throughout the day.

Description of Treatment Components

Behavioral therapy is the empirically supported treatment for behavioral difficulties with sleep initiation and maintenance (Meltzer and Mindell 2008). The specific treatment implemented will depend on the presenting concern; however, certain treatment components should be present in the treatment of most sleep difficulties. Treatment for children with sleep difficulties should begin by educating parents and the child or adolescent (depending on their age) about healthy sleep hygiene (see below), treatment options, and age-appropriate sleep habits (Meltzer and Crabtree 2015; Moturi and Avis 2010). In fact, parent education has one of the highest levels of research support as it increases families' understanding and commitment to treatment (Byars and Simon 2016; Meltzer and Mindell 2014; Taylor and Roane 2010). In addition to treatment elements that are commonly seen across presenting concerns, there are several treatment options for specific sleep difficulties.

Sleep Hygiene

Sleep hygiene includes increasing sleep promoting behaviors and decreasing sleep interfering behaviors (Moore 2012). Establishment of healthy sleep hygiene corresponds with fewer behavior problems, and the presence of these habits earlier in development increases the likelihood of these habits being present later in development (Stein et al. 2001). Sleep hygiene involves a number of factors. First, the sleeping environment should be cool, dark, and quiet (Moore 2012). Having a strong association between the bed and sleeping is essential. Children and adolescents should only use their bed for sleeping (Meltzer and Crabtree 2015). They should fall asleep in the same place every night and sleep in the location in which they fell asleep throughout the night (Stepanski and Wyatt 2003). When a child wakes up in the middle of the night, they seek out the conditions in which they fell asleep to return to sleep. Therefore, waking up in a different place than where they fell asleep will make returning to sleep difficult (Meltzer and Crabtree 2015). This concept also applies to caregivers who choose to co-sleep. In a large study of cross-cultural sleep habits in children from birth to 36 months of age, only 23% of parents reported that their child initiated sleep independently (Mindell et al. 2010). If caregivers choose to sleep with their child, they should consider doing so all night rather than for just a portion of the night to maintain consistent sleeping conditions (Ramos et al. 2007).

Additionally, children and adolescents should avoid stimulation before bed including caffeine, exercise, and electronic devices (Moore 2012). Such stimuli interfere with one's ability to fall asleep and return to sleep following night wakings (Calamaro et al. 2009; Moore 2012). Caffeine intake should be avoided or limited for children; however, it is especially important that they do not consume caffeine in the 3–7 h before bed as the effects of caffeine can last this long (see Arnaud 1987, and Meltzer and Crabtree 2015, for reviews). Further, using electronic devices at bedtime can delay sleep onset as the light emitted from these devices can suppress melatonin secretion and make it difficult for children to fall asleep (Green et al. 2017).

Another important element of healthy sleep hygiene is setting consistent sleep and wake times. These times should not fluctuate more than 1–2 h on the weekends (Meltzer and Crabtree 2015). It is recommended that children up to 12 years of age go to bed before 9:00 pm (Meltzer and Crabtree 2015) as problematic daytime behaviors are more common among children with later bedtimes (Yokomaku et al. 2008). The bedtime of adolescents depends on the time that they have to wake in the morning to ensure that they are getting a sufficient amount of sleep (Meltzer and Crabtree 2015).

Bedtime Routines

Another element of healthy sleep habits that should be incorporated into treatment for most sleep difficulties is a consistent bedtime routine. Children who have consistent bedtime routines tend to have earlier bedtimes, fall asleep more quickly, have fewer night wakings, and have increased sleep duration (Koulouglioti et al. 2014; Meltzer and Mindell 2014; Mindell et al. 2015). An early establishment of a bedtime routine is correlated with having a bedtime routine later in childhood (Mindell et al. 2015). Bedtime routines should consist of 3–5 simple steps and end in the child's bedroom (Meltzer and Crabtree 2015; Mindell et al. 2015). For younger children, charts or picture schedules may be helpful for remembering the steps of the routine (Meltzer and Crabtree 2015).

Extinction

Extinction is a commonly used behavioral treatment approach for children who present with bedtime resistance or behavioral insomnia of childhood-sleep-onset association type (Byars and Simon 2016). This approach is based on the theory that certain sleep problems are perpetuated by inappropriate parental attention or inappropriate sleep-onset associations (Meltzer and Crabtree 2015). Standard extinction involves completely ignoring all protests after the child is put to bed. If the child leaves his or her room, the caregiver guides the child back to his or her room while minimizing physical contact and verbal interactions. This technique has been shown to decrease bedtime resistance, sleep-onset latency, and night wakings (Kuhn and Elliott 2003; Mindell 1999; Taylor and Roane 2010).

While standard extinction is effective quickly if carried out consistently, some parents report fearing that it is harmful to their child and they have difficulty not responding to their crying child (Rickert and Johnson 1988). While no long-term negative effects of standard extinction have been found (Byars and Simon 2016; Price et al. 2012), graduated extinction is a technique that parents may be more comfortable with. Graduated extinction involves gradually decreasing parental presence at bedtime (Byars and Simon 2016). One way to implement this technique is by gradually moving the caregiver farther from the child's bed. For example, parents may start by sleeping in the bed with their child followed by sitting beside the bed, sitting in the room by the door, and sitting on the other side of the door, until parental presence is completely removed (Meltzer and Crabtree 2015). Graduated extinction can also be implemented by putting the child to bed and returning to check on them at increasing intervals. For both techniques, parents should be instructed to ignore protests and minimize their interactions with their child (Byars and Simon 2016). Both methods of graduated extinction have been shown to reduce night wakings, tantrums at bedtime, and bedtime resistance (Kuhn and Elliott 2003; Mindell 1999; Owens et al. 1999; Taylor and Roane 2010). However, the effects are less immediate than those obtained with standard extinction (France and Blampied 2005).

Bedtime Pass

The bedtime pass is a technique used to reduce the frequency of "curtain calls" and to increase the child's ability to sleep independently (Freeman 2006; Moore et al. 2007). The "bedtime pass" allows the child to come out of the room one time after being put to bed. When they do so, the caregiver responds to the child's request, and the child surrenders the pass. All subsequent "curtain calls" are ignored (Freeman 2006). Research has shown that this technique leads to children getting out of bed less frequently and decreases in sleep-onset latency and bedtime resistance (Freeman 2006; Friman et al. 1999; Moore et al. 2007). The bedtime pass is often used to treat the limit setting and combined types of behavioral insomnia of childhood (Byars and Simon 2014).

Bedtime Fading

As previously discussed, children and adolescents are more easily able to fall asleep in their bed if they have a strong association between their bed and falling asleep. Therefore, it is recommended that they do not stay awake in their bed for more than approximately 20 min (Meltzer and Crabtree 2015). Bedtime fading is a technique implemented by putting the child in bed close to the time they are naturally falling asleep to decrease the amount of time they are awake in their bed and strengthen the association between their bed and sleeping. Parents are asked to track the time at which their child falls asleep each night and then temporarily put the child to bed at that time. Once the child is able to fall asleep in 15–20 min, the bedtime is moved 15 min earlier until the child is falling asleep at the desired bedtime (Meltzer and Crabtree 2015). Bedtime fading is an empirically supported technique used to treat insomnia and bedtime resistance (Byars and Simon 2016). This technique has been associated with reduced night wakings, bedtime resistance, and sleep-onset latency (Byars and Simon 2016). When paired with bright light treatment in the morning, this approach may also be used to treat delayed sleep–wake phase disorder (Mindell and Owens 2015).

Chronotherapy

When the child is presenting with a significantly delayed sleep–wake phase (e.g., greater than 3 h), chronotherapy may be indicated (Mindell and Owens 2015). Because the natural circadian rhythm is slightly longer than 24 h, it is easier to go to bed later than to go to bed earlier as in bedtime fading (Piazza et al. 1997). With chronotherapy, the youth's bedtime and entire daily schedule is systematically moved later by 2–3 h each day until the desired bedtime is reached (Czeisler et al. 1981; Kuhn and Elliott 2003). Chronotherapy has been shown to be effective in treating delayed sleep phase in as little as 1–2 weeks (Lack and Wright 2007; Meltzer and Crabtree 2015; Weitzman et al. 1981). While this technique has been shown to be effective, it is likely to interfere with the youth's school schedule (Kuhn and Elliott 2003). Thus, Mindell and Owens (2015) recommended that implementation of chronotherapy occur during a school vacation. Additionally, it is very labor intensive and difficult for parents to implement as it disrupts the schedule of the entire family (Piazza et al. 1997). Additionally, when the youth presents with bedtime resistance or nighttime fears, chronotherapy is not likely to be the treatment of choice (Wiggs and France 2000). Due to these disadvantages, among others, chronotherapy may be a second-line treatment for youth with a delayed sleep–wake phase (Mindell and Owens 2015).

Scheduled Awakenings

Children who experience night wakings may develop a pattern in which they wake at the same time every night. Scheduled awakenings are used to break this pattern of habitual awakenings. This technique should only be used if night wakings occur around the same time every night, most nights during the week and medical causes have been ruled out (Johnson and Lerner 1985). Parents are asked to determine the times at which their child awakens during the night by tracking their sleep patterns for 1–2 weeks. Once this pattern is determined, the parents wake the child prior to this time every night and gradually increase the time between scheduled awakenings until the child sleeps through the night (Owens et al. 1999). While additional research is needed, there exists some research support for the effectiveness of this strategy in reducing night wakings (Byars and Simon 2016; Johnson et al. 1981; Taylor and Roane 2010). Scheduled awakenings may also be used in treatment for parasomnias (Kotagal 2009; Stores 2009).

Cognitive-Behavioral Therapy (CBT)

Many of the empirically supported treatments for sleep difficulties for young children are behavioral. However, when the child presents with dysfunctional beliefs about sleep or nighttime fears that make it difficult for them to initiate or maintain sleep, adding a cognitive component to treatment to address these dysfunctional beliefs and nighttime anxiety is indicated (Meltzer and Crabtree 2015). The most common elements of CBT for treating nighttime anxiety include systematic desensitization, cognitive self-instruction, and positive reinforcement (Gordon et al. 2007). Systematic desensitization is implemented by first identifying the component of nighttime that the child fears (e.g., the dark, being away from caregivers) and then assisting the child in gradually exposing themselves to the feared stimulus. Meltzer and Crabtree (2015) recommend creating game-like exposures for young children such as flashlight treasure hunts to expose them to being in their room in the dark. For older children with fears of the dark or fears related to separating from caregivers, staying in their room for increasing time intervals is recommended. Cognitive self-instruction or restructuring can be used with children or adolescents to challenge anxious thoughts or other maladaptive thoughts that interfere with sleep (Hendricks et al. 2014). Challenged thoughts will likely differ across development and may involve anxiety about the next day (e.g., a test, peer conflict) or related to being in the dark, separation from caregivers, or getting a sufficient amount of sleep. This technique can be used concurrently with exposures. During exposures, parents can praise brave behaviors and encourage children to engage in positive self-talk to build self-esteem (Meltzer and Crabtree 2015). Gordon et al. (2007) conducted a review of 29 studies that evaluated the efficacy of psychosocial treatments for nighttime fears in children. The majority of the studies reviewed utilized cognitive-behavioral techniques such as desensitization, imagery, positive self-talk, and positive reinforcement. Results indicated that cognitive-behavioral strategies are effective at reducing nighttime anxiety in as few as two to four sessions.

Benefits of CBT for reducing sleep problems and sleep-related anxiety have been shown in children as young as preschool age. Kahn et al. (2017) compared the effectiveness of cognitive-behavioral therapy with a play component and nondirective therapy in reducing nighttime fears in 4- to 6-year-old children. Children in the CBT condition were encouraged to work with their parents to think of strategies to reduce nighttime worries (e.g., thinking pleasant thoughts, holding a comfort item). Participants were encouraged to practice their techniques with dolls. Parents were also instructed to gradually move farther from their child's bed at night (i.e., graduated extinction with parental presence). Reinforcement was provided each morning after these exposures (Kahn et al. 2017). Children showed significant decreases in nighttime anxiety, bedtime resistance, and rates of co-sleeping after two 50-min sessions.

Preschool-aged children often have difficulties verbalizing the source of their worries. Furthermore, addressing children's nighttime fears is an important addition to behavioral sleep treatment protocols as it may decrease distress in both children and parents and, therefore, make treatment adherence and success more likely. Incorporating pretend play is a developmentally appropriate approach to introduce and practice cognitive-behavioral techniques with young clients. Fehr et al. (2016) piloted a brief cognitive-behavioral play intervention (CBPI) for children ages 4–6 years old. This intervention, adapted from cognitive-behavioral play therapy (Knell 1993), consisted of three 20- to 30-min sessions in which children were encouraged to play out stories about a child coping with sleep difficulties. Parents also received information about sleep and behavior management strategies. Coping with anxiety that may occur at night was targeted broadly by including stories about nighttime fears, separation, and worry about nightmares. The therapist was active in assisting the child in identifying and practicing coping strategies in play, and generalization was encouraged through playing out multiple stories with multiple themes. While further research is needed, children who received the CBPI demonstrated decreased levels of parent-reported anxiety following treatment.

Image Rehearsal Therapy When children present with recurrent nightmares, image rehearsal therapy can be used to replace the frightening aspects of their dreams with less fearful content. This approach often increases children's self-efficacy and feelings of control (Meltzer and Crabtree 2015). In particular, the child is encouraged to describe a recurrent nightmare in as much detail as possible (e.g., describe what they see, hear, feel, etc.). They are then encouraged to "be the boss of their dream" and replace the scary or sad parts of their dream with happy or benign content (Meltzer and Crabtree 2015: P. 138). The new content is scripted using mediums such as writing, drawing, and/or play, and the child is encouraged to rehearse the new dream to develop a sense of control over their dream (Krakow and Zadra 2006). For example, if a child is having nightmares about getting eaten by a monster, they may choose to rewrite the dream to give themselves the ability to shrink the monster so that they can stomp on it in their dream (Meltzer and Crabtree 2015). Image rehearsal therapy reduces the frequency and intensity of nightmares and amount of daytime anxiety associated with nightmares (Davis and Wright 2007; Krakow et al. 2001). This technique has also been shown to be effective at reducing trauma-related nightmares when coupled with exposure and relaxation (Fernandez et al. 2013).

Case Example

As James' sleep problems (presented earlier in this chapter) had not resolved 5 months after preschool started, his parents discussed their concerns with his pediatrician, who recommended treatment with a psychologist trained in behavioral sleep medicine. Consistent with empirical support, a comprehensive behavioral treatment with a primary parent management approach was initiated to address James' sleep difficulties. First, parent education about age-appropriate expectations for sleep habits and ways to optimize sleep hygiene were discussed. A consistent positive bedtime routine was established, and James' parents were able to successfully implement these changes. In addition, the psychologist requested that James' parents complete sleep diaries to further assess sleep habits and monitor treatment progress. Once these changes were made, behavioral strategies were incorporated.

Graduated extinction was used to address curtain calls and the negative sleep-onset association James had established with his parents' presence at bedtime. After discussing the two options for graduated extinction, James' parents decided to use the checking method at bedtime, providing James with brief check-ins every 5 min initially. His parents were instructed to keep these check-ins very brief and to avoid going through the bedtime routine again. They chose to use the consistent phrase, "You're doing a great job staying in your bed, James. I'll be back to check on you in 5 min." during check-ins. If he came out of his room, they were instructed to provide one reminder that it is bedtime and then to walk him back to his room with no further interactions. To strengthen positive sleep-onset associations, James' parents agreed to ensure that James would sleep in his bed each night. In particular, they agreed to walk him back to his bed if he came to their bed in the middle of the night. In addition, as the sleep diary indicated that James was being put to bed 2 h before he was regularly falling asleep, bedtime fading was introduced:

> In order to help James learn to fall asleep quickly, we want to put him to bed only when he is drowsy and likely to fall asleep soon. This will make sure that the cue of lying down in his bed is consistently paired with falling asleep and will limit time he spends in bed awake. To do that, we need to *temporarily* give him a later bedtime and put him to bed when his body is falling asleep. As he is currently falling asleep around 10 pm each night, this means you will start the bedtime routine shortly after 9 pm so that James is in bed by 9:30 pm. Once he is able to fall asleep quickly at that time for a few days in a row, you will move everything back by 15 minutes so his new bedtime will be 9:15 pm. Again, once he is falling asleep quickly for a few days, you may move it back again in 15-minute increments until you reach his target bedtime.

Finally, graduated extinction was paired with positive reinforcement (in this case, parental attention) as James was told that his parents would do a fun activity with him each morning that he was able to meet his goal, starting with staying in his own bed all night.

Implementation of these behavioral strategies was effective at helping James fall asleep quicker and decrease night wakings, thus increasing his total sleep duration. However, his parents reported that James continued to become distressed at bedtime and came out of his room multiple times per night. They reported that they struggled to remain consistent in minimizing responding to him during these times as they felt that he truly was struggling to cope with the adjustment to school and decreased time with them. They also reported that he had been consistently complaining about bad dreams. To address separation anxiety, fears about nightmares, child distress, and parental adherence, the clinician and James' parents agreed that adding a child-focused component to treatment would be beneficial. Thus, the CBPI was incorporated to assist James in learning coping strategies and to decrease his anxiety.

While continuing parent management, three sessions of CBPI were provided to James. As provided in the CBPI manual, standardized story stems about a child feeling anxious in specific scenarios were provided and played out (Fehr et al. 2016). Story stems provided at each session include practice coping with anxiety about (1) nighttime fears (e.g., the dark, monsters), (2) separation (e.g., a boy wanting to give his mother another kiss after being put to bed), and (3) bad dreams (e.g., worrying about having a bad dream). The therapist was active in the child's play modeling positive self-statements and a problem-solving approach and reinforcing coping strategies. Coping strategies were also directly practiced through the pretend play. After the first CBPI session, James' parents reported that they began reminding James to use the coping strategies when putting him in bed. For example, James reminded himself that if he needed his parents they would be down the hall and that he had his teddy bear to hug instead. They reported a significant decrease in James' anxiety, and subsequently their stress, after the second session. The majority of the treatment goals had been achieved by the third play session as James was now falling asleep within 15 min most nights, going calmly to bed at bedtime, and staying in his bed with consistent parental checks. He also was obtaining an age-appropriate amount of sleep, and his parents reported that they felt he was well rested during the day. Thus, the final CBPI session was used to reinforce coping strategies. James' progress was noticeable in the play narratives as well. During the first CBPI session, he had been unable to identify coping strategies that did not involve his parents. However, by the third session he was independently suggesting strategies like hugging his teddy bear if he missed his parents or reminding himself that he could give his parents another hug in the morning. His parents reported that he was using these strategies at bedtime consistently as well. At a 1-month check-in, James' parents reported that his nighttime anxiety and sleep difficulties were mainly resolved and that they felt confident in their ability to continue the strategies learned. They reported that the *coping strategies learned in CBPI had appeared to generalize to other areas of anxiety as James was using the strategies when he felt anxious before preschool as well, and they were pleased with the progress made in treatment.*

Conclusion

Difficulties with sleep initiation and maintenance are common in children and adolescents. In addition to families who may seek treatment directly for sleep problems, youth with emotional or behavioral concerns often experience comorbid sleep difficulties (see discussion in Meltzer and Crabtree 2015). Thus, therapists or other mental health professionals may be in an ideal position to recognize and treat sleep difficulties or make referrals to assist youth in obtaining effective treatment. There are a variety of empirically supported behavioral and cognitive-behavioral treatment strategies to address behavioral sleep difficulties. Comprehensive behavioral approaches can be highly effective, but many children's sleep difficulties remain unrecognized or untreated. Given the impact of insufficient sleep on a child's cognitive, academic, behavioral, and emotional development, it is imperative for those working with children and adolescents to be prepared to assess sleep difficulties and provide empirically supported treatments when needed.

References

Adams, L., & Rickert, V. (1989). Reducing bedtime tantrums: Comparison between positive routines and graduated extinction. *Pediatrics, 84*(5), 756–761.

Alison, J., Butler, J., & Estenne, M. (2008). Respiratory management. In L. Harvey (Ed.), *Management of spinal cord injuries* (pp. 205–226). New York: Elsevier Ltd.

American Academy of Sleep Medicine. (2014). *International classification of sleep disorders* (3rd ed.). Darien: American Academy of Sleep Medicine.

Arnaud, M. J. (1987). The pharmacology of caffeine. In *Progress in Drug Research/Fortschritte der Arzneimittelforschung/Progrès Des Recherches Pharmaceutiques* (pp. 273–313). Basel: Birkhäuser.

Astill, R. G., Van der Heijden, K. B., Van IJzendoorn, M. H., & Van Someren, E. J. (2012). Sleep, cognition, and behavioral problems in school-age children: A century of research meta-analyzed. *Psychological Bulletin, 138*(6), 1109.

Bélanger, M. È., Bernier, A., Simard, V., Desrosiers, K., & Carrier, J. (2018). Sleeping toward behavioral regulation: Relations between sleep and externalizing symptoms in toddlers and preschoolers. *Journal of Clinical Child & Adolescent Psychology, 47*(3), 366–373.

Bhushan, B., Maddalozzo, J., Sheldon, S. H., Haymond, S., Rychlik, K., Lales, G. C., et al. (2014). Metabolic alterations in children with obstructive sleep apnea. *International Journal of Pediatric Otorhinolaryngology, 78*, 854–859. https://doi.org/10.1016/j.ijporl.2014.02.028.

Blader, J., Koplewicz, H., Abikoff, H., & Foley, C. (1997). Sleep problems of elementary school children: A community survey. *Archives of Pediatrics & Adolescent Medicine, 151*, 473–480.

Boerner, K. E., Coulombe, J. A., & Corkum, P. (2015). Core competencies for health professionals' training in pediatric behavioral sleep care: A Delphi study. *Behavioral Sleep Medicine, 13*(4), 265–284.

Brietzke, S. E., & Gallagher, D. (2006). The effectiveness of tonsillectomy and adenoidectomy in the treatment of pediatric obstructive sleep apnea/hypopnea syndrome: A meta-analysis. *Otolaryngology—Head and Neck Surgery, 134*(6), 979–984.

Bruni, O., Violani, C., Luchetti, A., Miano, S., Verrillo, E., Di Brina, C., et al. (2004). The sleep knowledge of pediatricians and child neuropsychiatrists. *Sleep and Hypnosis, 6*, 130–138.

Bucks, R. S., Olaithe, M., Rosenzweig, I., & Morrell, M. J. (2017). Reviewing the relationship between OSA and cognition: W here do we go from here? *Respirology, 22*(7), 1253–1261.

Byars, K., & Simon, S. (2014). Practice patterns and insomnia treatment outcomes from an evidence-based pediatric behavioral sleep medicine clinic. *Clinical Practice in Pediatric Psychology, 2*(3), 337.

Byars, K. C., & Simon, S. L. (2016). Behavioral treatment of pediatric sleep disturbance: Ethical considerations for pediatric psychology practice. *Clinical Practice in Pediatric Psychology, 4*(2), 241.

Calamaro, C. J., Mason, T. B., & Ratcliffe, S. J. (2009). Adolescents living the 24/7 lifestyle: Effects of caffeine and technology on sleep duration and daytime functioning. *Pediatrics, 123*(6), e1005–e1010.

Czeisler, C. A., Richardson, G. S., Coleman, R. M., Zimmerman, J. C., Moore-Ede, M. C., Dement, W. C., et al. (1981). Chronotherapy: Resetting the circadian clocks of patients with delayed sleep phase insomnia. *Sleep, 4*(1), 1–21.

Davis, J. L., & Wright, D. C. (2007). Randomized clinical trial for treatment of chronic nightmares in trauma-exposed adults. *Journal of Traumatic Stress, 20*, 123–133. https://doi.org/10.1002/jts.20199.

DiFeo, N., Meltzer, L. J., Beck, S. E., Karamessinis, L. R., Cornaglia, M. A., Traylor, J., et al. (2012). Predictors of positive airway pressure therapy adherence in children: A prospective study. *Journal of Clinical Sleep Medicine, 8*(03), 279–286.

Epstein, L. J., Kristo, D., Strollo, P. J., Friedman, N., Malhotra, A., Patil, S. P., et al. (2009). Clinical guideline for the evaluation, management and long-term care of obstructive sleep apnea in adults. *Journal of Clinical Sleep Medicine, 5*(3), 263–276.

Fehr, K. (2015, October). Parent treatment-seeking behavior for childhood sleep problems. In R. Hazen (Chair), *Understanding the Family perspective in the medical setting: Ethical and clinical implications*. Symposium presented at the annual meeting of the Society for Developmental & Behavioral Pediatrics Annual Conference, Las Vegas.

Fehr, K. K., Russ, S. W., & Ievers-Landis, C. E. (2016). Treatment of sleep problems in young children: A case series report of a cognitive–behavioral play intervention. *Clinical Practice in Pediatric Psychology, 4*(3), 306–317. https://doi.org/10.1037/cpp0000153.

Fernandez, S., DeMarni Cromer, L., Borntrager, C., Swopes, R., Hanson, R. F., & Davis, J. L. (2013). A case series: Cognitive-behavioral treatment (exposure, relaxation, and rescripting therapy) of trauma-related nightmares experienced by children. *Clinical Case Studies, 12*(1), 39–59. https://doi.org/10.1177/1534650112462623.

France, K. G., & Blampied, N. M. (2005). Modifications of systematic ignoring in the management of infant sleep disturbance: Efficacy and infant distress. *Child & Family Behavior Therapy, 27*(1), 1–16. https://doi.org/10.1300/J019v27n01_01.

Frank, M. G., & Cantera, R. (2014). Sleep, clocks, and synaptic plasticity. *Trends in Neurosciences, 37*(9), 491–501. https://doi.org/10.1016/j.tins.2014.06.005.

Freeman, K. A. (2006). Treating bedtime resistance with the bedtime pass: A systematic replication and component analysis with 3-year-olds. *Journal of Applied Behavior Analysis, 39*(4), 423–428.

Friedman, M., Wilson, M., Lin, H. C., & Chang, H. W. (2009). Updated systematic review of tonsillectomy and adenoidectomy for treatment of pediatric obstructive sleep apnea/hypopnea syndrome. *Otolaryngology—Head and Neck Surgery, 140*(6), 800–808.

Friman, P. C., Hoff, K. E., Schnoes, C., Freeman, K. A., Woods, D. W., & Blum, N. (1999). The bedtime pass: An approach to bedtime crying and leaving the room. *Archives of Pediatrics & Adolescent Medicine, 153*(10), 1027–1029.

Goodday, A., Corkum, P., & Smith, I. M. (2014). Parental acceptance of treatments for insomnia in children with attention-deficit/hyperactivity disorder, autistic spectrum disorder, and their typically developing peers. *Children's Health Care, 43*(1), 54–71. https://doi.org/10.1080/02739615.2014.850879.

Goodwin, J. L., Kaemingk, K. L., Fregosi, R. F., Rosen, G. M., Morgan, W. J., Smith, T., et al. (2004). Parasomnias and sleep disordered breathing in Caucasian and Hispanic children–the Tucson children's assessment of sleep apnea study. *BMC Medicine, 2*(1), 1–9.

Gordon, J., King, N., Gullone, E., Muris, P., & Ollendick, T. H. (2007). Treatment of children's nighttime fears: The need for a modern randomized controlled trial. *Clinical Psychology Review, 27*, 98–113. https://doi.org/10.1016/j.cpr.2006.07.002.

Green, A., Cohen-Zion, M., Haim, A., & Dagan, Y. (2017). Evening light exposure to computer screens disrupts human sleep, biological rhythms, and attention abilities. *Chronobiology International, 34*(7), 855–865.

Gruber, R., Cassoff, J., Frenette, S., Wiebe, S., & Carrier, J. (2012). Impact on sleep extension and restriction on children's emotional lability and impulsivity. *Pediatrics, 130*, e1155–e1161. https://doi.org/10.1542/peds.2012-0564.

Guilleminault, C., & Pelayo, R. (1998). Narcolepsy in prepubertal children. *Annals of Neurology, 43*(1), 135–142.

Guilleminault, C., & Pelayo, R. (2000). Narcolepsy in children. *Pediatric Drugs, 2*(1), 1–9.

Hendricks, M. C., Ward, C. M., Grodin, L. K., & Slifer, K. J. (2014). Multicomponent cognitive-behavioural intervention to improve sleep in adolescents: A multiple baseline design. *Behavioural and Cognitive Psychotherapy, 42*(3), 368–373.

Johnson, C. M., & Lerner, M. (1985). Amelioration of infant sleep disturbances: II. Effects of scheduled awakenings by compliant parents. *Infant Mental Health Journal, 6*(1), 21–30.

Johnson, C. M., Bradley-Johnson, S., & Stack, J. M. (1981). Decreasing the frequency of infants' nocturnal crying with the use of scheduled awakenings. *Family Practice Research Journal, 1*, 98–104.

Kahn, M., Fridenson, S., Lerer, R., Bar-Haim, Y., & Sadeh, A. (2014). Effects of one night of induced night-wakings versus sleep restriction on sustained attention and mood: A pilot study. *Sleep Medicine, 15*, 825–832. https://doi.org/10.1016/j.sleep.2014.03.016.

Kahn, M., Ronen, A., Apter, A., & Sadeh, A. (2017). Cognitive–behavioral versus non-directive therapy for preschoolers with severe nighttime fears and sleep-related problems. *Sleep Medicine, 32*, 40–47.

Kataria, S., Swanson, M. S., & Trevathan, G. E. (1987). Persistence of sleep disturbances in preschool children. *The Journal of Pediatrics, 110*(4), 642–646.

Klackenberg, G. (1987). Incidence of parasomnias in children in a general population. In C. Guilleminault, (Ed.) *Sleep and its disorders in children* (pp. 99–113). New York, NY: Raven Press.

Knell, S. (1993). *Cognitive-behavioral play therapy*. Northvale: Jason Aronson Inc.

Koontz, K. L., Slifer, K. J., Cataldo, M. D., & Marcus, C. L. (2003). Improving pediatric compliance with positive airway pressure therapy: The impact of behavioral intervention. *Sleep, 26*(8), 1010–1015.

Kotagal, S. (2009). Parasomnias in childhood. *Sleep Medicine Reviews, 13*(2), 157–168.

Koulouglioti, C., Cole, R., Moskow, M., McQuillan, B., Carno, M., & Grape, A. (2014). The longitudinal association of young children's everyday routines to sleep duration. *Journal of Pediatric Health Care, 28*(1), 80–87. https://doi.org/10.1016/j.pedhc.2012.12.006.

Krakow, B., & Zadra, A. (2006). Clinical management of chronic nightmares: Imagery rehearsal therapy. *Behavioral Sleep Medicine, 4*, 45–70. https://doi.org/10.1207/s15402010bsm0401_4.

Krakow, B., Sandoval, D., Schrader, R., Keuhne, B., McBride, L., Yau, C. L., et al. (2001). Treatment of chronic nightmares in adjudicated adolescent girls in a residential facility. *Journal of Adolescent Health, 29*, 94–100. https://doi.org/10.1016/S1054-139X(00)00195-6.

Kuhn, B. R., & Elliott, A. J. (2003). Treatment efficacy in behavioral pediatric sleep medicine. *Journal of Psychosomatic Research, 54*(6), 587–597.

Lack, L. C., & Wright, H. R. (2007). Chronobiology of sleep in humans. *Cellular and Molecular Life Sciences, 64*(10), 1205.

Lange, T., & Born, J. (2011). The immune recovery function of sleep–tracked by neutrophil counts. *Brain, Behavior, and Immunity, 25*(1), 14–15. https://doi.org/10.1016/j.bbi.2010.08.008.

Lewandowski, A., Toliver-Sokol, M., & Palermo, T. (2011). Evidence-based review of subjective pediatric sleep measures. *Journal of Pediatric Psychology, 36*(7), 780–793. https://doi.org/10.1093/jpepsy/jsq119.

Marcus, C. L., Rosen, G., Ward, S. L. D., Halbower, A. C., Sterni, L., Lutz, J., et al. (2006). Adherence to and effectiveness of positive airway pressure therapy in children with obstructive sleep apnea. *Pediatrics, 117*(3), e442–e451.

Marcus, C. L., Brooks, L. J., Ward, S. D., Draper, K. A., Gozal, D., Halbower, A. C., et al. (2012). Diagnosis and management of childhood obstructive sleep apnea syndrome. *American Academy of Pediatrics, 130*(3), e3714–ee755.

Meltzer, L. J., & Crabtree, V. M. (2015). *Pediatric sleep problems: A clinician's guide to behavioral interventions*. Washington, DC: American Psychological Association.

Meltzer, L. J., & Mindell, J. A. (2008). Behavioral sleep disorders in children and adolescents. *Sleep Medicine Clinics, 3*, 269–279. https://doi.org/10.1016/j.jsmc.2008.01.004.

Meltzer, L. J., & Mindell, J. A. (2009). Pediatric sleep. In M. C. Roberts & R. G. Steele (Eds.), *Handbook of pediatric psychology* (pp. 491–507). New York: The Guilford Press.

Meltzer, L. J., & Mindell, J. A. (2014). Systematic review and meta-analysis of behavioral interventions for pediatric insomnia. *Journal of Pediatric Psychology, 39*, 932–948. https://doi.org/10.1093/jpepsy/jsu041.

Meltzer, L. J., Plaufcan, M. R., Thomas, J. H., & Mindell, J. A. (2014). Sleep problems and sleep disorders in pediatric primary care: Treatment recommendations, persistence, and health care utilization. *Journal of Clinical Sleep Medicine, 10*(4), 421. https://doi.org/10.5664/jcsm.3620.

Mindell, J. A. (1999). Empirically supported treatments in pediatric psychology: Bedtime refusal and night wakings in young children. *Journal of Pediatric Psychology, 24*(6), 465–481.

Mindell, J., & Owens, J. (2010). *A clinical guide to pediatric sleep: Diagnosis and management of sleep problems* (2nd ed.). Philadelphia: Lippincott Williams & Wilkins.

Mindell, J. A., & Owens, J. A. (2015). *A clinical guide to pediatric sleep: Diagnosis and management of sleep problems* (3rd ed.). Philadelphia: Wolters Kluwer.

Mindell, J., Sadeh, A., Kohyama, J., & How, T. H. (2010). Parental behaviors and sleep outcomes in infants and toddlers: A cross-cultural comparison. *Sleep Medicine, 11*, 393–399.

Mindell, J. A., Li, A. M., Sadeh, A., Kwon, R., & Goh, D. T. (2015). Bedtime routines for young children: A dose-dependent association with sleep outcomes. *Sleep, 38*(5), 717–722. https://doi.org/10.5665/sleep.4662.

Minges, K. E., & Redeker, N. S. (2016). Delayed school start times and adolescent sleep: A systematic review of the experimental evidence. *Sleep Medicine Reviews, 28*, 86–95.

Moore, M. (2012). Behavioral sleep problems in children and adolescents. *Journal of Clinical Psychology in Medical Settings, 19*(1), 77–83. https://doi.org/10.1007/s10880-011-9282-z.

Moore, B. A., Friman, P. C., Fruzzetti, A. E., & MacAleese, K. (2007). Brief report: Evaluating the bedtime pass program for child resistance to bedtime—A randomized, controlled trial. *Journal of Pediatric Psychology, 32*(3), 283–287. https://doi.org/10.1093/jpepsy/jsl025.

Moturi, S., & Avis, K. (2010). Assessment and treatment of common pediatric sleep disorders. *Innovations in Clinical Neuroscience, 7*(6), 24–37.

National Institute of Health. (2001). *Wake up America: A national sleep alert*. Washington, DC: U.S. Government Printing Office.

National Sleep Foundation. (2004). *Sleep in America poll*. Retrieved from https://sleepfoundation.org/sites/default/files/FINAL%20SOF%202004.pdf

National Sleep Foundation. (2015). *Sleep in America poll*. Retrieved from https://sleepfoundation.org/press-release/national-sleep-foundation-recommends-new-sleep-times

O'Donnell, A. R., Bjornson, C. L., Bohn, S. G., & Kirk, V. G. (2006). Compliance rates in children using noninvasive continuous positive airway pressure. *Sleep, 29*(5), 651–658.

Owens, J. A. (2001). The practice of pediatric sleep medicine: Results of a community survey. *Pediatrics, 108*(3), e51–e51. https://doi.org/10.1542/peds.108.3.e51.

Owens, J., & Adolescent Sleep Working Group, & Committee on Adolescence. (2014). Insufficient sleep in adolescents and young adults: An update on causes and consequences. *Pediatrics, 134*(3), e921–e932. https://doi.org/10.1542/peds.2014-1696.

Owens, J., & Jones, C. (2011). Parental knowledge of healthy sleep in young children: Results of a primary care clinic survey. *Journal of Developmental & Behavioral Pediatrics, 32*(6), 447–453.

Owens, L. J., France, K. G., & Wiggs, L. (1999). Behavioral and cognitive-behavioral interventions for sleep disorders in infants and children: A review. *Sleep Medicine Reviews, 3*(4), 281–302.

Owens, J. A., Rosen, C. L., & Mindell, J. A. (2003). Medication use in the treatment of pediatric insomnia: Results of a survey of community-based pediatricians. *Pediatrics, 111*, 628–635.

Owens, J., Jones, C., & Nash, R. (2011). Caregivers' knowledge, behavior, and attitudes regarding healthy sleep in young children. *Journal of Clinical Sleep Medicine, 7*(4), 345–350. https://doi.org/10.5664/JCSM.1186.

Petit, D., Pennestri, M. H., Paquet, J., Desautels, A., Zadra, A., Vitaro, F., et al. (2015). Childhood sleepwalking and sleep terrors: A longitudinal study of prevalence and familial aggregation. *JAMA Pediatrics, 169*(7), 653–658.

Piazza, C. C., Hagopian, L. P., Hughes, C. R., & Fisher, W. W. (1997). Using chronotherapy to treat severe sleep problems: A case study. *American Journal on Mental Retardation, 102*(4), 358–366.

Prashad, P. S., Marcus, C. L., Maggs, J., Stettler, N., Cornaglia, M. A., Costa, P., et al. (2013). Investigating reasons for CPAP adherence in adolescents: A qualitative approach. *Journal of Clinical Sleep Medicine, 9*(12), 1303–1313.

Price, A. H., Wake, M., Ukoumunne, O. C., & Hiscock, H. (2012). Five-year follow-up of harms and benefits of behavioral infant sleep intervention: Randomized trial. *Pediatrics, 130*(4), 643–651. https://doi.org/10.1542/peds.2011-3467.

Ramos, K. D., Youngclarke, D., & Anderson, J. E. (2007). Parental perceptions of sleep problems among cosleeping and solitary sleeping children. *Infant and Child Development, 16*(4), 417–431.

Rickert, V. I., & Johnson, C. M. (1988). Reducing nocturnal awakening and crying episodes in infants and young children: A comparison between scheduled awakenings and systematic ignoring. *Pediatrics, 81*(2), 203–212.

Robinson, A. M., & Richdale, A. L. (2004). Sleep problems in children with an intellectual disability: Parental perceptions of sleep problems, and views of treatment effectiveness. *Child: Care, Health & Development, 30*(2), 139–150.

Sadeh, A. (2005). Cognitive–behavioral treatment for childhood sleep disorders. *Clinical Psychology Review, 25*(5), 612–628.

Sadeh, A., Mindell, J. A., Luedtke, K., & Wiegand, B. (2009). Sleep and sleep ecology in the first 3 years: A web-based study. *Journal of Sleep Research, 18*(1), 60–73. https://doi.org/10.1111/j.1365-2869.2008.00699.x.

Scher, A. (2005). Crawling in and out of sleep. *Infant and Child Development, 14*(5), 491–500. https://doi.org/10.1002/icd.427.

Schreck, K., & Richdale, A. (2011). Knowledge of childhood sleep: A possible variable in under or misdiagnosis of childhood sleep problems. *Journal of Sleep Research, 20*, 589–597. https://doi.org/10.1111/j.1365-2869.2011.00922.x.

Slifer, K. J., Kruglak, D., Benore, E., Bellipanni, K., Falk, L., Halbower, A. C., et al. (2007). Behavioral training for increasing preschool children's adherence with positive airway pressure: A preliminary study. *Behavioral Sleep Medicine, 5*(2), 147–175.

Stein, M. A., Mendelsohn, J., Obermeyer, W. H., Amromin, J., & Benca, R. (2001). Sleep and behavior problems in school-aged children. *Pediatrics, 107*(4), e60–e60.

Stepanski, E. J., & Wyatt, J. K. (2003). Use of sleep hygiene in the treatment of insomnia. *Sleep Medicine Reviews, 7*(3), 215–225.

Stojanovski, S. D., Rasu, R. S., Balkrishnan, R., & Nahata, M. C. (2007). Trends in medication prescribing for pediatric sleep difficulties in US outpatient settings. *Sleep, 30*(8), 1013–1017.

Stores, G. (2009). Aspects of sleep disorders in children and adolescents. *Dialogues in Clinical Neuroscience, 11*(1), 81–90.

Stores, G., Montgomery, P., & Wiggs, L. (2006). The psychosocial problems of children with narcolepsy and those with excessive daytime sleepiness of uncertain origin. *Pediatrics, 118*(4), e1116–e1123.

Talbot, L., McGlinchey, E., Kaplan, K., Dahl, R., & Harvey, A. (2010). Sleep deprivation in adolescents and adults: Changes in affect. *Emotion, 10*, 831–841. https://doi.org/10.1037/a0020138.

Taylor, D. J., & Roane, B. M. (2010). Treatment of insomnia in adults and children: A practice-friendly review of research. *Journal of Clinical Psychology, 66*(11), 1137–1147. https://doi.org/10.1002/jclp.20733.

Vanderkerckhove, M., & Cluydts, R. (2010). The emotional brain and sleep: An intimate relationship. *Sleep Medicine Reviews, 14*, 219–226. https://doi.org/10.1016/j.smrv.2010.01.002.

Weitzman, E. D., Czeisler, C. A., Coleman, R. M., Spielman, A. J., Zimmerman, J. C., Dement, W., et al. (1981). Delayed sleep phase syndrome: A chronobiological disorder with sleep-onset insomnia. *Archives of General Psychiatry, 38*(7), 737–746.

Wiggs, L., & France, K. (2000). Behavioural treatments for sleep problems in children and adolescents with physical illness, psychological problems or intellectual disabilities. *Sleep Medicine Reviews, 4*(3), 299–314.

Yokomaku, A., Misao, K., Omoto, F., Yamagishi, R., Tanaka, K., Takada, K., et al. (2008). A study of the association between sleep habits and problematic behaviors in preschool children. *Chronobiology International, 25*, 549–564. https://doi.org/10.1080/07420520802261705.

Zepelin, H., & Rechtschaffen, A. (1974). Mammalian sleep, longevity, and energy metabolism. *Brain, Behavior and Evolution, 10*(6), 447–470. https://doi.org/10.1159/000124330.

Cognitive Behavioral Therapy for Pediatric Epilepsy and Psychogenic Non-epileptic Seizures

19

Karla K. Fehr, Julia Doss, Abby Hughes-Scalise, and Meghan M. D. Littles

Six months ago, Rachael[1] (age 13) began experiencing episodes of non-responsiveness. These episodes were first noticed by her teacher, who brought up concerns to Rachael's parents regarding Rachael uncharacteristically "daydreaming" in class. Although her parents and teachers attempted to gain her attention during these episodes, Rachael remained unresponsive. She reported that she did not know when these episodes were happening and did not remember them afterwards. In addition, she reported that they were concerning to her as she wants to do well in school and has been embarrassed when the teacher called on her and she either did not answer or was confused about what was asked. She also reported that some of her peers have been teasing her regarding these episodes. Her pediatrician referred her to a neurologist, who evaluated Rachael with electroencephalography (EEG) and identified that she was experiencing absence seizures, a type of seizure characterized by a brief loss of consciousness. She was diagnosed with epilepsy and started on an antiepileptic drug (AED) at that time. Rachel has not shared her diagnosis with any of her peers because she is concerned about how her peers will treat her. She also has been missing school any time she experiences somatic complaints, as she fears these symptoms could indicate another seizure will occur and she wants to avoid having a seizure at school. She attempts to stay close to her parents during these times, which can interfere with their work schedules as well.

More recently, Rachael began experiencing a second type of episode in which she is unresponsive, falls to the ground, and experiences full body shaking. These episodes have occurred 2–3 times per week over the past 6 weeks. They have only occurred at home so far, but Rachael is very anxious about these episodes occurring at school

---

[1] All cases in this chapter are confabulated.

K. K. Fehr (✉) · M. M. D. Littles
Department of Psychology, Southern Illinois University, Carbondale, IL, USA
e-mail: Kfehr@siu.edu

J. Doss
Minnesota Epilepsy Group and Children's Hospitals and Clinics, St Paul, MN, USA

A. Hughes-Scalise
United Family Medicine Residency, St. Paul, Eagan, MN, USA
e-mail: ahughes@unitedfamilymedicine.org

as well. Rachael's neurologist scheduled her to be admitted to the inpatient epilepsy monitoring unit for continuous EEG to determine the nature of these episodes.

Epilepsy

Epilepsy is a neurological disorder defined by the International League Against Epilepsy as two unprovoked seizures occurring greater than 24 h apart, one unprovoked seizure with a high recurrence risk for future seizures, or a diagnosis of an epilepsy syndrome (Fisher et al. 2014). Epilepsy can be diagnosed at any age, and its worldwide prevalence is estimated at 0.5–1% (Meyer et al. 2010; Russ et al. 2012). Epilepsy is considered to be a spectrum disorder, as the diagnosis includes a wide range of seizure types, presentations, severity, and comorbidity (Jensen 2011). Seizures may be categorized based on whether the seizures have a focal or generalized onset, the location in the brain of seizure onset, and/or the motor symptoms present. While structural abnormalities, tumors, or genetic markers can identify a cause for some children, approximately 50% of children are classified as having idiopathic epilepsy (Camfield and Camfield 2015). Idiopathic epilepsy represents presentations in which a child's background EEG is normal, brain scans are also normal, and there is no other known origin of the seizures.

There are a variety of epilepsy syndromes, each characterized by a specific group of features, prognosis, and behavioral/mood concerns (for an overview, see Guilfoyle et al. 2017). EEG, magnetic resonance imaging (MRI), or other testing may be used to diagnose specific types of epilepsy and assist in determining treatment. AEDs are the first line of treatment in managing epilepsy despite possible cognitive, behavioral, and emotional side effects (see Guilfoyle et al. 2017, for summary). Approximately 75% of children with epilepsy achieve seizure freedom within 2 years after initiating medication, although one-quarter of these children will experience seizures again either spontaneously or when medications are discontinued or in the process of being discontinued (Berg et al. 2001). Approximately 50% of youth with epilepsy (YWE) continue to have epilepsy as an adult (Camfield et al. 2012). Approximately 65% of people with epilepsy are well-controlled on AEDs, but one-third continue to experience seizures that are nonresponsive to medication or other treatment options (Brodie et al. 2012). Surgery or other options may be considered if seizure control is not achieved with AEDs. Epilepsy has been proposed as a systemic disorder due to the increased risk for a variety of medical and psychological comorbidities, which include neurological and non-neurological factors (Yuen et al. 2018). This conceptualization necessitates a comprehensive approach to treating individuals with epilepsy.

Biopsychosocial Conceptualization of Treatment

Pediatric epilepsy is a growing specialty within pediatric psychology as the biopsychosocial needs of this population are being increasingly recognized. Children and adolescents with epilepsy have lower adjustment (Malhi and Singhi 2007) and self-concept (Malhi and Singhi 2007; Scatolini et al. 2017) than their typically developing peers. Well-being is a particular area of concern in YWE as both self-esteem and HRQOL have been found to be lower in YWE than in youth with other chronic illnesses (Kwong et al. 2016; Wang et al. 2012). YWE also have an increased lifetime prevalence rate of behavioral, emotional, and social symptoms, including those associated with Attention-Deficit/Hyperactivity Disorder (ADHD), anxiety, and depression. The associated cognitive, behavioral, and/or emotional comorbidities may cause as much or more distress than the seizures (Jensen 2011). Thus, psychological functioning should be closely monitored so that treatment can be initiated as soon as symptoms are identified.

Adjustment Research has identified psychosocial impairment and specific psychosocial needs at the time of epilepsy diagnosis, including educational needs of parents and adjustment needs of children, adolescents, and their families. HRQOL is lower in youth who have experienced a single seizure and youth with new-onset epilepsy as compared to normative data (Modi et al. 2009). Without treatment, adjustment concerns appear to persist beyond the initial period of diagnosis. For example, HRQOL was found to be stable over 7 months after diagnosis, indicating an important possible treatment target (Modi et al. 2011b).

In addition to adjusting to a chronic medical condition, a recent review identified epilepsy-specific stressors at diagnosis including stigma regarding an epilepsy diagnosis, decreased autonomy due to increased parental monitoring or medical recommendations when concerns about safety during seizures are present (e.g., driving, swimming restrictions), and social concerns (Guilfoyle et al. 2017). Epilepsy stigma, reactions to seizures (i.e., fear in other children), and bullying or social isolation due to injury or incontinence during seizures often result in confusion or hesitation regarding sharing this diagnosis with peers, which is an important target of psychoeducation (Guilfoyle et al. 2017). In addition, children and adolescents often fear the possibility of experiencing another seizure (McNelis et al. 1998), particularly given the unpredictable nature of seizures. Therefore, treatment may focus on factors such as perceived control, self-esteem, self-efficacy, or coping (see review in Wagner and Smith 2006). Finally, parental stress and depressive symptoms have a negative impact on children's HRQOL, particularly during the first 12–24 months after diagnosis (e.g., Ferro et al. 2011; Wu et al. 2014), and this may be important to address in treatment as well.

Rachael appears to be experiencing many adjustment issues common to youth with newly diagnosed epilepsy. She has experienced embarrassment and bullying related to seizures at school. In addition, Rachael is experiencing anxiety about having future seizures, which is impacting her quality of life and attendance at school as well as her parents' ability to attend work. Thus, treatment would likely include psychoeducation regarding how to share this diagnosis with others should she have a desire to do so along with treatment focused on improving coping and supporting autonomy while ensuring safety.

Adherence While seizure control is associated with important medical and psychosocial outcomes, the effectiveness of AED treatment is impacted by a child's adherence to the prescribed medications. In youth with new-onset epilepsy, overall rates of adherence were approximately 80% in the first month, but only 23% of patients were completely adherent to their medications (Modi et al. 2008). Adherence appears to decrease over the first 6 months, as nonadherence rates of almost 60% have been found during this time period (Modi et al. 2011c), and over time as decreases in adherence were found in a 1-year study of adolescents (Smith et al. 2018). Clinically, it is important to be aware that parent report of adherence may indicate higher rates of adherence than those obtained by electronic monitoring (e.g., Modi et al. 2011a). Further, adherence monitoring must be ongoing, as early difficulties are likely to persist and adherence problems could be delayed (Modi et al. 2011c, 2014b).

Nonadherence is associated with a lower likelihood of achieving seizure freedom (e.g., Modi et al. 2014a). Nonadherence can also impact medical decision making as dosages may be increased or medication changes may be made unnecessarily (e.g., Modi et al. 2012). The most common barriers to adherence in children and adolescents include running out of medications, disliking the taste, parent forgetting, adolescent forgetting, child refusal, swallowing difficulties, embarrassment, and having competing activities (Gutierrez-Colina et al. 2018). Approximately 70–80% of children and adolescents experience at least one barrier to adherence (Gutierrez-Colina et al. 2018).

Rachael was initially adherent to her medication regimen despite reporting a bitter taste to the pills. However, as she began to experience fewer seizures, adherence concerns began to emerge. When asked, she reported that she intended to take her medication as prescribed but occasionally forgot when she was running late for school or was tired after a long day. Rachael also noted that there were a few situations in which she remembered her medication after leaving for school or getting in bed for the night but did not want to call her mother at work or get out of bed to get her medication. She noted that since her seizures had decreased, it wasn't "that big of a deal" if she missed an occasional dosage. Given that Rachael had initially been adherent to her medication, her epileptologist had planned to increase her AED dosage or initiate a new medication during her admission to the inpatient monitoring unit. Therefore, re-assessing medication adherence and identifying adherence difficulties was an important part of the hospitalization assessment process that prevented Rachael from being exposed to more medication than is necessary to control her seizures.

Psychosocial comorbidity It is well documented that YWE are at an increased risk of presenting with psychiatric comorbidities (McDermott et al. 1995). For example, in their review, Austin and Caplan (2007) reported that YWE were 4.7 times more likely to exhibit behavior problems compared to the general population and 2.5 times more likely compared to youth with chronic conditions that did not involve the central nervous system. A recent study of 6730 YWE aged 6–18 found that 29.7% exhibited a comorbid mental health diagnosis (e.g., anxiety, depression) and 30.8% presented with a neurodevelopmental comorbidity (e.g., ADHD, autism, intellectual disability; Wagner et al. 2015). It is important to note that while comorbid psychiatric difficulties are common, only a small portion of YWE who also present with mental health diagnoses receive psychological treatment (Ott et al. 2003).

There are high rates of comorbidity between epilepsy in children and externalizing disorders, including ADHD (17–23%), oppositional defiant disorder, and conduct disorder (Baca et al. 2011; Berg et al. 2011; Bilgiç et al. 2018; da Costa et al. 2015; Russ et al. 2012). In addition to rate of diagnosis, research examining behavior ratings has found that behavioral symptoms (e.g., aggression, rule-breaking) occur more frequently in YWE as compared to both typically developing peers and siblings (e.g., Cortesi et al. 1999; Eom et al. 2016). However, a meta-analysis found that effect sizes for these differences decreased when the comparison group was children with other chronic illnesses, suggesting that this pattern may not be specific to epilepsy (Rodenburg et al. 2005). In contrast, the meta-analysis found that attention problems were greater in YWE when compared to typically developing peers, peers with chronic illness, and siblings, suggesting that these concerns are likely specific to the diagnosis of epilepsy and not reflective of simply having a chronic illness or associated family factors (Rodenburg et al. 2005).

Current prevalence rates suggest that 4–19% of children with epilepsy meet diagnostic criteria for an anxiety disorder and approximately 8–21% present with depression (Baca et al. 2011; Berg et al. 2011; Russ et al. 2012; Wagner et al. 2015). In addition, up to 40–45% of YWE present with elevated depression and/or anxiety symptoms (Austin et al. 2011). The wide range of prevalence reported for internalizing disorders is thought to likely be influenced by both the child's age and chronicity of the condition, with older children, adolescents, and those with chronic epilepsy being more likely to receive a diagnosis and reporting greater severity of symptoms (Guilfoyle et al. 2012; Wagner et al. 2015). The fear and uncertainty associated with having future seizures has been cited as a key contributor in the relationship between these disorders (Guilfoyle et al. 2012; Rai et al. 2012). In addition, discrimination and misperceptions from others regarding epilepsy are thought to generate social isolation and low self-esteem, marked features of adolescent and childhood depression (Guilfoyle et al. 2012; Rai et al. 2012).

It has been proposed that psychiatric conditions present in those with epilepsy may be linked to the underlying pathology responsible for epileptic activity, rather than representing a neurological process distinct from epilepsy. While no consistent line of research supports a direct link between specific epileptic syndrome types and psychiatric problems (Almane et al. 2014), the importance of early detection and treatment of comorbid mental health conditions has been strongly asserted in the literature (Keezer et al. 2015). Untreated psychiatric conditions in YWE have been associated with lower reported HRQOL (Guilfoyle et al. 2015). In addition to decreased well-being, low HRQOL has been linked to increased healthcare charges in the year following initial diagnosis for YWE (Ryan et al. 2016). As such, effective assessment and treatment of comorbid psychiatric conditions can potentially lead to both improved psychosocial functioning and better utilization of healthcare resources. Further, the high rates of psychological comorbidity, negative sequelae associated with comorbidity, and chronicity of these difficulties may indicate that a lower threshold is warranted to initiate psychological treatment for YWE.

Given her diagnosis of epilepsy, Rachael is at increased risk for anxiety and depressive symptoms. Although Rachael was recently diagnosed with epilepsy, it would be important to further assess preexisting symptoms of anxiety and determine whether she meets diagnostic criteria for an anxiety disorder at this time. Furthermore, the social aspects and worries associated with epilepsy are hypothesized as factors in the development of anxiety disorders over time in YWE. Thus, even if Rachael is experiencing subclinical symptoms of anxiety currently, intervention for these symptoms would be warranted to attempt to prevent a future anxiety disorder diagnosis.

Developmental issues Cognitive deficits are present for some children with epilepsy, even at the time of seizure onset (Fastenau et al. 2009) and can be associated with some types of epilepsy or medication side effects. Approximately 25–50% of children with epilepsy are also diagnosed with an intellectual disability or developmental delay (Oh et al. 2017; Russ et al. 2012). Rates of learning disabilities (56%) and autism spectrum disorders (5–16%) are also higher in YWE compared to the general population (Berg et al. 2011; Russ et al. 2012). YWE often have below average adaptive functioning, which is associated with epilepsy-specific variables (i.e., number of AEDs, age of onset, duration of epilepsy, seizures that generalize) as well as parent anxiety (Kerne and Chapieski 2015). Developmental differences may exacerbate the child's psychosocial presentation, and parent education and management related to developmental concerns can be an important target of treatment. Neuropsychological evaluation can also be helpful with identifying specific cognitive profiles as well as accommodations or interventions that youth may qualify for in public schooling through an Individualized Education Plan (IEP) or under Section 504 of the Individuals with Disabilities Education Act (IDEA).

Other behavioral health issues YWE experience additional behavioral health issues that pediatric psychologists can assist with. For example, approximately 25–30% of YWE experience difficulties in social functioning (Carson and Chapieski 2016; Dal Canto et al. 2018). Social functioning concerns are elevated in YWE compared to youth with other chronic illnesses and compared to siblings, suggesting this is another area of concern specific to the diagnosis of epilepsy (Rodenburg et al. 2005).

Children and adolescents with epilepsy also experience greater sleep difficulties and daytime sleepiness than typically developing peers (Chan et al. 2011; Fehr et al. 2014; Larson et al. 2012; Maganti et al. 2006). In fact, research has shown that sleep disturbances in YWE are similar to those in youth with obstructive sleep apnea (Becker et al. 2003). In addition to the developmental importance of achieving sufficient sleep, impaired or insufficient sleep may impact seizure frequency for some children (see Malow 2004, for review). Unfortunately, sleep difficulties are not identified by standard clinic questioning in many YWE (Fehr et al. 2014). Thus, identifying and optimizing sleep habits and patterns may also be a goal of treatment (Please also see Chap. 18 of this volume).

Family stress, functioning, perceptions, and adjustment and parent–child interactions are common targets in the treatment of YWE as these factors are also related to child psychosocial and behavioral outcomes (see Austin and Caplan 2007, for review). In particular, maternal functioning may be important for pediatric psychologists to assess as mothers of children with epilepsy are more likely to experience elevated rates of parental stress and depression, even when compared to mothers of children with other neurological or neurodevelopmental concerns (Reilly et al. 2018). In addition, a study of 91 YWE found that family factors (including family problem-solving, family communication, parent fears and concerns, and parent life stress) predicted adherence trajectories in YWE (Loiselle et al. 2015). Across studies, it is clear that family factors impact psychosocial functioning above and beyond the impact of epilepsy.

Epilepsy-specific variables It is important to note that epilepsy-specific variables (e.g., underlying brain pathology, seizure frequency, seizure control, type of epilepsy including location and localization, AED side effects) can impact cognitive, behavioral, and socioemotional development (for a review see Austin and Caplan 2007; Lordo et al. 2017; Schraegle and Titus 2017). For example, youth who continue to experience seizures after initiation of AED treatment report lower self-esteem and quality of life than those who achieve seizure freedom (Chew et al. 2017; Modi et al. 2011b). Comorbid intellectual disability, nonidiopathic epilepsy, polytherapy, poor seizure control, earlier age of epilepsy onset, longer duration, and temporal predominance of EEG abnormalities have been associated with increased socioemotional or behavioral symptoms (Dal Canto et al. 2018). It is important to note that while optimizing seizure control is a primary goal for medical and psychosocial outcomes, modifiable variables such as perceived stress, negative illness perceptions, and family resilience have been found to mediate the relationship between seizure control and self-esteem (Chew et al. 2017). Thus, additional psychosocial support and intervention may be particularly important for youth who do not achieve seizure freedom with AEDs (Chew et al. 2017). Although a full review of the variability among these symptom profiles is outside the scope of this chapter, it is important for clinicians to be aware of these factors and to consider the impact of the child's unique medical presentation on his or her developmental and psychological functioning.

Description of Treatment Components

The broad goal of psychologists working with YWE is to maximize quality of life and psychosocial functioning (Michaelis et al. 2016). To do so, a psychologist must take into consideration the potential influences of the youth's seizures, antiepileptic medication, compliance/adherence to medical treatment, familial/social environment, and comorbid mood/behavioral difficulties when considering diagnosis and course of treatment. All of these factors may be potential treatment targets when working with YWE. They will each be described below, and treatment applications will be exemplified throughout this section as well as in the Case Example section at the end of this chapter. Of note, it is critical to keep in mind throughout this section the importance of consulting with the treating physician when questions related to the impact of seizure or medication-related variables arise.

Stress and seizures As noted above, previous research has shown that children who have more difficult to control or recurrent seizures are at increased risk for developing mood symptoms and behavior problems. Other research has looked at the potential for stress "triggering" seizures, as many patients retrospectively report stress as the most common precipitant to seizure activity (Novakova et al. 2013). Prospective research on the link between stress and seizure activity is inconclusive (Novakova et al. 2013). However, in clinical situations, parents often report concerns related to how stress may be impacting their child's seizures. Caregivers will assert that they become fearful of their children experiencing stress due to their worry that stress will make their child more vulnerable to experiencing a seizure. Often, concern about stress ultimately leads to avoidance of stress (or, in the case of behavior problems, giving in to demands to avoid stressful confrontation), rather than moving the child towards more active coping methods.

In these cases, it can be helpful to provide psychoeducation to families about the role of stress in everyday life, and the negative effects that avoidance can have on helping their child to learn effective stress management strategies. The goal of this psychoeducation is to shift families from a focus on avoiding stress to a goal of appropriately and effectively responding to stress using active coping strategies. Cognitive-behavioral therapy (CBT) techniques can be effective in helping families learn new strategies for responding to both everyday stress and stress specific to seizure activity. It has also been suggested that relaxation techniques such as visualization and deep breathing are useful tools when managing anxiety during pre-ictal or early ictal sensations (Michaelis et al. 2016).

Medication side effects When mood or behavioral difficulties arise in YWE, caregivers often ask whether these symptoms are the result of their child's AEDs. Research suggests that some AEDs put children at increased risk for psychiatric concerns. For example, Keppra was linked to behavioral difficulties in 10–15% of children enrolled in a multicenter open-label study (Opp et al. 2005). Further, common AED side effects such as fatigue and sleep disturbances overlap with symptoms of mental health conditions such as depression and anxiety (Kanner et al. 2012), making differential diagnosis complicated.

To tease out potential AED side effects from psychiatric distress, it is crucial to include consultation with the child's treating physician. It is also optimal to have baseline data on the child's psychosocial functioning prior to initiation of a new medication. If this is not possible, a thorough history of the child's psychological functioning prior to medication initiation from multiple perspectives (parents, teachers, etc.) can also be helpful. To ensure patient safety, it is important that the family, psychologist, and neurologist work closely together when concerns related to behavioral side effects of medications arise.

Of note, there are times that a child needs to stay on a medication that optimizes seizure control but results in mood or behavioral side effects. When this is the case, psychologists can still make meaningful strides in improving psychosocial functioning. Psychological interventions should focus on mood/behavior symptom management (see Comorbid Mood and Behavioral Difficulties below). It is also important to focus on adherence during this time, as mood and behavioral side effects can decrease family motivation to take medications as prescribed. Psychoeducation to caregivers on the risks and benefits of medication adherence from both the psychologist and physician can be helpful in these circumstances.

Compliance / adherence Epilepsy management can require significant effort on the part of the youth and family. In addition to adhering to AED regimens (which, for those with refractory or uncontrolled epilepsy, can involve multiple AED administrations per day), YWE are also often responsible for managing sleep hygiene and avoiding potential seizure triggers or situations in which it would be unsafe to have a seizure.

Research has shown that psychological treatment can positively impact medication adherence. A recent pilot randomized controlled clinical trial investigated the efficacy of a family-focused, multiple-session intervention that used psychoeducation and problem-solving techniques to address adherence and epilepsy knowledge in YWE (Modi et al. 2016). Results showed significant improvements in adherence during the active treatment phase but not at 3-month follow-up. These findings support the importance of continued monitoring and active problem-solving for families when adherence is a concern. Identification of the barriers to adherence can inform treatment as other specific interventions, such as behavioral treatment for pill swallowing anxiety, may also be indicated.

As in youth with other chronic conditions, adherence treatment needs to be individualized in order to address the specific barriers to adherence. In Rachael's case, a problem-solving approach may be effective to improve adherence even when seizure control is improved. For example, to address Rachael's compliance barriers, problem-solving facilitation may identify solutions such as ways to integrate taking her pill into her existing routine (e.g., taking her pills when she brushes her teeth) or allowing access to her medication in other settings (e.g., keeping medication at school in case she forgets to take it before leaving home). Problem-solving and discussion of how Rachael's mother could provide additional, age-appropriate support may include providing reminders and/or reinforcement for specific adherence-related goals.

Family environment Epilepsy is often stressful for the entire family, and family factors impact child psychosocial functioning and adherence. In this context, it is highly recommended that caregivers be included in any psychosocial treatment for YWE. Few epilepsy-specific family interventions exist (with the exception of Modi et al. 2016, as described above); however, there are many established therapies that address difficulties in the family system. A recent systematic review of family-based interventions for youth with chronic medical conditions concluded that while this research literature is still in its infancy, family therapy has potential to improve outcomes such as parent mental health and parent behavior (Law et al. 2014). These findings are particularly relevant given the bidirectional relationship between family factors and well-being in youth with chronic medical conditions (Knafl et al. 2017).

Rachael's parents noted daily difficulties in communicating with Rachael. While her parents described more general concerns (e.g., difficulty getting Rachael to tell them how school was going or how she was doing socially), they noted heightened stress related to communicating around Rachael's epilepsy management. They remarked that Rachael was frustrated at their "micro-managing" style but that they felt they were being appropriate and that they needed to ask Rachael questions and "stay on top of the epilepsy" for Rachael's own health. Rachael felt as though her parents were overly critical of her management, expecting her to be "perfect," and that she was not getting any credit for the times that she was taking care of herself (getting enough sleep, taking medications, avoiding swimming, etc.).

In these situations, solutions-focused family sessions addressing communication difficulties would likely be beneficial. An initial session could focus on collaboratively reframing and redefining the problem (e.g., Rachael doesn't want her parents to "back off" about her seizures, she wants more praise-focused communication related to her epilepsy management). Subsequent sessions could address how each family member might shift their own thinking and behavior to solve the problem. For example, Rachael's parents could start conversations about Rachael's epilepsy management with a positive statement about what they see her doing well. Rachael could choose a couple of days a week in which she initiates conversations with her parents about her seizure management, rather than parents always initiating the conversation.

Spotlight on adolescence/young adulthood Adolescence is a particularly vulnerable time for YWE. Adolescence in general is associated with an increased risk for the onset of psychological disorders (Kuehn 2005) as well as increased engagement in risky behaviors (Gardner and Steinberg 2005). In YWE, rebelliousness in adolescence has been associated with lower health-related quality of life (Smith et al. 2017). Adolescents with epilepsy are also facing a time of transition, both in terms of developmental stage as well as in their epilepsy care (Camfield et al. 2017). Specific to the transition period, YWE report issues with peer group and self-identity, as well as concerns related to body image and autonomy (Camfield et al. 2012).

Researchers have strongly advocated for a multidisciplinary approach when working with YWE at this stage (Carrizosa et al. 2014; Geerlings et al. 2016).

Psychologists are uniquely qualified to address issues that can negatively impact transition for YWE, such as comorbid psychological difficulties, issues related to independence and autonomy, and family stress. Very few epilepsy centers in the world have clinics focused on young adults and transition, and there are no documented interventions specific to young adults with epilepsy in the current literature. One notable exception is a multidisciplinary transition-age program that is currently being piloted at a Level 4 epilepsy center in the Midwest United States (Reger, Hughes-Scalise, & O'Connor, 2018). This transition program provides psychoeducation and brief psychosocial interventions across multiple appointments to patients and their caregivers as they transition from pediatric to adult medical care. While this program is in its pilot phase and its efficacy is still being determined, clinical guidelines endorsed by the Child Neurology Foundation and the American Academy of Pediatrics strongly advocate for a focus on acquiring skills in the domains of self-care and decision-making to maximize the potential for a successful medical transition (Brown et al. 2016). These recommendations assert the importance of continued research and clinical work focusing on the role of psychology in the transition process.

Comorbid mood and behavioral difficulties Screening for psychological comorbidities is an important component of understanding psychosocial functioning for YWE (Jones et al. 2016; Guilfoyle et al. 2015). Even with the use of validated psychological screening instruments, it is important that clinicians take into account seizure variables, potential medication side effects, and familial/social factors when interpreting elevated scores and routes for intervention.

Regarding treatment, there is a small but promising body of research suggesting the efficacy of therapeutic interventions for YWE and comorbid psychiatric concerns. Various interventions aimed at targeting improved epilepsy understanding and self-management have also shown positive impact on psychological distress and sleep problems (e.g., Rizou et al. 2017; Wagner et al. 2017). A small number of cognitive-behavioral interventions targeting anxiety in YWE have also been investigated in the literature. These interventions have varied in format, from computer-assisted approaches (Blocher et al. 2013) to individual therapy (Jones et al. 2014) to group therapy (Carbone et al. 2014). While none of these pilot programs were randomized or included a control group, all studies showed improvements in anxiety symptoms, suggesting CBT as a viable option for YWE who present with anxiety concerns. Given the high level of neurodevelopmental comorbidity (i.e., ADHD, intellectual disability) in YWE, it is important that treatment be tailored to the child's developmental level. Youth with borderline or impaired cognitive functioning are often referred to psychiatrists rather than psychologists, and even when they receive psychotherapy, it is often not adjusted to their cognitive ability (Wieland and Zitman 2016). It is possible for evidence-based behavioral and cognitive-behavioral therapies to be adapted for this population (e.g., Moskowitz et al. 2017). Further, it is highly recommended that caregivers and family members are involved in the therapy process when a child presents with intellectual disability and developmental risk (Crnic et al. 2017).

Challenging Treatment Scenarios

1. *"I don't want to take my medication. When I forget to take my meds, I don't have seizures, so I don't think I need meds anymore."*—teen with epilepsy.

    Many adolescents struggle with understanding the importance of medication adherence, particularly when their seizures are well controlled. Adolescents whose seizures are not well-controlled can also struggle with adherence, feeling as though it is not worth the effort of taking daily medication because they keep having seizures regardless of their compliance. When adherence issues arise, it is important to balance acknowledging/validating the burden of medication compliance while also providing psychoeducation regarding compliance. Motivation and commitment strategies with the adolescent can be helpful in these situations, as can incentive programs generated by the adolescent related to adherence behaviors.

2. *"Since her diagnosis, my daughter has stopped helping out at home. I know that chores make her stressed, and I don't want to stress her and make her have seizures, but I'm worried I'm doing too much for her and she's taking advantage of me."—parent of YWE*

Parents are often concerned that their own parenting instincts are no longer relevant in the context of a child's new epilepsy diagnosis. This can be especially challenging if parents view stress as a trigger for seizures. Therapists can respond to these concerns by reminding caregivers about the importance of teaching and modeling stress management (rather than stress avoidance). It is also helpful to remind families of the importance of attending to the new diagnosis (e.g., setting up new patterns related to medication management, seizure tracking, medical appointments) while not allowing the epilepsy diagnosis to become an "excuse" to avoid daily life responsibilities. Therapists can incorporate working on stress management strategies with the entire family, as well as facilitating family communication around developmentally appropriate expectations in the context of a new epilepsy diagnosis.

3. *"My child has epilepsy. Those that work with him need to understand that sometimes he gets overwhelmed, and he might hit when he is upset. He can't be punished for this because he can't control it and he needs to stay calm so he doesn't have more seizures"—parent of YWE*

At times, parental attribution of the causes of comorbid concerns or parents' own feelings regarding their child's epilepsy diagnosis or developmental concerns may impact their ability or desire to address the comorbid concerns. For example, parents may attribute concerns regarding disruptive behavior to medication side effects or developmental delays and thus accept these behaviors as part of their child's presentation. However, it is important that parents continue to encourage their child's development and teach developmentally appropriate behavioral and emotion regulation skills. Thus, a therapist may need to help parents identify developmentally appropriate expectations and assist the parent in coping with their own feelings regarding the child's diagnosis. Overall, research indicates that empirically supported treatments are effective for children with a comorbid epilepsy diagnosis, although the therapist may need to be sensitive to additional issues that can impact the course and rate of treatment.

Summary

As evidenced above, many factors influence psychosocial functioning in YWE, and a psychologist can play a unique role in helping youth and their families improve the quality of life. While the above factors were described individually, it is important to understand that these factors often influence each other. For example, mood symptoms can negatively impact an adolescent's compliance, which can then result in decreased seizure control. In turn, decreased seizure control may lead to an increased impact of the epilepsy on the adolescent's family functioning, which could further worsen mood symptoms. As such, a core task of a pediatric psychologist working with YWE is to understand the **links** between these various factors and to use this information to create an individualized path to improved functioning.

Psychogenic Non-Epileptic Seizures (PNES)

Psychogenic non-epileptic seizures (PNES) is a conversion disorder (Functional Neurological Symptom Disorder in DSM 5; American Psychiatric Association 2013) involving alterations in behavior, motor activity, consciousness, and sensation that resemble epileptic seizures (LaFrance Jr. et al. 2013). Unlike epilepsy, PNES are not associated with epileptiform activity in the brain as measured with EEG (Gates 2000). Several conceptual models describe the development of the physical symptoms in response to psychological stressors. A biopsychosocial model of conversion disorder theorizes that unresolved psychological stress creates both a physiological and emotional response, both of which impact each other and can perpetuate disruptive physical symptoms (Baslet 2011; Brown and Reuber 2016).

Biopsychosocial Conceptualization of Treatment

In youth, PNES are more common in adolescents but have been documented in children including those younger than 5 years of age (Vincentiis et al. 2006). PNES in children and adolescents is an understudied condition which can have significant psychological, familial, social, and financial consequences if not diagnosed and treated appropriately (Lancman et al. 1994; Plioplys et al. 2005, 2007). Diagnostic delay in children ranges from a few weeks up to 3.5 years on average (Patel et al. 2007). Delay in onset of symptoms to referral for appropriate treatment is likely due to multiple factors, including: access to resources and video EEG (vEEG), misdiagnosis of epilepsy, and/or the family or child not accepting the diagnosis as psychological rather than physical in origin (LaFrance Jr. et al. 2013; Reuber 2017).

Youth with PNES experience different risk factors than adults with the disorder, as examined in Plioplys et al. (2014). Specifically, a somatopsychiatric risk factor profile was discovered, with youth more likely than age-matched sibling controls to experience multiple psychiatric diagnoses at the time of PNES presentation (over 80%), learning difficulties (over 50%), and increased experience with childhood adversities (over 90%) (bullying, loss of parent/caregiver, witness to violence). Another study of youth with PNES found that a stressful home environment was a common risk factor (Vincentiis et al. 2006). Though histories of physical and sexual abuse are present in some youth with PNES, the prevalence is not greater than the rates found in the general population and they are not part of the somatopsychiatric profile.

While there are few treatment studies of PNES in children, delay in appropriate diagnosis is thought to hamper prognosis with regard to symptom remission, and the presence of ongoing episodes likely hinders normal developmental activities that the child would engage in (Valente et al. 2017). Several retrospective studies have speculated that diagnostic delay can have an impact on the emergence of other somatic complaints, making eventual treatment that much more challenging (Doss and Palmquist 2014; Gudmundsson et al. 2001; Wyllie et al. 1999).

Assessment The differential diagnosis between physiological non-epileptic events, such as complex tics, syncope, complex migraine headaches, sleep disorders, and PNES must include a thorough history, physical and neurological examination, and vEEG capturing the paroxysmal event without an ictal EEG epileptiform correlate (Patel et al. 2007). A detailed history is critical in the early PNES evaluation phase, whether the patient presents first to a pediatrician or to a neurologist. Necessary information to gather includes age of onset, semiology of events, and similarity between the events of interest (Davis 2004).

Psychiatric assessment is an essential part of the PNES evaluation. DSM 5 criteria (American Psychiatric Association 2013) outline key criteria of conversion disorder that aid in both diagnosis and treatment. Ideally, psychological evaluation occurs at the same time as the neurological assessment, because it provides information about the underlying stressors and emotional factors contributing to the patient's symptoms in question (Plioplys et al. 2007). Patients are frequently unaware of their distress or unable to understand the link between stressors and their symptoms, thus psychological evaluation aids in delivery of the PNES diagnosis and establishes a basis for psychological treatment (Caplan et al. 2017; Caplan and Plioplys 2010; Doss and Robbins 2017).

When Rachel initially presented for re-evaluation in the epilepsy monitoring unit, it was assumed that she was experiencing another epileptic seizure. The impact that her seizures and her medication had been having on her day-to-day life had been significant, and Rachel and her family struggled to identify other specific stressors. In fact, they felt that prior to her epilepsy diagnosis, "everything had been fine" and were unable to recall other emotional or behavioral struggles.

Rachel's assessment included a comprehensive epilepsy evaluation, with video EEG monitoring and an evaluation by a pediatric psychologist. During her stay, she had several "target" episodes and they were found to be non-epileptic in nature. It was explained to Rachel and her family that non-epileptic seizures are episodes often caused by emotional stressors. It is not uncommon for the person to be surprised and unaware of what the stressors could be at the time of diagnosis. This is because it is thought that the physical symptoms are the body's way of expressing the difficult emotions. It was explained that these symptoms are real and are not in her control currently.

Through the assessment process, Rachael and her family were able to recognize that there were both current and pre-existing stressors that likely contributed to the emergence of her non-epileptic symptoms. Though Rachel and her family initially denied any stressors other than her epileptic seizures, through the evaluation it was revealed that Rachel had been experiencing symptoms of anxiety and depression for a period of time prior to epilepsy onset. She had never had treatment for these symptoms, because her family was not aware of how much of an impact the emotional struggles were having on Rachel. There was a family history of anxiety in the maternal family, and Rachel's mother had experienced anxiety herself throughout her life.

Comorbidities Youth with PNES have high rates of co-occurring medical and psychiatric disorders. Plioplys et al. (2014) found that they more often seek medical care in the emergency department (6.1 vs 2 times compared to siblings), experience other types of somatic complaints, and report more physical illnesses than age-matched sibling controls, are more likely to have multiple psychological disorders at the time of onset of their PNES, and were more likely to have experienced significant childhood adversities (bullying, loss of parent, witness to violence) (Plioplys et al. 2014). In addition, epilepsy is the most commonly co-occurring neurological disorder and is present in about one-third of patients with PNES (Patel et al. 2007; Salpekar et al. 2010). In a study of youth with comorbid epilepsy and PNES, approximately half of the children had episodes that mimicked their own epileptic seizures and half had episodes similar to dissociation or panic attacks that did not resemble their epileptic seizures (Vincentiis et al. 2006).

Description of Treatment Components

Treatment for children with PNES should not only entail management of PNES symptoms but also the comorbid psychopathology (Plioplys et al. 2014). There are no known PNES treatment studies involving children that prospectively assessed the outcome of treatment. Several studies have reviewed PNES treatment in children and have found that 55–80% of the subjects have cessation in PNES symptoms after several treatment sessions (Doss and Palmquist 2014; Sawchuck and Buchhalter 2015).

There are a number of barriers to treatment of PNES, including difficulty communicating the PNES diagnosis to patients and their family members and various levels of acceptance of this diagnosis, ranging from full acceptance to full denial (Myers et al. 2017). Delay in time of onset of symptoms to treatment can pose a number of challenges, from managing the symptoms themselves to addressing issues of functioning which have been disrupted by the ongoing symptoms (Doss and Robbins 2017). Thus, management of PNES is thought to be best done with a multidisciplinary approach in which the treating physician (neurologist/pediatrician) continues to address medical questions while the treating psychologist or psychiatrist focuses initially on symptom management and return to function (Gates 2000). In addition, working with the family (parents or caregivers) is necessary to both manage symptoms but also work on any underlying family factors that contribute to the presentation of symptoms (Doss and Robbins 2017; Caplan et al. 2017). Due to lack of training and experience with conversion disorder, there are few psychiatrists and psychologists who feel competent to treat this disorder, resulting in one of the most significant barriers to successful treatment (Doss and Robbins 2017; Caplan et al. 2017).

Treatment of PNES is complex and requires both short- and long-term treatment goals. Initial management of physical symptoms is necessary in order to allow the child and family to return to "normal" functioning as quickly as possible; this is the first treatment goal initiated in PNES therapy (Doss and Robbins 2017). Consistency in symptom management is key; thus, a behavior plan aimed at managing symptoms is recommended (Caplan et al. 2017). Caplan provides a framework for the initial management of the PNES symptoms and the underlying emotional processes that caused the conversion symptoms. This approach recommends initially a behavioral approach to symptom management followed by working with the child individually and the parents separately to develop insight into emotional stressors and methods for coping with them. Comorbid school, learning, and peer struggles should be addressed early in treatment in order to enhance functioning and promote positive coping.

Long-term treatment of conversion disorder and the underlying psychopathology may also be necessary. While there are no studies of long-term outcomes of youth with PNES, high rates of new somatic symptoms, worsening comorbid psychopathology, and poor long-term functioning have been reported in studies of other forms of conversion disorder, especially when the underlying psychopathology is not treated (Walker et al. 1991; Plioplys et al. 2012). This has also been found in the few retrospective studies reported, noting that the longer from onset of symptoms to treatment, the longer it can take for symptoms to remit and the harder to address the underlying psychopathology (Plioplys et al. 2016).

Long-term treatment goals include improving communication between the caregiver and child and developing insight and then altered ways of coping with hard to express emotion. The long-term therapy portion of treatment often relies on methods utilized in cognitive-behavioral and psychodynamic/insight-oriented therapies. The patient and the caregivers each work individually with the therapist to explore stressors identified, actively problem solve those stressors, better understand their emotional reactions to stressors and develop ways of communicating about those stressors with others in adaptive ways (Caplan et al. 2017).

Prognosis has been postulated to be better in children than in adults with PNES (Gudmundsson et al. 2001), and symptom improvement is also expected to be quicker. This is especially true if diagnosis occurs close to the time of initiation of conversion symptoms, highlighting a significance of early recognition and diagnosis of PNES (Valente et al. 2017; Plioplys et al. 2007).

Challenging Treatment Scenarios

1. *"I'm not stressed, except about these episodes"—teen with PNES*

    This common statement following diagnosis and explanation of PNES can make initiating treatment challenging. Clinicians can manage these statements by validating the person's experience and explaining how conversion disorder tends to express itself (i.e., that individuals often are not aware that they are stressed in the moment of an episode because the body is expressing that emotion rather than the individual expressing it verbally). This can be confusing to patients. Therefore, it is helpful to review how stress can express itself (give examples of other situations in which the body may experience discomfort in response to something emotional such as heart racing before giving a speech in class, jittery excitement before a big game, headache after a long day at work).

2. *"I feel like they might have missed something, we are going to try to find another doctor"— parent of child with PNES*

It is very important to help the family assess whether they have had a good evaluation before initiating treatment. To do this, review what their evaluation entailed. Best practices for evaluation of PNES involve a video EEG with an episode recorded that does not have epileptiform correlate (Patel et al. 2007). If this did not occur, the child may need another evaluation. It is important to consult with the referring physician to determine this. If the child had a thorough evaluation, consulting with the referring physician can be helpful to explain why this diagnosis was made and how to move forward in treatment.

3. *"My PNES symptoms are better, so I don't need therapy anymore"—teen with PNES*

While there are certain circumstances where the underlying stressors are mild and do not require much treatment following PNES remission, this is often not the case (Doss and Palmquist 2014). Ongoing treatment for anxiety, depression and/or skills building to cope with stressors is often indicated and varies in length by individual. Helping the youth with PNES and their family remain engaged in treatment is an important component in treating their conversion disorder.

Case Example

After confirming diagnoses of epilepsy and PNES and differentiating seizures from episodes of PNES, Rachael began weekly outpatient therapy to address adjustment and anxiety related to epilepsy and PNES. Although the inpatient pediatric psychologist was not able to continue outpatient therapy, consultation with the outpatient therapist ensured continuity of care and treatment initiated on the epilepsy unit. Initial treatment goals were to assist the family in accepting the diagnosis, improve functioning, and decrease symptoms.

Given the importance of acceptance of the PNES diagnosis for commitment to psychological treatment, at the first treatment session the psychologist met with Rachael and her parents separately to assess their understanding and acceptance of the PNES diagnosis. When asked what each understood about the diagnosis, Rachael angrily reported that the diagnosis was incorrect as the episodes were not "in her head" and that she was not "making them up." Rachael's parents reported that while they were open to any treatment that would be effective, they still had concerns about the diagnosis. First, they stated that the episodes looked "real" and thus they were unsure that they could truly be psychological in nature. Second, they reported that they had read online that PNES is often caused by abuse and that Rachael had not experienced any significant stressor or trauma to cause PNES.

Identifying barriers to acceptance of the diagnosis, explaining the diagnosis, and collaborating with the neurologist to answer the family's medical questions is an important role of the treating psychologist. While some families are accepting of the diagnosis, other families struggle to accept a non-medical explanation for the symptoms. To address Rachael's concern the psychologist explained:

> You're right that these episodes are not "in your head." They are very real episodes, and I know you are very concerned about them happening. What we found out about these episodes while you were in the hospital is that the episodes are non-epileptic, meaning that by looking at the EEG we

could see that there was not a seizure happening when you had the episode. Even though they are not seizures, we know the episodes ARE real. When people have episodes that look like seizures but are not epileptic, we say that they are non-epileptic episodes. What we will be doing together is figuring out how to stop these episodes from getting in your way and, eventually, from occurring altogether. I know you don't have control over the episodes now, but we will be helping you learn when the episodes are going to occur and what to do to eventually prevent them from happening. How does that sound?

By calling the PNES "non-epileptic episodes" or "non-epileptic events," the psychologist validates the child's experience of the episodes as being real episodes but ensures there is no confusion by calling them a seizure. Furthermore, this explanation provides an introduction to what treatment will involve and the importance of the mind–body connection in resolving the episodes. In order to address Rachael's parents' concerns about the episodes seeming medical and "real" in nature as well as misconceptions about PNES being caused by abuse or trauma, the following explanation was provided:

> Rachael was monitored by video EEG while she was in the hospital. That allowed the neurologist to monitor her brain activity while she experienced the shaking episodes, and he determined that the episode was not a seizure or non-epileptic. Although it was non-epileptic, it was still a very real episode. Non-epileptic episodes are psychological in nature. However, unlike what you read online, in children these episodes can be caused by many different types of stressors and often it is a combination of a number of smaller stressors rather than just one stressor that causes them. What we want to do in treatment is to first help Rachael learn to gain control of the episodes to decrease and eventually prevent them from occurring. Later in treatment we will work on figuring out and addressing what caused the episodes.

After ensuring that Rachael and her parents were in agreement with the diagnosis and initiating psychological treatment, the primary treatment target became to create a behavioral plan to address episodes of PNES. Although these episodes had not yet occurred at school, the behavior management plan was developed to address symptoms at home, school, and in public to ensure that an episode that might occur in any setting could be calmly managed. In particular, in consultation with Rachael's parents and school, the behavior management plan included: instructions to caregivers about differentially responding to epileptic seizures versus PNES and where Rachael should go should she feel an episode may occur to practice her relaxation strategies learned in therapy (e.g., her bedroom at home, the school nurse's office at school). After discussing the plan together with Rachael and her parents, the psychologist met with Rachael's parents separately to discuss any concerns they had and to ensure that they understood the response plan for both epileptic seizures, as recommended by her neurologist, and PNES. Rachael's parents reported concern about needing to respond to Rachael's episodes to help her "come out of them" and due to concern over what would happen if the episode did not stop on its own and/or progressed. The psychologist reiterated how PNES differ from epileptic seizures and assisted Rachael's parents with understanding the importance of responding calmly and consistently to the non-epileptic episodes. Returning to normal functioning, including school, is an important component in the eventual treatment of these symptoms. Therefore, consultation with the school was completed following discussion with the family.

Over the next few sessions, the psychologist met with Rachael and her parents together and separately to discuss adherence to the behavior management plan, symptoms, and additional questions and concerns that arose while implementing the plan. The family was encouraged to speak with their neurologist about any medical questions they had at their follow-up appointment from the hospitalization, and the psychologist stayed in contact with the medical team and school personnel to ensure treatment continuity. In addition, Rachael was taught relaxation strategies, to monitor her level of distress, to identify "warning signs" that her distress is increasing, and to use relaxation strategies in those situations to eventually prevent episodes from occurring.

In addition, treatment began to incorporate psychoeducation related to the relatively recent *diagnosis of epilepsy. For example, Rachael and the psychologist discussed the challenges Rachael experienced with her peers and possible solutions. Given Rachael's embarrassment in school after experiencing absence seizures, Rachael and her mother agreed to speak with the teacher to explain the epilepsy diagnosis and ways to minimize Rachael's embarrassment, such as allowing Rachael to volunteer to respond rather than being called on unexpectedly or having the teacher repeat the question if Rachael is confused. Rachael and her therapist discussed whether Rachael was interested in sharing her epilepsy diagnosis with her peers, and Rachael decided to share it with a couple of close friends but not everyone in her class. However, Rachael felt it would be helpful to have school-wide education to reduce epilepsy stigma in general without identifying her own diagnosis. This option was discussed with her mother, who agreed to contact her state's epilepsy foundation or the Epilepsy Foundation of America to determine if this was a service they could assist with.*

Strategies from empirically supported CBT for anxiety were also incorporated in this stage of treatment. In addition to anxiety monitoring and relaxation strategies, cognitive strategies were introduced. Rachael learned to challenge automatic thoughts related to fears about having another seizure (e.g., "Even if I have another seizure at school, I know my teachers know what to do to keep me safe") and social worries (e.g., "It feels like everyone is looking at me after a seizure but I know people usually move on quickly"). Exposure was also used as Rachael was expected to attend school daily even if she was feeling somewhat anxious, although she was allowed to remove herself from the classroom whenever needed initially to practice relaxation.

Approximately 2 months into treatment, Rachael's PNES episodes began occurring significantly less frequently and less intensely. At this point, the psychologist began to shift to the second phase of PNES treatment: assisting Rachael with identifying and addressing the underlying stressors that resulted in the PNES. As the PNES episodes decreased, her anxiety related to epilepsy and school performance as well as her depressive symptoms and perceived lack of support from her family around the changes in her life related to the epilepsy diagnosis became more prominent. With the episodes no longer masking Rachael's psychological distress, the therapist could more directly approach Rachael's familial and social stressors and use evidence-based approaches to help Rachael cope more effectively.

Brief Conclusion

Epilepsy is a spectrum disorder (Jensen 2011) that can include psychological and developmental components in addition to the neurological symptoms. As such, a multidisciplinary approach to assessment and treatment of epilepsy and associated psychosocial difficulties is crucial to improve the quality of life for YWE. PNES is a complicated biopsychosocial disorder with significant functional morbidity due to the high cost in children's social, emotional, family and academic functioning, and healthcare service utilization. Misdiagnosis and diagnostic delay, resulting from both lack of access to approved standards for diagnosing and service providers comfortable with diagnosing and treating this disorder, impact prognosis. Treatment shortly following symptom onset is thought to provide the best chance for remission. Cognitive-behavioral treatment plays a central role in improving functioning and quality of life in both of these disorders. Although the research literature is still growing, there is a clear role for mental health professionals and empirically supported treatments in these pediatric populations.

References

Almane, D., Jones, J., Jackson, D., Seidenberg, M., & Hermann, B. (2014). The social competence and behavioral problem substrate of new- and recent-onset childhood epilepsy. *Epilepsy & Behavior, 31*, 91–96.

American Psychiatric Association. (2013). *Diagnostic and statistical manual of mental disorders* (5th ed.). Washington, DC.

Austin, J., & Caplan, R. (2007). Behavioral and psychiatric comorbidities in pediatric epilepsy: Toward an integrative model. *Epilepsia, 48*(9), 1639–1651.

Austin, J. K., Perkins, S. M., Johnson, C. S., Fastenau, P. S., Byars, A. W., deGrauw, T. J., et al. (2011). Behavior problems in children at time of first recognized seizure and changes over the following three years. *Epilepsy & Behavior, 21*(4), 373–381. https://doi.org/10.1016/j.yebeh.2011.05.028.

Baca, C. B., Vickrey, B. G., Caplan, R., Vassar, S. D., & Berg, A. T. (2011). Psychiatric and medical comorbidity and quality of life outcomes in childhood-onset epilepsy. *Pediatrics, 128*(6), 1532–1543. https://doi.org/10.1542/peds.2011-2045.

Baslet, G. (2011). Psychogenic non-epileptic seizures: A model of their pathogenic mechanism. *Seizure, 20*(1), 1–13.

Becker, D., Fennell, E., & Carney, P. (2003). Sleep disturbance in children with epilepsy. *Epilepsy & Behavior, 4*, 651–658.

Berg, A., Shinnar, S., Levy, S., Testa, F., Smith-Rapaport, S., Beckerman, B., et al. (2001). Two-year remission and subsequent relapse in children with newly diagnosed epilepsy. *Epilepsia, 42*(12), 1553–1562.

Berg, A. T., Caplan, R., & Hesdorffer, D. C. (2011). Psychiatric and neurodevelopmental disorders in childhood-onset epilepsy. *Epilepsy & Behavior, 20*(3), 550–555. https://doi.org/10.1016/j.yebeh.2010.12.038.

Bilgiç, A., Işık, Ü., Sivri Çolak, R., Derin, H., & Çaksen, H. (2018). Psychiatric symptoms and health-related quality of life in children with epilepsy and their mothers. *Epilepsy & Behavior, 80*, 114–121. https://doi.org/10.1016/j.yebeh.2017.12.031.

Blocher, J. B., Fujikawa, M., Sung, C., Jackson, D. C., & Jones, J. E. (2013). Computer-assisted cognitive behavioral therapy for children with epilepsy and anxiety: A pilot study. *Epilepsy & Behavior, 27*, 70–76.

Brodie, M. J., Barry, S. J. E., Bamagous, G. A., Norrie, J. D., & Kwan, P. (2012). Patterns of treatment response in newly diagnosed epilepsy. *Neurology, 78*, 1548–1554.

Brown, R., & Reuber, M. (2016). Towards an integrative theory of psychogenic non-epileptic seizures (PNES). *Clinical Psychology Review, 47*, 55–70.

Brown, L. W., Camfield, P., Capers, M., Cascino, G., Ciccarelli, M., de Gusmao, C. M., et al. (2016). The neurologist's role in supporting transition to adult health care: A consensus statement. *Neurology, 87*(8), 835–840.

Camfield, P., & Camfield, C. (2015). Incidence, prevalence, and aetiology of seizures and epilepsy in children. *Epileptic Disorders, 17*, 117–123.

Camfield, P., Camfield, C., & Pohlmann-Eden, B. (2012). Transition from pediatric to adult epilepsy care: A difficult process marked by medical and social crisis. *Epilepsy Currents, 12*, 13–21.

Camfield, P., Camfield, C., Busiah, K., Cohen, D., Pack, A., & Nabbout, R. (2017). The transition from pediatric to adult care for youth with epilepsy: Basic biological, sociological, and psychological issues. *Epilepsy & Behavior, 69*, 170–176.

Caplan, R., & Plioplys, S. (2010). Psychiatric features and management of children with psychogenic nonepileptic seizures. In S. C. Schachter & W. C. LaFrance (Eds.), *Gates and Rowan's nonepileptic seizures* (pp. 163–178). Cambridge: Cambridge University Press.

Caplan, R., Doss, J., Plioplys, S., & Jones, J. (2017). *Pediatric psychogenic non-epileptic seizures: A treatment guide*. Cham: Springer International Publishing.

Carbone, L., Plegue, M., Barnes, A., & Shellhaas, R. (2014). Improving the mental health of adolescents with epilepsy through a group cognitive behavioral therapy program. *Epilepsy & Behavior, 39*, 130–134.

Carrizosa, J., An, I., Appleton, R., Camfield, P., & Von Moers, A. (2014). Models for transition clinics. *Epilepsia, 55*(Suppl. 3), 45–51. https://doi.org/10.1111/epi.12716.

Carson, A., & Chapieski, L. (2016). Social functioning in pediatric epilepsy reported by parents and teachers: Contributions of medically related variables, verbal skills, and parental anxiety. *Epilepsy & Behavior, 62*, 57–61.

Chan, B., Cheong, E., Ny, S., Chan, Y., Lee, Q., & Chan, K. (2011). Evaluation of sleep disturbances in children with epilepsy: A questionnaire-based case-control study. *Epilepsy & Behavior, 21*, 437–440.

Chew, J., Haase, A., & Carpenter, J. (2017). Individual and family factors associated with self-esteem in young people with epilepsy: A multiple medication analysis. *Epilepsy & Behavior, 66*, 19–26.

Cortesi, F., Giannotti, F., & Ottaviano, S. (1999). Sleep problems and daytime behavior in childhood idiopathic epilepsy. *Epilepsia, 40*(11), 1557–1565.

Crnic, K. A., Neece, C. L., McIntyre, L. L., Blacher, J., & Baker, B. L. (2017). Intellectual disability and developmental risk: Promoting intervention to improve child and family well-being. *Child Development, 88*, 436–445.

da Costa, C. M., de Macêdo Oliveira, G., da Mota Gomes, M., & de Souza Maia Filho, H. (2015). Clinical and neuropsychological assessment of attention and ADHD comorbidity in a sample of children and adolescents with idiopathic epilepsy. *Arquivos De Neuro-Psiquiatria, 73*(2), 96–103. https://doi.org/10.1590/0004-282X20140219.

Dal Canto, G., Pellacani, S., Valvo, G., Masi, G., Rita Ferrari, A., & Sicca, F. (2018). Internalizing and externalizing symptoms in preschool and school-aged children with epilepsy: Focus on clinical and EEG features. *Epilepsy & Behavior, 79*, 68–74.

Davis, B. (2004). Predicting nonepileptic seizures utilizing seizure frequency, EEG, and response to medication. *European Neurology, 51*, 153–156.

Doss, J., & Palmquist, M. (2014, December). *Treatment of psychogenic non-epileptic seizures in the pediatric population*. Poster presented at the Annual Meeting of the American Epilepsy Society, Seattle.

Doss, J., & Robbins, J. (2017). The roles of the patient and family. In B. Dworetzky & G. Baslet (Eds.), *Psychogenic nonepileptic seizures: Toward the integration of care* (pp. 266–278). New York: Oxford University Press.

Eom, S., Caplan, R., & Berg, A. (2016). Behavioral problems and childhood epilepsy: Parent vs child perspectives. *The Journal of Pediatrics, 179*, 233–239.

Fastenau, P., Johnson, C., Perkins, S., Byars, A., deGrauw, T., Austin, J., et al. (2009). Neuropsychological status at seizure onset in children: Risk factors for early cognitive deficits. *Neurology, 73*, 526–534.

Fehr, K., Adams, E., Berg, K., & Frost, M. (2014, December). *Sleep problems, risk factors, and clinical implications among children at a tertiary care epilepsy center*. Poster session presented at the annual meeting of the American Epilepsy Society, Seattle.

Ferro, M., Avison, W., Campbell, M. K., & Speechley, K. (2011). The impact of maternal depressive symptoms on health-related quality of life in children with epilepsy: A prospective study of family environment as mediators and moderators. *Epilepsia, 52*(2), 316–325.

Fisher, R., Acevedo, C., Arzimanoglou, A., Bogacz, A., Cross, H., Elger, C., et al. (2014). A practical clinical definition of epilepsy. *Epilepsia, 55*(4), 475–482.

Gardner, M., & Steinberg, L. (2005). Peer influence on risk taking, risk preference, and risky decision making in adolescence and adulthood: An experimental study. *Developmental Psychology, 41*, 625–635.

Gates, J. (2000). Nonepileptic seizures: Time for progress. *Epilepsy & Behavior, 1*, 2–6.

Geerlings, R. P. J., Aldenkamp, A. P., Gottmer-Welschen, L. M. C., de With, P. H. N., Zinger, S., van Staa A. I., et al. (2016). Evaluation of a multidisciplinary epilepsy transition clinic for adolescents. *European Journal of Paediatric Neurology, 20*(3), 385–392.

Gudmundsson, O., Prendergast, M., Foreman, D., Foreman, D., & Cowley, S. (2001). Outcome of pseudoseizures in children and adolescents: A 6 year symptom survival analysis. *Developmental Medicine and Child Neurology, 43*, 547–551.

Guilfoyle, S. M., Wagner, J. L., Smith, G., & Modi, A. C. (2012). Early screening and identification of psychological comorbidities in pediatric epilepsy is necessary. *Epilepsy & Behavior, 25*, 495–500.

Guilfoyle, S. M., Monahan, S., Wesolowki, C., & Modi, A. C. (2015). Depression screening in pediatric epilepsy: Evidence for the benefit of a behavioral medicine service in early detection. *Epilepsy & Behavior, 44*, 5–10.

Guilfoyle, S., Wagner, J., Modi, A., Junger, K., Barrett, L., Riisen, A., et al. (2017). Pediatric epilepsy and behavioral health: The state of the literature and directions for evidence-based interprofessional care, training, and research. *Clinical Practice in Pediatric Psychology, 5*(1), 79–90.

Gutierrez-Colina, A., Smith, A., Mara, C., & Modi, A. (2018). Adherence barriers in pediatric epilepsy: From toddlers to young adults. *Epilepsy & Behavior, 80*, 229–234.

Jensen, F. (2011). Epilepsy as a spectrum disorder: Implications from novel clinical and basic neuroscience. *Epilepsia, 52*(Suppl. 1), 1–6.

Jones, J. E., Blocher, J. B., Jackson, D. C., Sung, C., & Fujikawa, M. (2014). Social anxiety and self-concept in children with epilepsy: A pilot intervention study. *Seizure, 23*, 780–785.

Jones, J. E., Siddarth, P., Almane, D., Gurbani, S., Hermann, B. P., & Caplan, R. (2016). Identification of risk for severe psychiatric comorbidity in pediatric epilepsy. *Epilepsia, 57*, 1817–1825.

Kanner, A. M., Schachter, S. C., Barry, J. J., Hesdorffer, D. C., Mula, M., Trimble, M., et al. (2012). Depression and epilepsy, pain and psychogenic non-epileptic seizures: Clinical and therapeutic perspectives. *Epilepsy & Behavior, 24*, 169–181.

Keezer, M. R., Sisodiya, S. M., & Sander, J. W. (2015). Comorbidities of epilepsy: Current concepts and future perspectives. *The Lancet Neurology, 15*, 106–115.

Kerne, V., & Chapieski, L. (2015). Adaptive functioning in pediatric epilepsy: Contributions of seizure-related variables and parental anxiety. *Epilepsy & Behavior, 43*, 48–52.

Knafl, K., Havill, N. L., Leeman, J., Fleming, L., Crandell, J. L., & Sandelowski, M. (2017). The nature of family engagement in interventions for children with chronic conditions. *Western Journal of Nursing Research, 39*, 690–723.

Kuehn, B. M. (2005). Mental illness takes heavy toll on youth. *Journal of the American Medical Association, 294*(3), 293–295. https://doi.org/10.1001/jama.294.3.293.

Kwong, K., Lam, D., Tsui, S., Ngan, M., Tsang, B., Sum Lai, T., et al. (2016). Self-esteem in adolescents with epilepsy: Psychosocial and seizure-related correlates. *Epilepsy & Behavior, 63*, 118–122.

LaFrance, W. C., Jr., Baker, G. A., Duncan, R., Goldstein, L. H., & Reuber, M. (2013). Minimum requirements for the diagnosis of psychogenic nonepileptic seizures: A staged approach: A report from the International League Against Epilepsy Nonepileptic Seizures Task Force. *Epilepsia, 54*(11), 2005–2018.

Lancman, M., Asconape, J., Graves, S., & Gibson, P. (1994). Psychogenic seizures in children: Long-term analysis of 43 cases. *Journal of Child Neurology, 9*, 404–407.

Larson, A., Ryther, R., Jennesson, M., Geffrey, A., Bruno, P., Anagnos, C., et al. (2012). Impact of pediatric epilepsy on sleep patterns and behaviors in children and parents. *Epilepsia, 53*(7), 1162–1169.

Law, E. F., Fisher, E., Fales, J., Noel, M., & Eccleston, C. (2014). Systematic review and meta-analysis of parent and family-based interventions for children and adolescents with chronic medical conditions. *Journal of Pediatric Psychology, 39*, 866–886.

Loiselle, K., Rausch, J. R., & Modi, A. C. (2015). Behavioral predictors of medication adherence trajectories among youth with newly diagnosed epilepsy. *Epilepsy & Behavior, 50*, 103–107.

Lordo, D., Van Patten, R., Sudikoff, E., & Harker, L. (2017). Seizure-related variables are predictive of attention and memory in children with epilepsy. *Epilepsy & Behavior, 73*, 3641.

Maganti, R., Hausman, N., Koehn, M., Sandok, E., Glurich, I., & Mukesh, B. (2006). Excessive daytime sleepiness and sleep complaints among children with epilepsy. *Epilepsy & Behavior, 8*, 272–277.

Malhi, P., & Singhi, P. (2007). Pediatric epilepsy: Psychosocial adaptation and family functioning. *Studia Psychologica, 49*, 265–274.

Malow, B. (2004). Sleep deprivation and epilepsy. *Epilepsy Currents, 4*(5), 193–195.

McDermott, S., Mani, S., & Krishnawami, S. (1995). A population-based analysis of specific behavior problems associated with childhood seizures. *Journal of Epilepsy, 8*, 110–118.

McNelis, A., Musick, B., Austin, J., Dunn, D., & Creasy, K. (1998). Psychosocial care needs of children with new-onset seizures. *Journal of Neuroscience Nursing, 30*(3), 161–165.

Meyer, A. C., Dua, T., Ma, J., Saxena, S., & Birbeck, G. (2010). Global discrepancies in the epilepsy treatment gap: A systematic review. *Bulletin of the World Health Organization, 88*, 260–266.

Michaelis, R., Tang, V., Wagner, J. L., Modi, A. C., LaFrance, W., Goldstein, L. H., et al. (2016). Psychological treatments for people with epilepsy (protocol). *Cochrane Database of Systematic Reviews, 2*, 1–16.

Modi, A., Morita, D., & Glauser, T. (2008). One-month adherence in children with new-onset epilepsy: Whitecoat compliance does not occur. *Pediatrics, 121*(4), e961–e966. https://doi.org/10.1542/peds.2007-1690.

Modi, A., King, A., Monahan, S., Koumoutsos, J., Morita, D., & Glauser, T. (2009). Even a single seizure negatively impacts pediatric health-related quality of life. *Epilepsia, 50*(9), 2110–2116.

Modi, A., Guilfoyle, S., Morita, D., & Glauser, T. (2011a). Development and reliability of a correction factor for parent-reported adherence to pediatric antiepileptic drug therapy. *Epilepsia, 52*(2), 370–376. https://doi.org/10.1111/j.1528-1167.2010.02789.x.

Modi, A., Ingerski, L., Rausch, J., & Glauser, T. (2011b). Treatment factors affecting longitudinal quality of life in new onset pediatric epilepsy. *Journal of Pediatric Psychology, 36*(4), 466–475. https://doi.org/10.1093/jpepsy/jsq114.

Modi, A., Rausch, J., & Glauser, T. (2011c). Patterns of nonadherence to antiepileptic drug therapy in children with newly diagnosed epilepsy. *JAMA, 305*(16), 1669–1676.

Modi, A., Wu, Y., Guilfoyle, S., & Glauser, T. (2012). Uninformed clinical decisions resulting from lack of adherence assessment in children with new onset epilepsy. *Epilepsy & Behavior, 25*(4), 481–484. https://doi.org/10.1016/j.yebeh.2012.09.008.

Modi, A., Rausch, J., & Glauser, T. (2014a). Early pediatric antiepileptic drug nonadherence is related to lower long-term seizure freedom. *Neurology, 82*, 671–673.

Modi, A., Wu, Y., Rausch, J., Peugh, J., & Glauser, T. (2014b). Antiepileptic drug nonadherence predicts pediatric epilepsy seizure outcomes. *Neurology, 83*, 2085–2090.

Modi, A. C., Guilfoyle, S. M., Mann, K. A., & Rausch, J. R. (2016). A pilot randomized controlled clinical trial to improve antiepileptic drug adherence in young children with epilepsy. *Epilepsia, 57*, e69–e75.

Moskowitz, L. J., Walsh, C. E., Mulder, E., McLaughlin, D. M., Hajcak, G., Carr, E. G., et al. (2017). Intervention for anxiety and problem behavior in children with autism spectrum disorder and intellectual disability. *Journal of Autism and Developmental Disorders, 47*, 3930–3948.

Myers, L., Mathur, V., & Lancman, M. (2017). Prolonged exposure therapy for the treatment of patients diagnosed with psychogenic non-epileptic seizures (PNES) and post-traumatic stress disorder (PTSD). *Epilepsy and Behavior, 66*, 86–92.

Novakova, B., Harris, P., Ponnusamy, A., & Reuber, M. (2013). The role of stress as a trigger for epileptic seizures: A narrative review of evidence from human and animal studies. *Epilepsia, 54*, 1866–1876.

Oh, A., Thurman, D., & Kim, H. (2017). Comorbidities and risk factors associated with newly diagnosed epilepsy in the U.S. pediatric population. *Epilepsy & Behavior, 75*, 230–236.

Opp, J., Tuxhorn, I., May, T., Kluger, G., Wiemer-Kruel, A., Kurlemann, G., et al. (2005). Levetiracetam in children with refractory epilepsy: A multicenter open label study in Germany. *Seizure, 14*(7), 476–484.

Ott, D., Siddarth, P., Gurbani, S., Koh, S., Tournay, A., Shields, W. D., et al. (2003). Behavioral disorders in pediatric epilepsy: Unmet psychiatric need. *Epilepsia, 44*, 591–597.

Patel, H., Scott, E., Dunn, D., & Garg, B. (2007). Nonepileptic seizures in children. *Epilepsia, 48*(11), 2086–2092.

Plioplys, S., Szwed, S., & Varn, M. (2005). Psychiatric problems in children with psychogenic nonepileptic seizures (NES). *Epilepsia, 46*, 159.

Plioplys, S., Asato, M., Bursch, B., Salpekar, J., Shaw, R., & Caplan, R. (2007). Multidisciplinary management of pediatric nonepileptic seizures. *Journal of the American Academy of Child and Adolescent Psychiatry, 46*, 1491–1495.

Plioplys, S., Doss, J., Siddarth, P., Birt, D., Bursch, B., Falcone, T., et al. (2012, December). *Risk factors for pediatric non-epileptic seizures (NES): Psychiatric and medical comorbidities*. Poster presented at the Annual Meeting of American Epilepsy Society, San Diego.

Plioplys, S., Doss, J., Siddarth, P., Bursch, B., Falcone, T., Forgey, M., et al. (2014). A multi-site controlled study of risk factors for pediatric psychogenic non-epileptic seizures. *Epilepsia, 55*(11), 1739–1747.

Plioplys, S., Doss, J., Siddarth, P., Bursch, B., Falcone, T., Forgey, M., et al. (2016). Risk factors for comorbid psychopathology in youth with psychogenic nonepileptic seizures. *Seizure, 38*, 32–37.

Rai, D., Kerr, M. P., McManus, S., Jordanova, V., Lewis, G., & Brugha, T. S. (2012). Epilepsy and psychiatric comorbidity: A nationally representative population-based study. *Epilepsia, 53*(6), 1095–1103. https://doi.org/10.1111/j.1528-1167.2012.03500.x.

Reger, K. L., Hughes-Scalise, A., & O'Connor, M. A. (2018). Development of the transition-age program (TAP): Review of a pilot psychosocial multidisciplinary transition program in a level 4 epilepsy center. *Epilepsy & Behavior, 89*, 153–158.

Reilly, C., Atkinson, P., Memon, A., Jones, C., Dabydeen, L., Das, K., et al. (2018). Symptoms of depression, anxiety, and stress in parents of young children with epilepsy: A case controlled population-based study. *Epilepsy & Behavior, 80*, 177–183.

Reuber, M. (2017). Communicating the diagnosis. In B. Dworetzky & G. Baslet (Eds.), *Psychogenic nonepileptic seizures: Toward the integration of care* (pp. 179–192). New York: Oxford University Press.

Rizou, I., De Gucht, V., Papavasiliou, A., & Maes, S. (2017). Evaluation of a self-regulation based pyschoeducational pilot intervention targeting children and adolescents with epilepsy in Greece. *Seizure, 50*, 137–143.

Rodenburg, R., Stams, G. J., & Meijer, A. M. (2005). Psychopathology in children with epilepsy: A meta-analysis. *Journal of Pediatric Psychology, 30*(6), 453–468.

Russ, S. A., Larson, K., & Halfon, N. (2012). A national profile of childhood epilepsy and seizure disorder. *Pediatrics, 129*(2), 256–264. https://doi.org/10.1542/peds.2010-1371.

Ryan, J. L., McGrady, M. E., Guilfoyle, S. M., Follansbee-Junger, K., Peugh, J. L., Loiselle, K. A., et al. (2016). Quality of life changes and health care charges among youth with epilepsy. *Journal of Pediatric Psychology, 41*, 888–897.

Salpekar, J., Plioplys, S., Siddarth, P., Bursch, B., Shaw, R., Asato, M., et al. (2010). Pediatric psychogenic nonepileptic seizures: A study of assessment tools. *Epilepsy and Behavior, 17*, 50–55.

Sawchuck, T., & Buchhalter, J. (2015). Psychogenic nonepileptic seizures in children: Psychological presentation, treatment and short-term outcomes. *Epilepsy and Behavior, 52*, 49–56.

Scatolini, F. L., Zanni, K. P., & Pfeifer, L. I. (2017). The influence of epilepsy on children's perception of self-concept. *Epilepsy & Behavior, 69*, 75–79.

Schraegle, W., & Titus, J. (2017). The relationship of seizure focus with depression, anxiety, and health-related quality of life in children and adolescents with epilepsy. *Epilepsy & Behavior, 68*, 115–122.

Smith, A. W., Mara, C., Ollier, S., Combs, A., & Modi, A. C. (2017). Rebellious behaviors in adolescents with epilepsy. *Journal of Pediatric Psychology, 43*, 52–60.

Smith, A., Mara, C., & Modi, A. (2018). Adherence to antiepileptic drugs in adolescents with epilepsy. *Epilepsy & Behavior, 80*, 307–311.

Valente, K., Alessi, R., Vincentiis, S., dos Santos, B., & Rzezak, P. (2017). Risk factors for diagnostic delay in psychogenic non-epileptic seizures among children and adolescents. *Neurology, 67*, 71–77.

Vincentiis, S., Valente, K., Thome-Souza, S., Kuczinsky, E., Fiore, L. A., & Negrao, N. (2006). Risk factors for psychogenic nonepileptic seizures in children and adolescents with epilepsy. *Epilepsy & Behavior, 8*, 294–298.

Wagner, J., & Smith, G. (2006). Psychosocial intervention in pediatric epilepsy: A critique of the literature. *Epilepsy & Behavior, 8*, 39–49.

Wagner, D. L., Wilson, D. A., Smith, G., Malek, A., & Selassie, A. W. (2015). Neurodevelopmental and mental health comorbidities in children and adolescents with epilepsy and migraine: A response to identified research gaps. *Developmental Medicine & Child Neurology, 57*(1), 45–52.

Wagner, J. L., Modi, A. C., Johnson, E. K., Shegog, R., Escoffery, C., Bamps, Y., et al. (2017). Self-management interventions in pediatric epilepsy: What is the level of evidence? *Epilepsia, 58*, 743–754.

Walker, L., Garber, J., & Greene, J. (1991). Somatization symptoms in pediatric abdominal pain patients: Relation to chronicity of abdominal pains and parent somatization. *Journal of Abnormal Child Psychology, 19*, 379–394.

Wang, J., Wang, Y., Wang, L. B., Xu, H., & Zhang, X. (2012). A comparison of quality of life in adolescents with epilepsy or asthma using the Short-Form Health Survey (SF-36). *Epilepsy Research, 101*, 157–165.

Wieland, J., & Zitman, F. G. (2016). It is time to bring borderline intellectual functioning back into the main fold of classification systems. *BJPsych Bulletin, 40*, 204–206.

Wu, Y., Follansbee-Junger, K., Rausch, J., & Modi, A. (2014). Parent and family stress predict health-related quality in pediatric patients with new-onset epilepsy. *Epilepsia, 55*(6), 866–877. https://doi.org/10.1111/epi.12586.

Wyllie, E., Glazer, J., Benbadis, S., Kotagal, P., & Wolgumuth, B. (1999). Psychiatric features of children and adolescents with pseudoseizures. *Archives of Pediatric and Adolescent Medicine, 153*, 244–248.

Yuen, A., Keezer, M., & Sander, J. (2018). Epilepsy is a neurological and a systematic disorder. *Epilepsy & Behavior, 78*, 57–61.

Cognitive Behavioral Therapy in Pediatric Oncology: Flexible Application of Core Principles

Christina G. Salley and Corinne Catarozoli

Introduction

Nearly 16,000 children and adolescents (birth–19 years) are diagnosed with cancer annually in the United States (Ward et al. 2014). Rates of survival have approached nearly 80% but, unfortunately, cancer remains the second leading cause of death for children (Ward et al. 2014). Cancer treatment varies widely by diagnosis and children may undergo surgery, radiation, chemotherapy, stem cell transplantation, and immunotherapies alone or in combination. It is not unusual for children to be enrolled in clinical trials while on treatment. For some, treatment can last many years and involve a substantial amount of time in outpatient and inpatient hospital visits.

The impact of a cancer diagnosis on a child and his or her family is significant. While the course of cancer treatment is highly individual, many children experience a number of physical side effects and significant symptom burden including hair loss or other changes in appearance, decreased immune function, reduced mobility, pain, fatigue, changes in appetite, nausea, and diarrhea (Miller et al. 2011; Levine et al. 2017), with "late effects" of treatment persisting well into survivorship (Dixon et al. 2018). Children often undergo repeated, invasive procedures which can be painful and distressing. Social isolation, inability to attend school regularly, role changes within the family, and cognitive changes are just some of the psychosocial challenges they experience. While many children with cancer are resilient and some even report positive changes as a result of their cancer experience (Wakefield et al. 2010), they remain at risk for social, emotional, and behavioral challenges.

Psychosocial support is imperative and has long been accepted as an important component of comprehensive care for children with cancer and their families. In December 2015, a large group of multidisciplinary experts published the first evidence and consensus-based psychosocial Standards of Care through the Psychosocial Standards of Care Project for Childhood Cancer (PSCPCC; Wiener et al. 2015). One of these standards addresses psychological intervention for children, indicating that "all youth with cancer and their family members should have access to psychosocial support and interventions throughout the cancer trajectory and access to psychiatry as needed" (Steele et al. 2015). In terms of psy-

C. G. Salley (✉)
Department of Child and Adolescent Psychiatry, NYU School of Medicine and Hassenfeld Children's Hospital at NYU Langone,
New York, NY, USA
e-mail: christina.salley@nyulangone.org

C. Catarozoli
Weill Cornell Medicine, New York, NY, USA
e-mail: cos2006@med.cornell.edu

chosocial providers, most pediatric oncology treatment programs in the United States have a social worker and a child life specialist or recreational therapist while approximately 60% have a psychologist and 19% have a psychiatrist on staff (Scialla et al. 2017a) to deliver support and intervention.

Biopsychosocial Assessment

Psychosocial assessment of children with cancer may take place at any time during the cancer journey with most programs offering assessment at the time of diagnosis, often by a social worker. Involvement of a pediatric psychologist may be routine or occur following a referral when problems arise (Selove et al. 2012). Comprehensive assessment should include review of relevant records, an interview with the child, an interview with the parents, and communication with the child's oncologist and other multidisciplinary providers involved in the child's care in order to fully understand the nature of the problem and how it is impacting the child's well-being and oncological treatment.

In order to appropriately evaluate the psychological functioning of a child with cancer, providers should equip themselves with an understanding of the normative distress response for children and parents at the time of diagnosis and also during special points of treatment including procedural distress, when the course of treatment changes due to poor response or toxicity, and transitioning from active treatment to palliative care or survivorship. It is important for clinicians to become familiar with common side effects of treatments (e.g., nausea, pain, fatigue) with special attention to those which may also be somatic symptoms indicative of psychological disorders. It may be difficult to discern if complaints and behavioral changes such as stomachaches or staying in bed more than usual may be expected responses to the treatment, indicators of psychological distress, or both. Similarly, some medical interventions commonly used in pediatric oncology can have a direct effect on emotional and behavioral functioning. For example, while some cancers require the use of corticosteroids, these drugs can cause mood lability and behavioral changes (Samsel and Muriel 2017). Unique consideration may also be required for children with brain tumors as their emotional, behavioral, and cognitive functioning can be particularly vulnerable given the sensitive location of their disease and treatment.

An important factor to assess during the clinical interview is the child and parents' prior experiences with cancer or serious illness (e.g., family member has died from cancer, the child had a teacher treated for cancer) as this often shapes beliefs about the ill child's circumstances. Similarly, religious, spiritual, or superstitious beliefs may also contribute to helpful or unhelpful assumptions and coping strategies given cancer's association with death and existential concerns. Finally, in addition to evaluating the child's functioning, an assessment of the family's risk factors and adjustment is recommended, given the impact of the illness on the entire family and bidirectional influences of parent and child functioning (Kazak et al. 2015).

Consider the following case which highlights some of these considerations. Anna, a 5-year-old female with neuroblastoma, was referred to the pediatric psychologist due to concerns regarding anxiety two months following her diagnosis.[1] The psychologist spoke with Anna's oncologist and social worker as a well as several nurses who had started to develop a relationship with the family. Anna's treatment course was typical thus far and she was experiencing anticipated side effects of chemotherapy. Providers were concerned about anxiety and emotional and behavioral regression around medical interventions such as physical examinations and blood draws. Anna's reaction was interfering with her care as she was not cooperative with nor speaking to providers and avoided eye contact. Her mother was concerned about Anna's adjustment and reactivity, often becoming tearful in front of Anna.

---

[1]This case is confabulated and is an amalgamation of several cases of fairly common presenting problems of children at this stage of development.

Regressive behaviors were noted including thumb sucking and co-sleeping.

In Anna's case, case conceptualization required information from multiple sources. It was clear that pre-existing anxiety and parental anxiety were exacerbating Anna's symptoms. It was likely that fatigue and nausea from treatment were also taxing her emotional resources even though Anna was unable to voice this. It became evident that Anna did not fully understand the purpose of procedures and that they were usually "sprung" on her last minute which contributed to a sense of lack of control resulting in regression and reactivity on Anna's part with underlying anxiety as a primary issue. Anna's treatment plan included developmentally appropriate education surrounding illness, medical play to increase Anna's exposure and comfort with medical interventions, a behavior plan with positive reinforcement to increase cooperation and appropriate communication with staff, collateral sessions with Anna's mother to teach positive attending and active ignoring skills, and finally a referral to a psychologist for Anna's mother to enhance her own coping skills.

Adapting Cognitive Behavioral Therapy to the Pediatric Cancer Setting

No single psychological treatment modality has been deemed superior for children with cancer, though most children and their families tend to receive supportive psychotherapy and crisis intervention soon after diagnosis to aid in adjustment (Steele et al. 2015). Providers delivering treatment to address ongoing distress or more marked psychopathology likely borrow from a variety of therapeutic approaches. Interventions rooted in Cognitive Behavioral Therapy are often utilized and 67% of respondents of a recent survey of pediatric oncology centers indicated that CBT was an intervention they used in their work with children with cancer (Scialla et al. 2017b). The use of CBT techniques is not surprising given strong evidence base for CBT to address concerns such as adjustment and behavioral problems or symptoms of anxiety and depression which are often reason for referral in the pediatric oncology setting.

There are few randomized controlled trials (RCTs) examining the use of CBT with children and adolescents with cancer. Coughtrey et al. (2018) conducted a systematic review and identified 12 RCTs which evaluated psychosocial interventions in children who had current or past treatment for cancer. Of these 12, four interventions used CBT and, overall, beneficial effects were noted on measures of depression and anxiety. The application of CBT to adult cancer populations and other pediatric illness groups with positive outcomes has been documented. Considerations for adapting CBT to the pediatric oncology setting follow.

Inclusion of Parents and Consideration of the Family

Decades of research has delineated the effects of a pediatric cancer diagnosis on the family. It is clear that the illness does not occur in vacuum; rather it affects each family member and adjustment of the ill child, parents, and siblings. In fact, nine of the 15 psychosocial standards of care for children with cancer and their families specifically mention siblings, parents, or families (Wiener et al. 2015). Parents are especially vulnerable to distress, as they grapple with the realization of their child's diagnosis while being required to digest complex medical information, make treatment decisions, and partner with the medical team in ensuring that their child cooperates with the treatment process. Parents with more chronic stress and who struggle to adjust to the cancer diagnosis early on are likely to have children with greater difficulties (Hamner et al. 2015; Kearney et al. 2015). While parents always exert a pronounced influence on children and their development, this is intensified in the pediatric cancer setting where emotions are especially strong and parents and children spend a significant amount of time with one another at the hospital and at home. At the extreme, this may result in co-dependency or regressions in the parent–

child relationship. While there is often at least some role of parents in manualized CBT with children, clinicians working within the pediatric oncology setting often have a considerable amount of face-to-face time with parents to help them progress in their own adjustment and to directly affect the course of the child's adjustment through parenting recommendations.

Psychoeducation and Rapport Building

Parents and children should receive psychoeducation regarding CBT and treatment targets (e.g., anxiety, mood, behaviors interfering with treatment). Integrating the context of the illness is critical as it provides a sympathetic framework through which to look at the problem. Explaining how preexisting difficulties can be exacerbated or how new, strong emotions can emerge with the stressors of cancer and its treatment can be validating and help foster a collaborative foundation from which to work on. This is particularly important as families may be referred to work with psychology without fully understanding the nature of the referral or believing that it is not only unnecessary but also a burden on top of their many demands. Normalizing the involvement of psychology in the family's cancer journey is essential as it can minimize resistance and lend to better outcomes.

Treatment Planning with Flexibility

Providing CBT to children with cancer requires flexibility. This can be particularly challenging to the well-trained CBT clinician who has learned to follow manualized treatments closely or at least build a systematic approach to achieving the treatment goals while maintaining the integrity of the treatment and to optimize outcomes. Clinicians working in pediatric oncology quickly learn that there is a constant state of tension in idealistic planning and unexpected disruption. Families experience this first hand as children become unexpectedly ill and may require hospitalizations lasting days to weeks or more. Children may feel too ill to participate in therapy sessions or be occupied with medical visits, leaving minimal time for psychological intervention even when there is urgent need for it. Therapy often occurs at the bedside while the child is receiving treatment in an outpatient clinic or inpatient setting. Privacy may not be possible and sessions may be interrupted when medical interventions must take priority.

The duration of the therapeutic relationship can vary widely from one session addressing a crisis situation to ongoing interactions over the course of many years. A clinician may be able to see a child several days in a row if the child is receiving a daily treatment or admitted to the hospital while, in other cases, many weeks may pass in between sessions. This affects, among other things, assigning "homework" which is an important component of CBT. Flexibility in planning and expectation management on the part of the provider is key. Finally, involvement of multidisciplinary providers is common where child life specialists or nurses may collaborate with the psychologist in developing and implementing behavior plans or exposure tasks.

Treatment Components

Cognitive Restructuring

A key treatment component of CBT is modifying thoughts that are inaccurate or maladaptive into those that are more positive and accurate in an effort to improve well-being. This is an important therapeutic tool in oncology where the diagnosis is unpredictable and the situation is uncontrollable, making the way that one thinks about the situation particularly essential to overall adjustment. Findings of a meta-analysis (Aldridge and Roesch 2007) regarding children's coping with cancer revealed that emotion-focused coping, which includes elements of cognitive restructuring such as reappraisal, was associated with positive adjustment. It was noted that this was especially evident earlier in the treatment process with less benefit over time. Others have also suggested that for children coping with chronic health conditions such as cancer, the uncontrollable aspects of the diagnosis and treatment are a good match for cognitive coping strategies such as cognitive restructuring, positive thinking, and acceptance (Compas et al. 2012). Compas et al. (2012) have labeled these cognitive strategies as "secondary control coping." This is in contrast to "primary control coping" in which efforts are made to change an individual's emotional response to the stressor or the stressor itself. In a study examining adjustment near the time of diagnosis, Compas et al. (2014) found that secondary control coping was negatively associated with symptoms of anxiety and depression. Furthermore, Jenkins et al. (2018) explored how coping strategies affected stress responses in children with cancer who underwent a cold pressor task as measured by salivary alpha amylase (sAA) levels. They found that children who were engaged in cognitive reappraisal or distraction had significantly lower sAA levels than children who were reassured during the task, suggesting that cognitive strategies may buffer the experience of pain in children with cancer.

Further support that adaptive cognitive strategies assist with adjustment to cancer and its demands lies in research identifying certain dispositional characteristics related to better outcomes. For example, children who have a more positive disposition are less distressed over time than children who are negative (Okado et al. 2016), more optimistic children with cancer have better psychological functioning (Howard Sharp et al. 2015), and those with greater dispositional resilience report less pain and distress during procedures (Harper et al. 2012).

Maladaptive cognitions arising within the pediatric oncology setting vary widely. Problematic thoughts near the time of diagnosis and during the early part of treatment may emerge as patients make attempts to understand and make sense of their illness. These perceptions can be elicited in early conversations by encouraging the child to share what they know about their illness, how their hospital experience has been so far, and their past experience with illness. Misattributions regarding the cause of the illness (e.g., "I got sick because I was bad), inaccurate understanding of the disease (e.g., describing their brain tumor as having "rocks in my head"), or negative assumptions with medical personnel (e.g., "going to the doctor is scary and always hurts") should be gently addressed in the moment through education. For example, work with Anna revealed that she was fearful of blood draws because she thought she was "getting cancer again" as she had associated early blood draws with the diagnosis. Assuring the patient that there is nothing anyone did to cause the disease, providing accurate and developmentally appropriate information regarding the diagnosis and treatment, and educating the patient and family on the roles of various providers and how the hospital system works can provide a framework for helpful ways to understand and think about this experience. Including parents in these conversations can be helpful as the information is new to them and they can independently engage in these helpful dialogues with their child. Online resources provided by the Children's Oncology Group (www.childrensoncologygroup.org), American Cancer Society (www.cancer.org), and American Society of Clinical Oncology (www.cancer.net) can be used as reference to support these conversations and address difficult questions.

Thoughts during treatment causing distress (e.g., "I'm going to be nauseous forever; my friends must think I've fallen off the face of the planet") can be altered through Socratic questioning and probability estimation. If the child has been in treatment for some time, psychologists can ask the child to tap into their prior experiences for evidence ("Nausea always ends at some point"). However, clinicians can anticipate that children and adolescents will struggle to provide responses to questioning as they have no prior experience with these concerns nor do they or their parents (typically) have medical expertise. Additionally, because the cancer experience is so overwhelming, encouraging the child to consider parallel situations (e.g., "Tell me how your friends have reacted in the past when you haven't been able to spend as much time with them.") is often deemed unacceptable to patients as they express that nothing can compare with their current situation. Here, the pediatric psychologist takes on an "expert" role and taps into information learned from working with many other children in similar circumstances ("Other kids with cancer feel isolated too but sometimes it turns out their friends worry they are bothering them if they text too much"). Similarly, including multidisciplinary team members who can provide more balanced, accurate stances from their expertise is useful. For example, pediatric nurses, may be able to say something like, "All kids on this type of chemotherapy feel crummy for the first three days, but by day four or five most start feeling a lot better."

One major challenge in doing this work is that many thoughts that are associated with negative feelings are not inaccurate. In their work with adult cancer patients, Levin and Applebaum (2014) speak of this "grain of truth" that is undeniable in thoughts such as, "I'm scared I might die" for the patient with a poor prognosis or "I'm missing out on everything important" for the teen whose illness does not allow them to participate in milestone events such as prom or graduation. Therapists must be careful to avoid sounding invalidating when suggesting that there may be other ways to think about the situation. Patients and parents may experience pressure from family and friends to "think on the bright side," and "stay positive." In fact, even children may have been told that staying positive is key to surviving the disease. For some, this type of talk is experienced as a burdensome, leads to the individual feeling they are not understood, and fosters resentment toward potential sources of social support. Therapists can avoid this pitfall by validating the emotional experience of the patient and acknowledge the difficult realities within their situation while also helping the patient identify any aspect of their thoughts that are unhelpful. When addressing an angry adolescent, one might say "Cancer has really shaken things up and there is no doubt it affects all parts of your life. You might expect that everything will be negatively impacted by having cancer. I wonder if we can be certain that will be the case? What might the best-case scenario be? What's most likely to happen?" Coping with realistic, yet distressing, thoughts may be addressed with strategies such as distraction, relaxation, and acceptance.

Behavior Change

Behavioral interventions are among the most effective approaches for addressing anxiety, distress, pain, and other somatic symptoms associated with pediatric cancer treatment. These strategies are often used in tandem and research studies have typically tested them combined into broader CBT packages. Much of the pediatric oncology literature focuses on applying behavioral interventions to procedural anxiety as cancer treatment often involves very painful medical procedures such as bone marrow aspiration and lumbar puncture (see Hockenberry et al. 2011 for review). Compliance with these treatments can be difficult, especially for young children who do not understand the purpose, and related distress can be high. In a number of studies, Jay and colleagues have tested a CBT intervention incorporating positive reinforcement, behavioral rehearsal, imagery, filmed modeling, and breathing exercises for children with cancer undergoing painful procedures. This program was found to be associated with lower observed behavioral distress, self-reported pain, and pulse rates than control conditions (Jay et al. 1985, 1987, 1991). CBT has also performed as well or better than pharmacological intervention, such as oral Valium, for pain management (Jay et al. 1987, 1991; Kuppenheimer and Brown 2002).

One of the core components of CBT for procedural anxiety is positive reinforcement, which involves the application of simple contingency management principles to increase desired behavior. Optimal targets for positive reinforcement are the difficult tasks that accompany these procedures, such as cooperating by holding still for a doctor or receiving an injection. Reinforcement is also effective for other unpleasant tasks, particularly those that require frequent repetition (e.g., blood draws, taking bad-tasting medication). Positive reinforcement and reward charts can be useful tools for managing oppositional, defiant, or regressive behavior. A reward chart should clearly display the target behaviors, framed in a positive manner (e.g., keep hands to self vs. no hitting). Ideally, children should be involved in choosing their prizes to maximize buy-in and ensure rewards are motivating. Potential reinforcers include concrete prizes like small toys, stickers, or points that can be exchanged for other prizes. Additionally, less tangible reinforcers, such as earning privileges or receiving special attention may be used in place of material prizes, particularly for older children or adolescents. Choosing rewards that can be consistently given within the confines of cancer treatment (i.e., are not contraindicated to medical recommendations, are readily available in the hospital) and are sustainable over time (i.e., not overly expensive, do not require excessive amounts of time) is critical to maintaining a behavior plan. Oftentimes these reward systems require coordination across parents and multidisciplinary providers to effectively and consistently apply reinforcers. For instance, a pediatric psychologist might need to communicate with a nurse, who is the main person interfacing with a child during the procedure, to award points or prizes. An example reward chart is provided below.

Charlie's reward chart

	Mon	Tues	Weds	Thurs	Fri
Keep hands to self					
Take medicine calmly					
Follow nurse's directions					

Charlie can earn 1 point per day for each target
Three points = 15 min of screen time

Children sometimes respond to the stress of cancer treatment by engaging in developmentally inappropriate behaviors such as clinging, tantruming, co-sleeping, or being overly dependent. Additionally, children taking corticosteroids as part of their cancer treatment can become atypically aggressive and difficult to manage. These behaviors can be compounded by parents who oftentimes become overly lenient or permissive because they feel uncomfortable being firm or punitive while their child is dealing with such a difficult illness. Pediatric psychologists should work with parents to normalize their feelings and reassure or give "permission" to set limits, along with teaching them a variety of management skills to reinforce independence and positive coping. Active ignoring is an effective parenting method for extinguishing regressive behavior (e.g., whining about taking medication, talking in a "baby voice").

Exposure is a relevant strategy for medical procedures that must be repeated frequently and can be used in tandem with rewards systems. As compared to traditional outpatient CBT, exposures in the context of cancer treatment tend to be more abbreviated and explicitly focused on a single situation (e.g., exposure to a needle stick vs. being in social situations). Thus, a fear hierarchy may not be as extensive and may only include a few items. For example, a child who is fearful of blood draws may generate a hierarchy containing watching a video of a child having blood drawn, sitting in the blood draw chair, watching another person have blood drawn in person, sitting in the chair while a nurse holds a syringe, and then having their own blood drawn. Prior to each exposure, the psychologist should prompt for anxious thoughts a child is having about the task (e.g., "the pain will be unbearable") and obtain an anxiety pre-rating. As the child engages in the task, the psychologist should prompt for ongoing anxiety ratings at brief intervals, such as every 30 s, and record these ratings. Once the task is completed, a debrief should occur, during which the child's anxious thoughts should be revisited and restructured using evidence from the exposure (e.g., "the pain was not as bad as I expected"). Multiple trials of an exposure can be tracked on the same chart to demonstrate how ratings drop with repetition. If a child is hospitalized, it is also possible that exposures may take place very close together over a brief period of time. When completing exposures, pain should be differentiated from anxiety, though a psychologist may prompt for both of these ratings in place of a traditional SUDs rating. Principles of exposure can also be used for avoidant behavior, including school refusal and social withdrawal. School exposures are particularly useful for patients following prolonged absences who may be nervous about re-entry. Similarly, exposures can be implemented in instances where a child is avoiding peers due to social anxiety (e.g., worry about their changed appearance or hair loss, anxiety that peers will find them depressing to be around).

Behavioral rehearsal is another strategy that can be used to manage expectancies and reduce anxiety related to medical procedures (Duff et al. 2012; Jay et al. 1985, 1987, 1991, 1995). The child is familiarized with the procedure and gains a sense of what to expect. For example, prior to a bone marrow aspiration, a child may first practice "administering" this treatment to a doll or stuffed animal. Then, they may lay in the required position as a provider pretends to complete the aspiration. Particularly for very young children who may not cognitively understand the implications of a given treatment, rehearsal provides a concrete explanation for the steps involved and specific outcomes to expect (i.e., showing a child that they will wear a cast following a surgery). Rehearsal also aids in communication between children, family members, and medical providers. Rehearsing an important conversation with a doctor in advance allows the child to formulate his or her thoughts, practice the language to use, and feel more comfortable and confident.

Lastly, mood symptoms in the context of cancer treatment are also appropriate targets for behavioral interventions. While some depressive symptoms may represent a normative reaction to coping with cancer, pediatric psychologists must differentiate these from more pathological presentations. Parents may also need support in distinguishing developmentally appropriate changes (e.g., a teenager who sleeps until noon and desires privacy) from those that are a cause for concern (e.g., a teenager who is increasingly withdrawn and isolated and has decreased interest in friends or activities). Behavioral activation and pleasant event scheduling should be used to target low mood, anhedonia, and fatigue associated with pathological depression. Here, psychologists must consider some of the real limitations facing adolescents with cancer diagnoses. Many typical pleasant events may not be feasible due to physical impairment or immuno-suppression, and will need to be tweaked to fit within treatment requirements.

Feelings and Somatic Complaints

While targeting emotions using CBT within pediatric oncology largely mimics this approach with other populations, several major differences should be taken into consideration. Namely, in addition to distressing feelings such as anxiety, treatment targets are often physical symptoms related to cancer treatment. Side effects to chemotherapy (e.g., nausea, vomiting, fatigue) and pain related to surgeries or other procedures can be extremely impairing to pediatric patients. Addressing these symptoms is critical and can be done using traditional CBT interventions with some adaptions.

Psychoeducation about the pain-stress connection is an important first step when addressing somatic symptoms with pediatric cancer patients. Helping children and families understand that stress in their body can trigger physical symptoms is important rationale for subsequent CBT interventions, rather than addressing symptoms medically. Attention to physical symptoms is a particular challenge when working with pediatric cancer patients. Children often become trained over time to be hypervigilant about changes in their body or somatic complaints as these can be indicative of disease progression. In fact, being perceptive to one's body is rather adaptive given the importance of early identification in cancer treatment. However, becoming overly attuned to bodily sensations can result in excessive attention to and distress about benign symptoms. Children will sometimes feel anxious about a symptom despite repeated reassurance from their doctor that it is not worrisome. Walking the fine line between reasonable vigilance and excessive hypervigilance is a difficult but important skill that pediatric psychologists can help foster. Incorporating input from the medical team is also critical to ensure important symptoms are not ignored.

Nausea and vomiting are common side effects of chemotherapy and are particularly impairing to children and adolescents, frequently leading to delayed or missed chemotherapy administrations (Dolgin et al. 1986; Miller et al. 2011). Children may also develop anticipatory nausea or vomiting prior to chemotherapy sessions as a conditioned side effect, making treatment even more aversive. Research suggests that relaxation strategies are effective in reducing chemotherapy-related nausea and vomiting in adult cancer patients (Figueroa-Moseley et al. 2007; Kamen et al. 2014), and several studies have shown the same effect among children (Zeltzer et al. 1991). Relaxation typically consists of diaphragmatic breathing, guided imagery, and progressive muscle relaxation and is utilized before and during chemotherapy administration. Belly breathing is a simple relaxation technique that can be taught by instructing children to take long, slow breaths, and fill their belly up with air like a balloon inflating. When they exhale, their belly should deflate like a balloon releasing air. Clinicians should demonstrate this strategy in vivo and lead the child in guided practice. Various apps and audio recordings are available for at-home practice as well.

Relaxation was also included as a component of Jay and colleague's studies on procedural distress among pediatric cancer patients (Jay et al. 1985, 1987, 1991, 1995), which found positive effects on pain indices. Similarly, an intervention incorporating muscle relaxation, deep breathing, pleasant imagery, and positive self-talk for children undergoing venipuncture showed reductions in self-reported distress, medical personnel reported distress, and observed behavioral distress (Dahlquist et al. 1985). Relaxation skills may also be taught via biofeedback so patients can be trained to regulate autonomic body function. Biofeedback for pain management has been examined in the pediatric chronic illness literature more broadly, but few studies have applied it specifically within pediatric oncology. Shockey et al. (2013) tested relaxation with biofeedback for children undergoing painful procedures and found this to be a beneficial combination treatment. Given these initial promising results, as well as positive findings within a variety of adult cancer populations (Burish and Jenkins 1992), biofeedback is an area that should be explored further in the future.

Case Example

Jonathan, a 12-year-old boy with Acute Lymphocytic Leukemia (ALL) was referred to the pediatric psychologist while admitted to the inpatient floor and undergoing initial diagnostic testing.[2] Jonathan's parents reported that they were concerned about his adjustment to cancer. His mother expressed excessive worry about her son's prognosis and his ability to cope and also revealed her own personal history of anxiety. Jonathan was a cooperative, friendly, and bright boy who reported feeling anxious about being in the hospital and missing school and friends. Early intervention by the pediatric psychologist included psychoeducation with all family members, introduction to Child Life staff to help familiarize him with his surroundings, and meeting individually with Jonathan's mother to help her manage her own anxiety. Over the course of the initial two months of treatment, Jonathan voiced concerns about isolation and no longer being able to participate in neighborhood basketball meet-ups with his friends.

Jonathan: I can't play basketball anymore, I'm stuck inside, and everybody is out there having fun without me!
Therapist: That's really tough. I am sure you miss getting to see your friends. I wonder if there is a way we can figure out how to keep you involved.
Jonathan: Mom won't let my friends come over!
Therapist: That's true. I know the doctors want to make sure you stay protected while your immune system is weak and so sometimes you won't be able to have friends inside the house. What are the rules about going outside?

---
[2]This case is confabulated and is an amalgamation of several cases of fairly common presenting problems of children at this stage of development.

Jonathan: I'm allowed to go outside but my friends hang out in the cul-de-sac and mom wants me to stay home.

Therapist: Is there anything you and your friends could do outdoors at your house?

Jonathan: Well, we do have the patio but that's boring.

Therapist: Why don't we ask your parents to help us come up with some ideas for getting your friends to come over and hang out on the patio?

In this example, the therapist acknowledges the real barriers (i.e., compromised immune system) that limit Jonathan's social participation while setting the stage for problem solving. The therapist then facilitated a solution-focused conversation with Jonathan and his mother. His mother suggested buying patio furniture and ordering pizza for the boys. Jonathan felt his friends would enjoy this. Further problem solving with the family led Jonathan's parents to purchase a video game system where he could virtually compete against his friends. Video games had previously been prohibited in the home but after discussion, his parents were willing to be more flexible in order to keep Jonathan connected with his friends.

Eight months into treatment, Jonathan developed anticipatory stress with stomach pain prior to appointments for major procedures. This was following one bad experience with a lumbar puncture in which Jonathan reported having more pain than usual. He started to fear further procedures which resulted in avoidant behavior. On mornings of procedures, he was refusing to get out of bed and the family was late arriving to the hospital. He was reluctant to admit to his doctors and nurses there was a problem as he wanted to maintain a "good patient" persona. The pediatric psychologist met with Jonathan on one of these mornings.

Therapist: What was going on in your mind this morning?

Jonathan: My stomach was really hurting so I just wanted to stay in bed and rest. The doctors say if I don't feel good then I'm supposed to rest.

Therapist: Sometimes belly pain can be a sign that we're stressed or worried. I wonder if that was going on for you this morning.

Jonathan: No! I'm not faking. My stomach really hurt.

Therapist: I believe you. You're not faking. Your mom had mentioned you were feeling nervous about your procedure. Can you tell me what you were thinking?

Jonathan: Well, last time I had that procedure, it hurt so bad! I'm sure it's gonna be the worst pain ever again.

Therapist: Let's take a look at that thought. How many times have you had procedures? Have they all been that bad?

Jonathan: Well I've had a lot. It's never fun but that one was the worst.

Therapist: Is there a chance it could be less this time too?

Jonathan: I'm not sure. Maybe.

Therapist: I've worked with lots of kids who have these types of procedures. They tell me that sometimes the pain is a 10 and sometimes it's a 2. But it's rarely a 10. So, what's the likelihood it will be a 10 for you this time?

Jonathan: I guess not very likely, but I'm still scared.

In addition to restructuring Jonathan's anxious thoughts through evidence gathering and probability estimation, the psychologist worked with Jonathan to learn relaxation strategies including diaphragmatic breathing and imagery to reduce his anxiety. Together, Jonathan and his psychologist also developed a plan for Jonathan to tell his doctors about that intense pain he had experienced in order to increase his self-efficacy about addressing his concerns with medical staff and practiced this through rehearsal.

Conclusion

Jonathan's case highlights how CBT provides a framework for conceptualizing psychological distress and developing appropriate interventions within the pediatric oncology setting. If all continues as planned, Jonathan and his family can expect to face the daily demands of treatment for a total of 2–3 years before transitioning into survivorship. While survivorship is a celebratory time, clinicians should be aware of special concerns that arise. Some share worries about the disconnect from their medical teams whom which they have relied on for years. New stressors may develop surrounding medical late effects of treatment that affect physical well-being as well as neurocognitive late effects which can cause difficulty in school and activities of daily living. Fear of recurrence and increased anxiety during surveillance scans may also occur. A combination of cognitive restructuring, acceptance, distraction, and problem solving are likely to be helpful to patients during this phase. Occasional "check-ins" by psychologists in association with medical follow-up visits may be useful.

Unfortunately, for some children and adolescents, there will come a point when their disease no longer responds to treatment and they will face the transition to palliative care and preparation for end-of-life. This sad and harsh reality is difficult for patients, families, and clinicians. Psychologists may feel an urgent pressure to help the patient and family feel better. Not surprisingly, certain cognitive restructuring strategies may be an inappropriate fit for the concerns reported by their patients. However, some CBT strategies can be helpful. For example, addressing somatic concerns and emotional angst through relaxation and imagery may alleviate distress. Note that in many cases, "active" relaxation strategies such as progressive muscle relaxation which includes tensing muscle areas may not be appropriate at this time. Supporting caregivers, who may feel helpless, by creatively identifying what they "can do" at this time may provide parents with some self-efficacy and help them remain an active support to their child. As a final step, contact should be made by some member of the child's psychosocial team to the child's family after death in order to offer condolences and assess the need for bereavement support.

There is a role for CBT from the time of diagnosis and across the illness trajectory for children and adolescents with cancer. Providers can adhere to the basic principles of CBT while making appropriate modifications in order to address early adjustment and normative distress responses as well as frank psychopathology in order to facilitate emotional and physical health. With flexibility, CBT strategies can be applied in outpatient and inpatient settings to this vulnerable and resilient population.

References

Aldridge, A. A., & Roesch, S. C. (2007). Coping and adjustment in children with cancer: A meta-analytic study. *Journal of Behavioral Medicine, 30*(2), 115–128. https://doi.org/10.1007/s10865-006-9087-y.

Burish, T. G., & Jenkins, R. A. (1992). Effectiveness of biofeedback and relaxation training in reducing the side effects of cancer chemotherapy. *Health Psychology, 11*(1), 17–23.

Compas, B. E., Jaser, S. S., Dunn, M., & Rodriguez, E. M. (2012). Coping with chronic illness in childhood and adolescence. *Annual Review of Clinical Psychology, 8*, 455–480. https://doi.org/10.1146/annurev-clinpsy-032511-143108.

Compas, B. E., Desjardins, L., Vannatta, K., Young-Salame, T., Rodriquez, E. M., Dunn, M., et al. (2014). Children and adolescents coping with cancer: Self- and parent reports of coping and anxiety/depression. *Health Psychology, 33*(8), 853–861. https://doi.org/10.1037/hea0000083.

Coughtrey, A., Millington, A., Bennett, S., Christie, D., Hough, R., Su, M. T., et al. (2018). The effectiveness of psychosocial interventions for psychological outcomes in pediatric oncology: A systematic review. *Journal of Pain and Symptom Management, 55*(3), 1004–1017. https://doi.org/10.1016/j.jpainsymman.2017.09.022.

Dahlquist, L. M., Gil, K. M., Armstrong, F. D., Ginsberg, A., & Jones, B. (1985). Behavioral management of children's distress during chemotherapy. *Journal of Behavior Therapy and Experimental Psychiatry, 16*(4), 325–329.

Dixon, S. B., Bjornard, K. L., Alberts, N. M., Armstrong, G. T., Brinkman, T. M., Chemaitilly, W., et al. (2018). Factors influencing risk-based care of the childhood cancer survivor in the 21st century. *CA: A Cancer Journal for Clinicians, 68*(2), 133–152. https://doi.org/10.3322/caac.21445.

Dolgin, M. J., Katz, E. R., Doctors, S. R., & Siegel, S. E. (1986). Caregivers' perceptions of medical compliance in adolescents with cancer. *Journal of Adolescent Health Care, 7*(1), 22–27.

Duff, A. J., Gaskell, S. L., Jacobs, K., & Houghton, J. M. (2012). Management of distressing procedures in children and young people: Time to adhere to the guidelines. *Archives of Disease in Childhood, 97*(1), 1–4.

Figueroa-Moseley, C., Jean-Pierre, P., Roscoe, J. A., Ryan, J. L., Kohli, S., Palesh, O. G., et al. (2007). Behavioral interventions in treating anticipatory nausea and vomiting. *Journal of the National Comprehensive Cancer Network, 5*(1), 44–50.

Hamner, T., Latzman, R. D., Latzman, N. E., Elkin, T. D., & Majumdar, S. (2015). Quality of life among pediatric patients with cancer: Contributions of time since diagnosis and parental chronic stress. *Pediatric Blood & Cancer, 62*, 1232–1236. https://doi.org/10.1002/pbc.25468.

Harper, F. W. K., Penner, L. A., Peterson, A., Albrecht, T. L., & Taub, J. (2012). Children's positive dispositional attributes, parents' empathic responses, and children's responses to pain pediatric oncology treatment procedures. *Journal of Psychosocial Oncology, 30*(5), 593–613. https://doi.org/10.1080/07347332.2012.703771.

Hockenberry, M. J., McCarthy, K., Taylor, O., Scarberry, M., Franklin, Q., Louis, C. U., et al. (2011). Managing painful procedures in children with cancer. *Journal of Pediatric Hematology/Oncology, 33*(2), 119–127. https://doi.org/10.1097/MPH.obo13e3181f46a65.

Howard Sharp, K. M., Rowe, A. E., Russell, K., Long, A., & Phipps, S. (2015). Predictors of psychological functioning in children with cancer: Disposition and cumulative life stressors. *Psychooncology, 24*(7), 779–786. https://doi.org/10.1002/pon.3643.

Jay, S. M., Elliott, C. H., Ozolins, M., Olson, R. A., & Pruitt, S. D. (1985). Behavioral management of children's distress during painful medical procedures. *Behaviour Research and Therapy, 23*(5), 513–520.

Jay, S. M., Elliott, C. H., Katz, E., & Siegel, S. E. (1987). Cognitive-behavioral and pharmacologic interventions for childrens' distress during painful medical procedures. *Journal of Consulting and Clinical Psychology, 55*(6), 860–865.

Jay, S. M., Elliott, C. H., Woody, P. D., & Siegel, S. (1991). An investigation of cognitive-behavior therapy combined with oral valium for children undergoing painful medical procedures. *Health Psychology, 10*(5), 317–322.

Jay, S., Elliott, C. H., Fitzgibbons, I., Woody, P., & Siegel, S. (1995). A comparative study of cognitive behavior therapy versus general anesthesia for painful medical procedures in children. *Pain, 62*(1), 3–9.

Jenkins, B. N., Granger, D. A., Roemer, R. J., Martinez, A., Torres, T. K., & Fortier, M. A. (2018). Emotion regulation and positive affect in the context of salivary alpha-amylase response to pain in children with cancer. *Pediatric Blood & Cancer, 65*(6), e26973. https://doi.org/10.1002/pbc.26973.

Kamen, C., Tejani, M. A., Chandwani, K., Janelsins, M., Peoples, A. R., Roscoe, J. A., et al. (2014). Anticipatory nausea and vomiting due to chemotherapy. *European Journal of Pharmacology, 722*, 172–179. https://doi.org/10.1016/j.ejphar.2013.09.071.

Kazak, A. E., Abrams, A. A., Banks, J., Christofferson, J., DiDonato, S., Grootenhuis, M., et al. (2015). Psychosocial assessment as a standard of care in pediatric cancer. *Pediatric Blood & Cancer, 62*, S426–S459. https://doi.org/10.1002/pbc.25730.

Kearney, J. A., Salley, C. G., & Muriel, A. C. (2015). Standards of psychosocial care for parents of children with cancer. *Pediatric Blood & Cancer, 62*, S632–S683. https://doi.org/10.1002/pbc.25761.

Kuppenheimer, W. G., & Brown, R. T. (2002). Painful procedures in pediatric cancer: A comparison of interventions. *Clinical Psychology Review, 22*(5), 753–786.

Levin, T. T., & Applebaum, A. J. (2014). Acute cancer cognitive therapy. *Cognitive and Behavioral Practice, 21*(4), 404–415. https://doi.org/10.1016/j.cbpra.2014.03.003.

Levine, D. R., Mandrell, B. N., Sykes, A., Pritchard, M., Gibson, D., Symons, H. J., et al. (2017). Patients' and parents' needs, attitudes, and perceptions about early palliative care integration in pediatric oncology. *JAMA Oncology, 3*(9), 1214–1220. https://doi.org/10.1001/jamaoncol.2017.0368.

Miller, E., Jacob, E., & Hockenberry, M. J. (2011). Nausea, pain, fatigue, and multiple symptoms in hospitalized children with cancer. *Oncology Nursing Forum, 38*(5), e382–e393. https://doi.org/10.1188/11.ONF.E383-E393.

Okado, Y., Howard Sharp, K. M., Tillery, R., Long, A. M., & Phipps, S. (2016). Profiles of dispositional expectancies and affectivity predict later psychosocial functioning in children and adolescents with cancer. *Journal of Pediatric Psychology, 41*(3), 298–308. https://doi.org/10.1093/jpepsy/jsv096.

Samsel, C., & Muriel, A. C. (2017). Risk factors and treatment for steroid-related mood and behavior symptoms in preschool children with leukemia: A case series. *Pediatric Blood & Cancer, 64*, 343–345. https://doi.org/10.1002/pbc.26220.

Scialla, M. A., Canter, K. S., Chen, F. F., Kolb, E. A., Sandler, E., Wiener, L., et al. (2017a). Implementing the psychosocial standards in pediatric cancer: Current staffing and services available. *Pediatric Blood & Cancer, 64*(11), e26634. https://doi.org/10.1002/pbc.26634.

Scialla, M. A., Canter, K. S., Chen, F. F., Kolb, E. A., Sandler, E., Wiener, L., et al. (2017b). Delivery of care consistent with the psychosocial standards in pediatric cancer: Current practices in the United States. *Pediatric Blood & Cancer, 65*(3), e26869. https://doi.org/10.1002/pbc.26869.

Selove, R., Kroll, T., Coppes, M., & Cheng, Y. (2012). Psychosocial services in the first 30 days after diagnosis: Results of a web-based survey of Children's Oncology Group (COG) member institutions. *Pediatric Blood & Cancer, 58*, 435–440. https://doi.org/10.1002/pbc23235.

Shockey, D. P., Menzies, V., Glick, D. F., Taylor, A. G., Boitnott, A., & Rovnyak, V. (2013). Preprocedural distress in children with cancer: An intervention using biofeedback and relaxation. *Journal of Pediatric Oncology Nursing, 30*(3), 129–138. https://doi.org/10.1177/1043454213479035.

Steele, A., Mullins, L. L., Mullins, A. J., & Muriel, A. C. (2015). Psychosocial interventions and therapeutic support as a standard of care in pediatric oncology.

Pediatric Blood & Cancer, 62, S585–S618. https://doi.org/10.1002/pbc.25701.
Wakefield, C. E., McLoone, J., Goodenough, B., Lenthen, K., Cairns, D. R., & Cohn, R. J. (2010). The psychosocial impact of completing childhood cancer treatment: A systematic review of the literature. *Journal of Pediatric Psychology, 35*(3), 262–274. https://doi.org/10.1093/jpepsy/jsp056.
Ward, E., DeSantis, C., Robbins, A., Kohler, B., & Jemal, A. (2014). Childhood and adolescent cancer statistics, 2014. *CA: A Cancer Journal for Clinicians, 64*, 83–103. https://doi.org/10.3322/caac.21219.
Wiener, L., Kazak, A. E., Noll, R. B., Patenaude, A. F., & Kupst, M. J. (2015). Standards for the psychosocial care of children with cancer and their families: An introduction to the special issue. *Pediatric Blood & Cancer, 62*, S419–S424. https://doi.org/10.1002/pbc.25675.
Zeltzer, L. K., Dolgin, M. J., LeBaron, S., & LeBaron, C. (1991). A randomized, controlled study of behavioral intervention for chemotherapy distress in children with cancer. *Pediatrics, 88*(1), 34–42.

Cognitive Behavioral Therapy for Children and Adolescents with Diabetes

Johanna L. Carpenter and Christina Cammarata

Introduction

Insulin-dependent diabetes mellitus (IDDM) is a term that encompasses type 1 diabetes and insulin-dependent type 2 diabetes, two diseases that require adherence to demanding and complicated daily medical regimens in order to prevent life-threatening conditions and long-term complications. Among children and adolescents with IDDM, psychosocial issues are common and intersect with biological and developmental factors that affect adherence and disease management. IDDM, particularly type 1 diabetes, has long been a focus within the field of pediatric psychology, with efforts focused on (a) refining a biopsychosocial model of disease management and (b) applying cognitive behavioral interventions to promote adjustment, coping, and adherence within the family and developmental context.

Type 1 diabetes is a complex autoimmune disease involving the destruction of the insulin-producing cells in the pancreas, which results in dysregulation of blood glucose, protein, and fat metabolism. Rates of type 1 diabetes are increasing by 2–5% worldwide, with 1 in 300 affected by age 18 (Maahs et al. 2011). Type 2 diabetes, closely linked to obesity, is characterized by a combination of resistance to peripheral insulin and inadequate insulin secretion by pancreatic beta cells. Once thought to be limited to adults, type 2 diabetes has steadily increased in prevalence among children and adolescents, with recent estimates approaching 1 in 500 (Dabelea et al. 2014), a subset of whom would be insulin-dependent. For type 1 diabetes, the Diabetes Control and Complications Trial (DCCT) suggests that intensive treatment focused on achieving a hemoglobin A1c (HbA1c) value as close to normal as possible without excessive hypoglycemia ($\leq$7–7.5%) can prevent or delay complications, such as cardiovascular disease, kidney damage, retinopathy, neuropathy, and premature death (Nathan and DCCT/EPIC Research Group 2014). Intensive treatment typically means a combination of multiple daily injections or an insulin pump, self-monitoring of glucose via finger pricks four to six times daily or the use of a continuous glucose monitor (CGM; worn subcutaneously on a continuous basis), correction of highs and lows, and monitoring and regulation of carbohydrate intake. Exercise can also play a role by helping to manage weight and by increasing sensitivity to insulin (Robertson et al. 2009). For youth with insulin-dependent type 2 diabetes, the insulin regimen and treatment goals are similar, with the possible addition of the oral hypoglyce-

J. L. Carpenter · C. Cammarata (✉)
Division of Behavioral Health, Department of Pediatrics, Nemours/Alfred I. duPont Hospital for Children and Sidney Kimmel Medical College, Thomas Jefferson University, Wilmington, DE, USA
e-mail: johanna.carpenter@nemours.org

mic agent metformin (American Diabetes Association 2016). Not surprisingly, this complex and multi-component regimen presents significant adherence challenges; as many as 75% of adolescents do not meet guidelines for glycemic control, placing them at risk for long-term complications (Kakleas et al. 2009).

Biopsychosocial Model of Diabetes Management

The biopsychosocial model of diabetes and its management is centered on the complex relations among glycemic control, adherence, and other psychosocial and biological variables—all embedded within the developmental context of childhood or adolescence. Broadly speaking, glycemic control refers to the degree to which the patient achieves in-range blood glucose levels, while minimizing hypoglycemia and hyperglycemia. This is typically assessed using the hemoglobin A1c (HbA1c) laboratory test, which measures the stability of blood glucose levels over the preceding 2–3 months by determining the percentage of glycosylated hemoglobin in the patient's blood. Individual blood glucose values from the patient's meter may also be examined to obtain a picture of recent glycemic control. Adherence, which refers to the completion of diabetes management tasks according to the prescribed medical regimen, is distinct from, but directly linked to, glycemic control, with better adherence associated with better glycemic control (Hood et al. 2009). Due to the complexity of the diabetes regimen, few patients and families consistently achieve optimal adherence. One study found that even a small difference in management task completion was associated with decrements in glycemic control over a 2-year period (Rausch et al. 2012). A number of biological and psychosocial variables have been associated with, or found to be predictive of, adherence and/or glycemic control.

Physiological Stress Response Activation

There is a complex interplay between glycemic control and the broad concept of psychological stress. Generally speaking, stress can raise blood sugar levels and negatively affect glycemic control through its activation of the sympathetic nervous system and the release of stress hormones, namely cortisol and catecholamines (Surwit and Schneider 1993). Among adolescent populations, several studies have supported the relation between stress and glycemic control (e.g., Seiffge-Krenke and Stemmler 2003). It should be noted, however, that the actual impact of stress on glycemic control can be highly individualized and variable (Riazi et al. 2004), which likely reflects the role of coping and variation in stress perception and reactivity across individuals.

Puberty

During puberty, insulin resistance increases in both diabetic and non-diabetic youth, which can contribute to significantly higher insulin doses in adolescents with IDDM and poorer glycemic control (Amiel et al. 1986). As a result, adolescents' insulin regimens need to be frequently adjusted, which may further complicate diabetes management for families.

Parenting and Family Conflict/Support

Effective diabetes management in children and adolescents is embedded in the context of the family; therefore, parenting and family-level variables are essential for the understanding of variability in diabetes-related outcomes. Adherence and/or glycemic control have been linked across multiple studies to family communication (e.g., Iskander et al. 2015), diabetes-specific conflict (e.g., Vaid et al. 2018), problem-solving (e.g., Wysocki et al. 2008b), and parent-adolescent relationship quality and parental monitoring (e.g., Berg et al. 2011). Also, key is achieving an appropriate balance of responsibility for diabetes tasks between youth with diabetes and caregivers, in accordance with the adolescent's developmental maturity rather than chronological age (Helgeson et al. 2008; Wysocki et al. 1996).

Executive Function

Executive function (EF) challenges have been linked to poorer adherence and glycemic control among adolescent with diabetes (Duke and Harris 2014), suggesting that EF issues may contribute to difficulty following complex diabetes regimens. One study found that approximately 11–18% of adolescents with diabetes had clinically significant EF deficits in one or more specific domains (Perez et al. 2017). EF weaknesses may be of particular concern in the context of other risk factors, such as lower levels of parental involvement or when diabetes responsibility has been fully transferred to the adolescent from the parent.

Diabetes Distress

Diabetes distress (DD) is a negative emotional response to having diabetes and the associated challenges of diabetes self-management, which could present as anger, hopelessness, sadness, apathy, and/or fearfulness (Hagger et al. 2016). Adolescents with significant DD (about one-third of adolescents with diabetes) are likely to perceive diabetes as burdensome and overwhelming; to struggle with diabetes self-efficacy, adherence, and glycemic control; and to experience guilt and/or frustration related to blood glucose management (Hagger et al. 2016). DD is distinct from, but could co-occur with, broader clinical disorders such as depression and anxiety (Hagger et al. 2016). One study found that diabetes distress is more strongly associated with glycemic control than depression and fully mediated the relation between depressive symptoms and HbA1c levels (Hagger et al. 2017).

Comorbid Mental Health Conditions

Youth with diabetes are disproportionately at risk for mental health conditions (Blanz et al. 1993). Multiple studies have documented increased risk of disorders including depression (e.g., Hood et al. 2006), anxiety (e.g., Herzer and Hood 2010); eating disorders (e.g., Pinhas-Hamiel et al. 2015); and externalizing problems (e.g., Holmes et al. 1998), as well as significant rates of needle phobia (Cemeroglu et al. 2015). The presence of psychiatric comorbidities increases the likelihood of repeat hospitalizations (Garrison et al. 2005); higher hemoglobin A1c levels (Pinhas-Hamiel et al. 2015); less frequent blood glucose monitoring (Herzer and Hood 2010; Hood et al. 2006), and recurrent diabetic ketoacidosis (Smaldone et al. 2005).

Case Example: Conceptualization

J[1] is a 14-year-old male with type 1 diabetes who was referred for consultation because of elevated HbA1c (10.0%). Due to nonadherence, he was recently transitioned to a multiple daily injection regimen after having used an insulin pump for 6 years. J was diagnosed with diabetes at age 5. He was a happy, typically developing boy prior to diagnosis. His HbA1c ranged from 7.2 to 8.2% until approximately age 13, at which time he began to struggle more with adherence.

Up until 4 weeks ago, J used an insulin pump and continuous glucose monitor (CGM). He rarely administered insulin boluses to cover for meals or correct high blood sugars and did not wear his CGM. Currently, he checks his blood sugar approximately twice per day and rarely covers meals with insulin appropriately. When his mother asks if he has completed diabetes

---

[1]This is an amalgamated case example from which unique identifying information has been removed.

tasks, he often lies and says yes. He dislikes his new regimen and wants to go back on a pump.

J lives with his biological parents. He is an only child. His mother has a high school education and works in retail. J's father works long hours as a laborer and has always had limited involvement in J's medical care. He has friends and enjoys playing sports. He reported that his favorite activity is playing video games and basketball. J is in the 11th grade and an average student. He described an indifferent attitude toward school and schoolwork. He hopes to attend a technical school after graduation. There is no history of learning or attention concerns.

J's parents used to be primarily responsible for reminding him to complete tasks but recently transitioned this responsibility to J. J and his mother often argue about his diabetes management, and he feels that she "just wants to control everything." J described not knowing when his mother will "start in on [him]" about his diabetes; he perceives that she "nags" or lectures him. He responds by eventually going to his room to ignore her, but sometimes they get into arguments and yell. He also finds endocrine appointments to be aversive because his mother scolds him afterwards and takes away his screen time privileges.

J expressed great dissatisfaction with his life and little sense of control over negative events related to his diabetes. When discussing his diabetes, J expressed apathy at times, as well as feeling frustrated and overwhelmed. He described diabetes as the cause of all the conflict in his house and believes that "everything would be fine" if he did not have it. He also mentioned that it seemed like nothing he did mattered, as he tends to "always" have high blood sugars and is "doomed" to have complications later in life. He also noted a tendency of his parents to "grill" him when his blood sugars were high.

His mother also expressed much frustration about her relationship with J and decreasing control over J's health. She expressed frequent worry about J's health and her perception that J does not care about his health. At his age, she does not believe that she should have to monitor him and his diabetes. She noted that when she attempts to talk to J, he is often surly or rude, or does not respond at all. She does not feel supported in her role as the primary diabetes caregiver.

> **Box 21.1 Treatment Targets for J's Case by Domain**
>
> Based on a family systems/CBT conceptualization, the following treatment targets were identified for J:
>
> **Cognitive**: Help J and his mother to reframe negative automatic thoughts. J's negative automatic thoughts included: *I can't do this; This isn't fair; What's the point since I'll never be cured*, whereas his mother's included: *He should be more independent; He doesn't care—why should I?*
>
> **Family**: Increase positive communication strategies and reduce conflict overall; strengthen parental family subsystem to help J's father increase his involvement and to reduce his mother's care burden; help family to balance parental supervision of diabetes with J's need for autonomy.
>
> **Affective**: Help J to reduce diabetes-related distress by linking diabetes with one or more identified values.
>
> **Behavioral**: Increase frequency of appropriate diabetes management tasks through problem-solving and an incentive system.

Biopsychosocial Conceptualization

A number of psychosocial variables appear to be underlying J's difficulty with adherence, including diabetes distress (resulting in avoidance of diabetes tasks); decreased parental support; and conflict with parents. These issues are all occurring in the developmental context of adolescence, which (a) likely led to J's parents prematurely transferring diabetes responsibility to J, and (b) is likely contributing to J feeling resentful of his mother's attempts to encourage task completion, due to normative autonomy-seeking. Stressful interactions with his mother and increased insulin resistance with pubertal onset may also be contributing to worse glycemic control.

Evidence-Based Treatment Approaches for Common Intervention Targets

Family Communication and Problem-Solving

Behavioral Family Systems Therapy for Diabetes (BFST-D) Behavioral Family Systems Therapy for Diabetes (BFST-D) is a well-established family-based intervention for adolescents with diabetes and their caregivers that has demonstrated positive effects on observed parent-adolescent communication (Wysocki et al. 2008a) and on treatment adherence and metabolic control (Wysocki et al. 2007). BFST-D consists of multiple components, including communication skills training, cognitive restructuring, structural family therapy, and problem-solving skills training, which are typically delivered in 12 sessions in single-family format. When it is possible to work with a family for 12 sessions, BFST-D is our treatment of choice, as it offers the most comprehensive approach to changing family dynamics, communication patterns, and diabetes task adherence in adolescents. Given that clinicians do not always have the luxury of time, we discuss some of these individual components in the sections below (i.e., problem-solving skills training, cognitive restructuring), so that clinicians might select the modules most appropriate for their patients.

The BFST-D communication skills training module presents many options to the clinician to help reshape family communication patterns. The manual provides a helpful summary of common communication "errors," including name-calling; giving the "silent treatment"; put-downs or shaming; lecturing or preaching; threatening; using sarcasm; eye-rolling, and making poor eye contact (Wysocki et al. 2001). We find it useful to begin by having each family member individually indicate which communication "errors" he or she may tend to engage in by completing a checklist—as well as which "errors" he or she has observed in other family members. This exercise forms the basis for identifying alternative, positive communication strategies and for self-monitoring of certain communication errors. Throughout the treatment, the clinician can provide feedback on observed communication skills, modeling, and even rehearsal to help family members engage in more adaptive communication. An additional goal of communication-focused work for adolescents and parents can be to figure out how to avoid communication "pitfalls" that are specific to their family. For example, if a reminder to check blood sugar almost always results in conflict, an adolescent might prefer that her father simply hand her the meter without actually saying anything. Similarly, if an adolescent felt that reporting a high blood sugar typically resulted in an argument or analysis about why the level was high, the family could make an agreement to respond to all blood sugar numbers without any judgment or commentary.

Diabetes Task Completion

Behavioral reward systems The token economy or reward system is a widely used, well-established behavioral intervention that makes a token or reward contingent on the demonstration of a desired behavior (Hackenberg 2009). Petry et al. (2015) found significant improvements in adolescents' blood glucose monitoring after they received a small monetary incentive for each blood glucose check. We frequently assist families in developing individualized reward systems based on specific diabetes goals, incentives, and family's reward system type preference (e.g., electronic, paper, or token; Table 21.1). We have found that the frequency of reinforcement and the immediacy/consistency with which incentives are provided are the most important concepts that dictate the success or failure of a home reward system. Thus, we always encourage families who wish to work toward less frequent, larger rewards (e.g., weekly or monthly) to also include more frequent, smaller rewards. If families are resistant to the idea of a reward system, we often discuss the role of rewards in helping to initiate and maintain new behaviors.

Table 21.1 Using behavioral reward systems for diabetes management

Ideas for diabetes goals	Ideas for incentives	Ideas for tracking
• Cooperating with blood sugar checks and injections • Checking blood sugar or giving injections independently • Adding one more blood sugar check per day • Following through on insulin administration after high blood sugar • Following recommended nutritional changes, such as increasing protein intake or eating breakfast • Dosing insulin before meals • *Asking* for food or a snack (instead of just helping himself/herself) • Having one or two sit-down snacks (instead of "grazing") • Measuring out food or using pre-packaged foods to help with carb-counting (instead of guessing) • Telling parents about highs/lows (instead of trying to hide them) • Recording numbers on a log • Wearing diabetes medical bracelet • Rotating insulin injection sites or using non-preferred sites • And more!	*Privileges:* • Screen time • Play dates, time with friends, sleepovers • Special outings (zoo, park, museum, movies, mall, restaurant, camping trip) • Extra one-on-one time with parents or other family members • Later bedtime on weekends • Driving practice (for teens) • Being allowed to control the remote/pick what is for dinner/pick the restaurant, etc. *Tangible rewards:* • Toys or gadgets • Gift cards • Small amounts of money, etc. Small rewards are given the same day or earned over the course of no longer than 1 week. Large rewards are earned over several weeks or months. Note: if using large rewards, make sure to have some privileges or small rewards sprinkled in there too. The definition of "small" vs. "large" rewards will vary by family	• *Electronic:* An electronic reward chart using a smart phone or tablet can help make it easier for parents to be consistent and to make the chart more engaging for children. One such smartphone/tablet reward chart "app" is called iReward chart, available either for one child and up to four tasks (free, Lite version) or for multiple children and more tasks (regular version, $3.99). iReward chart is available for multiple devices and platforms and allows for synchronization across two caregivers' devices • *Paper:* Points are recorded on a paper chart that is displayed in a central location, often on the refrigerator • *Token* (for children 5–8 years old): Tokens such poker chips or pennies are placed in a jar, box, coffee can, or other container every time that points are earned Points or tokens are awarded *each time* the behavioral goal is met (e.g., for each blood sugar check that the child cooperates with)

We typically prefer to begin the process of behavior modification using only positive reinforcement systems, but, in some cases, consequences are also helpful if the desired behavior is not demonstrated. We caution families that any removal of privileges should be relatively brief (e.g., no screen time after dinner that same day) so that the child or adolescent can try again later. The BFST-D manual includes a behavioral contract with both privileges and consequences (Wysocki et al. 2001).

Problem-solving skills training The challenges associated with diabetes are dynamic, and they may evolve rapidly as youth achieve new developmental tasks, are placed in new settings (e.g., after-school activities, sleepovers), and have seasonal changes in their diabetes care plan (e.g., summer or holiday breaks). Problem-solving skills training provides a structure for individuals and families to discuss and solve various diabetes-related issues using a series of clearly defined steps, which can then be applied flexibly to any diabetes challenge. Because problem-solving focuses on current and very specific behavioral goals, it may also help prevent conflict or breakdowns in family communication stemming from overly emotional responses or dwelling on past issues. Among children and adolescents, problem-solving skills interventions have been primarily associated with improvements in global adherence behaviors (Hill-Briggs and Gemmell 2007). Although less consistent, associations between problem-solving interventions and improved glycemic control have been found (e.g., Carpenter et al. 2014; Nansel et al. 2012).

Problem-solving skills training typically includes some instruction in the steps involved, as well as modeling, prior to the therapist guiding the family through the steps to solve an individualized problem. The precise steps may vary slightly but are as follows in our version: (1) Identify the problem to be solved; (2) Set a clear, specific, and measurable goal; (3) Identify an incentive that is contingent upon the goal's completion; (4) Brainstorm strategies that could help support the achievement of the goal; (5) Evaluate the strategies (from child/adolescent, parent, and endocrinologist perspective); (6) Choose one or more strategies to try for a specific period of time; (7) Evaluate how well the strategies worked to achieve the goal. If the strategies were not successful, pick a new strategy.

When modeling the problem-solving steps, we often use a non-diabetes example (someone who needs to leave the house imminently for a job interview but cannot find one of her shoes), but we may use a diabetes example as well if it seems that the family could benefit from a more explicit demonstration. The central challenge in teaching problem-solving tends to be the identification of a problem area and associated goal that are behavioral in nature (e.g., an identified problem such as "Snacking without covering" instead of "Too irresponsible") and sufficiently specific (e.g., a goal such as "Have larger snack at 4 p.m. everyday" instead of "Lower A1c"). The goal should be based on the current level of diabetes task completion (not optimal disease management) and reflect only a slight increase in responsibility beyond current task completion levels. This is essential in order to achieve initial success and to gradually build up new habits for long-term change. A final consideration, in step 4, is that the clinician should encourage the family to generate ideas without judging the ideas until the next step. A sample problem-solving worksheet is provided in Fig. 21.1.

Problem that we're working on: Checking blood sugar more frequently (currently 2x's/day)

Goal that we've set: Check blood sugar 3x's/day for 7 days in a row—add a.m. time

Reward for meeting the goal: More screen time (weekdays) or have friends over (Sat/Sun)

Solution	Evaluation – will this work…			Try it? If so, for how long?	Did it work? (If not, pick a new solution)
	…for you?	…for your parents?	…for your medical team?		
Keep meter on kitchen table in plain view	Yes +	Yes +	Yes +	Yes. For 2 days	Didn't help
Post-it note taped to breakfast foods	Yes +	Yes +	Yes +	Yes. For 2 days	Worked!
Do 3 checks in a row; get them out of the way!	Yes +	No –	No –		
Pair checking with routine activities	Yes +	Yes +	Yes +	Yes. For 1 week.	It worked!
Recurring cell phone alarm	So-So /	Yes +	Yes +		
Verbal reminder from parents	No –	So-So /	Yes +		
Log kept on fridge so that missing #'s are obvious	So-So /	So-So /	Yes +		
Have mom send 3 texts per day as reminder	Yes +	No –	Yes +		

Fig. 21.1 Sample problem-solving worksheet, filled in for blood sugar checking goal

Diabetes Distress (Hopelessness/Apathy/Lack of Acceptance)

Cognitive restructuring Cognitive restructuring is a technique central to cognitive behavioral therapy that helps individuals to recognize cognitive distortions and to reframe them into more adaptive or realistic thoughts (Please also see Chaps. 7 and 8 this volume). Cognitive distortions have been indirectly linked to worse glycemic control (Farrell et al. 2004). Cognitive behavioral interventions incorporating cognitive restructuring have shown some promise in addressing diabetes outcomes, including adherence and diabetes-related stress (e.g., Silverman et al. 2003). In our work, we have found the cognitive restructuring module within BFST-D to be helpful, as the manual provides examples of cognitive distortions or "strong beliefs" and ways to challenge these distortions, drawn from diabetes-specific and non-diabetes situations and encompassing both an adolescent and a parental perspective (Wysocki et al. 2001). Cognitive restructuring may be particularly helpful to cover in the context of strong family conflict, hopelessness about diabetes, and depressive symptoms. We recommend involving caregivers in order to identify distorted beliefs that they may have about parenting their adolescent with diabetes, as well as involving the adolescent.

Diabetes meaning-making Our approach to helping adolescents identify or make meaning out of having diabetes is not a specific approach that has been discussed in the literature, to our knowledge. It is related, however, to the process of values identification that is a core component of Acceptance and Commitment Therapy (ACT; Hayes et al. 2006), a third-wave behavior therapy focused on increasing psychological flexibility and living a meaningful life consistent with identified values. Although we are not aware of studies specific to pediatric diabetes, ACT is being studied in other adolescent chronic illnesses (e.g., Wicksell et al. 2009) and in adult diabetes samples (e.g., Gregg et al. 2007).

The first goal of a meaning-making intervention is to help the patient (usually an adolescent) to identify something that he or she values or that brings meaning to life (e.g., excelling at a sport, being a role model for a sibling or family member, an educational or career goal, an interest or hobby, a strong personal relationship, etc.). If the patient is able to do this, then the focus shifts to the second goal of exploring how diabetes management might be related to the patient's valued relationship, goal, or activity. The patient is asked to consider how taking care of diabetes might contribute to the patient's identified value(s). Similarly, the therapist guides the patient to question how not taking care of diabetes might hold the patient back from living the most meaningful, values-consistent life. It is important for the clinician to show a nonjudgmental and curious attitude and not convey an "agenda." If successful, the discussion helps the patient to see a connection between one or more personal values and diabetes management, thereby linking diabetes with meaning.

Motivational interviewing Motivational interviewing (MI) refers to the collaborative, client-centered process of promoting motivation for change through the use of guiding skills, effective responses to resistance, and listening for and leveraging change talk (Miller and Rollnick 2013) (Please see also Chap. 6 this volume). MI is a particularly useful approach for adolescent patients when the patient is so apathetic or ambivalent that he or she is not able to identify any pros of improving diabetes adherence. Two randomized controlled trials of interventions for adolescents with diabetes that included MI found variable impacts on glycemic control but improvements in other psychosocial variables, including quality of life (Channon et al. 2007; Mayer-Davis et al. 2018). A comprehensive overview of MI for diabetes management change is beyond the scope of this chapter, but we recommend further reading that focuses on MI in adolescence and emerging adulthood, such as Naar-King and Suarez (2011).

Injection Fear and/or Resistance

Injection routine chart A common concern among parents who perform blood glucose (BG) checks and insulin injections for their children is a lack of cooperation or active resistance when it is time for these tasks. If the issue is primarily that a child is successfully delaying the BG checks/injections—and not extreme distress with injections or finger sticks—then an injection routine chart and immediate incentive may be sufficient to improve diabetes task timeliness and cooperation while reducing parental frustration. The goal of an injection routine is to increase the child's comfort level and compliance by creating predictability and a habitual sequence of events. Ideally, an injection routine consists of about three to four steps, includes a regular location in the home for BG checks/injections, indicates any distractions or comfort objects to be used, specifies any necessary behaviors for which the child need prompts (e.g., sitting still), and includes an incentive or small reward (see Fig. 21.2 for an example). To encourage regular rotation of injection sites, one strategy is to write down all possible body parts on slips of paper and to allow the child to select one out of a jar or bowl (the selected slip of paper is not returned to the jar until all body parts have been used). Caregivers should be coached to follow the routine in a calm, matter-of-fact manner and to prepare the syringe out of the child's sight and have it completely ready before initiating the routine.

Graduated exposure For children or teens who display very high levels of distress when faced with BG checks and/or insulin injections, graduated exposure to the feared stimulus (the needle itself and/or the process of giving a shot or stick) is typically indicated. Graduated exposure is an essential "ingredient" within cognitive behavioral treatment of needle phobia or injection fear (McMurty et al. 2016) and is characterized by helping the child to gradually face or engage with needles/injections in imagined or real-world (in vivo) situations that increase in difficulty as the child is successful. Both imaginal and in vivo exposures have been successfully used with children with diabetes and needle fears (Rainwater et al. 1988). Exposure treatment begins with the development of a fear hierarchy, based on the patient's subjective distress ratings of various situations involving needles and injections/sticks. These situations are then rank-ordered from easiest to hardest, and rewards or privileges are associated with each step in the hierarchy. Relaxation training and/or cognitive restructuring can be integrated into the treatment plan prior to starting exposures.

Hierarchies will vary considerably across patients, both in terms of the starting point of the hierarchy and the patients' goals for the last step of the hierarchy. One patient might not be able to even tolerate the sight of a syringe and, thus, might start by imagining a syringe or imagining being given an injection. Another patient might

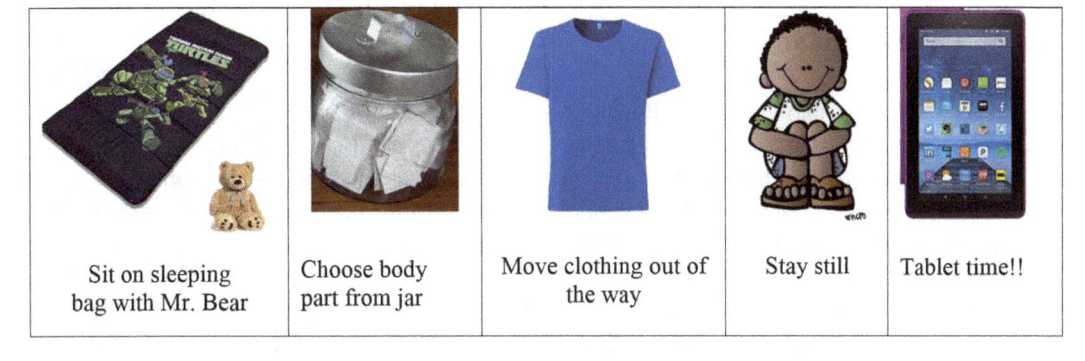

Sit on sleeping bag with Mr. Bear	Choose body part from jar	Move clothing out of the way	Stay still	Tablet time!!

Fig. 21.2 Sample injection routine chart

be able to start his hierarchy by tapping a capped needle against his skin or watching a video of an injection. A younger child whose caregivers will still be giving insulin injections might be working up to the point of being able to successfully follow an injection routine (as described above), whereas an adolescent might be working on being able to self-administer insulin. When working on the self-administration of insulin, it is very helpful to be able to co-treat for a few sessions with a diabetes educator or endocrinology nurse, which allows for the patient to practice with saline injections while receiving coaching on technique.

Other nonpharmacological interventions For a full review of interventions to reduce procedural pain and distress, the reader is referred to the recent chapter by Cohen et al. (2017). One intervention that may be used in combination with injection routines or exposure is Buzzy®, a small reusable thermomechanical device (buzzy-helps.com) that produces a strong vibrating sensation, with or without a concomitant numbing effect from a reusable ice pack, that can diminish patients' perception of needle pain (e.g., Moadad et al. 2016). Information about Buzzy® is now part of the psychoeducation that we provide in our inpatient setting to all patients and families with new diagnoses of IDDM. Distraction can also be a helpful adjunctive intervention when patients are not self-injecting and can effectively draw attention away from the injection and pain sensation (Koller and Goldman 2012).

Fear of Hypoglycemia

Fear of hypoglycemia may develop following a severe hypoglycemic event but may also emerge in youth and/or caregivers with high levels of trait anxiety (Shepard et al. 2014). Associated behaviors may include excessive BG checking or even purposely trying to maintain higher blood sugars, which may affect glycemic control as well as quality of life (Driscoll et al. 2016). The pediatric literature has focused exclusively on assessment of fear of hypoglycemia rather than intervention, but adult studies have revealed support for cognitive behavior therapy, as well as blood glucose awareness training to recognize hyperglycemia and hypoglycemia (Cox et al. 1988).

Fear of hypoglycemia is a challenging concern to treat because severe hypoglycemia is a very real possibility for patients with diabetes. Moreover, the physical symptoms of anxiety overlap somewhat with those of hypoglycemia (e.g., shakiness, sweating), making it potentially more challenging for patients to differentiate the two states. As an initial step, we have found it helpful to consult with the patient's endocrinology provider about the patient's risk for hypoglycemia, which may affect treatment strategies. We then request that the family log the patient's blood glucose values for the next 1–2 weeks until the next session. Before each blood glucose check, the patient and caregiver should each guess the meter reading and log their guesses, along with any physical symptoms that the patient experienced at the time. This exercise may reveal tendencies to underestimate blood glucose levels that are normal or high, or to be accurate about high levels but underestimate normal levels (which might suggest that the patient experiences high sugars as "normal"). Other specific treatment components may include additional education to differentiate anxiety symptoms from low blood glucose levels (perhaps with a diabetes educator), relaxation training, cognitive restructuring, and exposures (e.g., if a patient is reluctant to correct high BG).

Case Example: Treatment

Treatment for J's family used the BFST-D treatment framework. Sessions began with problem-solving skills training in order to work on containing conflictual interactions that often emerged during diabetes-related discussion while still addressing diabetes task completion.

Clinician: OK, let's think about how we can support J in his diabetes management. There are so many different things that someone with diabetes has to do that we want to focus on just one area at a time. But since it can be hard to focus on just one thing, many families have found it helpful to follow specific problem-solving steps—this helps us stay on track and can help the discussion be calmer and more productive. [Shows family problem-solving steps worksheet. Fig. 21.1] So I am going to walk us through each of the steps but also let the two of you discuss your ideas. Sounds okay? [They nod.]

Clinician: Great. Let's start with identifying the problem area that we want to focus on. We want this to be specific enough that we know what we need to be working on. For example, "A1c is too high" wouldn't be a helpful problem to identify, because it's too general.

Mom: OK. Well, in that case, I would start with his attitude. J needs to adjust his attitude about diabetes. Diabetes is here, and it's not going anywhere.

J: *You* try having diabetes, and we'll see what your attitude looks like.

Clinician: Let's see if we can narrow that down a little. If J had the type of attitude that you wanted him to have about his diabetes, what would he do to take care of his diabetes?

Mom: Well for starters, he would actually check his sugars when I ask him to! Not just pretend to and then feed me a bunch of lies. At first I believed him, but I wasn't born yesterday.

J: I told you, I don't lie to you anymore.

Mom: No, now you just don't do it! Your doctors want you to check your sugars at least five times!

Clinician: OK, so blood sugar checking could be a problem area to start with. I think that works well because it is very clear what we are working on. J, do you have any other ideas instead?

J: That's fine, whatever.

Clinician: OK, sounds good. So now we need a specific goal, related to the problem area of not checking sugars frequently enough. When we come up with this goal, we want it to be very clear and specific, so that you and J know whether or not the goal was met for the day. We also want the goal to be about one step up from where he is now, so that he's not trying to do too much all at once.

Mom: Well, I would say he needs to check at least five times a day. Maybe aim for seven.

Clinician: And right now you're checking about how often, J?

Mom: About twice per day.

J: No, Mom! You always assume the worst! Three times.

Mom: Well, two to three times, but two more often than three—usually lunch and bedtime.

Clinician: I see. So for two to three times per day, it may be too big of a leap to go straight to five or seven times. We want this goal to be attainable, and we also want to gradually build up the habit of checking so that it really sticks.

Mom: Hmm. Okay. I guess that means...we really need to do just three times? But his endocrinologist isn't going to like that. Remember, your doctor said that you need to check five times a day and if you don't it's going to be really unsafe. You don't want to end up in the hospital, do you?

Clinician: So, we are going to eventually get to the recommended number of daily checks, but we are getting there one step at a time. This is the first step. What do you think about the goal, J?

J: Easy. I could do so much more.

Mom: So then, why don't you?

Clinician: J, I know that you can; we'll get there soon. What check do you think you could add?

Mom: Definitely morning. Remember what Dr. G said!

J: Fine, morning, sure.

Clinician: That sounds perfect. OK, I think you're going to enjoy the next step, J. This is the step where you get to choose an incentive to work for, and you'll get it if you meet your goal. An incentive, or a reward, can really help get new habits going. It's also a way to recognize you for the hard work that you are doing taking care of diabetes. Let's talk about incentives that you could earn for meeting your goal. [J and his mother decide that he can earn screen time or outings with friends.]

Clinician: Nice work picking out some incentives. I think those sound great. The next step is the brainstorming step. With this step, you are going to be thinking of some ideas or strategies that should help you successfully add a morning check in every day. They could be strategies to help you remember, or just strategies to make it easier to get the check done. The important thing is to get all of your ideas out there, no matter how far-fetched they sound. You'll evaluate them later.

Mom: I'm not sure I understand what you mean by strategies. He just has to do it.

J: I don't need any strategies.

Clinician: What I mean by strategies are things that you and/or your mom can do that will increase the likelihood of successfully meeting your goal. I know that blood sugar checks are easy for you to do, but that doesn't mean that they are easy to fit into your life.

Mom: Oh, okay, I see. But what's an example?

Clinician: Well, if you'd like one to get you started, one strategy could be to put your meter in a really hard-to-miss spot that you are definitely going to see in the morning. Another is to start pairing your morning check with something else that is already part of your morning routine.

Mom: Oh, that could work, right J?

J: I don't know. Maybe.

Clinician: Right now, don't worry about whether they will work or not. Just try to come up with as many ideas as you can, and then you'll evaluate them in the next step.

[Mom and J discuss amongst themselves and come up with five ideas. They then complete the next step, which is to evaluate each idea from multiple perspectives: patient, caregiver, medical team.]

Clinician: You all are almost done. The last step that we can do here is to choose at least one strategy to try immediately for a certain period of time. Anything jumping out as one to try, J?

J: I don't really want to try any of them.

Mom: I really think that if we put the meter in your bathroom after your bedtime check that you'll remember better. You'll connect it with brushing your teeth.

J: No, that won't make a difference.

Mom: [sighs] "Okay, fine. What would you suggest if I said you have to pick one or else there will be no PS4 tonight?"

J: Seriously?! Ugh, fine, the meter one. In the kitchen.

Clinician: Keep the meter on the kitchen table so that you'll see it in the morning?

J: Yeah, sure. Is it time to go now?

Mom: Okay, so then I'll pick the Post-it notes on breakfast foods. We'll put them on your Honey Nut Cheerios since you're the only one who eats those.

J: Fine, whatever. I think it's time to go.

Clinician: Since we'll be seeing each other next week, why don't you try both of those strategies for 2 days and then reevaluate on Saturday to see how well they are working for you? If they are not working out, pick a new one from the list or think of a new strategy.

Mom: Okay, we'll do that.

Following the first problem-solving session, portions of the subsequent sessions were reserved for ongoing problem-solving work so that the family could continue to address diabetes goals in a gradual and stepwise fashion. Once J worked up to checking five times per day (adding one BG check per week), the focus of problem-solving shifted to calculating and taking his appropriate insulin dose. The majority of family work focused on reshaping negative communication patterns between J and his mother (some "errors" included blaming, lecturing, nagging, using sarcastic and rude tones, and withdrawal), as well as discussing and challenging automatic negative thoughts for both J and his mother, one example of when J used sarcasm and withdrawal from the transcript above, included saying "That's fine, whatever." and "Fine. Morning. Sure." J would often follow these with statements that he didn't really believe the strategy would be effective. In correcting these, J's primary communication goal was to use "I" statements instead of withdrawing to his room or saying, "Whatever." In the above session, J's mother often fell into patterns of nagging and blaming, for example "J needs to adjust his attitude about diabetes," and lecturing, "remember, your doctor said that you need to check five times a day and if you don't it's going to be really unsafe. You don't want to end up in the hospital, do you?" His mother's main goal was to reflect back what J said. J and his mother also found it helpful to conduct some of their diabetes communication by text message, which reduced conflict. Due to his work schedule, J's father was able to attend only two communication-focused sessions but agreed to take over responsibility for supervising J's 9 p.m. dose of long-acting insulin. Once conflict levels improved within the home, both parents were more amenable to the idea of shared parent-adolescent responsibility for diabetes tasks. J also stated that he "kind of liked" this idea now that his mother was no longer "on his back." Both parents also agreed to focus on J's completion of diabetes tasks rather than his blood glucose numbers, although this was a concept that required revisiting over the course of treatment. Finally, J was able to make a tenuous connection between wanting to be a mechanic and his diabetes management. At the conclusion of weekly treatment (13 sessions), J's A1c had dropped to 8.9%, and he is on track to return to insulin pump therapy with continued improvement.

Conclusion

IDDM is a complex chronic illness associated with a multitude of psychosocial challenges that can interact with physiological, familial, and developmental variables to affect adherence, glycemic control, and long-term health. Operating from a developmentally informed biopsychosocial conceptualization, clinicians can address intervention targets at the individual and family levels using a number of evidence-based treatment approaches that are drawn from a CBT or behavioral framework.

References

American Diabetes Association. (2016). Standards of medical care in diabetes: Children and adolescents. *Diabetes Care, 39*(Supplement 1), S86–S93. https://doi.org/10.2337/dc16-S014.

Amiel, S. A., Sherwin, R. S., Simonson, D. C., Lauritano, A. A., & Tamborlane, W. V. (1986). Impaired insulin action in puberty. A contributing factor to poor glycemic control in adolescents with diabetes. *New England Journal of Medicine, 315*, 215–219.

Berg, C. A., King, P. S., Butler, J. M., Pham, P., Palmer, D., & Wiebe, D. J. (2011). Parental involvement and adolescents' diabetes management: The mediating role of self-efficacy and externalizing and internalizing behaviors. *Journal of Pediatric Psychology, 36*, 329–339.

Blanz, B. J., Rensch-Riemann, B. S., Fritz-Sigmund, D. I., & Schmidt, M. H. (1993). IDDM is a risk factor for adolescent psychiatric disorders. *Diabetes Care, 16*, 1579–1587.

Carpenter, J. L., Price, J. E. W., Cohen, M. J., Shoe, K. M., & Pendley, J. S. (2014). Multifamily group problem-solving intervention for adherence challenges in pediatric insulin-dependent diabetes. *Clinical Practice in Pediatric Psychology, 2*, 101–115.

Cemeroglu, A. P., Can, A., Davis, A. T., Cemeroglu, O., Kleis, L., Daniel, M. S., et al. (2015). Fear of needles in children with type 1 diabetes mellitus on multiple daily injections and continuous subcutaneous insulin infusion. *Endocrine Practice, 21*, 46–53.

Channon, S. J., Huws-Thomas, M. V., Rollnick, S., Hood, K., Cannings-John, R. L., Rogers, C., et al. (2007). A multicenter randomized controlled trial of motivational interviewing in teenagers with diabetes. *Diabetes Care, 30*, 1390–1395.

Cohen, L. L., Blount, R. L., Chorney, J., Zempsky, W., Rodrigues, N., & Cousins, L. (2017). Management of pediatric pain and distress due to medical conditions. In M. C. Roberts & R. G. Steele (Eds.), *Handbook of pediatric psychology* (5th ed., pp. 146–160). New York: Guilford.

Cox, D. J., Carter, W. R., Gonder-Frederick, L. A., Clarke, W. L., & Pohl, S. L. (1988). Blood glucose discrimination training in insulin-dependent diabetes mellitus (IDDM) patients. *Biofeedback and Self Regulation, 13*, 201–217.

Dabelea, D., Mayer-Davis, E. J., Saydah, S., Imperatore, G., Linder, B., Divers, J., Bell, R., et al. (2014). Prevalence of type 1 and type 2 diabetes among children and adolescents from 2001 to 2009. *JAMA, 311*, 1778–1786. https://doi.org/10.1001/jama.2014.3201.

Driscoll, K. A., Raymond, J., Naranjo, D., & Patton, S. R. (2016). Fear of hypoglycemia in children and adolescents and their parents with type 1 diabetes. *Current Diabetes Reports, 16*, 77–79.

Duke, D. C., & Harris, M. A. (2014). Executive function, adherence, and glycemic control in adolescents with type 1 diabetes: A literature review. *Current Diabetes Reports, 14*, 532.

Farrell, S. P., Hains, A. A., Davies, W. H., Smith, P., & Parton, E. (2004). The impact of cognitive distortions, stress, and adherence on metabolic control in youths with type 1 diabetes. *Journal of Adolescent Health, 34*, 461–467. https://doi.org/10.1016/S1054-139x(03)00215-5.

Garrison, M. M., Katon, W. J., & Richardson, L. P. (2005). The impact of psychiatric comorbidities on readmissions for diabetes in youth. *Diabetes Care, 28*, 2150–2154.

Gregg, J. A., Callaghan, G. M., Hayes, S. C., & Glenn-Lawson, J. L. (2007). Improving diabetes self-management through acceptance, mindfulness, and values: A randomized controlled trial. *Journal of Consulting and Clinical Psychology, 75*, 336–343.

Hackenberg, T. D. (2009). Token reinforcement: A review and analysis. *Journal of the Experimental Analysis of Behavior, 91*, 257–586.

Hagger, V., Hendrieckx, C., Sturt, J., Skinner, T. C., & Speight, J. (2016). Diabetes distress among adolescents with type 1 diabetes: A systematic review. *Current Diabetes Reports, 16*, 9.

Hagger, V., Hendrieckx, C., Cameron, F., Pouwer, F., Skinner, T. C., & Speight, J. (2017). Diabetes distress is more strongly associated with HbA1c than depressive symptoms in adolescents with type 1 diabetes: Results from diabetes miles youth-Australia. *Pediatric Diabetes, 19*, 840–847.

Hayes, S. C., Luoma, J., Bond, F., Masuda, A., & Lillis, J. (2006). Acceptance and commitment therapy: Model, processes, and outcomes. *Behaviour Research and Therapy, 44*, 1–25.

Helgeson, V. S., Reynolds, K. A., Siminerio, L., Escobar, O., & Becker, D. (2008). Parent and adolescent distribution of responsibility for diabetes self-care: Links to health outcomes. *Journal of Pediatric Psychology, 33*, 496–508.

Herzer, M., & Hood, K. K. (2010). Anxiety symptoms in adolescents with type 1 diabetes: Association with blood glucose monitoring and glycemic control. *Journal of Pediatric Psychology, 35*, 415–425.

Hill-Briggs, F., & Gemmell, L. (2007). Problem solving in diabetes self-management and control: A systematic review of the literature. *Diabetes Education, 33*, 1032–1050.

Holmes, C. S., Respess, D., Greer, T., & Frentz, J. (1998). Behavior problems in children with diabetes: Disentangling possible scoring confounds on the child behavior checklist. *Journal of Pediatric Psychology, 23*, 179–185.

Hood, K. K., Huestis, S., Maher, A., Butler, D., Volkening, L., & Laffel, L. M. (2006). Depressive symptoms in children and adolescents with type 1 diabetes: Association with diabetes-specific characteristics. *Diabetes Care, 29*, 1389–1391. https://doi.org/10.2337/dc06-0087.

Hood, K. K., Peterson, C. M., Rohan, J. M., & Drotar, D. (2009). Association between adherence and glycemic control in pediatric type 1 diabetes: A meta-analysis. *Pediatrics, 124*, 1171–1179.

Iskander, J. M., Rohan, J. M., Pendley, J. S., Delamater, A., & Drotar, D. (2015). A 3-year prospective study of parent-child communication in early adolescents with type 1 diabetes: Relationship to adherence and glycemic control. *Journal of Pediatric Psychology, 40*, 109–120.

Kakleas, K., Kandyla, B., Karayianni, C., & Karavanaki, K. (2009). Psychosocial problems in adolescents with type 1 diabetes mellitus. *Diabetes & Metabolism, 35*, 339–350.

Koller, D., & Goldman, R. D. (2012). Distraction techniques for children undergoing procedures: A critical review of pediatric research. *Journal of Pediatric Nursing, 27*, 652–681.

Maahs, D. M., West, N. A., Lawrence, J. M., & Mayer-Davis, E. J. (2011). Epidemiology of type 1 diabetes. *Endocrinology and Metabolism Clinics of North America, 39*, 481–497.

Mayer-Davis, E. J., Maahs, D. M., Seid, M., Crandell, J., Bishop, F. K., Driscoll, K. A., et al. (2018). Efficacy of the flexible lifestyles empowering change intervention on metabolic and psychosocial outcomes in adolescents with type 1 diabetes (FLEX): A randomised controlled trial. *The Lancet Child & Adolescent Health, 2*, 635–646.

McMurty, C. M., Taddio, A., Noel, M., Antony, M. M., Chambers, C. T., Asmundson, G. J. G., et al. (2016). Exposure-based interventions for the management of individuals with high levels of needle fear across the lifespan: A clinical practice guideline and call for further research. *Cognitive Behaviour Therapy, 45*, 217–235.

Miller, W. M., & Rollnick, S. (2013). *Motivational interviewing: Helping people change* (3rd ed.). New York: Guilford Press.

Moadad, N., Kozman, K., Shahine, R., Ohanian, S., & Badr, L. K. (2016). Distraction using the BUZZY for children during an IV insertion. *Journal of Pediatric Nursing, 31*, 64–72.

Naar-King, S., & Suarez, M. (2011). *Motivational interviewing with adolescents and young adults*. New York: Guilford.

Nansel, R., Iannotti, R. J., & Liu, A. (2012). Clinic-integrated behavioral intervention for families of youth with type 1 diabetes: Randomized clinical trial. *Pediatrics, 129*, e866–e873.

Nathan, D. M., & DCCT/EDIC Research Group. (2014). The diabetes control and complications trial/epidemiology of diabetes interventions and complications study at 30 years: Overview. *Diabetes Care, 37*, 9–16.

Perez, K. M., Patel, N. J., Lord, J. H., Savin, K. L., Monzon, A. D., Whittemore, R., et al. (2017). Executive function in adolescents with type 1 diabetes: Relationship to adherence, glycemic control, and psychosocial outcomes. *Journal of Pediatric Psychology, 42*, 636–646.

Petry, N. M., Cengiz, E., Wagner, J. A., Weyman, K., Tichy, E., & Tamborlane, W. V. (2015). Testing for rewards: A pilot study to improve type 1 diabetes management in adolescents. *Diabetes Care, 38*, 1952–1954.

Pinhas-Hamiel, O., Hamiel, U., & Levy-Shraga, Y. (2015). Eating disorders in adolescents with type 1 diabetes: Challenges in diagnosis and treatment. *World Journal of Diabetes, 6*, 517–526.

Rainwater, N., Sweet, A. A., Elliott, L., Bowers, M., McNeill, J., & Stump, N. (1988). Systematic desensitization in the treatment of needle phobias for children with diabetes. *Child & Family Behavior Therapy, 10*, 19–31. https://doi.org/10.1300/J019v10n01_03.

Rausch, J. R., Hood, K. K., Delamater, A., Pendley, J. S., Rohan, J. M., Reeves, G., et al. (2012). Changes in treatment adherence and glycemic control during the transition to adolescence in type 1 diabetes. *Diabetes Care, 35*, 1219–1224.

Riazi, A., Pickup, J., & Bradley, C. (2004). Daily stress and glycaemic control in type 1 diabetes: Individual differences in magnitude, direction, and timing of stress-reactivity. *Diabetes Research and Clinical Practice, 66*, 237–244.

Robertson, D., Adolfsson, P., Scheiner, G., Hanas, R., & Riddell, M. C. (2009). Exercise in children and adolescents with diabetes. *Pediatric Diabetes, 10*, 154–168.

Seiffge-Krenke, L., & Stemmler, M. (2003). Coping with everyday stress and links to medical and psychosocial adaptation in diabetic adolescents. *Journal of Adolescent Health, 33*, 180–188.

Shepard, J. A., Vajda, K., Nyer, M., Clarke, W., & Gonder-Frederick, L. (2014). Understanding the construct of fear of hypoglycemia in pediatric type 1 diabetes. *Journal of Pediatric Psychology, 39*, 1115–1125. https://doi.org/10.1093/jpepsy/jsu068.

Silverman, A. H., Hains, A. A., Davies, W. H., & Parton, E. (2003). A cognitive behavioral adherence intervention for adolescents with type 1 diabetes. *Journal of Clinical Psychology in Medical Settings, 10*, 119–127.

Smaldone, A., Honig, J., Stone, P. W., Arons, R., & Weinger, K. (2005). Characteristics of California children with single versus multiple diabetic ketoacidosis hospitalizations (1998–2000). *Diabetes Care, 28*, 2082–2084.

Surwit, R. S., & Schneider, M. S. (1993). Role of stress in the etiology and treatment of diabetes mellitus. *Psychosomatic Medicine, 55*, 380–393.

Vaid, E., Lansing, A. H., & Stanger, C. (2018). Problems with self-regulation, family conflict, and glycemic control in adolescents experiencing challenges with managing type 1 diabetes. *Journal of Pediatric Psychology, 43*, 525–533. https://doi.org/10.1093/jpepsy/jsx134.

Wicksell, R. K., Melin, L., Lekander, M., & Olsson, G. L. (2009). Evaluating the effectiveness of exposure and acceptance strategies to improve functioning and quality of life in longstanding pediatric pain: A randomized controlled trial. *Pain, 141*, 248–257.

Wysocki, T., Taylor, A., Hough, B. S., Linscheid, T. R., Yeates, K. O., & Naglieri, J. A. (1996). Deviation from developmentally appropriate self-care autonomy: Association with diabetes outcomes. *Diabetes Care, 19*, 119–125.

Wysocki, T., Harris, M. A., Greco, P., Mertlich, D., & Buckloh, L. (2001). *Behavioral family systems therapy for adolescents (BFST) treatment and implementation manual*. Contact Dr. Tim Wysocki at twysocki@nemours.org.

Wysocki, T., Harris, M. A., Buckloh, L. M., Mertlich, D., Lochrie, A. S., Mauras, N., et al. (2007). Randomized trial of behavioral family systems therapy for diabetes: Maintenance of effects on diabetes outcomes in adolescents. *Diabetes Care, 30*, 555–560.

Wysocki, T., Harris, M. A., Buckloh, L. M., Mertlich, D., Lochrie, A. S., Mauras, N., et al. (2008a). Randomized controlled trial of behavioral family systems therapy for diabetes: Maintenance and generalization of effects on parent-adolescent communication. *Behavior Therapy, 39*, 33–36.

Wysocki, T., Iannotti, R., Weissberg-Benchell, J., Laffel, L., Hood, K., Anderson, B., et al. (2008b). Diabetes problem solving by youths with type 1 diabetes and their caregivers: Measurement, validation, and longitudinal associations with glycemic control. *Journal of Pediatric Psychology, 33*, 875–884. https://doi.org/10.1093/jpepsy/jsn024.

Cognitive Behavioral Therapy for Youth with Asthma: Anxiety as an Example

Ashley H. Clawson, Nicole Ruppe, Cara Nwankwo, Alexandra Blair, Marissa Baudino, and Nighat Mehdi

Introduction

Asthma is a chronic respiratory disease (National Asthma Education and Prevention Program 2007). Common asthma symptoms include wheezing, shortness of breath, coughing, chest tightness, and variable airway limitation. Asthma is characterized by a pattern of recurrent and intermittent symptoms, inflammation, airway obstruction, and bronchial hyperresponsiveness (National Asthma Education and Prevention Program 2007). There is substantial variability in the presentation of asthma, and multiple asthma phenotypes have been identified in the literature; however, often asthma can be characterized by chronic inflammation of the airways (Deliu et al. 2017; Global Initiative for Asthma 2018).

Approximately seven million children in the United States have asthma, making it the most common pediatric chronic medical condition in the USA (Global Initiative for Asthma 2018; National Heart Lung and Blood Institute 2007). In 2016, over 8% of children between the ages of 0 and 17 had asthma (Centers for Disease Control and Prevention 2016). According to the Centers for Disease Control (2016), asthma is more prevalent among non-Hispanic Black children (15.7%) and children of Hispanic descent (6.7%), with even higher rates among children of Puerto Rican descent (12.9%), compared to non-Hispanic White children (7.1%) (Centers for Disease Control and Prevention 2016). Additionally, individuals with lower socioeconomic statuses (10.5%) have higher rates of asthma compared to individuals above the Federal Poverty Level (7%) (Zahran et al. 2018). The health disparities seen with asthma are disheartening and complex; see this article for more detailed information on this issue (Canino et al. 2009).

For providers working with youth with asthma, it is important to understand the factors that influence the development and course of asthma. Asthma is thought to be caused by an interaction of biological and environmental factors; however, these causes remain not well understood. A recent report from the Global Initiative for Asthma identified several factors that are associated with risk for asthma onset, including biological and environmental factors; the strength of evidence varies across studied factors (Table 22.1).

A. H. Clawson (✉) · N. Ruppe · C. Nwankwo
A. Blair · M. Baudino
Department of Psychology, Oklahoma State University, Center for Pediatric Psychology, Stillwater, OK, USA
e-mail: ahum@okstate.edu

N. Mehdi
Department of Pediatrics, Pulmonary and Cystic Fibrosis Center, OU Children's Physician, Oklahoma City, OK, USA

Table 22.1 Factors associated with childhood asthma onset

Factors associated with increased risk for asthma onset in children	Factors associated with decreased risk for asthma onset in children
• Genetic predisposition • Maternal obesity and weight gain during pregnancy • Exposure to aeroallergens (mold, dust mites, etc.) • Exposure to irritants (maternal tobacco use during pregnancy, environmental tobacco smoke exposure, pollutants) • Certain medication use during pregnancy and by infants/toddlers (mixed evidence) • Poorer maternal psychosocial functioning • Sex (asthma is more prevalent among males during childhood and more prevalent among women in adulthood) • Preterm birth and low birth weight • Greater infant weight gain	• Maternal diet during pregnancy (mixed evidence) • Breastfeeding (mixed evidence) • Exposure to microbiota (often referred to as the hygiene hypothesis, microflora hypothesis, or biodiversity hypothesis): – Based on research that shows that individuals with early exposure to *some* microbiota (e.g., infections), with less antibiotic use, and who live on farms have lower rates of asthma. More specifically, individuals with early exposure to infections demonstrate increased levels of Th-1 cells, which are focused on fighting infection, and less Th-2 cell response (National Asthma Education and Prevention Program 2007)

Asthma is treated using a stepwise approach. Treatment is guided by the assessment of a child's asthma severity and asthma control (Mcmains 2015). Severity is defined as the intensity of symptoms for the individual (Global Initiative for Asthma 2018); asthma severity guides initial medical interventions (National Asthma Education and Prevention Program 2007). Asthma classification is broken down into intermittent or persistent asthma; those with persistent asthma are further categorized by intrinsic disease symptoms as having either mild, moderate, or severe persistent asthma. Asthma control is defined as an individual's response to medical intervention and guides adjustments to treatment (National Asthma Education and Prevention Program 2007). Both asthma severity and control require an assessment of asthma symptoms, medication use, functional impairment, lung functioning, and risk of future adverse events (e.g., asthma exacerbations) (Global Initiative for Asthma 2018; National Asthma Education and Prevention Program 2007). Asthma exacerbations (also called asthma attacks) are acute asthma events characterized by bronchoconstriction and worsening asthma symptoms. Exacerbations can be triggered by environmental factors (e.g., exposure to irritants, aeroallergens, and weather changes), poor asthma control (potentially because of inadequate medical management and/or poor medication adherence or improper techniques), emotional states (e.g., increased stress and laughing), and physiological factors (e.g., illness). Asthma symptoms, and especially asthma exacerbations, can be very frightening for children and their families, further highlighting the importance of understanding a child's asthma severity and control (Kean et al. 2006).

Multiple validated measures are available to aid in the assessment of asthma control among youth. For example, two brief measures that assess asthma control are the Asthma Control Questionnaire (Juniper et al. 2005) and the Asthma Control Test (Nathan et al. 2004)/Childhood Asthma Control Test (Liu et al. 2007). Lung function measures such as spirometry can be used to measure the volume and flow of air movement through the lungs (Global Initiative for Asthma 2018; National Heart Lung and Blood Institute 2007). Core outcome measures of lung functioning are forced expiratory volume (FEV_1), forced vital capacity (FVC), and the ratio of FEV_1/FVC (Tepper et al. 2012). Peak flow meters are also sometimes used in selected or high risk cases to measure objective lung functioning at home (Tepper et al. 2012).

Treatment

As mentioned earlier, the treatment of pediatric asthma is based on a stepwise treatment approach, with the goal of having well-controlled asthma using the least amount of medical intervention as possible. Medication for the treatment of asthma can be categorized into two categories: long-term controller medications and rescue or quick-relief medications. Long-term controller medications are used daily to prevent symptoms by reducing inflammation. Corticosteroids (often referred to as inhaled corticosteroids (ICS)), which are anti-inflammatory medications, are considered the one of the most effective long-term controller medications. Long-term controller medications help to reduce inflammation in the airways and long-term damage to the airways (National Asthma Education and Prevention Program 2007). Quick-relief medications are used to treat acute asthma symptoms and asthma exacerbations. Common quick-relief medications include bronchodilators (e.g., albuterol), systemic corticosteroids, and anticholinergics (National Asthma Education and Prevention Program 2007).

Understanding when to use these different types of medications can be confusing, and trying to identify which medications to use during asthma exacerbations can be especially stressful for families. In order to help families understand when their child should take the different types of medication, providers often use an asthma action plan to teach families when and how the child should take their controller and quick-relief medications. Asthma action plans are completed by a child's healthcare provider and aid families in managing a child's asthma at home and other places (e.g., school; example: http://allergist.aaaai.org/plan/index.php). Asthma action plans include information about the severity of the child's asthma, asthma triggers that affect the child, and graded instructions for what to do/what medications to take during different levels of asthma symptoms (e.g., no symptoms, some symptoms, severe problems). Some asthma action plans also include places to document peak flow meter readings.

Non-pharmacological interventions are also used in the management of childhood asthma. The evidence for the benefits of the different non-pharmacological interventions is varied (Global Initiative for Asthma 2018). Interventions with stronger research support include the following: parental and/or child smoking cessation, elimination of child environmental tobacco smoke exposure, physical activity (and information on how to manage asthma symptoms in order to engage in physical activity), healthy diet, weight reduction for patients with comorbid obesity, breathing exercises, and avoidance of asthma triggers. More research is needed to support clear recommendations for other non-pharmacological interventions (e.g., stress reduction, treatment of anxiety and depression). Clearly, mental health providers could play an important role in helping families manage childhood asthma.

This chapter focuses on the use of cognitive behavioral therapy (CBT) for youth with asthma; more specifically, the chapter will discuss the utilization of CBT to treat anxiety in youth with asthma. We use anxiety as an example to demonstrate how CBT can be tailored to target asthma-specific issues. Before we turn to CBT, we spend some time reviewing some common presenting problems that mental health providers might encounter when working with youth with asthma, including treatment nonadherence and emotional/behavioral difficulties.

Common Presenting Problems Relevant for Mental Health Providers

Treatment Nonadherence

Although good medication adherence is associated with lower risk of severe asthma exacerbations, the rates of asthma medication adherence are quite low among both children and adults

(Bender 2016; McQuaid et al. 2003). A growing body of literature has demonstrated that the rates of adherence are poor among children with asthma, with estimated mean adherence ranging from 48 to 58%, with even lower rates for individuals who experience exacerbations (13.7%) (Bender et al. 2000; McQuaid et al. 2003; Milgrom et al. 1996). Overall, data also suggest that youth and their caregivers tend to overestimate youth's medication adherence. Objective measures compared to self-report measures demonstrated that patients and caregivers tend to overreport medication adherence (94.5%) compared to actual use of medications (58.4%) (Milgrom et al. 1996). Another study found that youth self-reported over 89% adherence to medications such as inhaled corticosteroids, but objective measures (e.g., measuring canister weight) demonstrated lower adherence (69%) (Bender et al. 2000). Although adolescents are more aware of disease management, they are demonstrating lower rates of medication adherence compared to younger children (McQuaid et al. 2003).

We discuss nonadherence for three reasons. First, nonadherence results in poorer asthma control and health outcomes (Bauman et al. 2002; Global Initiative for Asthma 2018). Second, mental health providers who work with youth with asthma will likely encounter nonadherence as a common presenting problem. A meta-analysis of adherence-promoting interventions for youth with chronic medical conditions found a small effect size of interventions on adherence and disease outcomes (including pulmonary functioning); most of the examined interventions were multicomponent interventions that included cognitive and behavioral intervention components (Pai and McGrady 2014). See Chap. 25 in this book for more information about using CBT to promote adherence among youth with medical conditions. Lastly, adherence can be strongly influenced by an individual's psychosocial functioning, including cognitive (e.g., symptom perceptions, self-efficacy; Scherer and Bruce 2001), affective (anxiety, depression; DiMatteo et al. 2000), and behavioral factors (e.g., avoidance); some of these factors are discussed further in the below section.

Psychosocial Functioning

Overall, data suggest that youth with asthma are experiencing significant psychosocial difficulties, including higher rates of anxiety (Dudeney et al. 2017a, b; Lu et al. 2012; McQuaid et al. 2001), depression (Lu et al. 2012), behavioral difficulties (McQuaid et al. 2001), and similar or higher rates of engaging in deleterious health behaviors (e.g., tobacco; McLeish and Zvolensky 2010) and marijuana use (Jones et al. 2006) compared to youth without asthma.

More specifically, a meta-analysis found that about 27% of adolescents with asthma had depressive symptoms, almost double the rate of depressive symptoms among healthy adolescents (Lu et al. 2012). Prospective studies have also found that depression predicts adult-onset asthma (Gao et al. 2015). Among adults with asthma, an experimental design demonstrated that those with induced depressed mood showed an attentional bias toward health-threat pictures, with specific difficulty with disengaging from the stimuli, compared to those without asthma (Alexeeva and Martin 2018). The authors postulate that this attentional bias may impede accurate asthma symptom perceptions; something echoed in the broader literature (Janssens et al. 2009). Further, individuals with asthma who underwent a neutral mood induction demonstrated an avoidance of health-threat pictures. Avoidance coping styles have been associated with poorer health outcomes in the adult asthma literature (Adams et al. 2000) and with lower quality of life in adolescents with asthma (Van De Ven et al. 2007). Overall, data suggest that depressive symptoms among youth with asthma are associated with poorer health outcomes, including poor asthma control, increased length of hospital stays, frequent visits to healthcare providers, increased use of steroid medication, noncompliance with medical regimens, and impaired health-related quality of life (Strine et al. 2008).

A recent meta-analysis of cross-sectional studies found a similar pattern of findings with anxiety: The prevalence of anxiety disorders (23%) and symptomatology was higher among youth with asthma, and youth with asthma were over three times more likely to develop anxiety symptomology compared to youth without asthma (Dudeney et al. 2017a, b). There is a paucity of longitudinal studies on pediatric asthma and anxiety. One longitudinal study found that youth diagnosed with asthma by age 5 were more likely to develop later internalizing symptoms at age 14, but youth with internalizing symptoms in childhood were not more likely to develop asthma at age 14 (Alati et al. 2005). Another study examined the bidirectional, longitudinal associations between panic symptoms and asthma activity among young adults (Hasler et al. 2005). This study identified a bidirectional pattern: Individuals with asthma were more likely to meet diagnostic criteria for panic disorder and have panic symptoms at subsequent assessments, and individuals with panic disorder had more asthma symptoms at subsequent assessments. The comorbidity of asthma and anxiety among youth is also associated with poorer health outcomes: Individuals with asthma and anxiety experience increased asthma symptoms, poorer asthma control, increased functional impairment, and decreased quality of life (Richardson et al. 2006; Roy-Byrne et al. 2008). In their review of the literature, Goodwin et al. (2012) identified several potential pathways by which asthma and mental health difficulties might influence each other among youth. For example, having a chronic health condition may impact the development of mental health difficulties due to increased stress, impairment, or discomfort. On the other hand, having mental health difficulties may exacerbate current illness (e.g., avoidance of taking medications due to fears of side effects).

The remainder of the chapter will focus mainly on anxiety among youth with asthma. We chose to focus on anxiety because youth with asthma exhibit higher rates of anxiety compared to their healthy peers (Dudeney et al. 2017a), anxiety among youth with asthma is associated with poorer health outcomes (Richardson et al. 2006), and because the majority of the albeit limited literature on CBT among youth with asthma has focused on the treatment of anxiety (Pateraki et al. 2018).

Biopsychosocial Conceptualization of Anxiety for Youth with Asthma

Consistent with the CBT model, case conceptualization for treating youth with asthma includes an examination of the bidirectional relationships between individuals' thoughts, emotions, and behaviors (Kendall 2012b). Further, conceptualization requires an understanding of the environmental factors, or systems level factors, and the biological factors that may be impacting youth with asthma's functioning. Anxiety among youth with asthma could be asthma-specific (e.g., anxiety about symptoms, triggers, or medical treatment) or more generalized (ten Thoren and Petermann 2000). Anxiety in childhood is characterized by somatic/physiological, cognitive, behavioral, and emotional components (American Psychiatric Association 2013; Higa-McMillan et al. 2014; Kendall 2012a). The relationship between anxiety and asthma is complex; however, overall, the literature supports a CBT conceptualization (Yii and Koh 2013).

There is a paucity of information on why there are higher rates of anxiety among youth with asthma; however, biological, contextual, behavioral, cognitive, and affective factors likely play a role in the development and maintenance of anxiety among these youth. There appears to be a bidirectional relationship between asthma and anxiety symptoms: Asthma-related experiences may lead to increased anxiety (Goodwin et al. 2012; Yii and Koh 2013); on the other hand, emotional distress and poor health behaviors may also trigger worsening asthma symptoms (Global Initiative for Asthma 2018; National Asthma Education and Prevention Program 2007). An individual may experience anticipatory anxiety about having asthma symptoms (especially asthma exacerbations), hypervigilance regarding bodily sensations, anxiety while having asthma symptoms, anxiety surrounding their medical treatment, or posttraumatic stress type symptoms due to asthma events (Kean et al. 2006; Kew et al. 2016; Pateraki et al. 2018; ten Thoren and Petermann 2000). A vicious cycle could follow such that increased stress and arousal could then trigger worsening asthma symptoms or behaviors associated with poorer asthma outcomes (Global Initiative for Asthma 2018; National Asthma Education and Prevention Program 2007). In sum, there appears to be dynamic relations between anxiety and asthma.

Biological Factors

Asthma and anxiety are thought to be caused by gene and environment interactions (Global Initiative for Asthma 2018; Higa-McMillan et al. 2014). A study by Thomsen et al. (2011) identified an increase in the estimates of heritability for asthma from 1994 to 2003 based on twin studies. The authors suggest a potential epigenetic effect such that changes in environmental factors have led to changes in genetic expression, thereby increasing rates of asthma across time. Recent research supports the potential importance of investigating the impact of epigenetics on asthma (Yang et al. 2017). A few factors that have been implicated with epigenetic changes associated with asthma outcomes include exposure to allergens and irritants (e.g., pollution and tobacco smoke) and stress (Rosenberg et al. 2014; Yang et al. 2017). Data also support the role of genetics (Higa-McMillan et al. 2014), and more recently potentially epigenetics, in childhood anxiety (Bortoluzzi et al. 2018). In sum, genetics and epigenetics play important roles in the development of both pediatric asthma and anxiety.

As discussed earlier, asthma exacerbations can be triggered by stress and emotional states (Global Initiative for Asthma 2018; National Asthma Education and Prevention Program 2007). Peters and Fritz (2010) hypothesized that stress can induce asthma exacerbations due to the activation of the autonomous nervous system and resulting bronchorestriction. Further, the authors discuss how stress can impact asthma via the neuroendocrine systems' effects on lung inflammation, and how stress is related to increases in proinflammatory cytokines. The authors also implicate the brainstem's respiratory sensor system in the comorbidity between asthma and stress (Peters and Fritz 2010). Katon et al. (2004) reviewed potential theories on why there is high comorbidity between asthma and panic symptoms. The authors discussed several biological and physiological processes, including oversensitivity of the neural circuits responsible for fear responding to experiences of breathlessness among individuals with asthma, hypersensitivity to carbon dioxide, and higher levels of airway resistance (Katon et al. 2004). Psychopathology research that is not specific to youth with asthma supports the role of several neurobiological and physiological processes in development and maintenance of childhood anxiety disorders (Higa-McMillan et al. 2014; Rappaport et al. 2017). Lastly, it is also important to consider how asthma medications may impact anxiety. Overall, stress and anxiety seem to induce multiple biological processes that may exacerbate a child's asthma functioning, and there are biological factors that may make youth, including youth with asthma, more susceptible to developing anxiety symptoms.

Psychological Factors

There is significant overlap in the physiological symptoms of anxiety and asthma. Common symptoms of asthma include shortness of breath, wheezing, coughing, and chest tightness (Global Initiative for Asthma 2018; National Asthma Education and Prevention Program 2007). Individuals with asthma also have variable, and often unpredictable, difficulties with airflow limitations and may also experience an acute worsening of their asthma symptoms during asthma exacerbations. Some somatic symptoms of anxiety can manifest in similar ways, including shortness of breath, feelings of choking, chest pain or discomfort, dizziness/unsteadiness/lightheadedness, and numbness/tingling sensations (American Psychiatric Association 2013). The overlap between asthma and anxiety symptoms may lead to increased anxiety due to the difficulty disentangling whether the symptoms are indicative of asthma or anxiety.

Learning processes may contribute to increased anxiety among youth with asthma (Yii and Koh 2013). For example, previously neutral stimuli (e.g., going to school) may become associated with negative asthma experiences through classical conditioning and result in conditioned anxiety (e.g., anxiety about going to school due to a previous experience of having an asthma attack at school). Operant conditioning principles should also be considered (e.g., how escape and avoidance may be maintaining anxiety). When working with youth with asthma, there is a need for a comprehensive assessment to understand their asthma treatment regimen and the behavioral factors that might be impacting both their anxiety and asthma symptoms, including an assessment of their asthma self-management behaviors and functional behavioral analyses related to asthma and anxiety symptoms. Youth with asthma and anxiety may start to engage in avoidance (e.g., activity limitation) and escape behaviors (e.g., quick-relief medication use) in response to anxiety, thereby potentially maintaining their anxiety. For example, youth may overuse their quick-relief inhalers because they are using them in response to hyperventilation symptoms rather than asthma symptoms. Another behavioral response that could maintain anxiety would be avoidance or activity limitation due to fears of future asthma symptoms. Though youth are encouraged to avoid asthma triggers when possible (e.g., avoid irritants such as tobacco smoke), youth with comorbid anxiety may begin to overgeneralize what their asthma triggers are and avoid situations due to fears of potential asthma exacerbations (Sicouri et al. 2017a, b). Importantly, nonadherence to treatment regimens could also impact child anxiety due to poor asthma control.

Cognitive factors have also been investigated among youth with comorbid anxiety and asthma. One study identified several examples of negative thoughts identified by youth with asthma (Marriage and Henderson 2012): "I worry about going hot and blacking out," "I might die," "I don't like people watching me take my inhaler," "I might pass out," "I worry I might never get rid of my asthma," "The ambulance might not come in time," and "I am worried that one day I might collapse, have to have drips, have pipes in my lungs, and pass away." As this highlights, negative cognitions may be asthma-specific fears about health, mortality, social concerns, or the chronic nature of their illness. Of course, youth with asthma may also experience non-asthma-specific worries and fears (Sicouri et al. 2017a, b).

Park and colleagues identified a CBT model that focuses on the interrelations between panic symptoms and pediatric asthma (Park et al. 1996). The model posits that initial negative experiences with asthma may lead to cognitive interpretations of future bodily sensations that are similar to asthma symptoms as signals of impaired lung functioning and imminent threat. For example, a child may have experienced an asthma exacerbation and subsequently began interpreting bodily sensations that are similar to asthma symptoms (e.g., breathlessness from exercising) or actual asthma symptoms (e.g., shortness of breath) in a catastrophic manner (e.g., "I am going to die"). Catastrophic interpretations of bodily sensations may then lead to hyperventilation which in turn worsens anxiety. Further, youth may began engaging in avoidance or escape behaviors to reduce anxiety symptoms (Sicouri et al. 2017a, b). Overall, Park's model posits that youth with asthma's anxiety is largely impacted by their fears related to their asthma.

Little research has been done on the potential mechanisms contributing to high rates of comorbidity between anxiety and asthma in youth since Park's cognitive model. A meta-analysis including studies among the general child population found that children with anxiety demonstrated attentional biases toward threat-related stimuli (Dudeney et al. 2015). The authors later conducted a study to examine potential attentional biases toward asthma and other threat cues among youth with asthma (Dudeney et al.

2017b). The authors posited that based on Park's model, youth with asthma would demonstrate attentional biases toward asthma stimuli, with greater attentional biases among youth with asthma and anxiety. This hypothesis was not supported; however, attentional biases toward asthma stimuli were correlated with poorer asthma control. These results were not congruent with another study that examined anxiety among youth with moderate-to-severe asthma. This study found that youth with moderate-to-severe asthma demonstrated attentional biases toward asthma-related words but not anxiety or general negative emotion words (Lowther et al. 2016). Though the data are mixed, youth with anxiety may demonstrate attentional biases toward asthma-related stimuli, and these biases may be associated with poorer asthma control. This suggests that it may be beneficial to address attentional biases to asthma cues among youth with comorbid asthma and anxiety.

Another cognitive factor that has been shown to impact childhood anxiety is interpretation bias, including tendencies to perceive ambiguous scenarios as threatening, perceive more threat, and attend to threat more quickly (Higa-McMillan et al. 2014). Studies among adults with asthma have found that panic symptoms among individuals with asthma are influenced largely by an individuals' misinterpretation of nonthreatening bodily symptoms rather than actual current lung functioning (Carr et al. 1994). Sicouri et al. (2017b) examined if youth with comorbid asthma and anxiety showed interpretation biases related to asthma scenarios (consistent with Park's model) rather than interpretation biases to both ambiguous general scenarios (e.g., ambiguous social threat or physical threat scenarios) and ambiguous asthma scenarios (e.g., noticing a cough). Overall, the results suggested that youth with asthma perceived ambiguous asthma situations as threating and engaged in avoidant behavioral responding; youth with comorbid anxiety and asthma demonstrated similar interpretation biases and avoidance as youth with only anxiety, suggesting the need for interventions focused on general and asthma-specific contexts.

Lastly, another critical factor for case conceptualization among youth with comorbid anxiety and asthma is symptom perception: Data suggest that people with asthma's reports of their asthma symptoms are often discrepant from objectives measures of lung functioning (Janssens et al. 2009). In fact, estimates of rates of poor symptom perception among people with asthma vary from 15 to 60% (Janssens et al. 2009). Poor symptom perception is related to suboptimal asthma management (e.g., misuse of medications; Feldman et al. 2013) and increased healthcare utilization (Fritz et al. 1996). Poor symptom perception could present as symptom over-perception, with children perceiving more symptoms or more severe symptoms than objective measures of lung functioning, and/or as symptom under-perception, with children perceiving fewer or less severe asthma symptoms than objective measures (Janssens et al. 2009; Still and Dolen 2016). Janssens et al. (2009) proposed a working model of symptom perception and identified that a major risk for poor symptom perception is anxiety. Child anxiety, particularly the physiological symptoms of anxiety, has been found to be significantly related to a child perceptions of poorer lung functioning and overuse of quick-relief medications, even after controlling for asthma severity (Feldman et al. 2013).

Social and Environmental Factors

Poor family functioning, poor family health behaviors, socioeconomic disadvantage, and parental mental health difficulties have also been hypothesized to impact the comorbidity of anxiety and asthma among youth (Goodwin et al. 2012). Caregivers of youth with asthma exhibit higher rates of mental health difficulties compared to caregivers of children without asthma (Easter et al. 2015), and parental mental health is a strong predictor of child asthma functioning (Kaugars et al. 2004; Lim et al. 2011) and mental health functioning (Lim et al. 2011). Family functioning, and parenting difficulties, also significantly affect asthma outcomes and psychosocial functioning

```
         ┌─────────────────┐
         │ Negative Asthma │
         │     Event       │
         │  (e.g., asthma  │
         │  exacerbation)  │
         └─────────────────┘
```

Behavioral Response
- Use of quick relief inhaler
- Emergency room visit
- Avoidance of future similar situations
- Activity Limitation

Interpretations of Physiological Experiences
- Hypervigilance to bodily sensations
- Catastrophic misinterpretations of bodily sensations
- Attentional biases towards asthma related cues
- Symptom misinterpretation

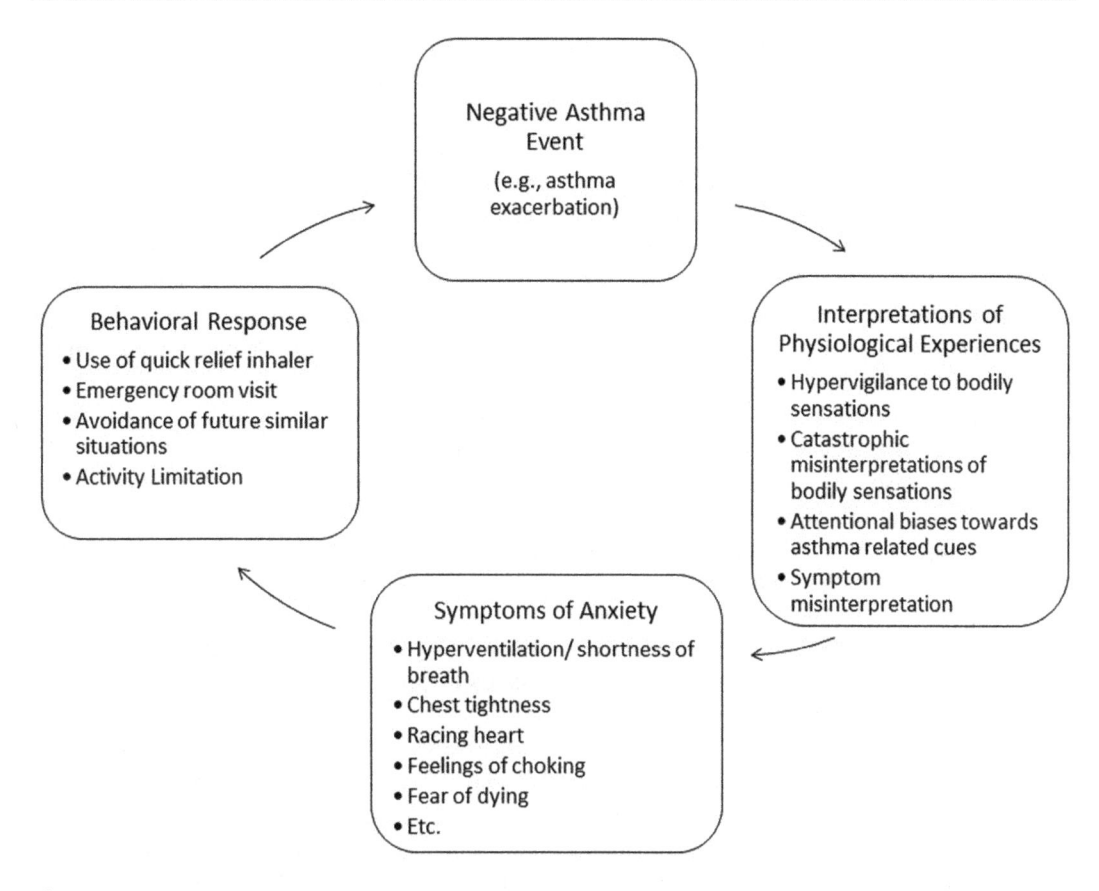

Symptoms of Anxiety
- Hyperventilation/ shortness of breath
- Chest tightness
- Racing heart
- Feelings of choking
- Fear of dying
- Etc.

Fig. 22.1 Example of potential pattern of anxiety among youth with asthma

among youth (Higa-McMillan et al. 2014; Kaugars et al. 2004; Wood et al. 2015). Therefore, understanding family functioning and parental mental health difficulties is an important component of treating anxiety among youth with asthma.

Overall, the literature supports the influence of multiple contextual, cognitive, affective, and behavioral factors on anxiety among youth with asthma. Figure 22.1 shows potential individual-level factors that may impact youth with asthma's anxiety.

We illustrate cognitive behavioral treatment approaches through the following case example[1]:

> Johnny is a 10-year-old African-American boy with persistent asthma. He is currently prescribed a controller medication and a quick-relief medication. Johnny is also supposed to take a pretreatment of albuterol via his inhaler and spacer before engaging in physical activity. Johnny lives at home with his mother and father.

Assessments

Asthma-Specific Assessments

Prior to initializing treatment, it is important to consult with the child's medical provider to discuss the child's asthma history and current functioning. Children with asthma may be followed by pediatricians and/or pulmonologists for their asthma, and it will be important to consult with all relevant medical providers. For example, it is recommended that clinicians get the following information about the child prior to starting treatment: general medical and developmental history, asthma control (including

---
[1] This case is completely confabulated.

an assessment of the frequency of asthma symptoms and exacerbations and resulting medical treatments; e.g., hospitalizations, emergency rooms visits), asthma severity, prescribed medications, asthma triggers, physician's perception of the child's medication adherence and symptom perception (i.e., does the child tend to accurately perceive their lung functioning compared to objectives lung functioning measures), asthma action plan, and physician's perceptions regarding the child's psychological functioning and ability to engage in psychological treatment given their asthma control. It is also important to discuss any potential differential diagnosis considerations that the child's medical provider is considering (e.g., asthma versus dyspnea due to exercise limitation or induced vocal cord dysfunction) (Abu-Hasan et al. 2005; Weinberger and Abu-Hasan 2007).

Assessments of factors related to the child's asthma functioning should also be completed with the family. Assessments of the family's perceptions of the child's asthma history, asthma control, asthma severity, prescribed medications, understanding of the asthma action plan, and medication adherence will be helpful in understanding the family's perceptions of the child's overall asthma functioning. It would also likely be beneficial to assess each family member's role in the child's asthma self-management. The Family Asthma Management Assessment System (FAMSS) is a semi-structured clinical interview that is completed with parents and children (or only with parents if the child is too young) and assesses the following key areas of asthma self-management: asthma knowledge, symptom assessment, response to symptoms and exacerbations, environmental control (child exposure to environmental triggers such as allergens or irritants), medication adherence, collaboration with healthcare providers, and balanced integration of asthma and family life (i.e., balance of attention to asthma by different family members, family functioning/issues, school attendance; McQuaid et al. 2005). The Asthma Trigger Inventory is a validated self-report measure of potential asthma triggers, including emotional triggers, animal allergens, pollen, physical activity, air pollution/irritants, and infections (Wood et al. 2007).

Asthma quality of life should be assessed among youth and their caregivers. The Pediatric Asthma Quality of Life Questionnaire is a reliable and valid clinical interview that assesses activity limitation due to asthma, asthma symptoms, and emotional functioning (Juniper et al. 1996a). Caregiver quality of life can be assessed with the Pediatric Asthma Caregiver's Quality of Life Questionnaire; this is a validated 13-item self-report measure that assesses how much a child's asthma has resulted in activity limitation for the caregiver and caregiver emotional functioning (Juniper et al. 1996b).

Psychological Functioning Assessments

Broad-band measures of a child's psychological functioning can be used to screen for various social, emotional, and behavioral difficulties. Examples of validated broad-band measures include the Behavior Assessment System for Children (BASC; Reynolds and Kamphaus 2016) and the Achenbach System of Empirically Based Assessment Child Behavior Checklist (CBCL; Achenbach 2009). Narrow-band band measures can then be used to more comprehensively assess specific constructs. Examples of validated anxiety self-report measures are described in Table 22.2. Self-monitoring logs, functional behavioral assessments, and thought logs will also be helpful in identifying the typical patterns surrounding the child's anxiety. Assessments should be given to inform diagnostic impressions, to facilitate case conceptualization (initially and as needed throughout treatment), and to monitor treatment progress.

Johnny's pediatrician referred the family to a psychologist because although Johnny's asthma is well-controlled overall, Johnny often reports that he feels that his lung functioning is more compromised than his objective lung functioning measurements indicate. Additionally, Johnny also tends to overuse his quick-relief inhaler.

Table 22.2 Examples of validated anxiety self-report measures

Self-report or parent-report measures		
The Multidimensional Anxiety Scale for Children™, Second Edition (MASC 2)	• Total score; anxiety probability score • Scales: separation anxiety/phobias, social anxiety, generalized anxiety, obsessions and compulsions, physical symptoms, harm avoidance (March et al. 1997)	• Parent and self-report • Ages 8–19 • Administration time: 15 min
Revised Children's Manifest Anxiety Scale™, second edition (RCMAS 2)	• Physiological anxiety • Worry • Social anxiety • Defensiveness (Reynolds and Paget 1983)	• Self-report • Ages 6–19 • Administration time: 10–15 min; <5 for short form
Screen for Child Anxiety Related Emotional Disorders (SCARED)	• Panic/somatic • Generalized anxiety • Separation anxiety • Social anxiety • Simple phobia/school phobia (Birmaher et al. 1999)	• Parent and self-report • Ages 8–18 • Administration time: 10 min; <5 for 5-item version
State-Trait Anxiety Inventory for Children™ (STAIC)	• State anxiety • Trait anxiety (Spielberger 1983)	• Self-report • Ages 6–14 • Administration time: 20 min
Fear Survey Schedule for Children-Revised (FSSC-R)	• Fear of failure and criticism • Fear of the unknown • Fear of minor injury and small animals • Fear of danger and death • Medical fears (Muris et al. 2014; Ollendick 1983)	• Self-report • Ages 7–16 • Administration time: 15–20 min; <10 for 25-item version
Clinical interviews		
Anxiety disorders interview schedule for DSM-IV: Child and Parent Version	• DSM-IV diagnoses (Silverman and Albano 1996)	• Parent and child versions • Ages 6–16

At the intake session, the psychologist met Johnny and his mother. During the initial session, Johnny's mother reported that Johnny quit participating in after school sports after his most recent asthma attack. Johnny reported significant fears surrounding having asthma exacerbations and avoidance of situations he feels might trigger an asthma attack (e.g., running during soccer practice). Johnny reported anxiety related to asthma and anxiety unrelated to his asthma. He reported that he avoided physical activity because he believed that exercising would cause him to have an asthma attack. He also endorsed catastrophic interpretations of bodily sensations (e.g., thoughts of imminent death when he gets winded from walking up stairs) and a lack of self-efficacy surrounding his ability to manage his asthma symptoms. Johnny's mother also reported anxiety surrounding Johnny's asthma management. Data from assessment and clinical interviews indicated that Johnny met criteria for Generalized Anxiety Disorder.

After the intake session, the therapist contacted Johnny's pediatrician to gather more information about his asthma history, current asthma control, asthma triggers, asthma treatment regimen, and discuss the pediatrician's concerns regarding Johnny's overuse of his quick-relief inhaler and symptom perception. The clinician also reviewed their diagnostic impressions with the pediatrician, discussed the proposed treatment plan (i.e., CBT for comorbid anxiety and asthma), and assessed if the pediatrician had any concerns regarding Johnny participating in CBT. The pediatrician supported the diagnosis of Generalized Anxiety Disorder and the treatment plan. The pediatrician also confirmed that is was safe for Johnny to engage in physical activity if he was using his controller medication as prescribed and completing his pretreatment of albuterol (delivered with his inhaler and spacer) before engaging in more rigorous physical activity (e.g., soccer practice).

Description of Treatment Components and Associated Empirical Support

CBT is effective for treating anxiety among youth (Butler et al. 2006). Given the morbidity and cost associated with comorbid asthma and mental health difficulties, several reviews on psychological interventions for individuals with asthma have been conducted over the past several years. Notably, there is a significant paucity of studies evaluating CBT for youth with asthma. In 2016, a Cochrane review on CBT for adults and adolescents with asthma identified nine randomized controlled trials (RCTs) evaluating CBT for adults with asthma; no RCTs for adolescents were identified (Kew et al. 2016). Among the few adult studies, there was significant variability in the methodology used across studies, significant risk for biases due to study design issues, and inconsistency across the results of the studies; therefore, the authors concluded that there was currently insufficient evidence to support more than low confidence in the results. The results of the review suggested that CBT may improve asthma quality of life, asthma control, and anxiety compared with usual care; CBT was not shown to have an impact on depression, asthma exacerbations, or medication adherence.

Due to the lack of RCTs evaluating CBT among individuals with asthma, a more recent systematic review included a wider range of study designs in their investigation of the efficacy of CBT for youth and adults with asthma (Pateraki et al. 2018). This review included RCTs, non-randomized controlled trials, and observational repeated measures designs. Overall, study quality was moderate. The authors identified 12 studies focused on adults (eight were RCTs) and four studies focused on youth (one was a RCT). Of the initially identified 12 adult studies, only five studies were included in the review as the other studies were excluded because of low study quality or because the intervention was not focused on treating individuals with clinical levels of anxiety. Of the remaining five adult studies, two studies found a significant positive effect of CBT on anxiety compared to controls. All studies that positively impacted anxiety included asthma-specific psychoeducation. All four studies evaluating CBT for youth with asthma found that CBT positively impacted anxiety; however, the authors found that only two studies were sufficiently methodologically rigorous. Further description of the common intervention components used in the child studies is discussed in more detail below.

Overall, the literature seems to support several key treatment components for addressing anxiety among youth with asthma, including behavioral, cognitive, affective, and systems level intervention components. Figure 22.2 presents a synthesis of the treatment components included in the studied interventions. Descriptions of these treatment components with some accompanying dialogue are provided in the below section. After we present a description of the common treatment components used in studies examining the efficacy or effectiveness of CBT for youth with comorbid asthma and anxiety, we provide an example of how asthma-specific information could be integrated into an existing empirically supported treatment for pediatric anxiety.

Behavioral Interventions

First, we will discuss behavioral treatment components from the studies focused on investigating CBT among youth with asthma and anxiety. Many of the studies included asthma skills training for youth. Skills training focused on concepts such as how to properly use inhalers, prevent and handle asthma exacerbations, cope with asthma symptoms at home and school, and talk to healthcare professionals about asthma (Colland et al. 1993; Marriage and Henderson

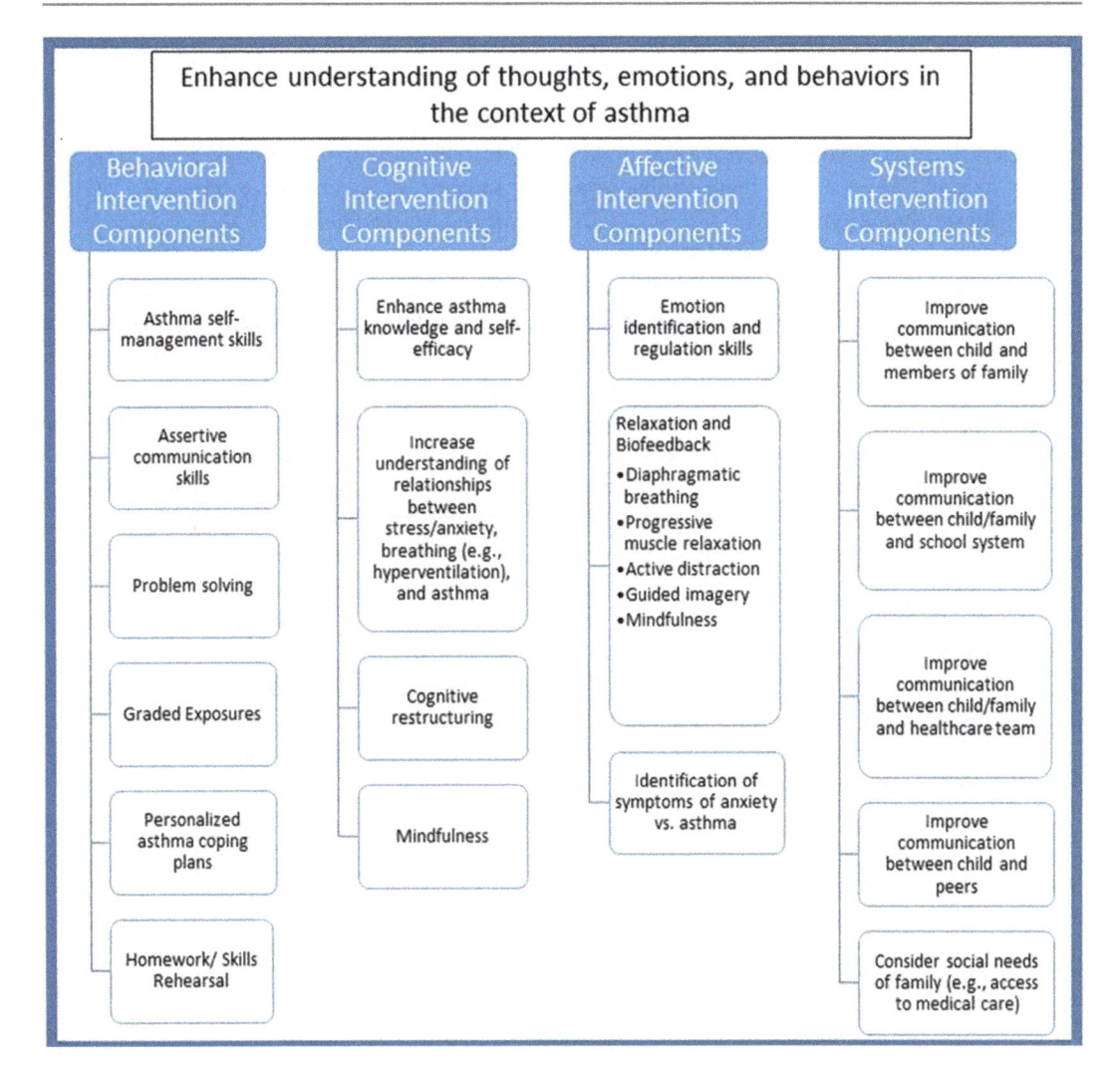

Fig. 22.2 Synthesis of the treatment components described in current literature

2012; Sicouri et al. 2017a, b). *An example of asthma-specific skills training is provided below*:

Therapist: So the last time we met we learned about the medicines that you take for your asthma, why it is important for you to take your controller medicine every day, and when to take your quick-relief inhaler. Today we are going to talk about asthma triggers. Do you know what an asthma trigger is?

Johnny: No, I'm not sure.

Therapist: A trigger is something that starts your asthma symptoms. Do you remember the last time that you had an asthma attack?

Johnny: My last asthma attack was at school during recess. It was really cold outside and I was racing this other boy in my class. In the middle of the race, I started feeling like I couldn't breathe so I went to my teacher and asked to go to the nurse so I could use my inhaler.

Therapist: Wow, that sounds like it could have been really scary! I'm glad that you told me about it and glad you asked to go to the nurse. Your doctor told me that very cold weather is one of your asthma triggers. That means that when it gets very cold outside, you are more likely to have asthma symptoms.

Johnny: Oh, I didn't know that. So what should I do?

Therapist: Once we figure out what your asthma triggers are, we can come up with a plan about how to avoid or cope with them so that you have fewer asthma symptoms.

Johnny: Oh... I guess that means I should stay inside during recess whenever it gets cold outside. And I should probably not race any more.

Therapist: Well, you could avoid playing outside when it gets cold, but it might be hard for you to always miss recess during the winter...and exercise is good for you! Sometimes doing physical activity like running when it is really cold outside can be an asthma trigger. What if you tried not to run outside during recess on cold days instead? And you could still race on days when it is warmer.

Johnny: I would be okay with that.

Therapist: Great! You can also wear scarves over your mouth when it is cold outside because it will help block some of the cold air. Have you and doctor talked about any other things that you can do to help with being able to exercise?

Johnny: I am supposed to take my albuterol in my inhaler before I exercise.

Therapist: That's right! Now let's talk more about what to do when it is cold outside and you want to play outside during recess. Are there other things that you like to do besides run during recess?

Johnny: Sometimes I like swinging on the swings.

Therapist: Okay, so what if you swing on the swings instead of run outside on days when it is below very cold outside?

Johnny: That sounds like a good plan!

Other key behavioral strategies that were included in previous studies were assertive communication skills training (e.g., how to talk to others about asthma), problem-solving, and creating individualized coping plans (Colland et al. 1993; Long et al. 2011). Multiple studies also provided patients with homework and/or opportunities to practice skills that they learned during sessions to practice and reinforce behavioral treatment components (Colland et al. 1993; Long et al. 2011). Graded exposures were also used in previous studies to reduce avoidance and fears in participants (Sicouri et al. 2017a, b). *An example of a graduated in vivo exposure script is described below.*

Therapist: Your mom told me that sometimes you don't want to play soccer because you're afraid that you'll have an asthma attack. Is that right?

Johnny: Yeah. I worry that if I run across the field, I'll start having trouble breathing.

Therapist: Okay, that's understandable, but do you remember what your doctor told you about your medicine? If you take your controller inhaler every day, you should be able to run across the soccer field without any problems.

Johnny: I know. I still worry about it though. I had an asthma attack the last time I was playing soccer. That's why I quit playing soccer.

Therapist: I know that must have been very scary. The last time we talked about that asthma attack, we acted like a detective to try and figure out some things you could start doing differently to help with not having more asthma attacks. What were some of these things?

Johnny: I didn't take my controller inhaler that day, and we said that if I work really hard to take my medicine every day it will help with preventing asthma attacks.

Therapist: That's right! How has that been going?

Johnny: Good.

Therapist: Great, taking your controller medications every day is great way to help keep your asthma symptoms under control. Anything else detective?

Johnny: Yah, I am supposed to take my albuterol 15 min before soccer practice, and I didn't do it that day I had an asthma attack. I'm still scared about running at soccer though.

Therapist: Hmmm...I know you really love soccer. So we know your doctor said it is safe for you to play soccer if you take your controller medicine every day and if you take your albuterol 15 min before playing soccer, and you are working hard to do that… but it seems like your anxiety is still getting in the way…. do you think that your fear might be taking over?

Johnny: I do love soccer… maybe my fear is getting in my way.

Therapist: I want us to do an exposure together to practice using your skills so you can start doing the things you love again. It's nice outside today. Did you take your controller medication this morning?

Johnny: Yes.

Therapist: Great. We're going to go out to the parking lot together and run across three times. I think that's about the length of a soccer field. I'm going to check in with you as we're running together to see how your anxiety and asthma are. If you start to feel your anxiety symptoms, practice your coping strategies. If you start to feel your asthma coming on, let me know. Before we start running, what should we do?

Johnny: I need to take my albuterol.

Therapist: Right! Your mom has it ready.

Before the exposure, Johnny reported that his anxiety was at a seven. The therapist and Johnny then ran across the parking lot three times. Johnny's therapist checked in after each lap to ask Johnny where his anxiety was. After each lap, Johnny's anxiety decreased.

Cognitive Interventions

All the studies incorporated cognitive components in treatment. The majority of studies provided youth with education about asthma (e.g., medication knowledge) in order to enhance self-efficacy (Colland et al. 1993; Long et al. 2011; Sicouri et al. 2017a, b). Additional cognitive interventions included learning about the relationships between stress, breathing (e.g., hyperventilating), and asthma (Long et al. 2011). Marriage and Henderson (2012) also incorporated mindfulness exercises into treatment to encourage youth to focus on the present moment rather than worrying about what has happened previously or what may happen in the future. The final cognitive component utilized in almost all the studies was cognitive restructuring (Long et al. 2011; Marriage and Henderson 2012; Papneja et al. 2016; Park et al. 1996; Sicouri et al. 2017a, b). *An example of cognitive restructuring is provided below:*

Therapist: When we met last we talked about some of the anxious thoughts that you have about your asthma. Do you remember what some of those are?

Johnny: One of them is that kids at school will think I'm weird if they see me using my inhaler.

Therapist: Right. Okay, so it sounds like you're expecting that something bad will happen if you have to use your inhaler at school.

Johnny: Yeah, kids might make fun of me.

Therapist: Remember when we talked about how you can be a detective and find evidence that supports your thoughts? Let's do that right now. Do you know for sure that kids are going to make fun of you if you use your inhaler?

Johnny: Well, no… but they might. I'm still worried that it might happen.

Therapist: You're right… that might happen. Remember though, we don't have a magic crystal ball that can predict the future and we don't know for sure what will happen. Let's keep looking for evidence. What has happened before when you had to use your inhaler in front of your friends at school?

Johnny: I had to use it in P.E. once and none of my friends even noticed because they were playing basketball.

Therapist: That's great! So let's say that you're at recess and you had to use your inhaler. What's the worst thing that could happen?

Johnny: Someone might see me using it and say something about it.

Therapist: Right, so let's figure out what you could do that would help you in that situation if it does happen. Do you have any ideas?

Johnny: I guess I could explain what my inhaler does and why I'm using it.

Therapist: That's a great idea! So now I want you to think back to the very first thought you had about kids making fun of you. Was that a helpful thought for you?

Johnny: No, it made me really nervous.

Therapist: Right. So let's come up with another thought that could have been more helpful for you in the moment.

Johnny: I guess I could think "Kids might notice my inhaler and if they do I can tell them what it's for."

Therapist: That's a great coping thought! Nice job!

Affective Interventions

Many studies also incorporated affective intervention components. For example, in a study by Long and colleagues (2011), youth were taught youth emotion identification and regulation skills (e.g., emotional expression and shifting attention). Several interventions also included relaxation training (e.g., diaphragmatic breathing, guided imagery, mindful body awareness scans, and progressive muscle relaxation) and biofeedback techniques to help children more easily recognize how relaxation impacted their respiration, muscle tension, and other signs of arousal (Long et al. 2011; Marriage and Henderson 2012; Papneja et al. 2016; Sicouri et al. 2017a, b). *A sample progressive muscle relaxation script is provided below:*

Therapist: Remember when we talked about where you feel anxiety in your body? Today we're going to practice relaxing those muscles. I know that you said sometimes you feel like your hands are shaking and tense. I want you to pretend that you have half of an orange in your right hand. Now I want you to squeeze your hand like you're trying to get all of the juice out. Squeeze as hard as you can. Feel how tight your muscles are. Now drop the orange and relax. Squeeze the orange again..... ok, now relax. Does your hand feel better now that it's relaxed?

Johnny: Yeah, I don't feel all tense anymore.

Therapist: That's awesome! We will learn to relax other parts of your body too and you can use this skill whenever you start to feel anxiety in your body to help you relax.

Another affective/cognitive intervention component utilized in many studies was teaching youth how to identify symptoms of anxiety (e.g., hyperventilation, tightness in the throat, nausea) and differentiate them from asthma symptoms (e.g., wheezing, coughing, difficulty breathing out; Park et al. 1996; Sicouri et al. 2017a, b). *Below is an example script that focuses on how to teach youth to differentiate asthma symptoms from anxiety symptoms:*

Therapist: Sometimes the way that you feel when you are anxious might feel the same as the way you feel when you are having asthma symptoms. Today, we're going to talk about how you can tell the difference between symptoms of anxiety and symptoms of asthma. Johnny, can you remember the last time that you were really worried about something?

Johnny: Yeah, last week I was afraid that I failed my math test.

Therapist: Okay, I want you to think back to that day. How did your body feel when you thought you might have failed your test?

Johnny: When my teacher started handing the tests back, I felt like there were butterflies in my stomach. I also felt my hands start to shake in my lap and my heart started to beat really fast. I started to breathe faster and faster, almost like I do when I have an asthma attack.

Therapist: It sounds like those are some of the physical symptoms of anxiety that you have when you get nervous. Those feelings are your body's way of telling you that you are anxious. Have you ever had those feelings other times when you were nervous or afraid about something?

Johnny: I never really thought about it before, but yeah, I guess I have. It happened once when I had to tell my mom I forgot my lunchbox at school. I thought she was going to be really mad. It happens when I think about playing soccer now too.

Therapist: And what kind of thoughts were you having in those situations?

Johnny: I guess I was thinking about how bad things could happen.

Therapist: Nice job finding those anxious thoughts detective! And how did those anxious thoughts change how you were feeling?

Johnny: Well, when I think about playing soccer and have thoughts about how I could have an asthma attack, I start to feel anxious in my body.

Therapist: Ok, so your brain was giving you anxious thoughts, and those anxious thoughts led you to have some physical anxiety symptoms in your body. Now I want you to think about the last time that you had an asthma attack and had to use your rescue inhaler. What did your body feel like then?

Johnny: At first, I felt like my chest was rattling because I was wheezing so much. Then, my chest started to get really tight and I started having trouble breathing. Pretty soon it felt like I couldn't get any air. That's when I used my albuterol.

Therapist: Okay, so now I want us to compare how you felt when you were nervous to how you felt when you were having asthma symptoms. Were any of the symptoms the same?

Johnny: Hmm. Well, both times my chest felt different from the way that it normally does. When I was nervous, my heart felt like it was racing. When I was having an asthma attack, it felt tighter and I was wheezing.

Therapist: Great work! What other differences did you notice?

Johnny: I never feel like there are butterflies in my stomach when I have asthma problems. I only ever feel that way when I get nervous.

Therapist: You are really becoming a great detective! So it seems like your body acts a little different when you are feeling anxious compared to when you are having asthma symptoms. I know we talked about how sometimes having trouble breathing makes you feel anxious too. What kind of thoughts do you have when you notice you are having trouble breathing?

Johnny: Sometimes when I notice I am having trouble breathing I start thinking that I could die.

Therapist: Those are some scary thoughts. And I bet when your brain gives you those anxious thoughts it makes your physical anxiety worse.

Johnny: Yah. I start to breathe faster and faster.

Therapist: It seems like those fearful thoughts make your body feel anxious. Next time, what might you do if your brain gives you an anxious thought like that?

Johnny: Well, I could just tell myself that I am going to be ok and take my deep breaths to help with my anxiety. And if I am still having trouble breathing after I take my deep breaths, I know I can use my rescue inhaler.

Therapist: Right! You can use your asthma coping plan to identify those anxious thoughts, use your coping thoughts, and use your coping strategies! And if you still feel like it is hard to breathe, you can use your rescue inhaler and talk to someone on your support team like it says on your asthma action plan that you and your doctor made together.

Systems Interventions

Systems level components, such as interventions aimed at improving communication among youth, family, the school system, and the healthcare team, are also an important area for treatment (Colland et al. 1993; Park et al. 1996). For example, therapists could help the family to develop a plan to talk to the school about a 504 plan, or role play with the child on how to ask their doctor questions about their asthma. Careful attention should also be paid to family factors, such as family functioning, family stress, and parental mental health difficulties, given their importance for understanding a child's functioning (Wood et al. 2015). Recent Cochrane reviews found preliminary support for family therapy for improving child asthma outcomes (Panton and Barley 2005) and for interventions focused on caregivers of youth with chronic medical conditions (Eccleston et al. 2015).

Further, a pilot study by Sicouri et al. (2017a) found that a CBT intervention that included a parental component resulted in improved child anxiety and asthma outcomes and improvements in caregiver quality of life; this finding is echoed in the general child anxiety literature (Kendall et al. 2017).

Summary of Relevant Intervention Components

Overall, there are limited data on the efficacy of CBT for anxiety among youth with asthma; however, it appears that CBT is effective for adults. The scant literature among youth with asthma provides preliminary support for the effectiveness of CBT for treating anxiety among youth with asthma. Based on the available data with youth with comorbid anxiety and asthma, a key feature of effective interventions seems to be tailoring CBT to include asthma-specific content (Pateraki et al. 2018). Further, incorporating asthma-specific content appears to be useful whether youth's anxiety is related to their asthma or not (Sicouri et al. 2017a, b). Clinicians can use their assessment and case formulations to tailor treatment. Comprehensive assessments of anxiety- and asthma-specific constructs prior to treatment initiation should be completed to inform a comprehensive case conceptualization that includes a description of the child's asthma and anxiety symptoms and hypotheses about the mechanisms maintaining a child's anxiety symptoms. The case formulation can then be used to tailor CBT to the child's needs. For more information about how to develop a case formulation and how to utilize a case formulation to inform CBT treatment, see Persons (2008).

In the earlier sections, we described elements of studied CBT interventions for comorbid anxiety and asthma and provided some sample dialogue. Many of the intervention components utilized in CBT interventions for youth with comorbid anxiety and asthma are elements of empirically supported treatments for pediatric anxiety. For example, many of these intervention components are included in Coping Cat (Kendall et al. 2017). The first half of this treatment focuses on teaching youth how to recognize feelings of anxiety, the CBT model, relaxation skills, cognitive coping skills, and reinforcing coping efforts. Children are also introduced to the concept of graduated exposures and build a fear hierarchy. Asthma-specific content could easily be integrated into this empirically supported treatment. During the first phase of treatment, youth could be provided with psychoeducation about asthma and appropriate asthma self-management skills (including when and how to take their different medications). Youth could also be taught the relationships between anxiety and asthma, taught to discriminate between asthma and anxiety symptoms, and taught to use coping skills to use in response to anxiety symptoms. The second half of treatment focuses on imaginal and in vivo graduated exposures; if the child is experiencing specific fears related to asthma, exposures may be tailored to include exposures to address these fears. Parents are involved in both parts of treatment. As noted earlier, family and parental factors are often linked to child asthma self-management and to child anxiety. During treatment, parents can be taught the same skills that the child is learning to help the parent to learn appropriate asthma self-management skills (including when and how the child should take their different medications), learn how to differentiate asthma symptoms from anxiety symptoms, and learn how they can help their child to use psychological interventions. Examples of how asthma could be integrated into existing empirically-supported treatments are provided below.

Johnny's graduated fear hierarchy mainly focused on engaging in physical activity. Johnny was taught to recognize his somatic symptoms of anxiety (e.g., accelerated breathing, heart racing) and if he was expecting bad things to happen (e.g., "I am going to die"). He was taught to use coping skills when he noticed he was feeling anxious (e.g., doing deep breathing, using progressive muscle relaxation). Johnny was also taught to use cognitive coping skills. For example, he would practice recognizing when he was having catastrophic thoughts (e.g., "I am going to die") and practice identifying more realistic and balanced thoughts ("My breathing seems to be faster. This is how my body tells me I am anxious sometimes. I am going to use my skills to reduce how nervous I feel because sometimes my anxiety seems like my asthma. If my breathing feels more like my asthma acting up after I try my skills, I will take my medication and tell another person so they can help me. I have got this."). Johnny was also taught to use communication skills to help him talk with his school, family, peers, and doctor about his anxiety and asthma, and problem-solving skills. The following is an example of an imaginal exposure that Johnny completed with his therapist.*

Therapist: When we met last time we talked about doing exposure exercises. Remember that during exposure exercises I want you to pay attention to how your body feels. If you start to feel anxiety symptoms, use some of your coping skills that we've been working on. Do you remember what those are?
Johnny: Deep breathing and distraction.
Therapist: Right. So if we start to do an exposure and you start to feel anxiety, practice your coping skills. If you start to feel like you are having asthma symptoms, I want you to let me know.
Johnny: Okay.
Therapist: So last time you came up with a list of all of the different places that you worry you might have an asthma attack. One of the places that you mentioned was the playground. On a scale from 1 to 10, how much do you worry about having asthma symptoms on the playground?
Johnny: Probably about a 4.
Therapist: Okay, this might sound silly, but we're going to imagine that you're on the playground at school. If you had to rate your anxiety on a scale from 1 to 10, where is it?
Johnny: A 2.
Therapist: Great. Now I want you to imagine that you cough. Where is your anxiety now?
Johnny: A 4.
Therapist: Okay, tell me what would happen next.
Johnny: I start to worry that I'm having trouble breathing.
Therapist: Where is your anxiety?
Johnny: A 5.
Therapist: Okay, then what happens?
Johnny: I start worrying that I am about to have an asthma attack.
Therapist: Where is your anxiety?
Johnny: A 7.
Therapist: Can you use your skills?
Johnny: I can take my deep breaths and tell myself I am going to be ok.
Therapist: Great, what else can you do? I can look around for an adult. I see a teacher on the other side of the playground.
Therapist: Where is your anxiety now?
Johnny: A 3.
Therapist: Then, what happens?
Johnny: Then, I have my friend go and get my teacher. My anxiety is back down to a 2 now.
Therapist: That's great! Let's talk about what happened with your anxiety. It started out at a 2, but how high did it get?
Johnny: It went up to a 7, then it came down again.
Therapist: Right! That's one of the neat things about anxiety. Sometimes it will go up and hit a high point, but then comes back down again.

After completing imaginal exposures, Johnny completed graduated in vivo exposures. Johnny's mother also learned how she could support Johnny and use similar skills to help differentiate Johnny's asthma versus anxiety symptoms; she also helped Johnny reward himself when he engaged in coping efforts.

Overall, a CBT model also fits with Janssens et al. (2009) working model of symptom perceptions. More specifically, CBT could help youth to discriminate between anxiety and asthma symptoms, use cognitive restructuring to address catastrophic thinking and threat evaluations, use relaxation strategies, and engage in graduated exposures. All these interventions could lead to improved symptom perceptions based on Janssens' model.

Conclusion

By the end of treatment, Johnny was using his controller medication and quick-relief medication appropriately (including taking his pretreatment of albuterol with his inhaler and spacer before doing physical activity) and engaging in physical activity (e.g., playing on the playground during recess, playing soccer). He was now able to identify his symptoms of anxiety and use coping skills to address his physiological anxiety symptoms and his catastrophic thinking patterns. He reported increased self-efficacy for managing his asthma and felt he was able to use his communication skills and problem-solving skills when his asthma symptoms did arise. Johnny's mother also reported improvements in her ability to manage Johnny's anxiety and asthma.

The available literature among youth with asthma provides preliminary support for the effectiveness of CBT for treating anxiety among youth with asthma. Tailoring CBT to include asthma-specific content appears to be an integral part of effective treatments. Key treatment components for addressing anxiety among youth with asthma include behavioral, cognitive, affective, and systems level intervention components.

References

Abu-Hasan, M., Tannous, B., & Weinberger, M. (2005). Exercise-induced dyspnea in children and adolescents: If not asthma then what? *Annals of Allergy, Asthma & Immunology, 94*(3), 366–371. https://doi.org/10.1016/S1081-1206(10)60989-1.

Achenbach, T. M. (2009). *The Achenbach System of Empirically Based Assessment (ASEBA): Development, findings, theory, and applications*. Burlington, VT: University of Vermont Research Center for Children, Youth, & Families.

Adams, R. J., Smith, B. J., & Ruffin, R. E. (2000). Factors associated with hospital admissions and repeat emergency department visits for adults with asthma. *Thorax, 55*(7), 566–573. https://doi.org/10.1136/thorax.55.7.566.

Alati, R., O'Callaghan, M., Najman, J. M., Williams, G. M., Bor, W., & Lawlor, D. A. (2005). Asthma and internalizing behavior problems in adolescence: A longitudinal study. *Psychosomatic Medicine, 67*(3), 462–470. https://doi.org/10.1097/01.psy.0000161524.37575.42.

Alexeeva, I., & Martin, M. (2018). Evidence for mood-dependent attentional processing in asthma: Attentional bias towards health-threat in depressive mood and attentional avoidance in neutral mood. *Journal of Behavioral Medicine, 41*(4), 550–567. https://doi.org/10.1007/s10865-018-9919-6.

American Psychiatric Association. (2013). *Diagnostic and statistical manual of mental disorders, 5th edition (DSM-5). Diagnostic and statistical manual of mental disorders* (5th ed.). Washington, DC: American Psychiatric Association.

Bauman, L. J., Wright, E., Leickly, F. E., Crain, E., Kruszon-Moran, D., Wade, S. L., et al. (2002). Relationship of adherence to pediatric asthma morbidity among inner-city children. *Pediatrics, 110*(1), e6. https://doi.org/10.1542/peds.110.1.e6.

Bender, B. G. (2016). Nonadherence to asthma treatment: Getting unstuck. *Journal of Allergy and Clinical Immunology: In Practice, 4*(5), 849–851. https://doi.org/10.1016/j.jaip.2016.07.007.

Bender, B., Wamboldt, F., O'Connor, S. L., Rand, C., Szefler, S., Milgrom, H., et al. (2000). Measurement of children's asthma medication adherence by self report, mother report, canister weight, and Doser CT. *Annals of Allergy, Asthma and Immunology, 85*(5), 416–421. https://doi.org/10.1016/S1081-1206(10)62557-4.

Birmaher, B., Brent, D. A., Chiappetta, L., Bridge, J., Monga, S., & Baugher, M. (1999). Psychometric properties of the screen for child anxiety related emotional disorders (SCARED): A replication study. *Journal of the American Academy of Child and Adolescent Psychiatry, 38*(10), 1230–1236. https://doi.org/10.1097/00004583-199910000-00011.

Bortoluzzi, A., Salum, G. A., da Rosa, E. D., Chagas, V., Castro, M. A. A., & Manfro, G. G. (2018). DNA methylation in adolescents with anxiety disorder: A longitudinal study. *Scientific Reports, 8*(1), 1–12. https://doi.org/10.1038/s41598-018-32090-1.

Butler, A. C., Chapman, J. E., Forman, E. M., & Beck, A. T. (2006). The empirical status of cognitive-behavioral therapy: A review of meta-analyses. *Clinical Psychology Review, 26*(1), 17–31. https://doi.org/10.1016/j.cpr.2005.07.003.

Canino, G., McQuaid, E. L., & Rand, C. S. (2009). Addressing asthma health disparities: A multilevel challenge. *Journal of Allergy and Clinical Immunology, 123*(6), 1209–1217. https://doi.org/10.1016/j.jaci.2009.02.043.

Carr, R. E., Lehrer, P. M., Rausch, L. L., & Hochron, S. M. (1994). Anxiety sensitivity and panic attacks in an asthmatic population. *Behaviour Research and Therapy, 32*(4), 411–418. https://doi.org/10.1016/0005-7967(94)90004-3.

Centers for Disease Control and Prevention. (2016). CDC—asthma—most recent asthma data. Retrieved October 29, 2018, from https://www.cdc.gov/asthma/most_recent_data.htm.

Colland, V. T. (1993). Learning to cope with asthma: A behavioural self-management program for children. *Patient Education and Counseling, 22*(3), 141–152.

Deliu, M., Belgrave, D., Sperrin, M., Buchan, I., & Custovic, A. (2017). Asthma phenotypes in childhood. *Expert Review of Clinical Immunology, 13*(7), 705–713. https://doi.org/10.1080/1744666X.2017.1257940.

DiMatteo, M. R., Lepper, H. S., & Croghan, T. W. (2000). Depression is a risk factor for noncompliance with medical treatment. *Archives of Internal Medicine, 160*(14), 2101. https://doi.org/10.1001/archinte.160.14.2101.

Dudeney, J., Sharpe, L., & Hunt, C. (2015). Attentional bias towards threatening stimuli in children with anxiety: A meta-analysis. *Clinical Psychology Review, 40*, 66–75. https://doi.org/10.1016/j.cpr.2015.05.007.

Dudeney, J., Sharpe, L., Jaffe, A., Jones, E. B., & Hunt, C. (2017a). Anxiety in youth with asthma: A meta-analysis. *Pediatric Pulmonology, 52*(9), 1121–1129. https://doi.org/10.1002/ppul.23689.

Dudeney, J., Sharpe, L., Sicouri, G., Lorimer, S., Dear, B. F., Jaffe, A., et al. (2017b). Attentional bias in children with asthma with and without anxiety disorders. *Journal of Abnormal Child Psychology, 45*(8), 1635–1646. https://doi.org/10.1007/s10802-017-0261-1.

Easter, G., Sharpe, L., & Hunt, C. J. (2015). Systematic review and meta-analysis of anxious and depressive symptoms in caregivers of children with asthma. *Journal of Pediatric Psychology, 40*(7), 623–632. https://doi.org/10.1093/jpepsy/jsv012.

Eccleston, C., Palermo, T. M., Fisher, E., & Law, E. (2015). Psychological interventions for parents of children and adolescents with chronic illness. *Cochrane Database of Systematic Reviews,* (4), CD009660. https://doi.org/10.1002/14651858.CD009660.pub3.

Feldman, J. M., Steinberg, D., Kutner, H., Eisenberg, N., Hottinger, K., Sidora-Arcoleo, K., et al. (2013). Perception of pulmonary function and asthma control: The differential role of child versus caregiver anxiety and depression. *Journal of Pediatric Psychology, 38*(10), 1091–1100. https://doi.org/10.1093/jpepsy/jst052.

Fritz, G. K., McQuaid, E. L., Spirito, A., & Klein, R. B. (1996). Symptom perception in pediatric asthma: Relationship to functional morbidity and psychological factors. *Journal of the American Academy of Child and Adolescent Psychiatry, 35*(8), 1033–1041. https://doi.org/10.1097/00004583-199608000-00014.

Gao, Y., Zhao, H., Zhang, F., Gao, Y., Shen, P., Chen, R., et al. (2015). The relationship between depression and asthma: A meta-analysis of prospective studies. *PLoS One, 10*(7), e0132424. https://doi.org/10.1371/journal.pone.0132424.

Global Initiative for Asthma. (2018). *Global strategy for asthma management and prevention, 2018.*

Goodwin, R. D., Bandiera, F. C., Steinberg, D., Ortega, A. N., & Feldman, J. M. (2012). Asthma and mental health among youth: Etiology, current knowledge and future directions. *Expert Review of Respiratory Medicine, 6*(4), 397–406. https://doi.org/10.1586/ers.12.34.

Hasler, G., Gergen, P. J., Kleinbaum, D. G., Ajdacic, V., Gamma, A., Eich, D., et al. (2005). Asthma and panic in young adults: A 20-year prospective community study. *American Journal of Respiratory and Critical Care Medicine, 171*(11), 1224–1230. https://doi.org/10.1164/rccm.200412-1669OC.

Higa-McMillan, C. K., Francis, S. E., & Chorpita, B. F. (2014). Anxiety disorders. In E. Mash & R. Barkley (Eds.), *Child psychopathology* (3rd ed., pp. 345–428). New York: The Guilford Press.

Janssens, T., Verleden, G., De Peuter, S., Van Diest, I., & Van den Bergh, O. (2009). Inaccurate perception of asthma symptoms: A cognitive-affective framework and implications for asthma treatment. *Clinical Psychology Review, 29*(4), 317–327. https://doi.org/10.1016/j.cpr.2009.02.006.

Jones, S. E., Merkle, S., Wheeler, L., Mannino, D. M., & Crossett, L. (2006). Tobacco and other drug use among high school students with asthma. *Journal of Adolescent Health, 39*(2), 291–294. https://doi.org/10.1016/j.jadohealth.2005.12.003.

Juniper, E., Guyatt, G., Feeny, D., Ferrie, P., Griffith, L., & Townsend, M. (1996a). Measuring quality of life in children with asthma. *Quality of Life Research, 5,* 35–46.

Juniper, E., Guyatt, G., Feeny, D., Ferrie, P., Griffith, L., & Townsend, M. (1996b). Measuring quality of life in the parents of children with asthma. *Quality of Life Research, 5*(1), 27–34. Retrieved from http://ovidsp.ovid.com/ovidweb.cgi?T=JS&PAGE=reference&D=emed4&NEWS=N&AN=1996095275.

Juniper, E. F., Svensson, K., Mörk, A. C., & Ståhl, E. (2005). Measurement properties and interpretation of three shortened versions of the asthma control questionnaire. *Respiratory Medicine, 99*(5), 553–558. https://doi.org/10.1016/j.rmed.2004.10.008.

Katon, W. J., Richardson, L., Lozano, P., & McCauley, E. (2004). The relationship of asthma and anxiety disorders. *Psychosomatic Medicine, 66*(3), 349–355. https://doi.org/10.1097/01.psy.0000126202.89941.ea.

Kaugars, A. S., Klinnert, M. D., & Bender, B. G. (2004). Family influences on pediatric asthma. *Journal of Pediatric Psychology, 29*(7), 475–491.

Kean, E. M., Kelsay, K., Wamboldt, F., & Wamboldt, M. Z. (2006). Posttraumatic stress in adolescents with asthma and their parents. *Journal of the American Academy of Child and Adolescent Psychiatry, 45*(1), 78–86. https://doi.org/10.1097/01.chi.0000186400.67346.02.

Kendall, P. (2012a). Anxiety disorders in youth. In P. Kendall (Ed.), *Child and adolescent therapy. Cognitive-behavioral procedures* (4th ed., pp. 143–189). New York, NY: The Guilford Press.

Kendall, P. (2012b). Guiding theory for therapy with children and adolescents. In P. Kendall (Ed.), *Child and adolescent therapy. Cognitive-behavioral procedures* (4th ed., pp. 3–24). New York, NY: The Guilford Press.

Kendall, P., Crawford, E., Kagan, E., Furr, J., & Podell, J. (2017). Child-focused treatment for anxiety. In J. Weisz & A. Kazdin (Eds.), *Evidence-based psychotherapies for children and adolescents* (3rd ed., pp. 17–34). New York, NY: The Guilford Press.

Kew, K. M., Nashed, M., Dulay, V., & Yorke, J. (2016). Cognitive behavioural therapy (CBT) for adults and adolescents with asthma. *Cochrane Database of Systematic Reviews*, (9). https://doi.org/10.1002/14651858.CD011818.pub2.

Lim, J., Wood, B. L., Miller, B. D., & Simmens, S. J. (2011). Effects of paternal and maternal depressive symptoms on child internalizing symptoms and asthma disease activity: Mediation by interparental negativity and parenting. *Journal of Family Psychology, 25*(1), 137–146. https://doi.org/10.1037/a0022452.

Liu, A. H., Zeiger, R., Sorkness, C., Mahr, T., Ostrom, N., Burgess, S., et al. (2007). Development and cross-sectional validation of the childhood asthma control test. *Journal of Allergy and Clinical Immunology, 119*(4), 817–825. https://doi.org/10.1016/j.jaci.2006.12.662.

Long, K. A., Ewing, L. J., Cohen, S., Skoner, D., Gentile, D., Koehrsen, J., Howe, C., Thompson, A. L., Rosen, R. K., Ganley, M., & Marsland, A. L. (2011). Preliminary evidence for the feasibility of a stress management intervention for 7- to 12-year-olds with asthma. *Journal of Asthma, 48*(2), 162–170.

Lowther, H., Newman, E., Sharp, K., & McMurray, A. (2016). Attentional bias to respiratory- and anxiety-related threat in children with asthma. *Cognition and Emotion, 30*(5), 953–967. https://doi.org/10.1080/02699931.2015.1036842.

Lu, Y., Mak, K. K., van Bever, H. P. S., Ng, T. P., Mak, A., & Ho, R. C. M. (2012). Prevalence of anxiety and depressive symptoms in adolescents with asthma: A meta-analysis and meta-regression. *Pediatric Allergy and Immunology, 23*(8), 707–715. https://doi.org/10.1111/pai.12000.

March, J. S., Parker, J. D. A., Sullivan, K., Stallings, P., & Conners, C. K. (1997). The Multidimensional Anxiety Scale for Children (MASC): Factor structure, reliability, and validity. *Journal of the American Academy of Child and Adolescent Psychiatry, 36*(4), 554–565. https://doi.org/10.1097/00004583-199704000-00019.

Marriage, D., & Henderson, J. (2012). Cognitive behaviour therapy for anxiety in children with asthma. *Nursing Children and Young People, 24*(9), 30–34. https://doi.org/10.7748/ncyp2012.11.24.9.30.c9392.

McLeish, A. C., & Zvolensky, M. J. (2010). Asthma and cigarette smoking: A review of the empirical literature. *The Journal of Asthma, 47*(4), 345–361. https://doi.org/10.3109/02770900903556413.

Mcmains, K. C. (2015). Assessment of asthma severity and control. *International Forum of Allergy and Rhinology, 5*(Suppl 1), S31–S34. https://doi.org/10.1002/alr.21559.

McQuaid, E., Kopel, S., & Nassau, J. (2001). Behavioral adjustment in children with asthma: A meta-analysis. *Journal of Developmental and Behavioral Pediatrics, 22*(6), 430–439.

McQuaid, E. L., Kopel, S. J., Klein, R. B., & Fritz, G. K. (2003). Medication adherence in pediatric asthma: Reasoning, responsibility, and behavior. *Journal of Pediatric Psychology, 28*(5), 323–333. https://doi.org/10.1093/jpepsy/jsg022.

McQuaid, E. L., Walders, N., Kopel, S. J., Fritz, G. K., & Klinnert, M. D. (2005). Pediatric asthma management in the family context: The family asthma management system scale. *Journal of Pediatric Psychology, 30*(6), 492–502. https://doi.org/10.1093/jpepsy/jsi074.

Milgrom, H., Bender, B., Ackerson, L., Bowry, P., Smith, B., & Rand, C. (1996). Noncompliance and treatment failure in children with asthma. *Journal of Allergy and Clinical Immunology, 98*(6), 1051–1057. https://doi.org/10.1016/S0091-6749(96)80190-4.

Muris, P., Ollendick, T. H., Roelofs, J., & Austin, K. (2014). The Short Form of the Fear Survey Schedule for Children-Revised (FSSC-R-SF): An efficient, reliable, and valid scale for measuring fear in children and adolescents. *Journal of Anxiety Disorders, 28*(8), 957–965. https://doi.org/10.1016/j.janxdis.2014.09.020.

Nathan, R. A., Sorkness, C. A., Kosinski, M., Schatz, M., Li, J. T., Marcus, P., et al. (2004). Development of the asthma control test: A survey for assessing asthma control. *Journal of Allergy and Clinical Immunology, 113*(1), 59–65. https://doi.org/10.1016/j.jaci.2003.09.008.

National Asthma Education and Prevention Program. (2007). *Guidelines for the diagnosis and management of asthma. National Asthma Education and Prevention Program Expert Panel Report 3*. Bethesda, MD. https://doi.org/NIH Publication Number 08-5846.

National Heart Lung and Blood Institute. (2007). *National Asthma Education and Prevention Program Expert Panel Report 3 (EPR-3): Guidelines for the diagnosis and Management of Asthma-Summary Report 2007*. Bethesda, MD.

Ollendick, T. H. (1983). Reliability and validity of the revised fear survey schedule for children (FSSC-R). *Behaviour Research and Therapy, 21*(6), 685–692. https://doi.org/10.1016/0005-7967(83)90087-6.

Pai, A. L. H., & McGrady, M. (2014). Systematic review and meta-analysis of psychological interventions to promote treatment adherence in children, adolescents, and young adults with chronic illness. *Journal of Pediatric Psychology, 39*(8), 918–931. https://doi.org/10.1093/jpepsy/jsu038.

Panton, J., & Barley, E. (2005). Family therapy for asthma in children. *Cochrane Database of Systematic Reviews*, (1), CD000089. https://doi.org/10.1002/14651858.CD000089.pub2.

Papneja, T., & Manassis, K. (2016). Characterization and treatment response of anxious children with asthma. *The Canadian Journal of Psychiatry, 51*(6), 393–396.

Park, S. J., Sawyer, S. M., & Glaun, D. E. (1996). Childhood asthma complicated by anxiety: An application of cognitive behavioural therapy. *Journal of Pediatrics and Child Health, 32*, 183–187.

Pateraki, E., Morris, P. G., Pateraki, E., Hons, B. S., & Sc, M. (2018). Effectiveness of cognitive behavioural therapy in reducing anxiety in adults and children with asthma: A systematic review children with asthma: A systematic review. *Journal of Asthma, 55*(5), 532–554. https://doi.org/10.1080/02770903.2017.1350967.

Persons, J. (2008). *The case formulation approach to cognitive-behavior therapy*. New York, NY: The Guilford Press.

Peters, T. E., & Fritz, G. K. (2010). Psychological considerations of the child with asthma. *Child and Adolescent Psychiatric Clinics of North America, 19*(2), 319–333. https://doi.org/10.1016/J.CHC.2010.01.006.

Rappaport, L. M., Sheerin, C., Carney, D. M., Towbin, K. E., Leibenluft, E., Pine, D. S., et al. (2017). Clinical correlates of carbon dioxide hypersensitivity in children. *Journal of the American Academy of Child and Adolescent Psychiatry, 56*(12), 1089–1096.e1. https://doi.org/10.1016/j.jaac.2017.09.423.

Reynolds, C., & Kamphaus, R. (2016). *Behavior assessment system for children, third edition (BASC-3)*. Bloomington, MN: Pearson.

Reynolds, C., & Paget, K. (1983). National normative and reliability data for the revised Children's Manifest Anxiety Scale. *School Psychology Review, 12*(3), 324–336. https://doi.org/10.1162/DRAM-a-00278.

Richardson, L. P., Lozano, P., Russo, J., McCauley, E., Bush, T., & Katon, W. (2006). Asthma symptom burden: Relationship to asthma severity and anxiety and depression symptoms. *Pediatrics, 118*(3), 1042–1051. https://doi.org/10.1542/peds.2006-0249.

Rosenberg, S. L., Miller, G. E., Brehm, J. M., & Celedón, J. C. (2014). Stress and asthma: Novel insights on genetic, epigenetic, and immunologic mechanisms. *Journal of Allergy and Clinical Immunology, 134*(5), 1009–1015. https://doi.org/10.1016/j.jaci.2014.07.005.

Roy-Byrne, P. P., Davidson, K. W., Kessler, R. C., Asmundson, G. J. G., Goodwin, R. D., Kubzansky, L., et al. (2008). Anxiety disorders and comorbid medical illness. *General Hospital Psychiatry, 30*(3), 208–225. https://doi.org/10.1016/j.genhosppsych.2007.12.006.

Scherer, Y. K., & Bruce, S. (2001). Knowledge, attitudes, and self-efficacy and compliance with medical regimen, number of emergency department visits, and hospitalizations in adults with asthma. *Heart and Lung: Journal of Acute and Critical Care, 30*(4), 250–257. https://doi.org/10.1067/mhl.2001.116013.

Sicouri, G., Sharpe, L., Hudson, J. L., Dudeney, J., Jaffe, A., & Hunt, C. (2017a). A case series evaluation of a pilot group cognitive behavioural treatment for children with asthma and anxiety. *Behaviour Change, 34*(1), 35–47. https://doi.org/10.1017/bec.2017.3.

Sicouri, G., Sharpe, L., Hudson, J. L., Dudeney, J., Jaffe, A., Selvadurai, H., et al. (2017b). Threat interpretation and parental influences for children with asthma and anxiety. *Behaviour Research and Therapy, 89*, 14–23. https://doi.org/10.1016/j.brat.2016.11.004.

Silverman, W., & Albano, A. (1996). *The anxiety disorders interview schedule for children for DSM-IV*. San Antonio, TX: Psychological Cooperation.

Spielberger, C. D. (1983). *Manual for the State-Trait Anxiety Inventory (STAI Form Y)*. Palo Alto: Consulting Psychologists Press. https://doi.org/10.1002/ana.22691.

Still, L., & Dolen, W. K. (2016). The perception of asthma severity in children. *Current Allergy and Asthma Reports, 16*(7), 1–6. https://doi.org/10.1007/s11882-016-0629-2.

Strine, T. W., Mokdad, A. H., Balluz, L. S., Berry, J. T., & Gonzalez, O. (2008). Impact of depression and anxiety on quality of life, health behaviors, and asthma control among adults in the United States with asthma, 2006. *Journal of Asthma, 45*(2), 123–133. https://doi.org/10.1080/02770900701840238.

ten Thoren, C., & Petermann, F. (2000). Reviewing asthma and anxiety. *Respiratory Medicine, 94*(5), 409–415. https://doi.org/10.1053/rmed.1999.0757.

Tepper, R. S., Wise, R. S., Covar, R., Irvin, C. G., Kercsmar, C. M., Kraft, M., et al. (2012). Asthma outcomes: Pulmonary physiology. *Journal of Allergy and Clinical Immunology, 129*(3 Suppl), S65–S87. https://doi.org/10.1016/j.jaci.2011.12.986.

Thomsen, S. F., van der Sluis, S., Kyvik, K. O., Skytthe, A., Skadhauge, L. R., & Backer, V. (2011). Increase in the heritability of asthma from 1994 to 2003 among adolescent twins. *Respiratory Medicine, 105*(8), 1147–1152.

Van De Ven, M. O. M., Engels, R. C. M. E., Sawyer, S. M., Otten, R., & Van Den Eijnden, R. J. J. M. (2007). The role of coping strategies in quality of life of adolescents with asthma. *Quality of Life Research, 16*(4), 625–634. https://doi.org/10.1007/s11136-006-9146-4.

Weinberger, M., & Abu-Hasan, M. (2007). Pseudoasthma: When cough, wheezing, and dyspnea are not asthma. *Pediatrics, 120*(4), 855–864. https://doi.org/10.1542/peds.2007-0078.

Wood, B. L., Cheah, P. A., Lim, J. H., Ritz, T., Miller, B. D., Stern, T., et al. (2007). Reliability and validity of the asthma trigger inventory applied to a pediatric population. *Journal of Pediatric Psychology, 32*(5), 552–560. https://doi.org/10.1093/jpepsy/jsl043.

Wood, B. L., Miller, B. D., & Lehman, H. K. (2015). Review of family relational stress and pediatric asthma: The value of biopsychosocial systemic models. *Family Process, 54*(2), 376–389. https://doi.org/10.1111/famp.12139.

Yang, I. V., Lozupone, C. A., & Schwartz, D. A. (2017). The environment, epigenome, and asthma. *Journal of Allergy and Clinical Immunology, 140*(1), 14–23. https://doi.org/10.1016/j.jaci.2017.05.011.

Yii, A. C. A., & Koh, M. S. (2013). A review of psychological dysfunction in asthma: Affective, behavioral and cognitive factors. *Journal of Asthma, 50*(9), 915–921. https://doi.org/10.3109/02770903.2013.819887.

Zahran, H. S., Bailey, C. M., Damon, S. A., Garbe, P. L., & Breysse, P. N. (2018). Vital signs: Asthma in children—United States, 2001–2016. https://doi.org/10.15585/mmwr.mm6705e1.

Cognitive-Behavioral Therapy for Pediatric Obesity

23

Carolina M. Bejarano, Arwen M. Marker, and Christopher C. Cushing

Introduction

Pediatric obesity is a chronic medical condition characterized by excess body weight. In children and adolescents, obesity is defined as a body mass index (BMI) at or above the 95th percentile (Centers for Disease Control and Prevention [CDC] 2017). BMI percentile is a metric that relates height, weight, age, and sex against population growth norms, which are represented using BMI growth charts (CDC 2015). Pediatric obesity currently affects 18.5% of children and adolescents. Stratified by age group, 13.9% of 2- to 5-year-olds, 18.4% of 6- to 11-year-olds, and 20.6% of 12- to 19-year-olds are obese (Hales et al. 2018). Rates of pediatric obesity have steadily increased from 5% in the 1970s, and rising trends have continued over the past decade (e.g., 16.9% of youth were obese in 2009–2010; Katzmarzyk et al. 2014; Ogden et al. 2012). In addition, 5.6% of these youth are severely obese, defined as a BMI at or above 120% of the 95th percentile (Hales et al. 2018).

These high rates of pediatric obesity are concerning because obesity is associated with a host of negative outcomes, including increased risk for cardiovascular disease, type 2 diabetes, sleep impairment, respiratory problems, low academic achievement, and depression (CDC 2017; Barlow and the Expert Committee 2007). For the 5% of youth who are severely obese, most already have at least one weight-related comorbidity, commonly dyslipidemia, hypertension, sleep apnea, asthma, and/or polycystic ovary syndrome (Ryder et al. 2018). Referral to a primary care practitioner, endocrinologist, sleep specialist, or gynecologist is indicated for these children.

Fortunately, empirically derived interventions exist to prevent and treat pediatric obesity. Behavioral interventions that target diet, physical activity, and behavior change techniques have demonstrated significant benefits for reducing weight, BMI, percent overweight, and improving metabolic outcomes in children and adolescents, with significantly larger weight reductions in moderate-to-high intensity interventions and some evidence that weight loss is maintained up to 1 year post-intervention (Whitlock et al. 2010; Wilfley et al. 2007). Pediatric obesity interventions have also demonstrated significant improvements in youth health-related quality of life (HRQOL), with or without weight loss (Tsiros et al. 2009). However, a recent review has quantified that reductions in BMI are associated with improvements in HRQOL indicating that as BMI goes down HRQOL goes up (Steele et al. 2016). Family-based behavioral interventions have

C. M. Bejarano · A. M. Marker · C. C. Cushing (✉)
Clinical Child Psychology Program and Life Span Institute, University of Kansas, 2011 Dole Human Development Center, Lawrence, KS, USA
e-mail: Christopher.cushing@ku.edu

demonstrated moderate-to-substantial reductions in weight and associated outcomes, and are recommended as a first-line treatment (Katzmarzyk et al. 2014).

Throughout this chapter, we present these evidence-based treatments for pediatric obesity within a cognitive-behavioral framework. We illustrate cognitive-behavioral treatment approaches through use of a case example, introduced here[1]:

> Amelia is a 9-year-old African American female who lives with her mother, Ms. Jones, and her 5-year-old brother. The family was referred from their pediatrician to the pediatric psychology clinic at the local hospital. At the intake session, Ms. Jones reported that Amelia has always been heavier than other girls of her age, that the family eats fast food frequently, and does not usually exercise. Ms. Jones expressed concern that Amelia has low self-esteem due to bullying she has experienced at school related to her weight. Her BMI at the intake was in the 97th percentile.

Biopsychosocial Conceptualization of Pediatric Obesity

Pediatric obesity is best explained using a biopsychosocial model that takes into account interactions among biological (e.g., genetic), psychological (e.g., mood, temperament), and social factors (e.g., culture, family environment) that lead to the development and maintenance of excess weight. It should be noted that these biopsychosocial factors may play a role as predisposing, precipitating, perpetuating, and/or protective of obesity.

Biological Factors

As stated above, pediatric obesity is diagnosed by anthropometric assessment of height, weight, and sex-specific BMI. Energy balance issues, or an imbalance in the relationship between energy in (from food and drink) and energy out (via exercise and daily energy requirements of the body), commonly underlie excess weight gain and can lead to the development of childhood obesity. Genetic factors play a predisposing role toward pediatric obesity, and there is about 77% heritability for both BMI and waist circumference (Wardle et al. 2008). Therefore, it can be beneficial for therapists to incorporate education about genetics into family-focused therapy for pediatric obesity. The therapist can provide the family with information about genetic predisposition for weight problems, while simultaneously empowering the family with tools to modify their diet and exercise habits in order to improve health and weight status.

Another biological factor in the presentation of pediatric obesity is the dysregulation of satiety hormones, which is commonly experienced subjectively as frequent and intense thoughts about food consumption and often an inability to fully recognize sensations of hunger and fullness (Balagopal et al. 2010). Additionally, taste preferences play a role in contributing to excess intake and weight concerns in children. Young children typically prefer foods with a high concentration of sweet taste and are more driven to consume these foods, although this preference typically declines during adolescence (Mennella et al. 2016).

Psychological Factors

A key psychological factor of interest pertaining to youth with obesity is HRQOL, which is defined as an individual's quality of life associated with well-being in physical, mental, and social domains, and is often assessed through both parent and child report in pediatrics (Tsiros et al. 2009). Children and adolescents of higher weight status consistently report lower HRQOL (Buttitta et al. 2014), which is associated with both physical symptoms, such as bodily pain, and lifestyle factors, such as quality of food intake, physical activity, and amount of screen time (Buttitta et al. 2014). Furthermore, children who are overweight or obese are more likely to be bullied, often contributing to low self-esteem and negative

---

[1]This case example was confabulated for this text and does not contain any identifiable patient information.

self-concept (Puhl et al. 2013). HRQOL is an important focus in the treatment of pediatric obesity, as low quality of life likely precipitates and perpetuates continued behavior that drives energy imbalance (e.g., not being active due to bodily pain associated with excess weight). While not typically rising to clinically disordered levels, subclinical symptoms of anxiety and depression in youth are often found to be comorbid with weight concerns due to the incidence of bullying, negative self-concept, and low self-esteem (Puhl et al. 2013). It is important to note that the normative differences in obesity are likely to be related to HRQOL, while clinically significant depression or anxiety affect only a subset of the population.

Problematic cognitions about self-concept, drive toward unhealthful behaviors, and low perceived ability to change behavior are prevalent in youth with obesity. Therefore, cognitive-behavioral approaches that teach children and adolescents to challenge and replace maladaptive thoughts can be effective in facilitating behavior change that is pertinent to treatment goals. Learned associations pertaining to unhealthful behaviors can also be a target for treatment progress. For example, emotional eating is common in the presentation of pediatric obesity, and is often driven by parental modeling and association of palatable or comforting foods with extreme emotions. Children may learn from family members that it is typical or appropriate to seek comfort with certain foods when they feel sad, angry, upset, or stressed. Children also usually learn to associate these foods with celebrations, such as having treats at birthday parties, holidays, or to celebrate accomplishments. Therefore, cognitive-behavioral therapy (CBT) approaches can be useful in breaking the associations between emotions (positive or negative) and food, challenging thoughts about the value of less healthful foods, and beginning to conceptualize food as a source of energy and nutrients to sustain activities of daily life. Similarly, this allows the opportunity to build coping strategies, such as relaxation techniques, to more effectively manage negative emotions, as well as begin to associate positive emotions with other concepts, such as building relationships with friends or family members.

Social and Environmental Factors

Social and environmental factors largely play into children and adolescents' dietary and physical activity habits, as well as the likelihood that they will follow recommendations for optimal health habits. These factors can be considered as affecting communities on a large scale (i.e., macro-environment), or affecting individual behavior (i.e., microenvironment) pertaining to weight status (Shaw et al. 2005). Additionally, cultural, socioeconomic, and familial factors largely affect health behavior (Bronfenbrenner 1977).

As noted, teasing from peers can have a substantial influence on the HRQOL of youth with obesity. Specifically, being teased during physical activity was associated with less engagement in physical activity, especially for girls with body dissatisfaction (Jensen and Steele 2009). Longitudinal associations indicate that children with overweight/obesity who experience teasing during physical activity report lower HRQOL later on (Jensen et al. 2013). Generally, weight-based victimization is prevalent in youth with obesity, especially from peers at school, and can take the form of verbal teasing, relational victimization, cyberbullying, and physical aggression (Puhl et al. 2013). The therapeutic process of a cognitive-behavioral approach can effectively target cognitions about weight-related behaviors and help children and adolescents challenge beliefs, manage emotions, and handle this experience in a more adaptive manner.

Modern society has developed into an environment that inhibits energy balance, often referred to as the obesogenic environment. Aspects of the home, school, and community environment interact to promote excess energy consumption and a lack of activity (Gorin and Crane 2008). Specifically, high-calorie, low-nutrient, low-cost food is widely available and convenient to acquire. Simultaneously, daily activities for work and leisure are predominantly sedentary; in children this translates to the school environment and activities such as watching television or playing video games. These factors overlap in specific contexts (e.g., fast food advertisements on television, the expectation of buying treat foods at the movie theater), further perpetuating energy imbalance.

Certain social and environmental factors may compound the likelihood that a child or adolescent develops a trajectory toward obesity. Indicators of socioeconomic status (SES), including parental education, parental occupation, family income, and neighborhood SES have been inversely associated with adiposity in children (Shrewsbury and Wardle 2008). For example, families of low SES are less likely to have the resources to purchase fresh produce and may therefore consume higher calorie, lower nutrient packaged foods. Related to SES, families that live in neighborhoods with more crime and lower traffic safety may have fewer opportunities to engage in outdoor physical activity. However, environmental factors can also be used to support change in dietary behavior and other health behaviors, such as in school and community contexts (Cushing et al. 2014b). Therefore, it is important to consider unique social and environmental barriers and facilitators in the case conceptualization of a child with obesity.

Assessing Pediatric Obesity

Pediatric obesity is often initially screened using body mass index (BMI), which is calculated with the formula weight in kilograms divided by height in meters squared. For adults, a BMI $\geq$ 30 kg/m^2 indicates a high level of body fatness which may be indicative of obesity, and a BMI $\geq$ 35 kg/m^2 indicates severe obesity. In children and adolescents who are still growing, a more accurate measure is BMI percentile, which relates an individual's BMI to typical levels of growth based on age and sex. BMI $\geq$85th and <95th percentile indicates overweight and BMI at or above the 95th percentile indicates obesity (CDC 2017). For children between 2 and 20 years old, BMI percentile can be plotted using growth charts or calculated using a child and teen BMI calculator (available online through the CDC). To most accurately assess BMI, providers should use a standard weight scale that measures weight in kilograms to the nearest 0.01 kg and a stadiometer that measures height in centimeters to the nearest 0.01 cm. Scales and stadiometers should be routinely calibrated, with the frequency of calibration depending on frequency of use. Standard practices include measuring a child in light clothing with shoes removed, repeating measurements two times (and a third time if the first two measurements do not match) to ensure accuracy, and using the average of these measurements to calculate BMI percentile. Although BMI may not be a perfect measure of body composition for youth who are very short, tall, or muscular, it is a user-friendly measure to initially assess obesity and to easily monitor treatment progress over time (e.g., weekly, pre-, and post-treatment). In cases where medical comorbidities are a concern, psychologists will need to receive consultation from medical professionals to evaluate biomarkers that could indicate life-threatening disease processes (e.g., hypertension).

In addition to anthropometric measures, it is important to assess psychosocial health due to the increased risks for depression, anxiety, low self-esteem, and impaired quality of life in youth with obesity. It may be useful to start with a broad-band screener such as the Behavior Assessment System for Children (BASC; Reynolds and Kamphaus 2016) or the Achenbach System of Empirically Based Assessment Child Behavior Checklist (CBCL; Achenbach 2009) to assess broad psychological, emotional, and behavioral symptoms. Each of these measures includes versions for a variety of ages and reporters (e.g., self, parent, teacher). Narrow-band screeners that are frequently used to assess quality of life in youth with obesity include the Pediatric Quality of Life Inventory (PedsQL; Varni et al. 2001), which measures HRQOL across physical, social, emotional, and academic domains; Sizing Me Up (Zeller and Modi 2009), which measures obesity-specific emotional, physical, social avoidance, positive social attributes, and teasing/marginalization; and the

Impact of Weight on Quality of Life-Kids (IWQOL; Kolotkin et al. 2006), which measures weight-specific quality of life pertaining to physical comfort, body esteem, social life, and family relations. Commonly used depression-specific screening measures include the Children's Depression Inventory (CDI; Kovacs 1985) and the Center for Epidemiological Studies Depression Scale-Revised (CESD-R; Eaton et al. 2004; Radloff 1977). Anxiety-specific screeners include the Screen for Child Anxiety Related Disorders (SCARED; Birmaher et al. 1999) and the Multidimensional Anxiety Scale for Children (MASC; March et al. 1997).

> *Ms. Jones reported a family history of type II diabetes. She indicated that she wanted to find ways for the family to eat healthier and for Amelia to feel better about herself. Assessment procedures included administration of a broad-band psychosocial screener, measures of quality of life and depressive symptoms based on the concerns about low self-esteem, and referral to a provider for a physical examination and blood work based on the family history of type II diabetes.*

Lifestyle behaviors related to pediatric obesity can be assessed using wearable devices and tracking logs. Accelerometers, such as those developed by the Actigraph Corporation, may be used to objectively measure the frequency, intensity, and duration of physical activity, as well as daily sleep patterns (Cushing et al. 2017). Food diaries and food recall (e.g., 24-h, 3-day, and 5-day recall) measures can be used to collect detailed information on energy intake, including portion sizes, micro-, and macronutrients. These self- and parent-recall methods can be problematic due to high burden associated with paper–pencil records, recall errors, or poor portion size estimation, but new technologies may help to overcome these difficulties. Food recall using personalized electronic devices or smartphones may be more acceptable for youth, and can harness features like alarms, text message prompts, or food photography apps to more accurately measure food intake (e.g., Cushing et al. 2010; Nicklas et al. 2012). These types of lifestyle behavior measures can be particularly helpful to identify behavior change targets and tailor multidisciplinary interventions. Finally, physiological measures, psychosocial symptoms, and lifestyle behaviors should be frequently re-assessed throughout treatment to assess progress and inform intervention adaptations or progression to more intensive care.

Treatment Components and Empirical Support

Clinical Interventions for Pediatric Obesity

Psychological interventions, such as behavioral and cognitive-behavioral weight-management strategies, have been widely used in the treatment of overweight and obesity (Shaw et al. 2005). Cognitive approaches include distraction from eating cues, recognizing and addressing negative thought patterns associated with poor health behavior, and coping skills to effectively manage situations and emotions pertaining to health behavior change. Meanwhile, the behavioral approaches include stimulus control, self-monitoring, goal setting, and reinforcement (Cushing et al. 2014a). Some of these behavioral approaches, such as goal setting and self-monitoring, are often additionally motivated within the context of a group therapy approach (Cushing et al. 2014a). This combination of cognitive and behavioral mechanisms appears to be effective in treating pediatric obesity (Janicke et al. 2014).

It is frequently necessary to include parents and family in treatment of pediatric obesity (Kitzmann et al. 2010; Kitzmann and Beech 2010). Comprehensive family lifestyle interventions have shown to be efficacious for improving weight status in treatment of pediatric obesity (Janicke et al. 2014). Moreover, family-based multidisciplinary cognitive-behavioral treatment was effective in reducing BMI and improving HRQOL for youth with obesity up to 12 months later (Vos et al. 2012). To date, it appears that both individual and group formats can be effective.

In practice, families are encouraged to use *stimulus control* (i.e., avoid having high fat high sugar food in the house, keep running shoes by the front door) to promote weight-management behaviors. In addition, families are strongly encouraged to heavily *self-monitor* relevant behaviors such as foods consumed and exercise performed. Sessions are used to set *Specific, Measurable, Attainable, Relevant, and Timely* goals. For instance, a goal might be to, "eat 5 servings of fruit and vegetables 6 out of 7 days this week." In session it is common to provide *feedback* on goal attainment and to teach formal *problem-solving* strategies to eliminate barriers to goal attainment. Some treatment approaches also attempt to identify maladaptive cognitions about diet or exercise (e.g., "If I exercise it will feel awful") and change them to more constructive thoughts about weight management (e.g., "If I do something active with someone I enjoy they can encourage me if it feels hard").

Nutrition and dietary interventions A key component of treatment for pediatric obesity is changes in diet. This involves nutrition education for both caregivers and children, and behavioral strategies to achieve change in dietary habits. A commonly used strategy for education and intake monitoring is the Stoplight Diet (Epstein and Squires 1988), a system in which families learn to identify the grams of sugar and fat in a serving of a food, use this information to categorize the food, and then make dietary decisions based on the categorization. In this way, the Stoplight Diet helps families learn skills that are both adaptable to the needs of their lifestyle and key to long-term lifestyle change. The Stoplight Diet specifies categories of Red, Green, and Yellow foods, based on the food's nutritional information. "Red" foods are those that have seven or more grams of fat per serving or 12 or more grams of sugar per serving, indicating high caloric density. "Green" foods are generally fresh fruits and vegetables, with the exception of some higher starch items. "Yellow" foods are those that are considered dietary staples, such as lean meats, low fat diary, and whole grain breads and starches. Families are instructed to limit "Red foods," which are commonly considered treats, usually to four times per week. This system is consistent with the *Go,* *Slow, Whoa* method also commonly used in pediatric health interventions, taking caution toward foods that are higher calorie and lower nutrient density (US Department of Health and Human Services and National Heart Lung and Blood Institute 2013). Practitioners should use a teach-back method with both parents and children to help them remember the relevant information for red, yellow, and green foods, and how often they should be eaten. It is usually most effective for a practitioner to teach families the Stoplight Diet with a hands-on activity of reading nutrition labels from common food items and labeling them as Red, Yellow, or Green foods. Families may also benefit from labeling foods in their home with red, yellow, and green stickers to assist in following the Stoplight Diet (Fig. 23.1).

At the second session, the psychologist talked further with the family about making dietary changes and provided nutrition education using the Stoplight Diet. Amelia expressed her concern that if she ate mostly "Green" foods, she would always be hungry. Below is a dialogue of how the psychologist helped challenge this belief:

Psychologist: Amelia, do you think you would be fuller if you ate an apple or drank a glass of apple juice?
Amelia: Definitely an apple, those take a while to eat, while I can just gulp down a glass of juice!
Psychologist: Ok, let's look at the nutrition information on an apple and apple juice. We know an apple is a fresh fruit, so what kind of food is that on the Stoplight Diet?
Amelia: It's a green one!
Psychologist: Good job. Now look at the grams of sugar on the apple juice. What kind of food is this one?
Amelia: It's a red food!
Psychologist: You're right. The fiber in fresh fruits and vegetables in "Green" foods help fill you up, and when you eat a balance of protein and whole grains with these, you will usually be satisfied. So, do you think it's true that you will be too hungry if you try to eat more green foods than red foods?
Amelia: No, that's true, the Green ones will help fill me up and are healthier.

The psychologist also provided education about how high sugar and high carbohydrate foods may often make people hungrier, which both Ms. Jones and Amelia thought about and realized these foods

Fig. 23.1 Stoplight diet

Stoplight Diet

Red Foods (limit to ≤4 servings per week): Candy, ice cream, fried foods, chips, soda, fast food

Yellow Foods (meals): Lean meats, low fat dairy, whole grains, nuts, corn, potatoes, peas, bananas

Green Foods (meals and snacks): Most fruits and vegetables

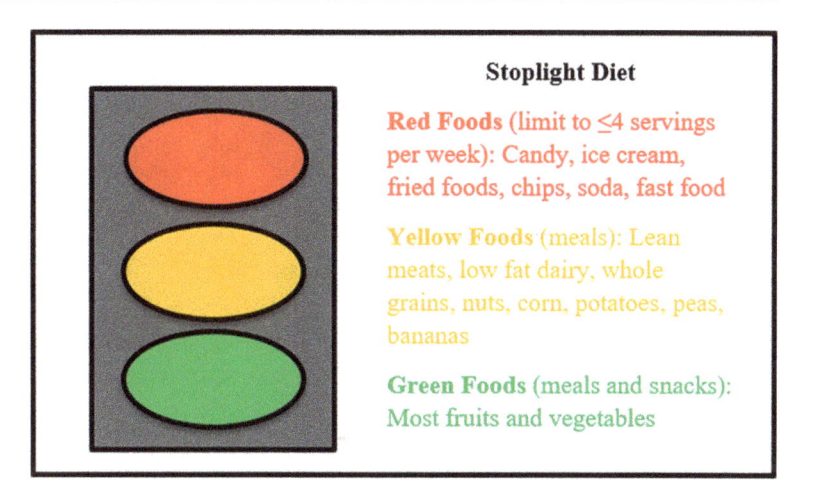

Fig. 23.2 Sample MyPlate

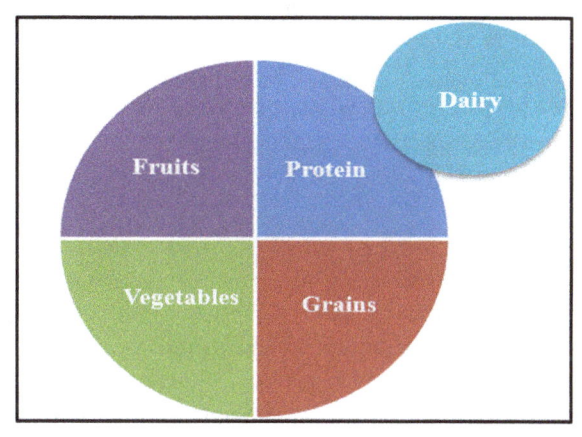

have indeed had that effect in the past. Generally, the psychologist highlighted the importance of cutting out sugar-sweetened beverages, such as juice, since they contribute both to empty calorie intake and cause spikes in blood glucose levels, which can contribute to risk for diabetes.

A method that can be used in conjunction with the Stoplight diet, the US Department of Agriculture *MyPlate* guidelines, is a popular strategy to help children and families create more healthful eating habits (www.choosemyplate.gov). Clinicians and dietitians use *MyPlate* to teach families about portion control and a balanced diet, focusing on the five food groups. Education focuses on identifying and categorizing foods as grains/starches, fruits, vegetables, lean dairy, and meat/protein. A small plate model is used, indicating that one half of the plate should consist of fruits and vegetables at a meal, one quarter should be lean protein, one quarter should be a starch/grain, and a serving of lean diary is included. This system is useful in helping families build awareness of their intake and portion sizes. When beginning to use this system, many families realize that they typically consume multiple servings of starch at a meal, and that portions are generally greater than a serving size. Therefore, using *MyPlate* is effective in helpful families make changes that improve their dietary intake by including sufficient protein, fruits, and vegetables, and limited starches and fats. It is often helpful to also use a teach-back method when introducing *MyPlate*, and have children and parents identify foods that go in each portion of the plate. Families may also like to use portioned plates that appear similar to *MyPlate* to facilitate this change during mealtime (Fig. 23.2).

Physical activity and sedentary behavior Education regarding physical activity and energy expenditure is another key area in treatment of pediatric obesity. Current physical activity guidelines recommend that children and adolescents engage in physical activity for 60 min a day, and limit screen time to less than 2 h per day (Katzmarzyk et al. 2016). Families should be educated about the health benefits of physical activity, and the health consequences of sedentary behavior, beyond weight-related health. It is important to provide ideas and resources for physical activities that are enjoyable for children, as well activities that can be done as a family. Additionally, caregivers and parents should be taught to identify different intensities of activity. For example, it is important to emphasize activity that is *moderate-to-vigorous*, which families can identify by their child breaking a sweat or moving vigorously enough to be too out of breath to sing.

Barriers to engaging in physical activity are commonly communicated by families. These barriers are often unique to the individual and the nature of one's lifestyle, and are best assessed in this way. For example, previous ecological momentary assessment studies have demonstrated that location, proximity of vegetation, weather, perceived safety, surrounding traffic, affect, and feeling states appear to be important predictors of activity in adolescents (Bejarano et al. 2019; Cushing et al. 2017). Moreover, there are likely individual differences that determine whether a given variable is a barrier or facilitator of physical activity (Cushing et al. 2017). Therefore, providers should ask patients and parents about the personal challenges they foresee in engaging in a physical activity regimen (and complement this information with technology-based assessments of physical activity and associated barriers/facilitators when possible) to provide personalized problem-solving to overcome physical activity barriers.

The activity component of an intervention also has families consider how they may choose to be active, rather than sedentary, during their leisure time. For example, discussing how hours spent watching television in the evening could be replaced by going on walks, bike riding, or playing outside, turns periods of sedentary screen time to opportunities for physical activity. It is often effective for the practitioner to talk with the family about their schedule and typical pasttimes, in order to identify specific time slots of sedentary behavior that can be replaced with a chosen physical activity. This use of activity scheduling and behavioral activation can help motivate and hold them accountable for this habit change that can be challenging. It is also helpful to provide families with a general idea of how many calories are burned during different activities, in order to continue to build awareness of the energy balance equation. Additionally, Table 23.1 provides ideas that practitioners may use to adapt physical activity interventions for different age groups.

Behavior change principles The approach of combining foci on diet and activity with behavior change principles is consistent with the CBT: misinformation or maladaptive beliefs about health are challenged and corrected, skills are taught and practiced, and the therapist adapts behavioral strategies as necessary to help families make changes that are consistent with the health education. There is strong evidence that behavioral strategies are the key change-inducing component of family-based interventions for pediatric obesity (Epstein and Squires 1988; Jelalian and Hart 2009). These behavioral strategies, including self-monitoring, goal setting, stimulus control, parent management, modeling, and social support, are described below (Martin and Pear 2002).

Self-monitoring is an integral part of cognitive-behavioral approaches to treatment for pediatric obesity. Self-monitoring for health behavior change involves a consistent awareness of targeted behaviors (e.g., eating fruits and vegetables, watching television), and tracking behaviors in a way that focuses on improvements from past habits (e.g., logging 30 min of activity per day when previously not engaging in any physical activity). In the context of the intervention

Table 23.1 Summary of pediatric obesity intervention adaptations by age group

	Toddlers and preschoolers	School-age children	Adolescents
Nutrition	• Parents responsible for purchasing and preparing food • Differential attention to ignore food complaints and praise healthy eating • One-bite rule for picky eaters to try new foods • Make healthy foods fun by cutting into shapes	• Parents still responsible for purchasing and preparing foods • Kids can be more involved in picking out foods and preparing foods with supervision • Household rules to ask permission before snacking	• Remove red foods from the home to decrease poor food choices when teens are home alone • Continue to monitor food intake • Be aware of food purchases outside the home
Physical activity	• 2- to 6-year-olds recommended to get 3 h of activity each day • Parents responsible for monitoring exercise • Parents schedule play-dates and outdoor activities • Focus on building motor skills	• Children older than 6 recommended to get 1 h of moderate-to-vigorous activity each day • Children may start organized sports • Parents and peers can be activity buddies • Focus on achieving all three types of exercise: aerobic, strength building, stretching • Focus on scheduling time for activity	• Watch for physical activity declines as gym/recess end and sports become more competitive • Adolescents take more ownership of self-monitoring • Transition from parent- to peer-supported exercise, like scheduling work-out times with a buddy and group activities
Behavior change principles	• Parent modeling of eating and exercise behaviors is key • Differential attention to reinforce healthy behaviors and ignore whining/complaints • Use of reward charts to reward healthy behaviors	• Differential attention to reinforce healthy behaviors and ignore whining/complaints • Use of reward charts to reward healthy behaviors	• Behavioral contracting to encourage healthy behaviors and autonomy • Increased communication about behavior expectations • SMART goals to achieve teen health values

components described above, self-monitoring can be an effective tool for children and caregivers to track the number of red foods eaten per week, log minutes of daily physical activity, and maintain awareness of their sedentary screen time in order to limit it. Engagement in self-monitoring, such as by the use of activity and diet logs, in itself encourages awareness and accountability, greatly contributing to modifications in usual behavior. Depending on the age and developmental level of the child, children may be able to take some autonomy for self-monitoring their health habits. In fact, there is evidence that sufficient recording of food consumption predicts better weight-management outcomes in adolescents (Saelens and McGrath 2003). Caregivers will lead the self-monitoring efforts for younger children, working toward building their own skills in this strategy.

Over the course of treatment, Amelia engaged in self-monitoring by using a wearable activity tracker that her grandparents gave her as a gift. She was enthusiastic about the feedback she received from the activity tracker, and she became motivated to count her steps daily and reach her goal of 60 min of activity per day. She made a friend in her neighborhood that she liked to go bike riding with, and in the clinic visits, reflected on how she now enjoyed physical activity because it was a fun time to spend with friends and family. She also reported having more energy than she did before.

Goal setting is a central piece of a cognitive-behavioral intervention for pediatric obesity, in both individual- and group-based treatment. Families are coached to set goals around nutrition and physical activity to maximize the chance they can successfully meet goals and it will result in meaningful change. Specifically, the sequential multiple assignment randomized trial (SMART) goal strategy is often used. In contrast to a commonly stated well-intentioned goal of "eating healthier" which does not specify exactly what behaviors will change, families learn to set goals that are specific, measureable, achievable, realistic, and time-framed (Locke 1996). To illustrate, an example of a goal-setting intervention with the Jones family is included below:

Mrs. Jones: Our goal this week will be to get more exercise.
Clinician: It is great that you want to be more active as a family. What kind of exercise will you do?
Mrs. Jones: I think we will all ride our bikes together.
Clinician: Good idea, when will be a good time to do that, and for how long will you ride?
Mrs. Jones: Well, we could do it in the evening, after dinner. We haven't been doing this very much so we could start by riding three evenings per week. I think 30 min would be good.
Clinician: That's a great goal! It is specific so that you will know whether or not you met it, it is reasonable based on your usual habits, but it is also a challenge to do more activity than you have been. We will check in next week to see how this went for you.

The clinician's next role in goal setting from a cognitive-behavioral perspective is to help the family evaluate whether they met their goal, and to problem-solve around any barriers. For example, if the family said they did not meet their goal because it rained most evenings last week, the clinician would challenge them to think of other activities they could do as a family, regardless of the weather.

Stimulus control in the context of pediatric obesity treatment generally means altering the environment in a way that supports healthful choices, and limits unhealthful choices. This often focuses on removing or limiting "Red" foods from the home environment so they are not available. In contrast, "Green" foods (fresh fruits and vegetables) can be readily available, in sight, and in reach. In this way, the healthy choice is the easy choice, as it would take family members more effort to access treat foods that are out of reach, or to leave the home in order to purchase treats. A common assignment to help with stimulus control is to have the family work together to read nutrition labels to remove the red foods from the home, and plan to dispose of them or donate them to a food pantry. There is often resistance to this assignment, especially if some family members do not have weight concerns. The practitioner can discuss how having planned treats on occasion, rather than a daily occurrence, is important for the health of the whole family.

The psychologist worked with the family to set SMART goals around increasing activity, decreasing red foods, and increasing fruit and vegetable consumption. The family reported on these goals weekly, and one week indicated that limiting red foods was hard because Amelia's younger brother really liked to eat cookies and candy. Ms. Jones said she thought it was unfair to not allow him to have these, since his weight is not a problem and she does not want to deprive him. The psychologist led a conversation to help Ms. Jones realize that the stimulus control efforts of removing the red foods would benefit the whole family, and be preventative for her brother's health in the long-run. The psychologist helped Ms. Jones plan a time once a week when the family could take a walk to go pick out a single portion of candy at the local convenience store.

Parenting strategies Lifestyle changes that allow for improved health and weight status entail effortful change for both parents and children. Parents typically experience their own resistance to changing habits, and this process of change is often even more difficult for children. Parents can benefit from parent management and behavioral strategies to manage children's reactions and possible noncompliance or misbehavior around these changes. For example, positive attention and praise for small health habits can be especially powerful, as well as talking positively about the new health behaviors that the family plans to start. In fact, there is evidence that parental praise of decreased sedentary behavior encouraged greater preference for high-intensity physical activity, engagement in these activities, and improved weight-management outcomes (Epstein et al. 1995). Communicating about the changes in diet and activity that the family will make, and what is expected of the child can help implement change more smoothly. Additionally, reinforcement beyond verbal praise, such as a reward chart for completing the planned physical activity for the day, has been shown to be effective in motivating children to comply with family changes. Parent-focused interventions appear to be especially effective, with evidence that targeting intervention efforts to parents exclusively was more effective for long-term weight-management goal as compared to interventions targeted to the children (Golan and Crow 2012). Parents and caregivers are the key facilitators and leaders of lifestyle changes, and modeling of healthful behaviors around diet and activity has been shown to help children more readily adopt the lifestyle that is essential for successful weight-management efforts.

Social support Children and adolescents are especially influenced by the perceptions and behaviors of their peers. For example, longitudinal associations have been found between being teased during physical activity with lower HRQOL in youth with overweight and obesity (Jensen et al. 2013). However, this influence can be used advantageously in the treatment of pediatric obesity. For example, perceived social support from same-age peers can improve obesity-specific health-related quality of life (Herzer et al. 2011). This further highlights the strengths of a group-based program, in which children are challenged to make the same lifestyle changes as their peers in the group, and experience solidarity in their challenges and successes. It can be helpful to have families identify friends, siblings, or family members who can schedule to engage in physical activity with the child or adolescent patient, as this often increases accountability and enjoyment.

Common Challenges with Clinical Intervention of Pediatric Obesity

Despite promising interventions for pediatric obesity, a number of challenges and barriers can reduce intervention effectiveness. First, lifestyle behavioral interventions for pediatric obesity historically have low enrollment rates. One contributing factor may be insufficient BMI screening or inadequate communication about youth weight status. Healthcare providers are identified as the first line of defense for weight screening and are recommended to assess child BMI at every well-check visit (Barlow and Expert Committee 2007; Spear et al. 2007). However, healthcare providers inconsistently document BMI and obesity in medical charts, infrequently order additional screening procedures (e.g., labs) for youth with obesity, and seldom refer families to specialists who can provide more intensive weight management (Chelvakumar et al. 2013; Higgins et al. 2014; Hillman et al. 2009; Walsh et al. 2013). When children and adolescents with obesity are appropriately identified, healthcare providers endorsed limited time or compensation to address obesity concerns, discomfort in communicating about weight status to the child's family, and limited knowledge about healthy lifestyle recommendations (Jelalian et al. 2003). In addition, referrals to more intensive weight-management services may be restricted by limited local access to evidence-based pediatric obesity interventions.

Furthermore, family-based pediatric obesity interventions typically use an opt-in approach where families of youth with obesity must consent to participate or even be contacted about weight-related interventions. Previous studies have found that only 12–16% of families expressed interest in a pediatric obesity intervention after referral by a healthcare provider, and only 6–9% of families enrolled in the intervention (Ghai et al. 2014; Markert et al. 2013). These low enrollment numbers are likely influenced by parent misperceptions about their child's weight, as almost 80% of parents fail to perceive their child as obese and inaccurate perceptions of child weight significantly reduce treatment-seeking behaviors (Towns and D'Auria 2009). However, parent concern about low child weight-related quality of life may be one factor related to greater treatment-seeking behaviors for obese youth (Cushing et al. 2013). Pediatric obesity interventions also demonstrate high attrition rates. Once a family enrolls in an intervention, a number of factors predict poor attendance, including higher baseline BMI (for both child and parent), minority race/ethnicity, further distance from intervention site, lower household income, and higher baseline depressive symptoms (Jelalian et al. 2008; Jensen et al. 2012). For families who are engaged in an intervention, additional environmental barriers such as limited access to safe spaces for exercise, limited healthy food access (e.g., "food desserts"), low social support for behavior change, inadequate cultural tailoring of interventions, and aversive consequences of health behaviors, such as feelings of discomfort during exercise, can attenuate effects of pediatric obesity interventions (Sallis et al. 2000). Thus, child and family characteristics can limit the effectiveness of available pediatric obesity interventions.

Conclusion

The family was seen for a total of 12 clinic visits. Amelia's BMI was tracked at each visit, and she and Ms. Jones completed the PedsQL as a measure of health-related quality of life at the intake, sixth visit, and at the last visit. Ms. Jones and Amelia recognized all the benefits of their work in eating healthier and being more active, including both having more energy, being in a better mood, feeling better about themselves, being able to focus more at work and at school, and Amelia having improved peer relations. At the last clinic visit, Amelia's weight was at the 95th percentile, the parent and child-reported health-related quality of life both improved significantly and Amelia's initially negative perception of treatment decreased significantly. At the end of the treatment, the family was referred to a group-based healthy lifestyles program, so that they could continue to have support for their successful changes.

Effective cognitive-behavioral treatment for this challenging medical condition involves education on nutrition and physical activity, with cognitive strategies and behavioral interventions that facilitate families' life-style changes to improve health and weight status. Commonly encountered challenges, innovative approaches, and application to a case example were included in the hopes that this information will be useful to practitioners treating pediatric obesity.

References

Achenbach, T. M. (2009). *The Achenbach System of Empirically Based Assessment (ASEBA): Development, findings, theory, and applications.* Burlington, VT: University of Vermont Research Center for Children, Youth, & Families.

Balagopal, P., Gidding, S. S., Buckloh, L. M., Yarandi, H. N., Sylvester, J. E., George, D. E., et al. (2010). Changes in circulating satiety hormones in obese children: A randomized controlled physical activity-based intervention study. *Obesity, 18*(9), 1747–1753.

Barlow, S. E., & the Expert Committee. (2007). Expert committee recommendations regarding the prevention, assessment, and treatment of child and adolescent overweight and obesity: Summary report. *Pediatrics, 120*(Supplement 4), S164–S192.

Bejarano, C. M., Cushing, C. C., & Crick, C. J. (2019). Does context predict psychological states and activity? An ecological momentary assessment pilot study of adolescents. *Psychology of Sport and Exercise, 41,* 146–152. https://doi.org/10.1016/j.psychsport.2018.05.008.

Birmaher, B., Brent, D. A., Chiappetta, L., Bridge, J., Monga, S., & Baugher, M. (1999). Psychometric properties of the Screen for Child Anxiety Related Emotional Disorders (SCARED): A replication study. *Journal of the American Academy of Child and Adolescent Psychiatry, 38*(10), 1230–1236.

Bronfenbrenner, U. (1977). Toward an experimental ecology of human development. *American Psychologist, 32*(7), 513.

Buttitta, M., Iliescu, C., Rousseau, A., & Guerrien, A. (2014). Quality of life in overweight and obese children and adolescents: A literature review. *Quality of Life Research, 23*(4), 1117–1139.

Centers for Disease Control and Prevention. (2015). About child & teen BMI. Retrieved May 15, 2018, from https://www.cdc.gov/healthyweight/assessing/bmi/childrens_bmi/about_childrens_bmi.html.

Centers for Disease Control and Prevention. (2017). Childhood overweight and obesity. Retrieved May 15, 2018, from https://www.cdc.gov/obesity/childhood/defining.html.

Chelvakumar, G., Levin, L., Polfuss, M., Hovis, S., Donahue, P., & Kotowski, A. (2013). Perception and documentation of weight management practices in pediatric primary care. *Wisconsin Medical Journal, 113*(4), 149–153.

Cushing, C. C. (2017). eHealth applications in pediatric psychology. In M. Roberts & R. Steele (Eds.), *Handbook of pediatric psychology* (5th ed., pp. 201–211). New York: Guilford Press.

Cushing, C. C., Bishop-Gilyard, C. T., Boles, R. E., Reiter-Purtill, J., & Zeller, M. H. (2013). Caregiver concern in adolescents with persistent obesity: The importance of quality of life assessment. *Journal of Developmental and Behavioral Pediatrics, 34*(1), 9.

Cushing, C. C., Borner, K., & Steele, R. G. (2014a). Pediatric obesity. In M. C. Roberts, B. S. Aylward, & Y. P. Wu (Eds.), *Clinical practice of pediatric psychology* (pp. 247–256). New York: Guilford Press.

Cushing, C. C., Brannon, E. E., Suorsa, K. I., & Wilson, D. K. (2014b). Systematic review and meta-analysis of health promotion interventions for children and adolescents using an ecological framework. *Journal of Pediatric Psychology, 39*(8), 949–962.

Cushing, C. C., Jensen, C. D., & Steele, R. G. (2010). An evaluation of a personal electronic device to enhance self-monitoring adherence in a pediatric weight management program using a multiple baseline design. *Journal of Pediatric Psychology, 36*(3), 301–307.

Cushing, C. C., Mitchell, T. B., Bejarano, C. M., Walters, R. W., Crick, C. J., & Noser, A. E. (2017). Bidirectional associations between psychological states and physical activity in adolescents: A mHealth pilot study. *Journal of Pediatric Psychology, 42*(5), 559–568.

Eaton, W. W., Muntaner, C., Smith, C., Tien, A., & Ybarra, M. (2004). Center for Epidemiologic Studies Depression Scale: Review and revision (CESD and CESD-R). In M. E. Maruish (Ed.), *The use of psychological testing for treatment planning and outcomes assessment* (3rd ed., pp. 363–377). Mahwah, NJ: Lawrence Erlbaum.

Epstein, L. H., & Squires, S. (1988). *The stoplight diet for children: An eight-week program for parents and children*. Pittsburgh: University of Pittsburgh Press.

Epstein, L. H., Valoski, A. M., Vara, L. S., McCurley, J., Wisniewski, L., Kalarchian, M. A., et al. (1995). Effects of decreasing sedentary behavior and increasing activity on weight change in obese children. *Health Psychology, 14*, 109–108.

Ghai, N. R., Reynolds, K. D., Xiang, A. H., Massie, K., Rosetti, S., Blanco, L., et al. (2014). Recruitment results among families contacted for an obesity prevention intervention: The obesity prevention tailored for health study. *Trials, 15*, 163. https://doi.org/10.1186/1745-6215-15-463.

Golan, M., & Crow, S. (2012). Targeting parents exclusively in the treatment of childhood obesity: Long-term results. *Obesity Research, 12*(2), 357–361.

Gorin, A. A., & Crane, M. M. (2008). The obesogenic environment. In E. Jelalian & R. Steele (Eds.), *Handbook of childhood and adolescent obesity* (pp. 145–161). New York: Springer.

Hales, C. M., Fryar, C. D., Carroll, M. D., Freedman, D. S., & Ogden, C. L. (2018). Trends in obesity and severe obesity prevalence in US youth and adults by sex and age, 2007–2008 to 2015–2016. *Journal of the American Medical Association, 319*(16), 1723–1725.

Herzer, M., Zeller, M. H., Rausch, J. R., & Modi, A. C. (2011). Perceived social support and its association with obesity-specific health-related quality of life. *Journal of Developmental and Behavioral Pediatrics, 32*(3), 188.

Higgins, A., McCarville, M., Kurowski, J., McEwen, S., & Tanz, R. R. (2014). Diagnosis and screening of overweight and obese children in a resident continuity clinic. *Global Pediatric Health, 1*, 2333794X14559396. https://doi.org/10.1177/2333794X14559396.

Hillman, J. B., Corathers, S. D., & Wilson, S. E. (2009). Pediatricians and screening for obesity with body mass index: Does level of training matter? *Public Health Reports, 124*(4), 561–567. https://doi.org/10.1177/003335490912400413.

Janicke, D. M., Steele, R. G., Gayes, L. A., Lim, C. S., Clifford, L. M., Schneider, E. M., et al. (2014). Systematic review and meta-analysis of comprehensive behavioral family lifestyle interventions addressing pediatric obesity. *Journal of Pediatric Psychology, 39*(8), 809–825.

Jelalian, E., Boergers, J., Alday, C. S., & Frank, R. (2003). Survey of physician attitudes and practices related to pediatric obesity. *Clinical Pediatrics, 42*(3), 235–245. https://doi.org/10.1177/000992280304200307.

Jelalian, E., & Hart, C. N. (2009). Pediatric obesity. In M. C. Roberts & R. G. Steele (Eds.), *Handbook of pediatric psychology* (4th ed., pp. 446–463). New York: Guilford Press.

Jelalian, E., Hart, C. N., Mehlenbeck, R. S., Lloyd-Richardson, E. E., Kaplan, J. D., Flynn-O'Brien, K. T., et al. (2008). Predictors of attrition and weight loss in an adolescent weight control program. *Obesity, 16*, 1318–1323. https://doi.org/10.1038/oby.2008.51.

Jensen, C. D., Aylward, B. S., & Steele, R. G. (2012). Predictors of attendance in a practical clinical trial of two pediatric weight management interventions. *Obesity, 20*, 2250–2256. https://doi.org/10.1038/oby.2012.96.

Jensen, C. D., Cushing, C. C., & Elledge, A. R. (2013). Associations between teasing, quality of life, and physical activity among preadolescent children. *Journal of Pediatric Psychology, 39*(1), 65–73.

Jensen, C. D., & Steele, R. G. (2009). Brief report: Body dissatisfaction, weight criticism, and self-reported physical activity in preadolescent children. *Journal of Pediatric Psychology, 34*(8), 822–826.

Katzmarzyk, P. T., Barlow, S., Bouchard, C., Catalano, P. M., Hsia, D. S., Inge, T. H., et al. (2014). An evolving scientific basis for the prevention and treatment of pediatric obesity. *International Journal of Obesity, 38*(7), 887.

Katzmarzyk, P. T., Denstel, K. D., Beals, K., Bolling, C., Wright, C., Crouter, S. E., et al. (2016). Results from the United States of America's 2016 report card on physical activity for children and youth. *Journal of Physical Activity and Health, 13*(11 Suppl 2), S307–S313. https://doi.org/10.1123/jpah.2016-0321.

Kitzmann, K. M., & Beech, B. M. (2010). Family-based interventions for pediatric obesity: Methodological and conceptual challenges from family psychology. *Journal of Family Psychology, 20*(2), 175.

Kitzmann, K. M., Dalton, W. T., III, Stanley, C. M., Beech, B. M., Reeves, T. P., Buscemi, J., et al. (2010). Lifestyle interventions for youth who are overweight: A meta-analytic review. *Health Psychology, 29*(1), 91.

Kolotkin, R. L., Zeller, M., Modi, A. C., Samsa, G. P., Quinlan, N. P., Yanovski, J. A., et al. (2006). Assessing weight-related quality of life in adolescents. *Obesity (Silver Spring), 14*, 448–457.

Kovacs, M. (1985). The children's depression inventory (CDI). *Psychopharmacology Bulletin, 21*(4), 995–998.

Locke, E. A. (1996). Motivation through conscious goal setting. *Applied and Preventive Psychology, 5*(2), 117–124.

March, J. S., Parker, J. D., Sullivan, K., Stallings, P., & Conners, C. K. (1997). The Multidimensional Anxiety Scale for Children (MASC): Factor structure, reliability, and validity. *Journal of the American Academy of Child & Adolescent Psychiatry, 36*(4), 554–565.

Markert, J., Alff, F., Zschaler, S., Gausche, R., Kiess, W., & Bluher, S. (2013). Prevention of childhood obesity: Recruiting strategies via local paediatricians and study protocol for a telephone-based counselling programme. *Obesity Research and Clinical Practice, 7*, e476–e486. https://doi.org/10.1016/j.orcp.2012.07.008.

Martin, G., & Pear, J. (2002). *Behavior modification: What is it and how to do it* (7th ed.). Upper Saddle River, NJ: Prentice Hall.

Mennella, J. A., Bobowski, N. K., & Reed, D. R. (2016). The development of sweet taste: From biology to hedonics. *Reviews in Endocrine and Metabolic Disorders, 17*(2), 171–178.

Nicklas, T. A., O'Neil, C. E., Stuff, J., Goodell, L. S., Liu, Y., & Martin, C. K. (2012). Validity and feasibility of a digital diet estimation method for use with preschool children: A pilot study. *Journal of Nutrition Education and Behavior, 44*(6), 618–623.

Ogden, C. L., Carroll, M. D., Kit, B. K., & Flegal, K. M. (2012). Prevalence of obesity and trends in body mass index among US children and adolescents, 1999-2010. *Journal of the American Medical Association, 307*(5), 483–490.

Puhl, R. M., Peterson, J. L., & Luedicke, J. (2013). Weight-based victimization: Bullying experiences of weight loss treatment–seeking youth. *Pediatrics, 131*(1), e1–e9.

Radloff, L. S. (1977). The CES-D scale: A self-report depression scale for research in the general population. *Applied Psychological Measurement, 1*, 385–401.

Reynolds, C. R., & Kamphaus, R. W. (2016). *Behavior assessment system for children, third edition (BASC-3)*. Bloomington, MN: Pearson.

Ryder, J. R., Fox, C. K., & Kelly, A. S. (2018). Treatment options for severe obesity in the pediatric population: Current limitations and future opportunities. *Obesity (Silver Spring), 26*(6), 951–960.

Saelens, B. E., & McGrath, A. M. (2003). Self-monitoring adherence and adolescent weight control efficacy. *Children's Health Care, 32*(2), 137–152.

Sallis, J. F., Prochaska, J. J., & Taylor, W. C. (2000). A review of correlates of physical activity of children and adolescents. *Medicine & Science in Sports & Exercise, 32*(5), 963–975.

Shaw, K. A., O'Rourke, P. K., Del Mar, C., & Kenardy, J. (2005). Psychological interventions for overweight or obesity. *Cochrane Database of Systematic Reviews, 2*, 1–62.

Shrewsbury, V., & Wardle, J. (2008). Socioeconomic status and adiposity in childhood: A systematic review of cross-sectional studies 1990–2005. *Obesity, 16*(2), 275–284.

Spear, B. A., Barlow, S. E., Ervin, C., Ludwig, D. S., Saelens, B. E., Schetzina, K. E., et al. (2007). Recommendations for treatment of child and adolescent overweight and obesity. *Pediatrics, 120*(Supplement 4), S254–S288.

Steele, R. G., Gayes, L. A., Dalton, W. T., III, Smith, C., Maphis, L., & Conway-Williams, E. (2016). Change in health-related quality of life in the context of pediatric obesity interventions: A meta-analytic review. *Health Psychology, 35*(10), 1097–1109.

Towns, N., & D'Auria, J. (2009). Parental perceptions of their child's overweight: An integrative review of the literature. *Journal of Pediatric Nursing, 24*(2), 115–130. https://doi.org/10.1016/j.pedn.2008.02.032.

Tsiros, M. D., Olds, T., Buckley, J. D., Grimshaw, P., Brennan, L., Walkley, J., et al. (2009). Health-related quality of life in obese children and adolescents. *International Journal of Obesity, 33*(4), 387.

US Department of Health and Human Services, & National Heart Lung and Blood Institute. (2013). We can! Go, slow and whoa foods. Retrieved May 15, 2018, from https://www.nhlbi.nih.gov/health/educational/wecan/tools-resources/eatplaygrow-gsw.htm.

Varni, J. W., Seid, M., & Kurtin, P. S. (2001). PedsQL 4.0: Reliability and validity of the pediatric quality of life inventory, version 4.0 generic core scales in healthy and patient populations. *Medical Care, 39*, 800–812.

Vos, R. C., Huisman, S. D., Houdijk, E. C., Pijl, H., & Wit, J. M. (2012). The effect of family-based multidisciplinary cognitive behavioral treatment on health-related quality of life in childhood obesity. *Quality of Life Research, 21*(9), 1587–1594.

Walsh, C. O., Milliren, C. E., Feldman, H. A., & Taveras, E. M. (2013). Factors affecting subspecialty referrals by pediatric primary care providers for children with obesity-related comorbidities. *Clinical Pediatrics, 52*(8), 777–785. https://doi.org/10.1177/0009922813488647.

Wardle, J., Carnell, S., Haworth, C. M., & Plomin, R. (2008). Evidence for a strong genetic influence on childhood adiposity despite the force of the obesogenic environment. *The American Journal of Clinical Nutrition, 87*(2), 398–404. https://doi.org/10.1093/ajcn/87.2.398.

Wilfley, D. E., Tibbs, T. L., Van Buren, D., Reach, K. P., Walker, M. S., & Epstein, L. H. (2007). Lifestyle interventions in the treatment of childhood overweight: A meta-analytic review of randomized controlled trials. *Health Psychology, 26*(5), 521.

Whitlock, E. P., O'Connor, E. A., Williams, S. B., Beil, T. L., & Lutz, K. W. (2010). Effectiveness of weight management interventions in children: A targeted systematic review for the USPSTF. *Pediatrics, 125*, e396–e418.

Zeller, M. H., & Modi, A. C. (2009). Development and initial validation of an obesity-specific quality-of-life measure for children: Sizing me up. *Obesity, 17*, 1171–1117. https://doi.org/10.1038/oby.2009.47.

Working with Transgender and Gender Expansive Youth

24

Andrea Carolina Tabuenca
and Krista Hayward Basile

Introduction

Increased visibility of diverse gender identities over the past several decades has shed greater light on the needs of these communities. Clinicians are now better understanding how chronic minority stress has contributed to the vulnerabilities, psychosocial adversities, and poor mental health outcomes of this population. Fortunately, there is a growing body of research identifying effective treatment modalities for reducing risk and enhancing resilience with transgender and gender expansive (TGE) youth. Interventions are based on a professional consensus that supports gender-affirmative models of care. Within a Cognitive Behavioral Therapy (CBT) theoretical framework, formulations acknowledge how minority stress can foster maladaptive thinking patterns that contribute to psychosocial impairments. Treatment is focused on restructuring unhelpful cognitive and behavioral patterns in a manner that supports youth in affirming their authentic selves and promotes resilience in the face of adversity.

Language

Gender identity refers to an aspect of a person's intrinsic sense of self that often reflects an interaction of biological, cultural, and environmental factors. The term "transgender" is used to denote an individual whose personal sense of gender identity does not correspond with their sex assigned at birth (natal sex). In contrast, the term "cisgender" denotes someone whose personal sense of gender is congruent with their sex assigned at birth. Although the term transgender is often understood to imply cross-gender identification as either male or female, it can also represent a range of gender identities that exist outside of this binary. As we progress through an era with greater social awareness of the diversity of gender experiences, additional language has developed to allow people to better express their authentic sense of self. Currently, some commonly used terms to denote gender identity include non-binary, gender fluid, gender non-conforming, and gender expansive. This terminology is not exhaustive and will likely continue evolving along with our understanding of gender and identity. In this chapter, the term TGE will be utilized to reflect the most contemporary literature on this population.

TGE individuals are often considered within the context of a greater Lesbian Gay Bisexual Transgender and Queer (LGBTQ) population.

A. C. Tabuenca (✉)
Stanford University, Stanford, CA, USA
e-mail: atabu@stanford.edu

K. H. Basile
Palo Alto University, Palo Alto, CA, USA

Collectively, LGBTQ groups share a common experience of exposure to minority stress regarding deviations from common societal expectations for gender and sexuality. However, there is a distinct difference between those represented as "T" and those represented as "LGB." While LGB identities refer to the attractions or romantic interests between people, trans and gender expansive identities refer to an individual's intrinsic sense of gender. The letter "Q" is often added to this acronym as well, to denote "Queer" identities that are diverse through the spectrum of both gender and sexuality.

Diagnosis

Changes in diagnostic terminology While diagnostic labels can increase access to healthcare through billing codes that grant insurance coverage, they may also carry stigma that hurt the very population they are intended to aid. There continues to be controversy regarding the terminology and criteria used to identify TGE youth within standard clinical tools including the *Diagnostic and Statistical Manual of Mental Disorders Fifth Edition* or DSM-5 and the *International Classification of Diseases* (ICD-11) (Cohen-Kettenis and Pfäfflin 2010; Meyer-Bahlburg 2010; Winters 2006; Drescher 2010; Drescher et al. 2016). Concerns were raised that previously used diagnostic classifiers such as "Gender Identity Disorder" (APA 1980, 1987) characterize gender diverse identities as inherently pathological. In response, the diagnostic term "Gender Dysphoria" was introduced through the DSM-5 (APA 2013) with the intent to classify the distress associated with experiences of gender diverse identities rather than pathologizing the identities themselves. In applying this diagnosis, it is key to acknowledge that clinically significant distress in trans and gender expansive individuals commonly results from social responses to the expressed identity rather than stemming from the identity in and of itself (Vasey and Bartlett 2007). Ongoing concerns about stigmatization from classification of gender dysphoria as a mental health disorder have influenced recent changes within ICD-11. TGE experiences will now be classified with the label "Gender Incongruence" and listed under Conditions Related to Sexual Health (Reed et al. 2016). With a growing scientific knowledge base of gender, approaches to diagnosis are likely to continue evolving in future iterations of diagnostic manuals and classifications systems.

Gender Dysphoria In many individuals, the experience of incongruence between one's gender identity and their sex assigned at birth can lead to clinically significant distress and functional impairment in daily life. The label "Gender Dysphoria" formally captures this experience through diagnostic criteria outlined in the DSM-5 (APA 2013). However, this term is more often attributed to the various multidimensional experiences of gender incongruence that can be related to physical anatomy, external gender expression, and adherence to socially ascribed gender roles. Keo-Meier and Ehrensaft (2018, p. 11) denote the difference between these two uses of the term in the following way: "Gender Dysphoria, capitalized, is a diagnosis in the DSM-5, and gender dysphoria, lowercase, is the experience that 'something is not right' regarding one's gender. This can include body dysphoria—commonly chest dysphoria and genital dysphoria—as well as distress related to being [trans or gender expansive]."

Regardless of whether DSM-5 criteria for Gender Dysphoria are met, experiences of gender dysphoria are unique and diverse among children. For many, dysphoria may be most intensified when faced with social expectations for gender norms, including clothing selection and choice of activities for recreation or play. This often leaves the child with a very difficult decision between two potentially painful outcomes. If the child chooses to align their expression or gender role with their authentic sense of identity, they may be exposed to isolating and damaging social rebuke. Conversely, conforming to norms that are incongruent with their internal sense of identity can expose the child to a devastating sense of dysphoria that impacts mood and anxiety throughout the activity.

Experiences of gender dysphoria can also be felt very personally with regard to anatomical development. In some cases, dysphoria may be felt early on due to a sense of incongruence with primary sex characteristics such as genitalia. Other times, dysphoria may become noticeable when secondary sex characteristics such as breast enlargement, hip widening, facial hair, and Adam's apple are either noticed or expected to develop. This sense of dysphoria can impact daily self-care. Tasks such as showering and changing clothing might be avoided, as they expose the individual to these parts of the body and increase dysphoria.

The prevalence of children struggling with gender dysphoria is difficult to report due to challenges in capturing the various identities and presentations that may reflect this experience. The DSM-5 asserts prevalence ranges between 0.0005 and 0.014% for natal adult males and 0.002 and 0.003% for natal adult females. However, readers are cautioned that these are "likely modest underestimates" (American Psychiatric Association 2013). The 2011 National School Climate Survey in the United States reported substantially higher rates for youth, including approximately 8% of middle and high school students who identified as transgender and 7% of students who identified as another gender, genderqueer, or androgynous (Kosciw et al. 2012). Prevalence rates recorded will likely continue to vary as we become more attuned to the diverse experiences of this population.

Vulnerabilities Due to Minority Stress

A population of children at risk It is imperative to consider the mental health risks of TGE youth within a framework of minority stress. "Focusing too narrowly on mental health outcomes may serve to over-pathologize a vulnerable population who may be experiencing a normative response to pervasive discrimination, violence, and exclusion" (Valentine and Shipherd 2018, p. 12). Meyer (2003, p. 5) describes a model that differentiates three processes by which minority stress is experienced by sexual and gender minorities:

(a) external, objective stressful events and conditions (chronic and acute)
(b) expectations of such events and the vigilance this expectation requires
(c) the internalization of negative societal attitudes

Valentine and Shipherd (2018) further explored analyses of this stress model through a systematic review of social stress and mental health among TGE individuals. Studies have consistently found that TGE people were commonly exposed to social stigma and discrimination that impacted their mental health (Valentine and Shipherd 2018).

Minority stress and poor access to care can contribute to poor mental health across all LGBTQ identities (Williams and Mann 2017), yet transgender individuals remain at the highest risk for a myriad of poor outcomes within this group (Reisner et al. 2015; Connolly et al. 2016; Testa et al. 2012, 2014, 2017). In comparison to same-aged cisgender peers, TGE children and adolescents are two to three times more likely to experience clinical levels of depression and anxiety (Becerra-Culqui et al. 2018; Reisner et al. 2015). TGE youth are also at increased risk of requiring inpatient hospitalization, with higher prevalence of self-injury, suicidal ideation, and greater risk of engaging in dangerous and life-threatening behaviors (Grossman and D'Augelli 2007; Reisner et al. 2015).

Resilience through empowerment Resilience should not only be viewed as a child's ability to survive in the face of adversity but to "grow and flourish because of the experience" (Malpas et al. 2018, p. 141). Fortunately, there has been a growing effort towards identifying ways in which mental health professionals and families can help enhance resilience among TGE children. This often involves the promotion of skills that facilitate navigation through a world that is ill equipped to accommodate and respect TGE individuals (The World Professional Association for Transgender Health 2011). Allan and Ungar (2014) highlight seven resilience factors that can be enhanced through direct intervention. These include: access to material resources, supportive relationships with significant others, a sense of identity that fuels a sense of satisfaction or pride and purpose, experiences of power and control, cultural adherence fostering a connection with community, social justice providing a sense of fairness and equality, and sense of social cohesion often found through spiritual identity (Allan and Ungar 2014). Foundationally, interventions that promote these seven factors will utilize multidimensional approaches aimed at strengthening the supports available to the child through individual intervention, family-based interventions, and facilitated connections to community resources and supports.

Professional Consensus on Standards of Care

Several professional associations have acknowledged and asserted a responsibility for ensuring that providers are appropriately meeting the healthcare needs of TGE individuals. The World Professional Association of Transgender Health (WPATH) provides Standards of Care that promote the gender-affirmative model of treating TGE individuals in both medical and psychosocial contexts (WPATH 2011). This includes competent use of gender-affirmative treatments such as hormone therapy and surgical intervention (Anton 2009; WPATH 2011). These standards are upheld by the American Psychological Association, which acknowledges evidence that "appropriately evaluated individuals benefit from gender transition treatments" (Anton 2009, p. 442; APA 2015; Colizzi et al. 2014). Furthermore, the APA encourages affirmation of gender diverse groups through legal and social recognition that is consistent with their gender identities (Anton 2009; APA 2015). The American Psychiatric Association echoes these assertions in their Position Statement on Access to Care for Transgender and Gender Variant Individuals, acknowledging the benefits of medical and surgical affirmative treatments and advocating for the removal of barriers that impact access to care (Drescher and Haller 2012). Affirmative interventions are also supported by the Association for Behavioral and Cognitive Therapies (2018).

These positions are based on emerging evidence that gender-affirmative efforts promote more positive mental health, reduce symptoms of depression and anxiety, and increase self-esteem and life satisfaction (Colizzi et al. 2014; Travers et al. 2012). Conversely, therapies offering "reparative" or "conversion" techniques that make efforts to change a person's gender identity have repeatedly been shown to be coercive, harmful, and increase the risk of poor psychological outcomes (Substance Abuse and Mental Health Services Administration 2014). The American Medical Association (AMA) has published a health policy (H-160.991) that strongly opposes any such approaches (AMA 2017, p. 1). Lawmakers have also acted to protect individuals from this harmful practice by making reparative therapies illegal in several states (Ludwig 2016).

Historically, practices have also implemented a "wait and see" approach that suggests delaying a child's transition until adolescence or adulthood; these approaches were often well-intentioned toward allowing children more time to develop certainty about their gender prior to making changes to their expression. However, it is imperative to understand that ignoring a child's sense of urgency to affirm their gender is not a passive intervention (Murchison et al. 2016). Rather, clinical experience has shown that delayed transition can lead to a prolonged and worsening experience of gender dysphoria that disrupts psychosocial aspects of development (Murchison et al. 2016; D'Augelli et al. 2006; Garofalo et al. 2006; Roberts et al. 2012; Skidmore et al. 2006; Toomey et al. 2010; Travers et al. 2012). Studies show that when trans and gender expansive children are supported in their identities, mental health outcomes are more positive with little psychosocial distinction from cisgender peers (Olson et al. 2016; Connolly et al. 2016). This has also been shown to be true for affirmation through earlier medical interventions that are approached with thoughtfulness and maturity (Smith et al. 2001; De Vries et al. 2014).

Biopsychosocial Considerations in Conceptualization of Care: Case Conceptualization Through the Gender-Affirmative Lens

Referral Information

The following case was confabulated to illustrate common clinical presentations among TGE youth. The information provided is not that of any real individual.

Jay is a 12-year-old Indian American gender expansive child who was assigned female at birth. Jay identifies as non-binary and has been using they/them/their pronouns for the past 3 months. Jay was referred for therapy services by their pediatrician due to concerns of persistently depressed mood beginning 6 months ago and worsening over the past several weeks. Additional symptoms reported include disrupted sleep, crying spells, anhedonia, difficulties concentrating, and increasing social withdrawal. Their parents have also noticed superficial cuts across Jay's arms, though self-injury was denied. Jay's pediatrician notes that these symptoms are occurring alongside Jay's expressed discomfort with bodily changes. Jay is currently in Tanner stage III of puberty and has complained of noticeable breast development. They have expressed an urgent desire to stop these changes and hope that they will "never actually have to get a period." As these symptoms progress, Jay has also exhibited frequent school refusal which is significantly affecting classwork and grades. Following clinical interviews with the child and family, Jay's symptoms were confirmed as meeting DSM-5 criteria for Major Depressive Disorder of moderate severity as well as Gender Dysphoria (APA 2013).

Child interview During their interview, Jay presented as a soft spoken, yet articulate child. They wore a hoodie and jeans. Their hair was half shaven with the remainder tied up in what Jay described as "my man bun." Thick eyeliner was noted around their eyes and purple nail polish was worn on their fingernails. Jay was somewhat guarded, but confirmed the symptoms described in the referral. Although suicidal ideation was denied, they endorsed a chronic sense of "wishing I hadn't been born." They expressed feeling "like something was off" since early childhood and experiencing a worsening sense of isolation from family and peers around the age of 10. Jay became somewhat less guarded when invited to discuss their considerations about gender, beginning with "it's all just confusing I guess." They described initially wondering about their sense of attraction to others, stating "I guess some people think I look like a lesbian. Maybe. I'm not sure. I've had crushes on boys before, so I don't know. I think I kind of look like a boy, but that doesn't mean I'm a boy either I guess." Jay reported researching their experience more thoroughly online for the past several months and self-diagnosing with Gender Dysphoria. Jay resonated with the sense of discomfort others had expressed about their developing bodies, stating "I would hate to look like a woman. Unless it was Halloween or something." Jay described this experience as initially confusing "because I feel totally wrong as a girl, but I really don't want to become a guy either. Can I just be me and everyone just be quiet?"

In continuing to explore media related to gender dysphoria, Jay encountered videos discussing non-binary and gender fluid identities. They found these descriptions as closely matching their experience and consequently asserted their identity as non-binary to parents and peers. Jay's school offers support through a Gay Straight Alliance (GSA) student organization. However, Jay reported feeling uncomfortable during GSA meetings after fellow LGBTQ peers frequently misgendered them using he/him/his pronouns. Jay recalled one peer stating, "Using 'they' is too confusing! When are you finally going to transition?" In addition, Jay expresses discomfort with restroom use, describing a perception that "everyone always thinks I'm in the wrong bathroom no matter which I use." When questioned about school refusal, Jay expressed feeling "too tired" to get up in the morning for school. They added, "I just want to be alone so I can figure things out. Everyone seems to have themselves figured out except me. I'm not sure I'll ever grow up to be normal."

Parent interview The parent interview revealed family history of postpartum depression following Jay's birth and the birth of their younger sister. Jay's father endorsed a history of substance abuse during Jay's early childhood. Although these issues led to temporary parental separation when Jay was 2 years old, the family reunited within the year. Both parents have received treatment and the family remains intact. Aside from concerns about Jay's current presentation, parents denied any recent significant psychosocial stressors to the family. Jay's parents expressed acceptance of Jay's gender exploration, while describing ambivalence about a non-binary identity. Both parents described themselves as "very progressive and pro LGBTQ rights." Nevertheless, they expressed concern that "Jay is choosing a hard path" and "things would just be easier if Jay could just decide who he is so we can make the changes." Jay's mother acknowledged difficulties using Jay's requested pronouns of they/them because "I look at him, I mean them, and I see a trans boy. I wonder if something is stopping him from really expressing this." She then expressed specific concerns that Jay's "uncertainty" about gender could be related to early family disruption and history of maternal depression.

Biopsychosocial Conceptualization

Various biological factors of Jay's history must be considered in formulating this case. Some of these are non-modifiable biological factors, such as Jay's family history of depression and their sex assigned at birth. Furthermore, Jay is experiencing clinically significant distress due to initial development of secondary sex characteristics that are incongruent with their personal sense of gender identity. Without intervention (i.e., implementing a "wait and see" approach), Jay's gender dysphoria and sequelae of psychological symptoms are likely to intensify. Intervention with puberty blockers can attenuate risk, providing relief from the anticipation of irreversible bodily changes that do not align with Jay's gender.

Jay's example also highlights how daily experiences can expose non-binary individuals to chronically harmful social messages that result in pressures to conform to an inauthentic cisnormative identity. These pressures are salient across different environments, even permeating networks intended to lend support and affirmation. Despite the various protective factors typically offered by GSA communities, social biases within this group are apparent and exclusionary of Jay's identity. Commentary that Jay's pronouns are too difficult to use sends the message that non-binary identities are less deserving of affirmative efforts, creating a context of risk for low self-worth. Parental expectations that Jay should eventually conform to binary standards further invalidate Jay's identity, subsequently invalidating an inherent aspect of their sense of self.

Consistent with empirical perspectives, all cases should be considered with competency that attends to factors of cultural context. This involves thoroughly assessing for cultural factors that might influence how Jay's family and community considers ideas related to gender identity, gender roles, and gender fluidity. Many families of Indian heritage belong to communities that value adherence to traditional gender roles, which may feel reinforcing of a gender binary that does not align with Jay's experience. However, some Indian traditions also recognize the existence of a third gender that some consider to be neither completely male nor female. This view may be more supportive of Jay's non-binary identity, thereby reducing pressures to conform to a binary expectation.

Cognitive Behavioral Considerations

Jay's concern that "I'm not sure I'll ever grow up to be normal," is a clear example of a distorted self-regard perpetuated by minority stress. Jay perceives themselves as "abnormal" or pathological in the context of their cisnormative surroundings. They support these beliefs with perceived evidence that "everyone else seems to have themselves figured out except for me." Rather than acknowledging the externally imposed hardships associated with identities that are not yet readily understood or accepted, Jay attributes their sense of otherness to an intrinsic failure. This manner of distorted thinking creates serious injury and fosters lasting depression.

The cycle of thinking patterns that drive psychological distress in Jay's situation is likely reinforced by the daily external messages. Jay's chronic exposure to these messages promotes behavioral responses that are less adaptive and create cycles that sustain depression. For example, Jay's reaction of isolating themselves from others to "just be alone so I can figure things out" is likely impacting school attendance, affecting peer relationships, reducing opportunities for behavioral activation, and reducing help-seeking behaviors. Jay's presentation is also suspect for self-injury, suggesting they are currently lacking more adaptive strategies for more effectively tolerating distress. Isolative behaviors are likely to further impact Jay's ability to utilize more adaptive coping strategies that rely on plans for appropriate help seeking.

Treatment Components and Associated Empirical Support

Gender-Affirmative Family Behavior Interventions

Considering TGE youth within a family context is paramount to understanding the mechanisms that impact risk and resiliency. When children come out at home, family reactions can range from highly accepting to highly rejecting of that child's identity. Many families' responses fall somewhere along the middle of this continuum, expressing ambivalence through a mix of accepting and rejecting behaviors (Substance Abuse and Mental Health Services Administration 2014). A range of responses can include outright rejection, tolerance, acceptance, and celebration of the child's identity (Malpas 2018). The level of rejection perceived by the child is directly linked with the level of risk to their mental health outcomes. Ryan (2009) reported that youth from families considered to be *highly* rejecting were eight times more likely to attempt suicide. Those from *moderately* rejecting families were more than twice as likely to attempt suicide as those from families with *minimal* rejecting behaviors (Ryan 2009). Similar findings were reported for youth regarding risk of clinical depression, anxiety, substance use, and HIV infection (Ryan et al. 2010).

It is essential to recognize that families perceived as rejecting of gender and sexual minority youth can be motivated by care and concern for that child (Substance Abuse and Mental Health Services Administration 2014). Rejecting behaviors are often driven by an underlying cultural context that aims to make youth successful within our existing heteronormative and cisnormative society (Ryan and Diaz 2011). Consequently, caregivers may attempt to change a child's identity and gender expression toward conformity to protect a child from victimization, help their child fit in, and promote a happier life (Substance Abuse and Mental Health Services Administration 2014). While well intentioned, these actions send a dangerous message of invalidation to TGE youth, who are often asked to challenge or hide a core aspect of their identity on a daily basis.

Interventions that enhance family support Prior to initiating a family intervention, clinicians should privately assess the child's status as "out" within the family. Careful consideration must be given to potential family disruption and subsequent risk to the child's physical and emotional safety prior to proceeding with family-based interventions (Keuroghlian et al. 2014; Quintana et al. 2010; Durso and Gates 2012). When safe, affirmative interventions such as The Family Acceptance Project (Ryan and Diaz 2011) and Multidimensional Family Approaches (Malpas 2011) can help promote resilience by enhancing family affirmation. Clinicians should emphasize to caregivers that these approaches do not aim to change family values or deeply held beliefs. Rather, they seek to clarify these values, acknowledge them as strengths, and explore their alignment with research findings that promote the well-being of gender and sexual minority youth (Ryan and Chen-Hayes 2013; Hill et al. 2010).

Treatment begins by assessing family behaviors along the continuum of acceptance as well as the impact these behaviors have on the child. This baseline information is then used to inform the goals and strategies that can help families move toward the more accepting end of this continuum. See Table 24.1 for examples of parent behaviors along a supportive continuum. Clinicians should meet with parents individually to explore perceptions about the child's identity and concerns regarding the implications of this identity.

Oftentimes, parents feel overwhelmed by fears of a potentially bleak future for their child if a gender expansive identity persists. Fears may be expressed in behaviors that are perceived as rejecting despite being rooted in caring concern and protectiveness. Parents may delay efforts to affirm their child by refusing to use the child's asserted name and pronoun, managing the child's wardrobe, and encouraging the child to participate in activities that are socialized to align with their sex assigned at birth. In doing so, they might maintain hopefulness that opportunities remain for the child to embrace a cisgender identity and be shielded from the stigmatizing responses of society at large.

Clinicians should help parents understand how these behaviors may be driven by the *faulty* belief that withholding affirmation or encouraging conformity creates a natural context for TGE identities to passively dissipate over time. An

Table 24.1 Family behaviors along a continuum of support

Family behaviors	Level of support			
	Rejecting	Tolerating	Accepting	Celebrating
Using name and pronouns	Refusing to use the name/pronoun asserted by the child and encouraging others to do the same	Inconsistently using the child's asserted name and pronoun Tolerating use of the child's asserted name and pronoun	Actively attempting to use the child's asserted name and pronoun (e.g., correcting mistakes)	Actively using the child's asserted name and pronoun Making statements that reflect pride in the child's identity
Respecting gender expression	Disallowing or punishing the child for attempting to align their gender expression with their identity	Allowing the child to express in a preferred manner, despite apparent discomfort or disapproval from parent	Allowing or encouraging the child to express in a preferred manner Avoiding messages of discomfort or disapproval	Taking pride in the child's expression Actively encouraging the child to continue exploring their individuality through expression
Respecting gender role	Actively placing the child in social roles that do not align with the child's gender identity	Allowing the child to abstain from activities that represent gender roles that do not feel right to them	Supporting the child in seeking out opportunities to participate in activities that align with gender identity	Actively seeking out and advocating for the child to connect with opportunities to express gender role in an affirming manner
Supporting medical intervention	Communicating absolute refusal to support child with medical intervention	Expressing willingness to passively accept medical intervention once the child is of age to legally consent for themselves	Acknowledging the potential benefits of medical affirmation and proceeding with appropriate precaution relevant to the child's individual needs	Expressing commitment to proceed with this intervention if indicated for the child and sharing in the child's joy of milestones through medical affirmation

This table was developed as a modified representation of ideas discussed in Malpas (2011)

example of this faulty belief as expressed by a parent may include, "my child is still young and can't really know who they are yet. If I use the new name, I could be encouraging an idea that will lead to a lot of confusion, regret, and bullying." Clinicians can support parents in challenging these beliefs by emphasizing two critical points. First, there is no evidence that affirmation will promote persistence of an inauthentic gender identity. Second, there *is* evidence that non-affirmation can be perceived as rejection by the child. This can embitter family relationships, exacerbate a child's self-concept, and reduce resilience overall. Thus, parents should be made aware that rejecting behaviors can exacerbate the very hardships that many families are intending to prevent (Ryan and Diaz 2011).

These messages can be reinforced with families by sharing data collected through various research initiatives including online booklets provided by the Family Acceptance Project along with findings from the Trans PULSE Project. These findings demonstrate that strong parental support of a child's gender identity and expression is directly linked with greater self-esteem, higher life satisfaction, reduced depression, and fewer suicide attempts in youth when compared to peers who did not perceive parents as strongly supportive (Ryan et al. 2010; Travers et al. 2012). Links to these tools can be found in the reference section. Psychoeducation can help families challenge attributions about their roles in protecting the child by understanding that acceptance is a critical protective tool for strengthening resilience. The previously stated faulty belief may thus be reframed as "Gender exploration can be a process. Regardless of the outcome, acceptance is the best form of protection along the way. By listening and affirming the identity that my child shares, I can create an emotionally safe environment at home that lowers the risks of being different in society." Clinicians can then help families apply this message practically by identifying affirming behaviors that facilitate this process as outlined in Table 24.1.

It is also important to attend to the supportive needs of parents and other family members who often have their own complex emotional reactions to a child's transition. It is not uncommon for families to feel a sense of grief or "ambiguous loss" that is confusing and overwhelming for both parents and children (Ryan and Diaz 2011; Coolhart et al. 2018). Clinicians should normalize and validate for parents this sense of a having lost the narratives associated with having a son or daughter. However, they should also highlight that this experience inevitably brings an opportunity for the child to thrive within a new narrative that aligns with their authentic self. Efforts should also be made to facilitate connections to family support networks that can provide the therapeutic benefits of processing shared experiences. Online resources such as CenterLink are designed to facilitate the identification of nearby LGBTQ community centers that can offer supportive networks ("Community of LGBT" 2018).

Gender-Affirmative Cognitive Behavioral Therapy

Acknowledging Current Gaps in the Literature

Research studies that incorporate contemporary views on gender identity into CBT approaches are still in their nascent stages. Clinical recommendations often focus on adapting existing treatment models with modifications that acknowledge minority stress, cultural factors, body dysphoria, and transition processes in a competent manner (Busa et al. 2018a, b; Ryan 2014; Collazo et al. 2013; Balsam et al. 2006; Pachankis 2014). However, empirical literature assessing the efficacy of specifically modified interventions is scant (Busa et al. 2018a). Given these limitations, interventions should be implemented with caution. Treatments should be aligned with the WPATH (2011) Standards of Care and utilize consultation with gender specialists and/or trans-affirming organizations.

Promising interventions in trans-affirmative CBT Some emerging studies suggest effective adaptations of trans-affirmative cognitive behavioral frameworks or TA-CBT

(Austin and Craig 2015; Craig and Austin 2016; Austin et al. 2017). Among these interventions is Affirmative Cognitive Behavioral Therapy (AFFIRM), which has demonstrated promising outcomes specific to TGE youth (Austin et al. 2018). These approaches aim to address the negative thinking patterns developed by sexual and gender minority youth in the context of continual exposure to transphobic and homophobic attitudes, beliefs, and behaviors (Austin et al. 2018; Bockting et al. 2013; Mizock and Mueser 2014). With support, children can develop more effective strategies for managing their responses to transphobia and build resilience in the face of stigma.

Implementing trans-affirmative CBT interventions Initial sessions must focus on providing standard psychoeducation on the skills necessary for the child to engage in CBT intervention. These include identifying and labeling feelings, distinguishing thoughts from feelings, and understanding the existence of counterproductive thinking patterns (Sburlati et al. 2014). Additionally, psychoeducation should be provided on concepts related to gender identity, gender dysphoria, and cisnormativity. A few examples of developmentally sensitive vocabulary that can be used to explain relevant terminology can be found in Table 24.2. Educating children on these issues allows them to better conceptualize their experiences within a model of minority stress, disarming the effects of transphobic stigmas that are otherwise internalized (Austin et al. 2018; Craig and Austin 2016; Austin and Craig 2015).

Once the child demonstrates a strong grasp of these concepts, emphasis can be shifted toward exploring thought patterns that may be developing under exposure to minority stress specific to the child. Clinicians should support the child in sharing their experiences across several settings, including in the home, at school, at places of worship, and during extracurricular activities. In

Table 24.2 Developmentally sensitive definitions relevant to gender identity

Term	Definition
Gender identity	What a person knows is true about who they are inside, whether their identity is a boy, a girl, a mix of both, or neither
Assigned sex	An assumption that others make about what a person's gender identity will be based on their bodies when they are born
Transgender	When someone's gender identity *does not* match their assigned sex. This word is usually used by people whose gender identity is seen as the "opposite" of their assigned sex
Cisgender	When someone's gender identity *does* match their assigned sex
Non-binary identities	People do not identify as either a boy or a girl. They can identify as a mix of both or as neither
Gender fluid identities	People whose gender identities change
Gender expression	The ways we choose to show our gender identity by how we dress, how we play, or how we act
Gender expansive	When someone's gender identity or expression does not fit with what people would expect of them based on their assigned sex
Gender binary	The idea that there are only boys and girls. This is wrong because it leaves out people who are non-binary or gender fluid
Cisnormativity	When people assume that everyone is cisgender. This means that sometimes people make decisions or treat others in a way that leaves out people who are not cisgender. This is unfair and feel hurtful
Sexual orientation	This a term used to describe how people feel about others. It is a way of understanding who we might have romantic feelings for or see as more than just friends. This is different from our gender identity, which is about how we see ourselves instead of how we feel about others

Note: Table 24.2 is not an exhaustive list of terms that represent the extensive diversity of gender and sexual identities. Moreover, it is important to consider that these are terms that are continuously evolving as we progress in our understanding of them. Our explanations of these terms may change as we learn more about the complexities of identity reviewing the child's daily exposure to narratives about gender and sexuality, clinicians must remain alert to the messages the child may be internalizing and how these may affect thoughts about the self, others, and the future. Attention should be given to maladaptive thinking patterns that develop in relation to the child's self-concept, which may be expressed through negative self-talk. For example, children may perceive themselves as "disordered" or "pathological" due to daily messages that are covertly expressed or overtly taught (Austin and Craig 2015). These self-perceptions can perpetuate feelings of shame and guilt and increase risk for clinical levels of depression and anxiety (Austin et al. 2017).

The case of "Jay" discussed earlier in this chapter provides one example of how maladaptive thinking patterns may develop within the context of problematic social messages. After chronic exposure to social pressures to conform to either side of a gender binary, Jay's authentic experience of an identity that falls outside of this binary was internalized as "abnormal." Consistent with common patterns of distorted thinking, Jay viewed this label as accurate, pervasive to their identity, and assumed that it will persist into the future. These aspects were reinforced by overt messages by those who invalidated their identity and bathroom options that reinforced a gender binary. Covert messages that also reinforce maladaptive self-views include a lack of representation and education on identities that exist outside of a gender binary.

While Jay is clearly aware of the overt social messages that are causing them distress, more support may be needed to call out the problematic nature of these messages as well as the mechanisms by which they directly impact thinking. The child should be thoroughly educated on the connection between social attitudes, negative self-perceptions, maladaptive thinking patterns, and the subsequent emotional distress that accompanies them. Support is provided for the child to eventually learn to identify and diffuse these thoughts through cognitive restructuring. Traditional CBT strategies targeting depression and anxiety can be applied, including the use of techniques for labeling and describing thought distortions, engaging in thought stopping, and selecting adaptive replacement thoughts.

However, a TA-CBT framework does more than support the child in challenging common distortions. It also emphasizes affirmation and validation of the hardships associated with experiences that promote distorted thinking (Craig and Austin 2017; Austin and Craig 2015). Jay's perception of non-binary identities as abnormal or pathological must be identified as a distortion. The chronic stigmatizing experiences that have reinforced this distortion should be called out and validated as a significant hardship. In doing so, Jay can begin to understand how hardships contextualized within societal misconceptions can directly affect thinking patterns that entrench them in distressing emotions. Providing guidance for Jay to arrive at this formulation of their experience can then allow them to begin exploring information available to dispute these thoughts. To facilitate interventions in challenging and restructuring negative thinking patterns, Austin et al. (2018) support use of the ABCD model detailed by Ellis (1991) within a TA-CBT framework that incorporates real-world considerations for TGE youth. This model guides patients through exploring an Activating event, related Beliefs, resulting Consequence, and the Dispute of faulty cognitions. See Fig. 24.1 for a sample thought diary that illustrates an application of this intervention with Jay. This model is also used with the case example discussed below.

Applied Case Example

Case History

The following case was confabulated to illustrate common clinical presentations among TGE youth. The information provided is not that of any real individual.

Lisa is a 16-year-old African American transgender girl. She was referred by her pediatric endocrinologist for therapeutic services following worsened anxiety and depression after switching to a new school. Lisa's earliest symptoms were noted around the age of eight. Her distress peaked at age 13 after coming out to her parents as transgender and expressing worsening dysphoria with pubertal onset. Initially, Lisa's

Activating Event	A kid at the GSA told me that "using 'they' is too confusing!" and asked me when I'm going to "finally transition."
Belief	Being non-binary isn't a real thing. I have to make up my mind about being a boy or a girl because otherwise I'll never be normal.
Consequence	I feel sad and angry that I'll never be normal. It makes me want to stay home from school and be alone so I don't have to face everyone else who does have it figured out.
Dispute	Non-binary identities are real and important. I am not confused about who I am. Others feel confused about me sometimes because they haven't learned enough about non-binary people to understand. This makes life really hard sometimes. There are people out there who do understand and lots of ways for me to connect with them to get support. Me, my family, and others can also work together to help change things at school that support a binary.

Fig. 24.1 Cognitive restructuring of internalized transphobic attitudes: Jay's example

family was hesitant to support social transition and adamantly against medical intervention. Although they allowed Lisa to express herself through feminine clothing in the home, they discouraged her from wearing these styles in public. They disclosed a strong fear that feminine expression would place Lisa at risk for bullying or other forms of stigmatization.

Although Lisa was eager to begin transitioning socially, she experienced substantial anxiety about the implications of this decision. She often found herself trying to guess what others were thinking about her and assuming they were labeling her as "that boy in the dress." Concurrently, she experienced chronic worry about whether others would refuse to date her because of her gender. She mourned that she would "never have a typical high school girl experience." Lisa's depressive symptoms also appeared to be perpetuated by fatalistic thinking patterns. For example, Lisa often made comments such as "unless I can change my DNA, I doubt I'll ever be ok." She expressed bouts of intense sadness, drew minimal pleasure from previously preferred activities, and lacked motivation to increase participation in social activities "because what's the point if I can't do them as the true me." When her parents expressed a desire to see Lisa pick up old hobbies again, Lisa endorsed an overwhelming sense of guilt for "putting my parents through all of this."

Through supportive family intervention, Lisa's parents could acknowledge the set of risks associated with preventing Lisa from affirming her identity in her desired manner. In time, the family moved positively along the continuum of acceptance. They also began to identify community allies that could help facilitate Lisa's social transition in a safe manner. By age 14, Lisa took her first steps to socially transition. Fortunately, Lisa attended a public school in a highly progressive area at that time. The school was already equipped with experience in facilitating social transitions of past students and able to support the family in navigating this process. These environmental supports helped create a context that fostered evidence against many of Lisa's thought distortions. With sensitive education for students and opportunities for allyship through student support organizations, Lisa was exposed to consistently supportive responses to her social transition. Teachers and students acknowledged her courage in becoming her authentic self and made every effort to support her. As Lisa's mental health improved through affirmation, her parents' motivation to continue strengthening their support increased in tandem. Although they remained hesitant to support medically affirming treatments, they demonstrated efforts to continue informing themselves on this process.

Lisa's situation appeared to be progressing in a very promising direction. Unfortunately, the family was soon met with significant hardship as Lisa's father lost his job. The family was forced to relocate, placing Lisa in a new school with no previous experience in supporting TGE students. Despite her parents' anticipatory efforts to educate the school on the benefits of gender-affirmative practices, her experience has felt frustrating and stigmatizing. Lisa describes her school as "putting no effort at all into supporting me." She reported often being referred to by the wrong name due to school rosters continuing to display her previously used legal name. During gym class activities, a teacher loudly implied confusion that her gender expression did not align with the information provided on the roster. Classmates who heard this exchange began discussing Lisa's identity with peers throughout the school. Soon after, a subset of students' parents expressed discomfort with Lisa using the girls' bathroom out of safety concerns for their daughters. As a result, Lisa was asked to use the gender-neutral bathroom at the nurse's office. Lisa is struggling to cope with this striking transition and experiencing an intense resurfacing of depression and anxiety.

Biopsychosocial Considerations

Lisa is a 16-year-old adolescent who is progressing through major physical pubertal changes. Depending on the trajectory of masculinization experienced, Lisa is at elevated risk for several serious implications related to body dysphoria. Moreover, if Lisa expresses as female but is taken as male by others, her risk of exposure to stigmatization, discrimination, and violence increases substantially. Coupled with her intersecting identity as a person of color, Lisa's risk of social and physical victimization is tremendously high. As a result, the family's hesitation to support medically affirming treatments is a point of significant concern, particularly in the context of a new and rejecting environment.

Lisa's history of struggling with anxiety and depression makes her more vulnerable to experiencing a significant recurrence of these symptoms. Her tendency to ruminate on self-deprecating and fatalistic thoughts places her at risk for further entrenchment in her depressive symptoms. This pattern can subsequently impact her ability to identify supports in a difficult environment. Social attitudes have also greatly impacted Lisa's ability to cope with gender dysphoria. Previously, Lisa had begun to manage her anxious thoughts and depressive symptoms with the help of a well-informed and progressive support network. This opportunity is a privilege that is sadly not afforded to many TGE youth. In contrast to responses from her previous community, Lisa may be exposed to social encounters that verify rather than challenge anxious thoughts. These may subsequently reinforce a low self-concept and increase hopelessness about the future. In these contexts, the avenue to resilience holds additional barriers that require a higher degree of self-reliance with access to internal resources.

Intervention

Lisa began seeing a new clinician who employed a trans-affirmative model of cognitive behavioral therapy. As such, the clinician acknowledged that Lisa's emotional reaction to her transition is exacerbated and maintained by persistent exposure to discriminatory practices and stigmatization. The clinician also remained attentive to attitudes about gender and sexuality that were intertwined with cultural norms in Lisa's new community. The intervention must be delivered with strong attention to the reality of how these cultural ideas create a risky context for Lisa to openly express her authentic self. Lisa's sense of emotional and physical safety is prioritized when exploring avenues to continue progress toward affirmation. The following exchange illustrates how the clinician uses a strength-based cognitive restructuring approach to help Lisa. The clinician works to reduce negative self-perception by understanding her experience through contextual factors of minority stress and taking inventory of her current supports. Finally, the clinician can enhance resilience by fostering a sense of empowerment through developing strategies to establish connections with additional supports.

Sample Exchange 1: Targeting the Impact of Minority Stress on Thoughts Related to Self, Others, and the Situation

Lisa: Deep down I always knew the world would be this way. I guess it was only a matter of time until I had to leave that progressive bubble and face the facts.

Clinician: The world is definitely harder for transgender people. It must be really painful for you to have to leave such a supportive school and suddenly have to face all of this discrimination over basic rights like using the bathroom.

Lisa: Yeah, being here just reminds me that this will always be my life. I'll never be welcomed in girl spaces. I'll never actually be like other girls.

Clinician: I can see how everyone's actions at school send this awful message to you. From everything you've shared, people seem to have pretty negative attitudes about your gender identity. Where do you think these attitudes come from?

Lisa: I don't know. Probably their parents? Maybe their church? They all just agree with each other. It makes me feel like I'm the one that's completely crazy.

Clinician: It sounds like you're saying that the way people were brought up or the communities they live in can affect the way they think and act, which is very true. When people spend their whole lives around others who are just like them, it's hard for them to know how to respond to someone who is different. They start to think that their way is the only "normal" way to be, and they make the mistake of treating others as if they were "abnormal" or wrong for being different. This is why transphobia can be so bad in small places where there isn't a lot of diversity.

Lisa: There's no diversity here! I feel so different all the time. At my old school, there were a lot of LGBTQ people and a lot of ethnicities. I was different but still normal. Here, I'm just a freak.

Clinician: We've talked about how the world can be harder for trans kids, but it also sounds like you've had two really different experiences in the world so far. Does who you are change depending on where you live?

Lisa: Well, no. I'm still the same. But I *feel* abnormal here.

Clinician: So, the way you are treated doesn't change who you are. It *can* change the way you think about yourself, which can change the way you feel.

Lisa: What's the difference?

Clinician: When someone is different than others around them, they can feel extra stressed because they are constantly treated differently or unfairly. We call this "minority stress." This experience means that you're constantly exposed to bad information about yourself, like that you are different and don't deserve the same respect as others. When we get those messages over and over again, we can start to believe them too. Do you think that's happened to you?

Lisa: Well, when they treat me like a freak all the time, I feel like it must be true.

Clinician: So, it sounds like you've started to believe the bad information. That's pretty common. It's hard to shield against it when it keeps getting thrown at you in different ways.

Lisa: Yeah, that sucks. Is it even possible to shield against it?

Clinician: Sometimes it can be helpful to catch these thoughts when you notice them. Once you catch them, you can have a plan for switching them out with the true information. What would you consider the true information?

Lisa: The information from my old town, which I guess is that I'm not a freak. I *am* a girl. I'm just also transgender, but that doesn't mean I'm not normal.

Clinician: Those are excellent facts to have. How do we keep these facts in reach for you when you're facing the bad information every day?

In this exchange, the clinician notes that Lisa is labeling herself in the same way she perceives others to be labeling her. In this way, she is unwittingly conceding to transphobic views and internalizing these messages. Psychoeducation is provided on concepts relevant to minority stress in order to make Lisa aware of this connection. The impact of discriminatory messages on her self-concept is highlighted. Lisa is encouraged to explore how cognitions about herself have been impacted by chronic exposure to adversity. The clinician supports her in questioning these messages by relying on strengths that were fostered by previously affirming environments. Strategies can then be identified to apply these strengths toward increasing access to affirming and supportive self-talk. Some strategies may include keeping a "truth journal" where Lisa challenges daily misinformation individually. The journal can be processed in therapy where the clinician can further reinforce an internal dialogue of resilience. See Fig. 24.2 to illustrate the ABCDs relevant to this exchange.

Sample Exchange 2: Establishing Cognitions that Promote Agency and Empowerment to Manage Current Adversity

Lisa: I give up! They can't understand. They make it sound like it's a good thing I can't use the girl's bathroom. Like I should be happy because I get access to a private one all to myself.

Clinician: I hear you. It must be so frustrating and hurtful to be singled out daily for something as basic as using the bathroom.

Lisa: It sucks! And no one gets it! I'm the only trans kid they've ever seen. They just want me to go away.

Clinician: I see why you feel so alone as the only identified trans kid at school. Especially since your school doesn't have any experience or information on how to support you.

Activating Event	My new school discriminates against me. They don't believe I deserve the same rights as other girls
Belief	I'm not like other girls. They treat me like a freak because I am a freak.
Consequence	I feel depressed all the time. I feel hopeless that I will ever feel normal.
Dispute	The way others treat me doesn't say anything about my truth. Being discriminated against is awful for a lot of reasons. It can make me start to think things about myself that aren't true. I need to take care of myself by stopping these unhelpful thoughts and keeping the helpful thoughts alive.

Fig. 24.2 Cognitive restructuring of internalized transphobic attitudes: Lisa's example

Lisa: I wish I could change it. I wish I could be like those kids we talked about on the news who are suing their school, but I just don't have the energy.

Clinician: I don't blame you. This is exhausting, but those examples are evidence that you are not the only person going through this right now. People are working very hard to make changes so that this type of discrimination stops.

Lisa: Not fast enough.

Clinician: That's true. In the meantime, you and a lot of others are still struggling. Sometimes the best way to deal with that struggle is to connect with others going through similar experiences so that you remember you aren't alone. I can give you some safe online resources where you can meet other trans kids going through similar issues.

Lisa: I guess it'd be nice to hear from someone else that is actually dealing with this. I can't be the only one in this freaking state.

Clinician: Definitely not, and there are some things we can learn from how others have handled this situation. For example, one step would be to have a meeting with your school to establish a gender support plan. We can work together to make an exact plan for how you can remove yourself from a tough situation and find support from someone you trust at school. We can make this part of your 504 plan, to be sure that everyone is instructed to follow it.

Lisa: That could be better than what I have now at least.

Clinician: Who are the people in your life we can ask to help us with this plan?

Lisa: Well, my parents will definitely want to help. The art teacher in my school is the only person that seems to listen to me there. Maybe she can help?

Clinician: Great. We'll make sure everyone is at this meeting. I can also come and share information with the school from organizations that specialize in creating gender support plans.

Lisa: I guess the more people the better. It basically feels like me against the world.

In this exchange, the clinician responds affirmatively by acknowledging Lisa's pain in the face of unfair discrimination. The clinician *avoids* attempting to positively reframe this experience by focusing on "the bright side" such as highlighting advantages to using a single occupancy restroom in the nurse's office. While well intentioned, a "bright side" approach would invalidate Lisa's experience of being stigmatized. The clinician must acknowledge that systems that exclude or police the use of public restrooms by TGE youth send a strong message of social rejection to that child. Lisa's description of this experience illustrates first-hand the impact of chronic systemic ostracization on a child's self-view.

Lisa also alludes to previously provided examples of other students undergoing similar hardships. Clinicians can educate patients and families on several initiatives for social justice powered by communities advocating to change faulty systems (Davis et al. 2009; Craig 2013). Highlighting these struggles is not meant to offer a specific solution for Lisa, whose trans identity should not automatically require her to become a vocal advocate for social justice. However, she may benefit from acknowledging membership within a community committed to fighting on her behalf. Progress made by such communities in recent decades can be reviewed as well, fostering hopefulness for a generally upward trajectory of social progress. Membership in a trans-affirming community can also help Lisa challenge her assertions that she will never be seen for who she is or will always feel out of place among others.

The clinician should be diligent in providing Lisa with local resources that can connect her with supportive networks and social opportunities within trans-affirming settings. The clinician also works to help Lisa learn of additional supports at her disposal. This includes providing psychoeducation about an option for creating a gender support plan and organizational information that is available to continue educating Lisa's school ("Gender Spectrum Education" 2017). Guidance is also provided for Lisa to take inventory of the supports that she is already aware of; these include any allies that may be staffed in her

Activating Event	I am emotionally and physically unsafe at my school.
Belief	I am alone in this fight and powerless to stop it.
Consequence	I feel isolated and want to give up on trying to make this better.
Dispute	Even if I'm the only trans kid facing this at my school right now, I am not the only one who has ever gone through this. Kids in other schools are dealing with this too and there are organizations working to help their schools make positive changes. I have a team of people supporting me who can help me make a plan to keep me safe and make me more comfortable at school.

Fig. 24.3 Cognitive restructuring to promote a sense of community

school as well as acknowledging her increasingly supportive family. By offering their own advocacy with the school, the clinician provides additional support by challenging Lisa's view that she is alone in this hardship. This approach empowers Lisa to rely on an existing network of supports so that she does not have to face adversity in isolation. See Fig. 24.3 to illustrate the ABCDs relevant to this exchange.

Sample Exchange 3: Targeting Predictions about the Future to Promote Hopefulness and Agency to Manage Anticipated Adversity

Lisa: I'm exhausted. How am I going to keep up this fight for my whole life?

Clinician: You have good reason to feel exhausted and good reason to think that things will always be harder for you in some ways. But let's consider some things that might make these challenges easier to manage. Do you think your last school was always as accepting as it is now? Even 20 or 30 or 40 years ago?

Lisa: Well, no. I'm pretty sure things were much harder for everyone back then.

Clinician: It seems like a lot of communities and schools have made some progress, though some more than others. I wonder what your current school will be like in 10 years.

Lisa: I guess a little better at least. But I'll be out of this school by then.

Clinician: True. Things might be better for other trans students in the future, even though that doesn't benefit you now. So, where will you be in the future?

Lisa: Hopefully somewhere like my old town. Hopefully I get into a college like that school.

Clinician: That would make some of these challenges easier to manage because you would be in a supportive community again. How can we use the time we have now to make sure that the next time you move somewhere feels better than this?

Lisa: I should definitely research schools and make sure I make a good choice for myself.

Clinician: What kinds of things could you plan for?

Lisa: Well, there have to be LGBTQ student groups so I can hopefully meet other trans people. I should also find out about how they place trans students in dorm rooms. And also look into what the cities are like.

Clinician: I wonder if we could find current trans students who might be able to help you get more information from schools and give us tips on making a plan?

Lisa: I bet I could look at school websites and find an email.

Activating Event	Simple things like using the bathroom and staying safe require incredible effort and energy.
Belief	Things will be like this forever. I may not have the energy to keep this up for the rest of my life.
Consequence	I feel exhausted and wonder how I will ever get through life. The future feels bleak and I get very depressed.
Dispute	Things may never be as easy for me as they are for cisgender people, but that doesn't mean they will always be this hard. The world is slowly getting better and the tough stuff I deal with today may be easier in the future. My community can also make a big difference. Whenever possible, I can focus on finding ways to keep myself in spaces where these changes are more obvious and things feel easier.

Fig. 24.4 Cognitive restructuring to promote hopefulness and agency to manage adversity

In this exchange, the clinician explores how Lisa's current assessment of her situation affects her predictions about the hardships she may experience in the future. Lisa's belief that being transgender will expose her to greater challenges is reasonable. However, the intensity of these challenges will depend on Lisa's environments and ongoing social progress. Guiding Lisa through thought exercises that have her consider evidence for ongoing social change can promote hopefulness for the future. Lisa can be empowered to begin making her own changes in the present by exploring options where she has agency over changing her environment. See Fig. 24.4 to illustrate the ABCDs relevant to this exchange.

Conclusion

Examples of TGE voices as well as culturally diverse frameworks of gender are ubiquitous throughout history. However, only in recent decades have we begun to better understand the intersection of identity development and mental health in youth. Although research on this population is in its nascent stages, awareness of the unique considerations for TGE children and their families is growing exponentially. Findings consistently support the use of gender-affirmative intervention models to reduce negative mental health outcomes and enhance resilience. Chronic exposure to adversity can create a context for youth to develop negative thinking patterns that internalize transphobic stigmas and maintain symptoms of depression and anxiety. Behavioral family interventions aim to increase acceptance and affirmation in a manner that enhances supportive environments to foster improved self-concept, sense of safety, and resilience. Trans-affirmative CBT can also be implemented to restructure negative thinking patterns by contextualizing distorted thinking within a framework of minority stress. By providing education, affirmation, and connections to community support, providers can help TGE youth create the opportunities to live within their authentic identities and the space to thrive in this process.

Acknowledgement The authors would like to extend a special thanks to Diane Ehrensaft, PhD, for her review and consultation on this chapter. Dr. Ehrensaft's dedication to transgender and gender expansive youth has been invaluable to the progress of this field. Her longstanding support and advocacy for gender-affirmative care have been foundational to our current understanding of best practices and essential to the concepts covered in this chapter.

References

Allan, R., & Ungar, M. (2014). Resilience-building interventions with children, adolescents, and their families. In S. Prince-Embury & D. H. Saklofske (Eds.), *Resilience interventions for youth in diverse populations* (pp. 447–462). New York: Springer.

American Medical Association (2017). Policy H-160.991: Health care needs of lesbian, gay, bisexual, and transgender populations. Retrieved August 12, 2018, from https://policysearch.ama-assn.org/policyfinder/detail/transgender?uri=%2FAMADoc%2FHOD.xml-0-805.xml.

American Psychiatric Association. (1980). *Diagnostic and statistical manual of mental disorders* (3rd ed.). Washington, DC: American Psychiatric Association.

American Psychiatric Association. (1987). *Diagnostic and statistical manual of mental disorders* (3rd ed., rev. ed.). Washington, DC: American Psychiatric Association.

American Psychiatric Association. (2013). *Diagnostic and statistical manual of mental disorders* (5th ed.). Arlington, VA: American Psychiatric Association.

American Psychological Association. (2015). Guidelines for psychological practice with transgender and gender nonconforming people. *American Psychologist, 70*(9), 832–864.

Anton, B. S. (2009). Proceedings of the American Psychological Association for the legislative year 2008: Minutes of the Annual Meeting of the Council of Representatives, February 22–24, 2008, Washington, DC, and August 13 and 17, 2008, Boston, MA, and minutes of the February, June, August, and December 2008 meetings of the Board of Directors. *American Psychologist, 64*, 372–453. https://doi.org/10.1037/a0015932.

Association for Behavioral and Cognitive Therapies. (2018). Fact sheets: Transgender and gender nonconforming youth. Resource document. Association for Behavioral and Cognitive Therapies. Retrieved August 20, 2018, from http://www.abct.org/Information/?m=mInformation&fa=fs_TRANSGENDER.

Austin, A., & Craig, S. L. (2015). Transgender affirmative cognitive behavioral therapy: Clinical considerations and applications. *Professional Psychology: Research and Practice, 46*(1), 21.

Austin, A., Craig, S. L., & Alessi, E. J. (2017). Affirmative cognitive behavior therapy with transgender and gender nonconforming adults. *Psychiatric Clinics, 40*(1), 141–156.

Austin, A., Craig, S. L., & D'Souza, S. A. (2018). An AFFIRMative cognitive behavioral intervention for transgender youth: Preliminary effectiveness. *Professional Psychology: Research and Practice, 49*(1), 1.

Balsam, K. F., Martell, C. R., & Safren, S. A. (2006). Affirmative cognitive-behavioral therapy with lesbian, gay, and bisexual people. In P. A. Hays & G. Y. Iwamasa (Eds.), *Culturally responsive cognitive behavioral therapy: Assessment, practice, and supervision* (pp. 223–243). Washington, DC: American Psychological Association.

Becerra-Culqui, T. A., Liu, Y., Nash, R., Cromwell, L., Flanders, W. D., Getahun, D., et al. (2018). Mental health of transgender and gender nonconforming youth compared with their peers. *Pediatrics, 141*. https://doi.org/10.1542/peds.2017-3845.

Bockting, W. O., Miner, M. H., Swinburne Romine, R. E., Hamilton, A., & Coleman, E. (2013). Stigma, mental health, and resilience in an online sample of the US transgender population. *American Journal of Public Health, 103*, 943–951. https://doi.org/10.2105/AJPH.2013.301241.

Busa, S., Janssen, A., & Lakshman, M. (2018a). A review of evidence-based treatments for transgender youth diagnosed with social anxiety disorder. *Transgender Health, 3*, 27–33. https://doi.org/10.1089/trgh.2017.0037.

Busa, S. M., Leibowitz, S., & Janssen, A. (2018b). Transgender adolescents and the gender-affirming interventions: Pubertal suppression, hormones, surgery, and other pharmacological interventions. In A. Janssen & S. Leibowitz (Eds.), *Affirmative mental health care for transgender and gender diverse youth* (pp. 49–62). Cham: Springer.

CenterLink, Inc. (2018). CenterLink. The Community of LGBT Centers. Retrieved November 4, 2018, from https://www.lgbtcenters.org/LGBTCenters.

Cohen-Kettenis, P. T., & Pfäfflin, F. (2010). The DSM diagnostic criteria for gender identity disorder in adolescents and adults. *Archives of Sexual Behavior, 39*, 499–513. https://doi.org/10.1007/s10508-009-9562-y.

Colizzi, M., Costa, R., & Todarello, O. (2014). Transsexual patients' psychiatric comorbidity and positive effect of cross-sex hormonal treatment on mental health: Results from a longitudinal study. *Psychoneuroendocrinology, 39*, 65–73. https://doi.org/10.1016/j.psyneuen.2013.09.029.

Collazo, A., Austin, A., & Craig, S. L. (2013). Facilitating transition among transgender clients: Components of effective clinical practice. *Clinical Social Work Journal, 41*, 228–237. https://doi.org/10.1007/s10615-013-0436-3.

Connolly, M. D., Zervos, M. J., Barone, C. J., II, Johnson, C. C., & Joseph, C. L. (2016). The mental health of transgender youth: Advances in understanding. *Journal of Adolescent Health, 59*, 489–495. https://doi.org/10.1016/j.jadohealth.2016.06.012.

Coolhart, D., Ritenour, K., & Grodzinski, A. (2018). Experiences of ambiguous loss for parents of transgender male youth: A phenomenological exploration. *Contemporary Family Therapy, 40*, 28–41. https://doi.org/10.1007/s10591-017-9426-x.

Craig, S. L. (2013). Affirmative supportive safe and empowering talk (ASSET): Leveraging the strengths and resiliencies of sexual minority youth in school-based groups. *Journal of LGBT Issues in Counseling, 7*, 372–386. https://doi.org/10.1080/15538605.2013.839342.

Craig, S. L., & Austin, A. (2016). The AFFIRM open pilot feasibility study: A brief affirmative cognitive behavioral coping skills group intervention for sexual and gender minority youth. *Children and Youth Services Review, 64*, 136–144.

D'Augelli, A. R., Grossman, A. H., & Starks, M. T. (2006). Childhood gender atypicality, victimization, and PTSD among lesbian, gay, and bisexual youth. *Journal of Interpersonal Violence, 21*, 1462–1482. https://doi.org/10.1177/0886260506293482.

Davis, T. S., Saltzburg, S., & Locke, C. R. (2009). Supporting the emotional and psychological well being of sexual minority youth: Youth ideas for action. *Children and Youth Services Review, 31*, 1030–1041. https://doi.org/10.1016/j.childyouth.2009.05.003.

De Vries, A. L., McGuire, J. K., Steensma, T. D., Wagenaar, E. C., Doreleijers, T. A., & Cohen-Kettenis, P. T. (2014). Young adult psychological outcome after puberty suppression and gender reassignment. *Pediatrics, 134*, 696–704. https://doi.org/10.1542/peds.2013-2958.

Drescher, J. (2010). Queer diagnoses: Parallels and contrasts in the history of homosexuality, gender variance, and the diagnostic and statistical manual. *Archives of Sexual Behavior, 39*, 427–460. https://doi.org/10.1007/s10508-009-9531-5.

Drescher, J., & Haller, E. (2012). *Position statement on access to care for transgender and gender variant individuals*. Washington, DC: American Psychiatric Association.

Drescher, J., Cohen-Kettenis, P. T., & Reed, G. M. (2016). Gender incongruence of childhood in the ICD-11: Controversies, proposal, and rationale. *The Lancet Psychiatry, 3*, 297–304. https://doi.org/10.1016/S2215-0366(15)00586-6.

Durso, L. E., & Gates, G. J. (2012). *Serving our youth: Findings from a national survey of service providers working with lesbian, gay, bisexual, and transgender youth who are homeless or at risk of becoming homeless*. Los Angeles: The Williams Institute, True Colors Fund & The Palette Fund.

Ellis, A. J. (1991). The revised ABC's of rational-emotive therapy (RET). *Rational-Emotive and Cognitive-Behavioral Therapy, 9*, 139–172.

Garofalo, R., Deleon, J., Osmer, E., Doll, M., & Harper, G. W. (2006). Overlooked, misunderstood and at risk: Exploring the lives and HIV risk of ethnic minority male-to-female transgender youth. *Journal of Adolescent Health, 38*, 230–236. https://doi.org/10.1016/j.jadohealth.2005.03.023.

Gender Spectrum. (2017). Gender spectrum. Education. Retrieved November 4, 2018, from https://www.genderspectrum.org/resources/education-2/.

Grossman, A. H., & D'Augelli, A. R. (2007). Transgender youth and life-threatening behaviors. *Suicide and Life-threatening Behavior, 37*, 527–537. https://doi.org/10.1521/suli.2007.37.5.527.

Hill, D. B., Menvielle, E., Sica, K. M., & Johnson, A. (2010). An affirmative intervention for families with gender variant children: Parental ratings of child mental health and gender. *Journal of Sex & Marital Therapy, 36*, 6–23. https://doi.org/10.1080/00926230903375560.

Keuroghlian, A. S., Shtasel, D., & Bassuk, E. L. (2014). Out on the street: A public health and policy agenda for lesbian, gay, bisexual, and transgender youth who are homeless. *American Journal of Orthopsychiatry, 84*, 66. (2014). https://doi.org/10.1037/h0098852.

Keo-Meier, C., & Ehrensaft, D. (2018). Introduction to the gender affirmative model. In C. Keo-Meier & D. Ehrensaft (Eds.), *The gender affirmative model: An interdisciplinary approach to supporting transgender and gender expansive children* (pp. 3–19). Washington, DC: American Psychological Association.

Kosciw, J. G., Greytak, E. A., Bartkiewicz, M. J., Boesen, M. J., & Palmer, N. A. (2012). *The 2011 National School Climate Survey: The experiences of lesbian, gay, bisexual and transgender youth in our Nation's schools*. New York: Gay, Lesbian and Straight Education Network (GLSEN).

Ludwig, C. (2016). Conversion therapy, its detrimental consequences, and its place in the national spotlight. *Rutgers Journal of Law and Religion, 18*, 121.

Malpas, J. (2011). Between pink and blue: A multidimensional family approach to gender nonconforming children and their families. *Family Process, 50*(4), 453–470.

Malpas, J. (2018). *Family therapy*. Presentation at the Annual Meeting of the World Professional Association for Transgender Health, Buenos Aires, Argentina.

Malpas, J., Glaeser, E., & Giamettei, S. (2018). Building resilience in transgender and gender expansive children, families, and communities: A multidimensional family approach. In C. Keo-Meier & D. Ehrensaft (Eds.), *The gender affirmative model: An interdisciplinary approach to supporting transgender and gender expansive children* (pp. 141–156). Washington, DC: American Psychological Association.

Meyer, I. H. (2003). Prejudice, social stress, and mental health in lesbian, gay, and bisexual populations: Conceptual issues and research evidence. *Psychological Bulletin, 129*, 674–697. https://doi.org/10.1037/0033-2909.129.5.674.

Meyer-Bahlburg, H. F. (2010). From mental disorder to iatrogenic hypogonadism: Dilemmas in conceptualizing gender identity variants as psychiatric conditions. *Archives of Sexual Behavior, 39*, 461–476. https://doi.org/10.1007/s10508-009-9532-4.

Mizock, L., & Mueser, K. T. (2014). Employment, mental health, internalized stigma, and coping with transphobia among transgender individuals. *Psychology of Sexual Orientation and Gender Diversity, 1*(2), 146.

Murchison, G., Adkins, D., Conard, L.A., Ehrensaft, D., Elliott, T., Hawkins, L.A., et al. (2016). Supporting and caring for transgender children. Resource document. Human Rights Campaign. Retrieved August 30, 2018, from https://assets2.hrc.org/files/documents/SupportingCaringforTransChildren.pdf?_ga=2.166331386.558525591.1532827416-214163977.1531751536.

Olson, K. R., Durwood, L., DeMeules, M., McLaughlin, K. A. (2016). Mental health of transgender children who are supported in their identities. *Pediatrics, 137*(3), https://doi.org/10.1542/peds.2015-3223.

Pachankis, J. E. (2014). Uncovering clinical principles and techniques to address minority stress, mental health, and related health risks among gay and bisexual men. *Clinical Psychology: Science and Practice, 21*, 313–330. https://doi.org/10.1111/cpsp.12078.

Quintana, N. S., Rosenthal, J., & Krehely, J. (2010). *On the streets: The federal response to gay and transgender homeless youth*. Washington, DC: Center for American Progress.

Reed, G. M., Drescher, J., Krueger, R. B., Atalla, E., Cochran, S. D., First, M. B., et al. (2016). Disorders related to sexuality and gender identity in the ICD-11: Revising the ICD-10 classification based on current scientific evidence, best clinical practices, and human rights considerations. *World Psychiatry, 15*, 205–221. https://doi.org/10.1002/wps.20354.

Reisner, S. L., Vetters, R., Leclerc, M., Zaslow, S., Wolfrum, S., Shumer, D., et al. (2015). Mental health of transgender youth in care at an adolescent urban community center: A matched retrospective cohort study. *Journal of Adolescent Health, 56*, 274–279. https://doi.org/10.1016/j.jadohealth.2014.10.264.

Roberts, A. L., Rosario, M., Corliss, H. L., Koenen, K. C., & Bryn Austin, S. (2012). Childhood gender nonconformity: A risk indicator for childhood abuse and posttraumatic stress in youth. *Pediatrics, 129*, 410–417. https://doi.org/10.1542/peds.2011-1804.

Ryan, C. (2009). *Supportive families, healthy children: Helping families with lesbian, gay, bisexual & transgender children*. San Francisco, CA: Family Acceptance Project, San Francisco State University.

Ryan, C. (2014). Generating a revolution in prevention, wellness, and care for LGBT children and youth. *Temple Political & Civil Rights Law Review, 23*(2), 331–344.

Ryan, C., & Chen-Hayes, S. (2013). Educating and empowering families of LGBTQ K-12 students. In E. S. Fisher & K. Komosa-Hawkins (Eds.), *Creating school environments to support lesbian, gay, bisexual, transgender, and questioning students and families: A handbook for school professionals* (pp. 209–227). New York, NY: Routledge.

Ryan, C., & Diaz, R. (2011). *Family acceptance project: Intervention guidelines and strategies*. San Francisco: Family Acceptance Project.

Ryan, C., Russell, S. T., Huebner, D., Diaz, R., & Sanchez, J. (2010). Family acceptance in adolescence and the health of LGBT young adults. *Journal of Child and Adolescent Psychiatric Nursing, 23*, 205–213. https://doi.org/10.1111/j.1744-6171.2010.00246.x.

Sburlati, E. S., Lyneham, H. J., Schniering, C. A., & Rapee, R. M. (2014). *Evidence-based CBT for anxiety and depression in children and adolescents: A competencies based approach*. West Sussex, UK: John Wiley & Sons, Ltd..

Skidmore, W. C., Linsenmeier, J. A. W., & Bailey, J. M. (2006). Gender nonconformity and psychological distress in lesbians and gay men. *Archives of Sexual Behavior, 35*, 685–697. https://doi.org/10.1007/s10508-006-9108-5.

Smith, Y. L., Van Goozen, S. H., & Cohen-Kettenis, P. T. (2001). Adolescents with gender identity disorder who were accepted or rejected for sex reassignment surgery: A prospective follow-up study. *Journal of the American Academy of Child & Adolescent Psychiatry, 40*, 472–481. https://doi.org/10.1097/00004583-200104000-00017.

Substance Abuse and Mental Health Services Administration. (2014). *A practitioner's resource guide: Helping families to support their LGBT children*. HHS publication no. PEP14-LGBTKIDS. Substance Abuse and Mental Health Services Administration: Rockville, MD.

Testa, R. J., Sciacca, L. M., Wang, F., Hendricks, M. L., Goldblum, P., Bradford, J., et al. (2012). Effects of violence on transgender people. *Professional Psychology: Research and Practice, 43*, 452–459. https://doi.org/10.1037/a0029604.

Testa, R. J., Jimenez, C. L., & Rankin, S. (2014). Risk and resilience during transgender identity development: The effects of awareness and engagement with other transgender people on affect. *Journal of Gay & Lesbian Mental Health, 18*, 31–46. https://doi.org/10.1080/19359705.2013.805177.

Testa, R. J., Michaels, M. S., Bliss, W., Rogers, M. L., Balsam, K. F., & Joiner, T. (2017). Suicidal ideation in transgender people: Gender minority stress and interpersonal theory factors. *Journal of Abnormal Psychology, 126*, 125–136. https://doi.org/10.1037/abn0000234.

The World Professional Association for Transgender Health, Inc. (2011). Standards of care for the health of transsexual, transgender, and gender nonconforming people, seventh version. Resource document. The World Professional Association for Transgender Health. Retrieved July 30, 2018, from https://www.wpath.org/media/cms/Documents/SOC%20v7/SOC%20V7_English.pdf.

Toomey, R. B., Ryan, C., Díaz, R. M., Card, N. A., & Russell, S. T. (2010). Gender-nonconforming lesbian, gay, bisexual, and transgender youth: School victimization and young adult psychosocial adjustment. *Developmental Psychology, 46*, 1580–1589. https://doi.org/10.1037/a0020705.

Travers, R., Bauer, G., Pyne, J., Bradley, K., Gale, L., Papadimitriou, M. (2012). Impacts of strong parental support for trans youth: A report prepared for Children's Aid Society of Toronto and Delisle Youth Services. Resource document. Trans Pulse Project. Retrieved August 12, 2018, from http://transpulseproject.ca/wp-content/uploads/2012/10/Impacts-ofStrong-Parental-Support-for-Trans-Youth-vFINAL.pdf.

Valentine, S. E., & Shipherd, J. C. (2018). A systematic review of social stress and mental health among transgender and gender non-conforming people in the United States. *Clinical Psychology Review, 66*, 24–38. https://doi.org/10.1016/j.cpr.2018.03.003.

Vasey, P. L., & Bartlett, N. H. (2007). What can the Samoan "fa'afafine" teach us about the Western concept of gender identity disorder in childhood? *Perspectives in Biology and Medicine, 50*, 481–490. https://doi.org/10.1353/pbm.2007.0056.

Williams, S. L., & Mann, A. K. (2017). Sexual and gender minority health disparities as a social issue: How stigma and intergroup relations can explain and reduce health disparities. *Journal of Social Issues, 73*, 450–461. https://doi.org/10.1111/josi.12225.

Winters, K. (2006). Gender dissonance: Diagnostic reform of gender identity disorder for adults. *Journal of Psychology & Human Sexuality, 17*, 71–89. https://doi.org/10.1300/J056v17n03_04.

Noncompliance and Nonadherence

25

Kathleen L. Lemanek and Heather Yardley

Medical Noncompliance and Nonadherence

Medical noncompliance and nonadherence have been identified as a healthcare challenge for decades. Nonadherence varies across and within medical conditions and individuals, with negative consequences to patients, families, and society, including inadequate disease management or treatment outcome, increased morbidity and mortality, and escalating healthcare costs (DiMatteo 2004b; Rapoff 2010). This chapter will review the literature on pediatric medical nonadherence in terms of defining adherence, providing prevalence estimates, describing factors affecting adherence and models of adherence, and outlining assessment measures and intervention strategies. A case example will be presented that highlights these issues, especially assessment and intervention strategies based on conceptualization of relevant factors. The chapter will conclude with recommendations for clinical practice and research to promote adherence.

Case Introduction

We will use the case of Mark to demonstrate principles discussed throughout the chapter. Mark[1] (a pseudonym) was an 18-year-old male with a 3-year history of type 1 diabetes (T1D). He was currently in high school, involved in sports, and reportedly had several friends. Although Mark was referred to psychology primarily for nonadherence, school attendance was also of concern. Avoidance of tasks related to diabetes management had increased over the 2 months before the referral. Mark reported being concerned about his diabetes management because he was worried about having long-term consequences, going low at school and not being able to get help, impact on his future career, and early death. Mark was avoiding his diabetes-related tasks because he did not want to see evidence of his blood sugar on his meter. He was also avoiding school because of his concerns of going low and limited motivation because of his perception that he could not achieve his career goals.

K. L. Lemanek (✉)
The Ohio State University, Nationwide Children's Hospital, Columbus, OH, USA
e-mail: Kathleen.lemanek@nationwidechildrens.org

H. Yardley
Department of Pediatric Psychology and Neuropsychology, The Ohio State University and Nationwide Children's Hospital, Columbus, OH, USA

[1] Case has been deidentified and is shared with permission.

Definition of Compliance/Adherence

One of the original definitions of medical compliance was proposed by Haynes (1979), "the extent to which a person's behavior (in terms of medications, following diets, or executing lifestyle changes) coincides with medical or health advice" (pp. 1–2). This definition emphasizes patients following the instructions and recommendations of medical providers, with minimal input or questions from the patients and families. Adherence replaced the term compliance as models of health care focused on disease management and shared decision-making (Bauman 2000). Murphy and Coster (1997) provided the following definition of adherence: "the willingness and ability of a person to follow health instructions, to take medications as prescribed, to attend scheduled clinic appointments, and to complete recommended investigations" (p. 797). This definition supports the partnership between patients and medical providers, with reciprocal and regular interactions. Modi et al. (2012) recently detailed a model of self-management and differentiated it from adherence. In this model, self-management is a broader construct that includes both behaviors and processes patients and families follow to manage a medical condition. However, the constructs are related in that poor self-management can result in nonadherence and, subsequently, inadequate clinical outcomes (Modi et al. 2012).

Prevalence of Nonadherence

Adherence to medical recommendations and regimens is far below 100% (e.g., 75%, Hommel et al. 2009; less than 50%, Rapoff 2010) and can lead to serious direct (i.e., hospitalizations; Benjamin 2012) and indirect (i.e., incorrect prescribing of medication; Lemanek et al. 2001) consequences including excessive healthcare utilization (Quittner et al. 2002) or death.

Researchers have begun to look at adherence to many aspects of medical regimens including medication management, exercise, monitoring of biological markers, and nutrition. Two types of nonadherence are routinely discussed in the literature, unintentional nonadherence (e.g., carelessness/forgetfulness; Gadkari and McHorney 2012) and intentional nonadherence in which an individual chooses not to follow recommendations. In addition, nonadherence can be classified as chronic (consistently not following recommendations) and acute (periodic nonadherence). Cost-related nonadherence includes delaying refills or changing doses in order to reduce health-related costs (Gibson et al. 2005). Interventions may vary based on the type and classification of nonadherence.

Factors Related to Adherence

Numerous factors have been associated with adherence or nonadherence, but fewer predictive factors have been identified partly due to the complexity of the relationships among factors. In general, studies support an association between greater number of risk factors and poorer adherence (Logan et al. 2003). These factors have been grouped into one of four board categories: (1) patient/family factors, (2) disease factors, (3) regimen factors, and (4) healthcare system-related factors (Goh et al. 2017; Rapoff 2010).

Patient factors center on demographic variables, knowledge and psychological functioning. Adolescents, patients with deficits in executive functioning skills, and patients/families from minority or lower socioeconomic status have lower rates of adherence than other groups (e.g., Killian et al. 2018; McQuaid et al. 2012; Perez et al. 2017). Patients' and parents' knowledge of the disease and regimen components have been consistently related to adherence (e.g., Carbone et al. 2013). Rapoff (2010) has distinguished between patients and parents "knowing that" (having knowledge) and "knowing how" (having specific skills to implement the regimen). La Greca and Bearman (2003) extended this conceptualization of "knowing" to include decision-making about completing regimen components in daily situations. Decision-making may be related to executive functioning skills in which forgetting/poor planning is the number one reason for nonadherence (e.g., Mehta et al. 2017). Adherence is worse in patients with comorbid emotional and behavioral problems, such as anxiety and depression (e.g., Gray et al. 2012) and conduct problems and hyperactivity (e.g., Malee et al. 2011).

Parent distress, family conflict and disorganization, level of parent support/monitoring, and poor communication within families and with medical providers are associated with poor adherence (e.g., DiMatteo 2004a; Killian et al. 2018; Landers et al. 2016). The differential impact of these factors within families of diverse cultural and ethnic backgrounds has been explored minimally. Greater adherence has been found in families who recently immigrated to the United States (Hsin et al. 2010) and in patients younger than 10 years old and of non-Caucasian ethnicity, who are following a gluten-free diet for celiac disease (Mager et al. 2018).

The second category of factors focuses on aspects of the medical condition. Adherence declines over time, especially with earlier age of onset (e.g., Hilliard et al. 2013). Patients who are not experiencing symptoms or perceive symptoms as occurring less often or severe show poorer adherence (e.g., Adams et al. 2004). Finally, patient and family health beliefs about the severity and susceptibility of the disease and benefits of the regimen are correlated with adherence, while barriers to care hinder adherence (e.g., Riekert and Drotar 2002).

The third category is factors related to the medical regimen. Poor adherence is associated with multicomponent regimens (e.g., Chandwani et al. 2010) and regimens that disrupt schedules and activities (e.g., Modi and Quittner 2006) or include frequent and/or aversive hospital-based procedures (Goh et al. 2017). Finally, physical and cosmetic side effects and ingestion issues (e.g., taste of medication) are associated with poor adherence (e.g., Simons et al. 2010).

Health system-related factors pertain to perceptions of patients/families' communication with medical providers and hospital experiences, with positive communication about the medical condition and its treatment (e.g., DiMatteo 2004a) and perception of support (e.g., Cohen and Wamboldt 2000) associated with adherence. Medical providers' compliance with clinical guidelines may influence medical outcomes for patients, which may then indirectly affect patient adherence (Drotar 2009). Barriers to providers' compliance involve lack of knowledge or awareness of current treatments and flexibility or accuracy in implementing guidelines (Cabana et al. 2001). Insufficient health insurance, availability of medications, and financial problems are other system-level factors related to nonadherence (Goh et al. 2017).

Theoretical Models Related to Adherence

There are many models of adherence, each focusing on a slightly different aspect of adherence behaviors. Three of the most prominent are presented here. The health belief model (HBM) proposes that perceived susceptibility (risk of having/contracting an illness), severity of the illness/treatment, benefits to engaging in health behaviors, barriers (perceived or actual) to care, and cues (internal or external) to action work in concert to influence adherence to a medical regimen or recommendation. HBM accounts for a large portion of the variance in adherence behaviors (Jones et al. 2014).

Second, the theory of planned behavior (TPB; Ajzen 1991) extends the theory of reasoned action by adding that behaviors can be planned, thus adding perceived behavioral control to the model. Reasoned action theory suggests that how we evaluate a behavior (attitude), the subjective norm, and motivation work together to change the likelihood that a behavior is completed. The addition of perceived behavioral control allows for evaluation of self-efficacy to complete a task and may be related to adherence (Downs and Hausenblas 2005).

Finally, the transtheoretical model (Prochaska and DiClemente 1983) proposes stages of change. They are pre-contemplation (no intent to take action), contemplation (evaluating pros and cons of changing behavior), preparation (preparing to take action in the immediate future), action (taking specific actions to change behavior), and maintenance (sustained changes and relapse prevention). Each is a separate step in behavior change that involves internal and external motivation, behavior, and self-efficacy. Identifying where a person is in terms of their stage in the change process can influence interventions to improve adherence (Guite et al. 2014).

Adherence Measures

Adherence measure can be classified along a continuum of directness to indirectness (Rapoff 2010) or objective to subjective (Duncan et al. 2014). Each measure has distinct advantages and disadvantages that affect clinical and research reliability, validity, and utility. In general, objective measures are more reliable and valid than subjective measures, and are more easily administered by medical providers and mental health professionals (DiMatteo 2004b). Objective measures also provide lower rates of adherence than subjective measures. Subjective measures can be given by professionals and other individuals who have experience with them, such as school personnel and parents. Treatment outcomes, such as clinical symptoms and quality of life, have been assessed along with adherence, but are not measures of adherence per se. The following section summarizes literature reviews on adherence measures by Duncan et al. (2014), Quittner et al. (2008), and Rapoff (2010).

Bioassays directly measure drug levels (e.g., opiates, growth hormone), metabolic products of drugs (e.g., THC-COOH, amphetamine), or clinical marker (e.g., A1C, viral loads) in bodily fluids, such as blood, urine, and saliva. Therapeutic drug monitoring is used clinically to measure drugs at specific time points to individualize therapy, avoid toxicity, detect drug interactions, and monitor adherence (Kang and Lee 2009). The rate of absorption depends on the dose administered and the route of administration, such as orally through the mouth or injected into the skin. Data from assays are quantifiable, which may foster optimal clinical outcomes. However, they are not available for all medications, are costly, and are less reliable due to pharmacokinetic variations based on drug metabolism factors and individuals' absorption rates.

Automated measures refer to electronic monitoring of regimen components where information of data are recorded and stored by date and time ("timestamping"). Such regimen components may include tablet or liquid medication removed from standard vials, pills taken from blister packages, actuation of metered dose inhalers, blood glucose test results, and performance of chest physiotherapy. Electronic monitors, such as the medication event monitoring system (MEMS) bottle caps and the metered dose inhaler (MDI), are often considered the "gold standard" when assessing adherence because these devices provide continuous and dosing-specific data at the time of administration, thus allowing for patterns of adherence to be determined. Technically sophisticated providers, patients, and families may be drawn to these automated systems, but they often experience mechanical failures, are costly, and do not measure actual consumption of medications or completion of other adherent behaviors (Hommel et al. 2017). The cost may be equalized by a reduction in unnecessary healthcare services, such as hospitalizations, laboratory tests, and medication changes (Urquhart 1997).

Pharmacy refill data, pill counts, and canister weights (e.g., inhaled medications) are objective measures of adherence, with refill data also being more direct. Refill records can be used to arrive at a medication possession ratio (MPR) to determine the percentage of time a patient has medication available. This ratio is calculated by dividing the sum of days of a medication for all refills during a specific period of time by the number of days during that time. Pharmacy refill data are inexpensive, if fees are not charged by pharmacies, and seem to be accurate in terms of prescriptions being filled. However, obtaining such data can be difficult, if several pharmacies are used, or not possible, if medications are filled through automatic medication programs. Although pill counts and canister weights are also inexpensive and easy to collect, actual consumption of medication is not measured.

Subjective reports from patients and parents are the most common methods to assess adherence and include structured interviews, questionnaires, and diaries or self-monitoring of regimen components. Many questionnaires and interviews are disease specific, such as for epilepsy (e.g., Pediatric Epilepsy Medication Self-Management Questionnaire; Gutierrez-Colina et al. 2018) and asthma (e.g., Family Asthma Management System Scale; McQuaid et al. 2005). Diary data on adherence can be obtained from written logs, hand-held computers (PDAs), or phone interviews. The 24-h Recall is a well-known phone-based diary of daily activities and adherence that completed at least three times (two weekdays and one weekend) (Johnson et al. 1992). Unstructured interviews can be administered during clinic visit, but questions should focus on discrete behaviors and within a brief time frame (e.g., day or week before visit). Likert-type rating scales, if added to the interview, should be more specific than a simple 0 (*not adherent*)–10 (*very adherent*) scale. Behavior anchors reflecting points along this continuum and a time frame would improve specificity, such as did not complete any chest physiotherapy for cystic fibrosis the past week to completed one therapy a day to completed two therapies a day as prescribed. Advantages of these methods include being inexpensive and available for multiple informants, and potentially providing details about adherence and factors influencing adherence. A major disadvantage is adherence may be overestimated due to self-reports, perhaps, being subject to recall bias and social desirability factors.

Provider estimates involve global ratings of adherence to regimen components by medical providers. Ratings are considered indirect and subjective, and can be dichotomous (yes/no) for overall adherence or for each regimen component, or based on a Likert-type scale, ranging from, for example, 4 (*almost always adherent*)–0 (*rarely adherent*). Provider estimates are cost-effective and feasible, but adherence can be overestimated, perhaps due to ratings being unreliable as they are based on perceptions of individual providers.

Treatment outcomes are not direct measures of adherence but are indicators of health status and, thus, related to adherence. Health status indicators include clinical signs obtained through instrumentation, such as blood pressure or limited joint range of motion, and symptoms based on patient or parent report, such as pain or fatigue. Another measure of treatment outcome is the subjective perception of quality of life across domains of physical, emotional, social, and academic/work functioning. Quality-of-life measures can be general or specific, depending on the degree to which the impact of illness, injury, or medical treatment on daily functioning is referenced. Treatment outcome measurement can be useful in tracking treatment goals, but should not be sole measure of adherence for clinical or research purposes.

Treatment of Nonadherence

There are many adherence improvement strategies that each address a specific aspect of nonadherence. Educational strategies are used to provide information to the patient and family about the condition and its management. Research has demonstrated that while this is initially helpful, education alone is not sufficient to maintain adherence (Dean et al. 2010). Including organizational strategies (e.g., increasing access to care, simplifying regimens; improving communication) has been shown to assist in maintaining adherence (DiMatteo 2004a).

Cognitive behavioral therapy (CBT) is the foundation for many interventions to improve adherence. The cognitive component aims to increase positive or more realistic thoughts from maladaptive thoughts regarding adherence. Reframing can also help to improve one's acceptance of their illness by seeing it as only one aspect of themselves. The behavioral component seeks to increase adherence-related behaviors across the spectrum (i.e., taking medication, lifestyle modifications). Behavioral interventions can also address barriers to adherence by increasing self-monitoring and use of technology. Using behavioral interventions is related to increased effectiveness for improving adherence (Dean et al. 2010). Research has shown that a multicomponent intervention is the most effective (Kahana et al. 2008). Combining education and cognitive behavioral strategies is important to improving adherence in multiple settings (DiMatteo 2004a; Gould and Mitty 2010).

Treatment Course for Case Example

Mark participated in 15 sessions of cognitive behavioral therapy with a pediatric psychologist specializing in adherence promotion. Treatment included several types of adherence promoting interventions including psychoeducation, cognitive restructuring, and behavioral activation training. Several factors related to adherence were crucial to Mark's treatment. These factors include Mark's knowledge about his diabetes (targeted first in treatment), Mark's parents' desire to increase independence and success, the many components of his diabetes regimen, and communicating with the medical team regarding what he was actually doing. To measure progress, we monitored number of days he attended school, number of blood glucose checks per day, and his and parents' subjective report of his progress.

Psychoeducation was used first to provide information about T1D and its management. Psychoeducation was provided during sessions based on knowledge from the therapist's extensive experience working with youth with T1D. Additionally, *Understanding Diabetes* (Chase 2006) is recommended to all patients. The goal was to provide Mark with knowledge about how managing his illness could prevent any long-term sequelae and early death. In addition, discussion of possible limitations on his career choices was employed. For example, Mark wished to be a physician but was concerned that T1D would prevent that, he was assured that T1D would not necessarily prevent him from achieving this.

Following improved understanding of his T1D, Mark learned cognitive restructuring to help ameliorate anxiety regarding treatment and concerns about his health during the school day. Mark was encouraged to examine what safety factors were in place (i.e., knowledgeable adults at school, 504 plan in place) to help him manage. Mark also talked with friends about his diabetes and its management for additional social support.

Behaviorally, Mark worked on goal setting (increasing blood glucose checks) with aids to help him (i.e., phone reminders). Mark found an app that allowed him to electronically track and submit blood glucose values to his physician (i.e., mySugr). This tracking allowed the medical team to provide him with intermittent praise and ability to make adjustments more quickly giving Mark peace of mind about his care. Mark's second goals were around reentering school on a regular basis. Thus, Mark would set goals of attending a number of days per week and receive recognition for those days. Parents were willing to provide him with additional incentives or privileges for attending school. Mark was instrumental in choosing these rewards. In the beginning, Mark received small incentives (e.g., extra videogame time) for attending 1 day of school. Rewards were increased in terms of desirability as the number of days increased.

At the end of treatment, Mark had accomplished the identified goals. He was checking blood glucose the assigned number of times per day (i.e., 4–6) and had returned to school (0 days absent). Mark was able to easily communicate with the medical team regarding blood glucose values and make adjustments as needed. Mark indicated improved acceptance and understanding of his illness. Parents and Mark reported subjective improvement in his diabetes care and attitude toward diabetes. This case demonstrates the importance of a multi-factored intervention to improve adherence. Using only one of the components (psychoeducation, cognitive restructuring, behavioral techniques) would have not addressed all concerns around nonadherence. For example, an educational approach alone would not have addressed his worries and maladaptive thoughts around his diabetes management. However, not including education would have left him without the needed information to improve his care and better understand his illness. Finally, incorporating all stakeholders in Mark's care (family, school, and medical providers) allowed consistency in implementing strategies and provided him with additional support.

Conclusions and Future Directions

Kravitz and Melnikow (2004) drew five conclusions in their commentary on the comprehensive review on adherence by DiMatteo (2004b): (1) nonadherence will always be with us, (2) the method of assessment matters, (3) mean adherence is higher for some conditions than others, (4) correlations between adherence and sociodemographic factors, while statistically significant, are quite modest in magnitude, and (5) the field of adherence research is ready for a multitrait multimethod approach (i.e., different regimen components measured by at least two assessment methods). Kravitz and Melnikow (2004) add that reliable and valid assessment measures should be based on clinically grounded adherence models. The self-management model proposed by Modi et al. (2012) supports the development of measures grounded in theory, as well as effective and individually tailored interventions.

Electronic monitoring and diaries are considered the two most accurate measures of adherence in terms of agreement across informants (Duncan et al. 2014; Quittner et al. 2008). Self-report questionnaires and interviews may, though, provide more qualitative information about barriers to adherence. An increased attention to electronic methods of measurement and technology has been recommended and include the development of brief, patient-reported adherence measures that can be incorporated into electronic health records given at each clinic visit, and inexpensive electronic measures (Steiner 2012). Electronic medical records can also be used to provide patients and families with written comprehensive treatment plans (Quittner et al. 2008) or "dashboards" to monitor specific intervention steps (Steiner 2012). Miscommunication about aspects of the medical condition and its treatment may be lessened by referring to these written plans during medical appointments (Quittner et al. 2008). Treatment outcome measurement should also be incorporated into clinical practice and research when assessing adherence, along with the impact of nonadherence on healthcare costs to families and to society (Rapoff 2010). The relationship between adherence and health outcomes based on models, such as linear or threshold, will need to be explored for specific regimen components within the context of the individual, family, and healthcare system (Kravitz and Melnikow 2004; Modi et al. 2012).

Multiple risk factors correlate with adherence/nonadherence, but the predictive ability of these sociodemographic or clinical characteristics is minimal. The sensitivity and specificity of assessment measures should be examined to delineate individual differences related to racial, ethnic, cultural, and economic factors that influence adherence (Quittner et al. 2008; Steiner 2012). Health literacy is one specific sociodemographic characteristic that has been found to predict health outcomes (Miller 2016). Health literacy is defined as the ability to read, understand, and act on health information (Department of Health and Human Services 2000). Verbal and written communication between patients, families, and medical providers using terminology understood by patients and families is one recommended education tool (Miller 2016). Cultural competency training for all providers has also been suggested due to findings that communication problems with patients and families with limited English proficiency and implicit biases pertaining to cultural differences affect direct patient care, adherence, and subsequently, health outcomes (McQuaid 2018).

Multicomponent adherence intervention strategies should be emphasized in future clinical and research efforts (Rapoff 2010; Wu et al. 2013). Rapoff (2010) has recommended targeting patients: (a) whose adherence drops below some acceptable level (80%) and (b) who experience compromised healthcare outcomes. Clinicians will then need to decide which assessment/intervention strategy to use, how these strategies are tailored to individual differences of patients and families, what treatment materials to implement, how assessment and intervention are carried out within multidisciplinary teams, and how interventions are evaluated in real-world practices (Duncan et al. 2014; Wu et al. 2013).

A distillation and matching model has been proposed by Duncan et al. (2014) to employ in future research to identify aspects of effective and tailored adherence promotion strategies across pediatric populations. This model posits that it is possible to identify the core effective elements in evidence-based practice (distillation) and apply them based on how they fit with client/patient characteristics (i.e., matching; Chorpita et al. 2005). Another critical element of practice implementation is treatment integrity. Treatment integrity refers to the degree to which individuals conducting interventions adhere to specific intervention protocol in a consistent manner (Rapoff 2010). Adherence research in terms of designing and implementing intervention strategies may be enhanced using this outcome within both quality improvement projects and clinical trials.

The complexity of adherence requires assessment and interventions efforts involve a partnership between patients, families, and healthcare providers within the larger context of communities and society. This partnership will support consideration of factors at multiple levels to ensure individually tailored interventions that result in optimal adherence and health outcomes.

References

Adams, C. D., Dreyer, M. L., Dinakar, C., & Portnoy, J. M. (2004). Pediatric asthma: A look at adherence from the patient and family perspective. *Current Allergy and Asthma Reports, 4*, 425–432.

Ajzen, I. (1991). The theory of planned behavior. *Organizational Behavior and Human Decision Processes, 50*, 179–211.

Bauman, I. J. (2000). A patient-centered approach to adherence: Risks for nonadherence. In D. Drotar (Ed.), *Promoting adherence to medical treatments in chronic childhood illnesses. Concepts, methods, and interventions* (pp. 71–94). Mahwah, NJ: Erlbaum.

Benjamin, R. M. (2012). Medication adherence: Helping patients take their medicines as directed. *Public Health Reports, 127*, 2–3.

Cabana, M. D., Rand, C. S., Becher, O. J., & Rubin, H. R. (2001). Reasons for pediatrician nonadherence to asthma guidelines. *Archives of Pediatrics & Adolescent Medicine, 155*, 1057–1062.

Carbone, L., Zebrack, B., Plegue, M., Joshi, S., & Shellhaas, R. (2013). Treatment adherence among adolescents with epilepsy: What really matters? *Epilepsy and Behavior, 27*, 59–63.

Chandwani, S., Koenig, L. J., Sill, A. M., Abramowitz, S., Conner, L. C., & D'Angelo, S. (2010). Predictors of antiretroviral medication adherence among a diverse cohort of adolescents with HIV. *Journal of Adolescent Health, 51*, 242–251.

Chase, H. P. (2006). *Understanding diabetes*. Denver, CO: Children's Diabetes Foundation.

Chorpita, B. F., Daleiden, E. L., & Weisz, J. R. (2005). Identifying and selecting the common elements of evidence based interventions: A distillation and matching model. *Mental Health Services Research, 7*, 5–20.

Cohen, S. Y., & Wamboldt, F. S. (2000). The parent-physician relationship in pediatric asthma care. *Journal of Pediatric Psychology, 25*, 69–77.

Dean, A. J., Walters, J., & Hall, A. (2010). A systematic review of interventions to enhance medication adherence in children and adolescents with chronic illness. *Archives of Disease in Childhood, 95*, 717–723.

Department of Health and Human Services. (2000). *Healthy people 2010* (2nd ed.). Washington, DC: U.S. Government Printing Office.

DiMatteo, M. R. (2004a). The role of effective communication with children and their families in fostering adherence to pediatric regimens. *Patient Education and Counseling, 55*, 339–344.

DiMatteo, M. R. (2004b). Variation in patients' adherence to medical recommendations: A quantitative review of 50 years of research. *Medical Care, 42*, 200–209.

Downs, D. S., & Hausenblas, H. A. (2005). The theories of reasoned action and planned behavior applied to exercise: A meta-analytic update. *Journal of Physical Activity and Health, 2*, 76–97.

Drotar, D. (2009). Physician behavior in the care of pediatric chronic illnesses: Association with health outcomes and treatment adherence. *Journal of Developmental and Behavioral Pediatrics, 30*, 246–254.

Duncan, C. L., Mentrikowski, J. M., Wu, Y. P., & Fredericks, E. M. (2014). Practice-based approach to assessing and treating nonadherence in pediatrics regimens. *Clinical Practice in Pediatric Psychology, 2*, 322–336.

Gadkari, A. S., & McHorney, C. (2012). Unintentional non-adherence to chronic prescription medications: How unintentional is it really? *Health Services Research, 12*, 98.

Gibson, T. B., Ozminkowski, R. J., & Goetzel, R. Z. (2005). The effects of prescription drug cost sharing: A review of the evidence. *American Journal of Managed Care, 11*, 730–740.

Goh, X. T., Tan, Y. B., Thirumoorthy, T., & Kwan, Y. H. (2017). A systematic review of factors that influence treatment adherence in paediatric oncology patients. *Journal of Clinical Pharmacy and Therapeutics, 42*, 1–7.

Gould, E., & Mitty, E. (2010). Medication adherence is a partnership, medication compliance is not. *Geriatric Nursing, 31*, 290–298.

Gray, W. N., Denson, L. A., Baldassano, R. N., & Hommel, K. A. (2012). Treatment adherence in adolescents with inflammatory bowel disease: The collective impact of barriers to adherence and anxiety/depressive symptoms. *Journal of Pediatric Psychology, 37*, 282–291.

Guite, J. W., Kim, S., Chen, C. P., Sherker, J. L., Sherry, D. D., Rose, J. B., et al. (2014). Pain beliefs and readiness to change among adolescents with chronic musculoskeletal pain and their parents before an initial pain clinic evaluation. *The Clinical Journal of Pain, 30*, 17–26.

Gutierrez-Colina, A., Smith, A., Mara, C., & Modi, A. C. (2018). Adherence barriers in pediatric epilepsy: From toddlers to young adults. *Epilepsy & Behavior, 80*, 229–234.

Haynes, R. B. (1979). Introduction. In R. B. Haynes, D. W. Taylor, & D. L. Sackett (Eds.), *Compliance in health care* (pp. 1–7). Baltimore, MD: Johns Hopkins University Press.

Hilliard, M. E., Mann, K. A., Peugh, J. L., & Hood, K. K. (2013). How poorer quality of life in adolescence predicts subsequent type 1 diabetes management and control. *Patient Education and Counseling, 91*, 120–125.

Hommel, K. A., Davis, C. M., & Baldassano, R. N. (2009). Objective versus subjective assessment of oral medication adherence in pediatric inflammatory bowel disease. *Inflammatory Bowel Diseases, 15*, 589–593.

Hommel, K. A., Ramsey, R. R., Rich, K. L., & Ryan, J. L. (2017). Adherence to pediatric treatment regimens. In M. C. Roberts & R. Steele (Eds.), *Handbook of Pediatric psychology* (5th ed., pp. 119–133). New York: Guilford.

Hsin, O., La Greca, A. M., Valenzuela, J., Moine, C. T., & Delamater, A. (2010). Adherence and glycemic control among Hispanic youth with type 1 diabetes: Role of family involvement and acculturation. *Journal of Pediatric Psychology, 35*, 156–166.

Johnson, S. B., Kelly, M., Henretta, J. C., Cunningham, W., Tomer, A., & Silverstein, J. (1992). A longitudinal analysis of adherence and health status in childhood diabetes. *Journal of Pediatric Psychology, 17*, 537–553.

Jones, C. J., Smith, H. E., Frew, A. J., Du Toit, G., Mukhopadhyay, S., & Llewellyn, C. D. (2014). Explaining adherence to self-care behaviours amongst adolescents with food allergy: A comparison of the health belief model and the common sense self-regulation model. *British Journal of Health Psychology, 19*, 65–82.

Kahana, S., Drotar, D., & Frazier, T. (2008). Meta-analysis of psychological interventions to promote adherence to treatment in pediatric chronic health conditions. *Journal of Pediatric Psychology, 33*, 590–611.

Kang, J.-S., & Lee, M.-H. (2009). Overview of therapeutic drug monitoring. *The Korean Journal of Internal Medicine, 24*(1), 10.

Killian, M. O., Schuman, D. L., Mayersohn, G. S., & Triplett, K. N. (2018). Psychosocial predictors of medication non-adherence in pediatric organ transplantation: A systematic review. *Pediatric Transplantation, 22*, e13188. https://doi.org/10.1111/petr.13188.

Kravitz, R. L., & Melnikow, J. (2004). Medical adherence research. Time for a change in direction? *Medical Care, 42*, 197–199.

La Greca, A. M., & Bearman, K. J. (2003). Adherence to pediatric treatment regimens. In M. C. Roberts (Ed.), *Handbook of pediatric psychology* (3rd ed., pp. 119–140). New York: Guilford Press.

Landers, S. E., Friedrich, E. A., Jawad, A. F., & Miller, V. A. (2016). Examining the interaction of parental involvement and parenting style in predicting adherence in youth with type 1 diabetes. *Families, Systems, & Health, 34*, 41–50.

Lemanek, K. L., Kamps, J., & Chung, N. B. (2001). Empirically supported treatments in pediatric psychology: Regimen adherence. *Journal of Pediatric Psychology, 26*, 253–275.

Logan, D., Zelikovsky, N., Labay, L., & Spergel, J. (2003). The illness management survey: Identifying adolescents' perceptions of barriers to adherence. *Journal of Pediatric Psychology, 28*, 383–392.

Mager, D. R., Marcon, M., Brill, H., et al. (2018). Adherence to the gluten-free diet and health-related quality of life in an ethnically diverse pediatric population with celiac disease. *Journal of Pediatric Gastroenterology and Nutrition, 66*, 941–948.

Malee, K., Williams, P., Montepiedra, G., et al. (2011). Medication adherence in children and adolescents with HIV infection: Associations with behavioral impairment. *AIDS Patient Care and STDs, 25*, 191–200.

McQuaid, E. L. (2018). Barriers to medication adherence in asthma. The importance of culture and context. *Annals of Allergy, Asthma and Immunology, 121*, 37–42.

McQuaid, E. L., Walders, N., Kopel, S. J., Fritz, G. K., & Klinnert, M. D. (2005). Pediatric asthma management in the family context: The family asthma management system scale. *Journal of Pediatric Psychology, 30*, 492–502.

McQuaid, E. L., Everhart, R. S., Seifer, R., Kopel, S. J., Mitchell, D. K., Eseban, C. A., et al. (2012). Medication adherence among Latino and non-Latino white children with asthma. *Pediatrics, 129*, e1404–e1410.

Mehta, P., Steinberg, E.A., Kelly, S.L., Buchanan, C., & Rawlins, A.R. (2017). Medication adherence among adolescents solid-organ transplant recipients: A surgery of healthcare providers. *Pediatric Transplantation, 21*. https://doi.org/10.1111/petr.1308.

Miller, T. A. (2016). Health literacy and adherence to medical treatment in chronic and acute illness: A meta-analysis. *Patient Education and Counseling, 99*, 1079–1086.

Modi, A. C., & Quittner, A. L. (2006). Barriers to treatment adherence for children with cystic fibrosis and asthma: What gets in the way? *Journal of Pediatric Psychology, 31*, 846–858.

Modi, A. C., Pai, A. L., Hommel, K. A., Hood, K. K., Cortina, S., Hilliard, M. E., et al. (2012). Pediatric self-management: A framework for research, practice, and policy. *Pediatrics, 129*, e473–e485.

Murphy, J., & Coster, G. (1997). Issues in patient compliance. *Drugs, 54*, 797–800.

Perez, K. M., Patel, N. J., Lord, J. H., Savin, K. L., Monzon, A. D., Whittemore, R., et al. (2017). Executive function in adolescents with type 1 diabetes: Relationship to adherence, glycemic control, and psychosocial outcomes. *Journal of Pediatric Psychology, 42*, 636–646.

Prochaska, J. O., & DiClemente, C. C. (1983). Stages and processes of self? Change of smoking: Toward an integrative model of change. *Journal of Consulting and Clinical Psychology, 51*, 390–395.

Quittner, A. L., Espelage, D. L., Ievers-Landis, C., & Drotar, D. (2002). Measuring adherence to medical treatment in childhood chronic illness: Considering multiple methods and sources of information. *Journal of Clinical Psychology in Medical Settings, 7*, 41–54.

Quittner, A. L., Modi, A. C., Lemanek, K. L., Ievers-Landis, C. E., & Rapoff, M. A. (2008). Evidenced-based assessment of adherence to medical treatments in pediatric psychology. *Journal of Pediatric Psychology, 33*, 916–936.

Rapoff, M. A. (2010). *Adherence to pediatric medical regimens* (2nd ed.). New York: Springer.

Riekert, K. A., & Drotar, D. (2002). The beliefs about medication scale: Development, reliability, and validity. *Journal of Clinical Psychology in Medical Settings, 9*, 177–184.

Simons, L. E., McCormick, M. L., Devine, K., & Blount, R. L. (2010). Medication barriers predict adolescent transplant recipients' adherence and clinical outcomes at 18-month follow-up. *Journal of Pediatric Psychology, 35*, 1038–1048.

Steiner, J. F. (2012). Rethinking adherence. *Annals of Internal Medicine, 157*, 580–585.

Urquhart, J. (1997). The electronic medication event monitor. Lessons for pharmacotherapy. *Clinical Pharmacokinetics, 32*, 345–356.

Wu, Y. P., Rohan, J. M., Martin, S., Hommel, K., Greenley, R. F., Loiselle, K., et al. (2013). Pediatric psychologist use of adherence assessments and interventions. *Journal of Pediatric Psychology, 38*, 595–604.

Part III

Special Topics

26 Training Issues in Pediatric Psychology

Ryan R. Landoll, Corinn A. Elmore, Andrea F. Weiss, and Julia A. Garza

Training Issues in Pediatric Psychology

Integrated behavioral health care in primary care is a growing subspecialty within the field of psychology (Vogel et al. 2017). With this increased focus, there has been an emergence of training programs, but these have historically focused on practice with the adult population (Dobmeyer et al. 2016). There is a growing need for behavioral health care in the pediatric primary care population. However, there is a lack of standard training and development of expertise in the subspecialty of pediatric primary care. The application of general competencies and training programs for work in primary care may not account for critical differences and unique complexities in caring for children and adolescents. In this chapter, we first review the competency guidelines for working in primary care, covering both generalist guidelines and efforts made to create competencies for the pediatric population. We then describe and address the current state of the literature on training for integrated primary care and where we are lacking in providing this training specifically for pediatric psychologists. Finally, we address the challenges faced in the development of future training programs and provide recommendations for the continued evolution of these training programs.

Competencies for Practice in Primary Care Psychology

Given the increasing need for and integration of psychological services in primary care, competencies for providing mental health treatment in primary care are critical in formulating an approach to primary care practice. In addition, they provide a framework for building competencies in the practice of primary care psychology in pediatrics. Factors initially thought to be important to such practice were discussed by Hunter and Goodie (2010) and expanded upon

---

This chapter was authored in part by the employees of the United States government. Any views expressed herein are those of the authors and do not necessarily represent the views of the United States government or the Department of Defense.

R. R. Landoll (✉) · J. A. Garza
Uniformed Services University of the Health Sciences, Bethesda, MD, USA
e-mail: Ryan.landoll@usuhs.edu

C. A. Elmore
Pediatric and Adolescent Primary Care Medical Homes, Walter Reed National Military Medical Center, Bethesda, MD, USA

A. F. Weiss
Malcolm Grow Medical Clinics and Surgery Center, Joint Base Andrews, MD, USA

and codified most recently in 2015 by the American Psychological Association (APA). The APA has put forth several competencies for the practice of primary care psychology over the last several years (APA 2015). There are six competency areas in the APA report on this topic (APA 2015). These cluster areas include science, systems, professionalism, relationships, application, and education. Each competency area is further broken down into specific knowledge, skills, and behaviors expected of a psychologist practicing in primary care and assume that basic competencies for the practice of general psychology are met by those practicing in this setting (APA 2015). More recently, there has been recognition of the need for competencies specifically for pediatric primary care (Hoffses et al. 2016; Spirito et al. 2003; Njroge et al. 2017). A recent effort to codify pediatric specific primary care competencies built upon existing generalist primary care competencies as well as emphasized the need for crosscutting knowledge in pediatric psychology (Palermo et al. 2014).

Training Programs in Pediatric Primary Care

Many practitioners in primary care have been practicing in this setting for less than a decade (Hoffses et al. 2017). As such, it is not surprising that there are few well-established training programs for primary care psychology, even fewer for pediatric settings (Briggs et al. 2016). Most training in this domain occurs at internship or postdoctoral levels and is roughly evenly divided between these two training levels (Hoffses et al. 2017). The field of pediatric primary care has traditionally lagged behind integrated primary care more generally in regard to the establishment of clear models of care as well as robust evaluation of outcomes (Briggs et al. 2016). This is in contrast to a clear recognition of the importance of behavioral health in pediatrics, particularly in reaching vulnerable youth and preventing negative long-term sequelae (Stancin and Perrin 2014).

For this reason, where training programs do exist, they often do not focus exclusively on psychologists. Some focus on training behavioral health providers more broadly across various levels of training. The HealthySteps program, for example, has been well established as a prevention program aimed at early developmental screening. This program has relied on a wide variety of behavioral health professionals to serve as early developmental specialists and is incorporated across several training programs (Zuckerman et al. 2004; Talmi et al. 2016; Briggs et al. 2016). Like Healthy Steps, training also often focuses on specific processes or populations, for example, communication about autism spectrum disorder (Kawamura et al. 2016). Finally, another unique feature of literature in this area is that training in pediatric primary care tends to focus on either physician training (cf. Foley et al. 2015) or interprofessional education opportunities (cf. Kawamura et al. 2016; Pisani and Siegel 2011; Ragunanthan et al. 2017). This broad and inclusive focus in training is generally reflective of the growing importance of interprofessional health care, particularly in primary care (Fiscella and McDaniel 2018).

While there are few large-scale, well-established training programs, in part driven by the wide variety and poor articulation of pediatric primary care models, there are several pilot programs that are particularly noteworthy. In addition, the codification of specific competencies endorsed by the Society for Pediatric Psychology (Palermo et al. 2014) represents an important standard for unique training programs that have not been established in the empirical literature but nonetheless promote a consistency in training and establishing competency. Furthermore, successful training programs and practitioners have worked to enhance their reach through a variety of workshops and conferences. Finally, established primary care training programs from the adult literature are beginning to recognize the importance of pediatrics and explore this population. The following section will explore each of these training themes.

Pilot Training Programs

In addition to the empirical literature, there are several pilot programs that have been established to train clinicians in pediatric primary care. The following section will review some example programs and their training models. Of note, the competencies developed which are reviewed above are utilized as a foundation for evaluation of skill for each of the programs (Palermo et al. 2014; Hoffses et al. 2016). Of note, these programs were selected as examples and are not meant to be an exhaustive list of pilot training programs. However, they provide a good overview of the kinds of programs that currently exist and some key elements of successful training programs.

Children's Hospital of Philadelphia The Healthy Minds, Healthy Kids Program (HMHK) services children and their families receiving medical care within a large pediatric primary care clinic affiliated with the Children's Hospital of Philadelphia (Njroge et al. 2017). Approximately 15,000, mostly ethnic minority patients with public insurance, are served in a designated medically underserved area of Philadelphia, Pennsylvania. Staff include 22 primary care physicians, 3 pediatric nurse practitioners, and 30–40 pediatric medical residents. The HMHK team includes licensed pediatric psychologists, social workers, child psychiatrists, and trainees completing their psychology doctoral internship or child psychiatry fellowship. Psychology interns spend 16 h per week in the clinic for 1 year, while psychiatry fellows rotate through the clinic for 6 h per week for 6 months.

In the training program, trainees are first oriented to the pediatric primary care culture and are then taught skills such as documentation in the medical record, strategies for communication with primary care medical staff, and cultural competencies specific to the patient population. Trainees receive the majority of referrals through warm handoffs where the patient meets and is provided brief consultation on the same day following a primary care visit. In addition, patients may receive referrals after visits. Trainees are expected to maintain a caseload for intake appointments and follow-up care in eight sessions or fewer in order to aid in access to care.

Clinical training focuses on enhancing integrated care skills through emphasis on assessment, diagnosis, and evidenced-based practices for common presenting problems in primary care (e.g., elimination disorders, obesity, ADHD). In addition to didactic training, trainees engage in several experiential learning activities including observing well-child visits across child developmental stages, case presentations, as well as shadowing medical and ancillary staff. Trainees also have opportunities to provide seminars on behavioral interventions in primary care to medical staff to facilitate interprofessional communication and professionalism. Finally, trainees work with the multidisciplinary staff to do case-based discussion. At three times during training, trainees are assessed on their competency using the competency guidelines discussed previously (Palermo et al. 2014). The expectation is that trainees will move from "competent with support" to "competent without support" at the conclusion of training.

Montefiore Medical Center/Albert Einstein School of Medicine Another pilot program of interest is the psychology internship program of Montefiore Medical Center/Albert Einstein School of Medicine in Bronx, New York (Briggs et al. 2016). Interns provide services at assigned pediatric primary care sites associated with the Montefiore Medical Network. Staff include approximately one full-time psychologist for every 5000 children and one psychiatrist for every 20,000 children, and service approximately 90,000 children and families. The majority of the patient population is ethnically diverse and lives below the federal poverty line. Interns in the Child and Adolescent and Combined Specialization tracks of the program may select the pediatric Behavioral Health Integration Program (BHIP) as an elective rotation and receive training in integrated pediatric primary care 1 day per week for 11 months. Two programs comprise the BHIP program: the Healthy

Steps (HS) program and the Child and Adolescent Psychology and Psychiatry (CAPP) program.

Healthy Steps is a national model of care aimed at preventative efforts through screening, assessment, and intervention for patients of ages 0–5. At Montefiore, pregnant mothers are universally screened during their last trimester with the Adverse Childhood Experiences Study (ACES) questionnaire. Families who are identified "at risk" based on screening are selected to receive intensive Healthy Steps services. These services include ongoing screening and consultation from clinicians designated as Healthy Steps specialists who attend all well-child visits for these families. Briggs et al. (2016) report that approximately 5–10% of their patient population for this age group meet criteria for the intensive Healthy Steps services. The CAPP program provides services for children of ages 5–18. Patients are universally screened with the Pediatric Symptom Checklist-17 (PSC-17) and the Youth Pediatric Symptom Checklist-17 (PSC-17Y; Gardner et al. 1999) during the well-child visits. Identified families are then referred to trainees through warm handoffs or traditional referrals.

Interns provide direct care through screeners and assessments and then conduct intake appointments and provide brief evidence-based interventions for four to six 30-min appointments. Patients who receive care through the BHIP program generally exhibit mild-to-moderate health problems that are suited for the brief consultation model of care. Trainees refer families who could benefit from more intensive services to behavioral health services in the community. Training is provided through several avenues. Interns are not only assigned individual supervisors for weekly hour-long supervision, but also meet with staff who serve as "content experts" for particular areas of intervention (e.g., trauma) through consultations and group training. Interns are also trained didactically in coordination of care with primary care physicians. Interns attend monthly professional development and BHIP trainings as well as weekly didactic training with the larger internship cohort. To ensure competence, trainees are formally assessed twice per year using the benchmark competencies for pediatric psychologists (Palermo et al. 2014).

MetroHealth The MetroHealth system is located in Northeast Ohio and is affiliated with Case Western University School of Medicine (MetroHealth Medical Center Psychology Internship Training Faculty n.d.). The psychology residency program began 4 years ago and has three primary care tracks including pediatric psychology, neurodevelopmental disabilities, and trauma and community health tracks. MetroHealth includes several primary care clinics as part of their health system including resident continuity clinics, adolescent medicine clinics, Spanish-speaking clinics, and family medicine clinics. Patients receiving services in these clinics are typically ethnically diverse and receive public medical assistance. All trainees dedicate 30% of their training time to a primary care clinic and are placed on an interdisciplinary team. Trainees provide brief solution-focused interventions with children and train medical residents in behavioral health interventions for primary care.

Psychology residents receive 2 h weekly of individual supervision with a licensed psychologist and 1 h of group supervision in weekly primary care rounds. Trainees also receive supervision from members of the interprofessional team in the primary care clinic (physicians, psychiatrists, social workers, etc.). Monthly case conferences are held with the team to review specific cases. In addition, trainees receive "on-the-spot" supervision with the assigned licensed psychology "Supervisor of the Day." Didactic training is provided 2 h a week and focuses on understanding the primary care culture, enhancing collaboration with medical providers, and brief interventions for common presenting concerns in pediatric primary care. Interns are formally evaluated twice per year on their integrated pediatric primary care skills through an evaluation packet informed by the Competencies Benchmark document with specific behavioral anchors for competency (Palermo et al. 2014).

Unique to this training program is the training focus on collaborative psychotropic medication management between primary care psychologists and primary care physicians. Due to the limited child psychiatry resources, psychology residents are able to use their knowledge of the biological basis of behaviors and diagnostic assessment to supplement the medical knowledge of physicians. Trainees develop these skills through attending didactic sessions led by psychiatrists on topics such as psychopharmacology, pathophysiology, and evidence-based treatment for common primary care presenting problems. This training is done along with medical residents to provide uniformity in training across the two disciplines. In these seminars, interns learn how to monitor medication treatment effects and are able to provide insight on possible adjustments to medications. Psychology residents conduct diagnostic assessments with patients and then collaborate with the attending psychiatrist to review findings. The psychiatrist will then forward the recommendation to the whole team through the electronic health record system. Following this initial consultation, the psychology trainee aids in monitoring medication response while the medical resident prescribes the medication. The aim is to increase comfort of medical staff in prescribing psychotropic medication and to provide more knowledge to psychology residents on medication treatment and management.

Seminars, Workshops, and Conferences

In addition to formal training programs at the predoctoral and postdoctoral levels, there are several avenues for continuing education and brief training opportunities. Although there are numerous trainings designed to target and address commonly seen diagnoses within a primary care setting more generally for behavioral health professionals, there has been less emphasis on integration within the pediatrics. Similarly, in workshops and conferences designed for medical professions (e.g., nurse practitioners, physicians, etc.) topics of discussion are primarily focused on physical medical conditions with less emphasis on mental health conditions and integration with other disciplines in a primary care setting. The following sections will describe in more detail the areas of intersection to establish competency in addressing mental health concerns and multidisciplinary integration in pediatric primary care through workshops, trainings, and conferences.

There are several different workshops and trainings available online for medical and mental health professionals to further develop competencies in working with children and adolescents. The Society of Clinical Child and Adolescent Psychology offers various online trainings designed to improve competency in the treatment of children and adolescents, such as adherence to treatment, cognitive behavioral treatment for depression, and assisting children in transitioning after a divorce, among others (http://effectivechildtherapy.fiu.edu/professionals/workshops; Society of Clinical Child and Adolescent Psychology 2018). However, a limitation of these various trainings offered by the Society of Clinical Child and Adolescent Psychology is that they are not adapted for a primary care setting. The University of Michigan's School of Social Work also offers a certification program to train social workers, nurses, case managers, physicians, and psychologists to work within a pediatric primary care setting (The Regents of the University of Michigan 2018). Montefiore Medical Group and Pediatric Behavioral Health Services also offer training to providers in the previously mentioned BHIP program (Montefiore: The University Hospital for Albert Einstein College of Medicine 2018).

The American Academy of Pediatrics similarly offers online workshops that focus on a range of medical conditions, as well as managing depression in primary care settings, diagnosing and treating ADHD, utilizing the Medical Home model (i.e., coordinating care for a patient through a primary medical provider) to address mental health concerns in primary care, and aiding primary care providers in addressing mental health concerns within the school setting, etc. (American Academy of Pediatrics 2018). The Washington Chapter of the American Academy of Pediatrics (WCAAP) also offers periodic workshops for medical providers to further enhance patient care within a pediatric primary care setting, to include workshops with an emphasis on early attachment and relationships, screening for depression in adolescents, and the promotion of multidisciplinary care in the pediatric primary care setting (WCAAP 2018).

In addition, there are a several conferences available annually that focus on training for pediatric medical conditions and pediatric mental health concerns. The Maryland Department of Health and Mental Hygiene Behavioral Health Integration in Pediatric Primary Care (BHIPP) program (http://www.mdbhipp.org/) offers training in pediatric primary care to behavioral health providers through grand-round topics on communication within primary care and a variety of presenting concerns as well as consultation and conferences (Maryland BHIPP 2018). Although some conferences are similarly meant for particular disciplines (e.g., pediatric nurse practitioners, family medicine practitioners, pediatric primary care physicians), there is overlap in the relevance of topics discussed and the type of workshops being offered at these various conferences. A summary of these conferences is presented in Table 26.1.

Additional Resources In addition to various workshops and trainings offered for both medical

Table 26.1 Pediatric primary care psychology training conferences

Sponsoring organization/conference title	Provider specialty	Notes
National Association of Pediatric Nurse Practitioners (https://www.napnap.org/national-conference)	Nurse practitioners	Conference focuses on sleep medications in pediatric primary care, utilizing motivational interviewing to minimize risk behaviors (e.g., smoking, lack of physical activity) in adolescents, and improving interprofessional collaborative practice in primary care settings
Annual Pediatric Primary Care Conference (VCU Health) (https://vcu.cloud-cme.com/aph.aspx?EID=6342&P=5)	Family practice, general practice, nurse practitioner, nursing, pediatrics, physician assistant, social work	Focuses primarily on common medical conditions seen in pediatric primary care settings, but there are also workshops on utilizing cognitive behavioral therapy, improving sleep, and treating anxiety within the primary care setting
Society of Pediatric Psychology (https://www.societyofpediatricpsychology.org/node/726)	Pediatric psychologists	Annual conferences that have emphasized the need to further integrate care within primary care settings to increase accessibility of mental health services to children and adolescents, focused on examining the role of a pediatric psychologist, and emphasized treating children with health conditions
Miami International Child and Adolescent Mental Health Conference (FIU Center for Children and Families, The Children's Trust, the Society of Clinical Child and Adolescent Psychology, and Miami-Dade County Public Schools) (https://ccf.fiu.edu/training-and-education/professionals/continuing-education/micamh-conference/index.html)	Psychologists, counselors, school psychologists, social workers	Offers trainings on various treatments and common concerns to utilize within a clinic setting and training for parents
National Conference in Clinical Child and Adolescent Psychology (University of Kansas, Society of Clinical Child and Adolescent Psychology) (https://ccpp.ku.edu/conferences)	Psychologists	Offered training in treating children and adolescents with ADHD, addressing child maltreatment, and identifying risk factors for depression and suicide, treating chronic pain in pediatric setting

providers and mental health professionals, it is pertinent for providers to be aware of various resources available to assist children and adolescents in a pediatric setting, as connecting families to resources can be an important primary care intervention. A few examples include programs and nonprofit organizations such as the Colorado Housing and Finance Authority (CHFA). CHFA aids children by helping to increase the availability of housing to lower income families and further support additional organizations to ensure children obtain clean bedding (CHFA 2018). The DREAM program also aids children from lower income families by providing them with mentors, increasing access to educational opportunities, preparing adolescents to transition to college, and enabling children to participate in outdoor recreation activities (Dream Program n.d.). Other large organizations, such as the Consortium for Science-Based Information on Children, Youth and Families (CSICYF), provide online resources for parents and families on developmental milestones and how to enhance educational opportunities (CSICYF 2019).

Pediatric Adaptations of Generalist Primary Care Psychology Training

As integrated mental health in primary care has increased in the civilian sector, the military has a long history of primary care behavioral health (Hunter and Goodie 2010). The United States Air Force (USAF) primary care behavioral health program embeds psychologists and social workers as behavioral health consultants located in primary care clinics (Landoll et al. 2019). They provide focused, timely encounters in a consultative fashion to primary care providers, consistent with the Primary Care Behavioral Health (PCBH) model (Dobmeyer et al. 2016). In regard to training, the USAF uses a competency-based system with robust phased training (Dobmeyer et al. 2016). For active duty USAF psychologists, this is completed by the integration of a training model into each of the three residency sites, which train and graduate approximately 24 psychologists in the USAF per year. Unfortunately, while this is an example of a well-established training program, like many established programs, there is a focus on generalist care. While there is a recommendation that provision of care to pediatric patients should only be done by a provider with previous training or competence in the area (AFMOA USAF 2014), there remains a need for guidance and training on adapting this model of training or care to the pediatric population.

Challenges in Training and Future Directions

Despite the many exciting opportunities for training in integrated pediatric primary care, several challenges exist. Common themes in the literature were identified in the following areas: curriculum, personnel, and integration.

Curriculum Challenges

As a relatively new area in psychology, few child-focused graduate programs provide specific training in integrated care. Graduate training programs may struggle to add more coursework to an already loaded training curriculum (Dobmeyer et al. 2003). As a result, in many child-focused training programs, students are likely to be trained in providing traditional psychotherapy over the brief, consultative model of treatment required in primary care. Once students enter their practicum experiences, they may struggle with this paradigm shift (Rozensky and Janicke 2012). If students do not receive their initial training in integrated care until their clinical internship or postdoctoral fellowship, there exists less time for building a professional identity as leaders while learning new skills (Stancin 2016). Therefore, there is a particular need for a unified framework for training in psychology graduate programs (McDaniel et al. 2002). In evaluating proficiency in skill, the specific behavioral anchors for competency in integrated pediatric primary care were only recently developed (Hoffses et al. 2016). As a result, the long-term implications and practicality of using these anchors are not fully understood. Finally, the unique role psychologists play in the integrated care teams compared to other related fields (e.g., behavioral health coordinator, case manager, social worker, etc.) has not been clearly defined (Stancin and Perrin 2014).

Another training curriculum concern is in the lack of information on adapting care to diverse patient populations. Many primary care clinics service patient populations that are diverse in not only their ethnic background, but also in income, access to care, and ideas around health and wellness. While virtually all training programs reviewed for this chapter mentioned training in diversity, there was little information on how this diversity training is conducted, maintained, and evaluated. Pediatric psychologists working in primary care not only need to be aware of cultural diversity in a general sense, but also need to understand the context in which their specific primary care site operates. Both trainees and supervisors should be regularly assessed for their own biases and how to bring this understanding to the rest of the interdisciplinary team. Psychologists should also be trained in understanding the intersection between physical and mental illness for the patient population and how to incorporate spiritual and cultural beliefs into their approach with patients (Spirito et al. 2003). Finally, an understanding of the differences in access for various cultural groups is important. For example, a child of a military service member may struggle with continuity of care due to frequent moves.

Personnel Challenges

With the existing challenges in developing a standardized training curriculum, it may be difficult to identify trainees who would best implement an integrated care model. Traditional behavioral health training is not sufficient for working in integrated care. Trainees providing integrated care must be flexible, able to take quick feedback, and adapt to primary care culture. The pediatric primary care environment is exceptionally fast paced. Behavioral health providers must deliver care in 15–30 min rather than the 45- to 60-min expectation in specialty behavioral health settings. First, rapport building and assessment occur within the first few minutes of the appointment rather than over several appointments as in specialty behavioral health care. Trainees may overestimate the importance of building rapport before delivering assessment and intervention and then rush through the visit, which impacts quality of care. Identifying presenting concerns quickly and then providing solution-focused intervention is a skill to be developed. Trainees may be tempted to use the same intervention for every patient with the same presenting problem due to trying to manage these expectations. They may also select interventions prematurely and/or over-rely on referral to specialty behavioral health care (Dobmeyer et al. 2003). Communicating the findings and clear treatment recommendations to the family within these time constraints may be a challenge. Complicating the matter is the expectation to complete documentation while completing the aforementioned tasks. Documentation associated with primary care behavioral health should be concise and easily understood by the patient and interdisciplinary team. When beginning training, students may tend to overdocument, making the information more difficult to be easily accessed and integrated by physicians. Verbal feedback to physicians is preferred, fitting in with the primary care culture (Dobmeyer et al. 2003). In selecting trainees, those who have direct experience with medical teams are better prepared to work in this environment and may have more professional confidence to establish themselves as competent to the physicians (Blount and Miller 2009).

Direct training in pediatric integrated care is relatively new, which results in few available faculty supervisors. Faculty mentors and supervisors must not only have direct clinical experience in primary care, but must also have training in supervising and teaching this information to trainees. Specifically, training in providing evidence-based care in a brief model, working in a fast-paced unpredictable environment, and integrating into interdisciplinary teams is critical to providing adequate supervision. Very often, seasoned specialty care providers rely on their past training experiences and eventually fail to properly integrate or provide brief enough interventions for primary care (Blount and Miller 2009). Unfortunately, there is limited availability in training for faculty transitioning from specialty behavioral healthcare settings into integrated primary care. Certificate and postgraduate programs are available (e.g., University of Michigan School of Social Work), but few are pediatric focused and are often costly. Continuing and remediation education will be necessary to facilitate these transitions.

Integration Challenges

When integrating behavioral health into an existing medical team, there will be growing pains. In order to best facilitate integration, it is critical to ensure stakeholder buy-in for an integrated program before placing trainees at a primary care site (Godoy et al. 2017). The interdisciplinary team must not only be open to including behavioral health services, but also they must be willing to take active steps in training and ensuring access for behavioral health trainees to be included in team huddles and trainings. To aid with this buy-in, it is important to provide education to medical providers on the types of problems that integrated behavioral health trainees can provide. When beginning integration, there is often variability in medical staff triage strategies, where integrated behavioral healthcare providers are underutilized or only used for provider consultation rather than during warm handoffs incorporated into the medical visit (Blount and Miller 2009). Differences in terminology, training background (biomedical versus psychosocial), and expectations for treatment further compound these issues (Bray 2004). It is important to remember that psychologists have distinct skills in diagnosis and assessment, which are critical for triage and delegating appropriate treatments. Understanding the unique skills psychologists provide is critical in enhancing professional identity while also working within interdisciplinary teams.

Another challenge for training is in the unpredictable nature of pediatric primary care. The patient need for behavioral health services may fluctuate daily based on a variety of external factors (e.g., academic schedule) making it difficult to predict the workload for trainees. Some days there may be several referrals, while other days there may be few children presenting with behavioral health concerns. Oftentimes, trainees may have unscheduled downtime. The training program must be equipped to utilize that time for additional didactic training, shadowing opportunities, supervision, etc. to ensure that students receive adequate training in both circumstances.

Future Directions

Although the field of integrated pediatric primary care has grown exponentially in the past 20 years, there still remains several opportunities for growth. One of these areas is creating more structured training in child-focused integrated care in graduate programs in psychology. This includes predoctoral clinical experiences, focused course work in the area, and specific training on delivering evidence-based interventions in a brief model of care. Coursework should place particular emphasis on foundational skills in health psychology, pediatric psychology, interdisciplinary collaboration, and an understanding of pediatric primary care culture. During clinical internship and postgraduate training, the development of more dedicated training tracks in integrated behavioral health is needed. Finally, creating more opportunities for seasoned mental health professionals to receive training in delivering and supervising integrated care is crucial to addressing the workforce limitations described previously.

Another future direction for training is in securing and sustaining funding for training programs. Training grants for graduate medical education (GME) funding may be secured through the Department of Health and Human Services (HHS); however, these funds are limited in availability. In many healthcare systems, a set amount of money is allocated to the system per patient. Although the research is clear in its assertion that inclusion of behavioral health services in primary care actually reduces overall costs over time (Landoll et al. 2019), it may be difficult to convince institutions of the value of paying staff psychologists for supervision purposes (Garcia-Shelton and Vogel 2002). It will be important for training in programs to have several avenues to sustain the training program financially.

Access to care and stigma in receiving behavioral health care continues to be a problem. Telehealth is an emerging way to provide population-based health care and may be especially important for parents with limited resources or in less populated areas (Godoy et al. 2017). While there is burgeoning literature on the provision of integrated care services through telehealth means in the integrated adult population, there is very limited information on the effectiveness of these services in pediatric primary care.

Finally, shared training between psychology trainees and pediatric medical residents could help better facilitate integration of behavioral health into the pediatric care clinic. In this model of training, psychology and pediatric trainees would have shared didactic training, shared faculty, and mentoring from both psychology and pediatrician staff. This allows psychology trainees to learn about the primary care culture and physician needs directly from medical providers, while medical residents learn from psychologists. Mutual training opportunities could better enable a team environment and provide opportunity for direct observation of skills for training (Stancin 2018). Furthermore, it would facilitate using shared language as well as shared understanding of the culture of each discipline. Stancin (2018) conducted preliminary satisfaction surveys at MetroHealth in Cleveland, Ohio and found that both psychology and pediatric medicine residents "valued having more than one discipline in training" which highlights satisfaction for cross-discipline mentoring (Stancin 2018).

Recommendations for Establishing Training Programs

By examining the existing training programs, the following recommendations should be considered in establishing a training program in pediatric primary care:

1. *Start with Defined Competencies.* One advantage of the pediatric literature in this area is the establishment of competencies for practice in primary care (Palermo et al. 2014; Njroge et al. 2017). Using these competencies and operationalizing them for your specific training program is a critical first step in establishing the learning objectives.
2. *Consider the Training Level of the Learner.* Graduate programs are currently limited in their training in primary care, though this is improving (Hall et al. 2015). Opportunities for predoctoral training in pediatric populations may be further limited. This is consistent with the medical literature where training at the level of undergraduate medical education (UME) is fairly limited. Fortunately, the APA's competencies delineate levels of skill designed for readiness for internship as well as independent practice, so these can be adapted for all training levels. However, it is important that this is considered when establishing your program, particularly in light of the next recommendation.
3. *Build Your Team.* Another advantage the pediatric literature demonstrates is its embrace of interdisciplinary practice and interprofessional education. In fact, in the pediatric primary care competency movement, there has even been efforts to establish interprofessional competencies (Njroge et al. 2017). Many of the training programs reviewed involved learners from other healthcare backgrounds outside psychology (Bunik et al. 2013). While some training models work with learners who are at developmentally similar stages professionally (cf. Pisani and Siegel 2011), others do not (Kawamura et al. 2016). Thus, when considering your trainee's level of expertise and the interprofessional team to incorporate

into your training program, many different combinations are possible, but the advantages and disadvantages of these combinations should be considered.
4. *Be Intentional in Your Curriculum.* Hopefully, the above recommendations have helped to focus your learning objectives and promoted careful consideration of your learners and their environment. These factors are included as pre-considerations in the interprofessional education literature (Reeves et al. 2016) and set the stage for informed curriculum development. Intentional, planned curriculum is an important, yet often overlooked, aspect of healthcare education (Thomas et al. 2015). Using an established curriculum design method can help ensure that appropriate stakeholders are included in implementation decisions and that good pedagogical process are included for the context. Ultimately, this will maximize the likelihood of your program's success in educating learners.
5. *Share Your Story.* Part of well-informed, intentional curriculum design is a consideration of the assessment process (Thomas et al. 2015). As such, good educational methodology also lends itself to meaningful systematic evaluation. This is the foundation of empirical knowledge, and considering how your curriculum can inform the broader literature, and then working to disseminate that knowledge, including pedagogical details, is a crucial final step of your individual process.
6. *Build Consensus.* Hopefully, if more programs that are competency based, informed, and intentional are disseminated, it can spur consensus within the field on models of pediatric primary care. This provides evidence for important debates within the field. Attempts to "downward extend" models of adult integrated primary care create debate about whether or not there are qualitative differences in practicing within a pediatric setting, what they are, and how they should be addressed.

In conclusion, pediatric primary care is an area of incredible growth and great importance. Like many new areas of practice, initial efforts to provide training rely on evidenced-based strategies but further evaluation and standardization is needed. There are no easy answers, and attempting to provide any is beyond the scope and expertise of this chapter. However, these debates need to be had, and providing data to do so can only enrich the quality of scientific decision-making.

References

American Academy of Pediatrics. (2018). *Webinars*. Retrieved from https://www.aap.org/en-us/professional-resources/webinars/Pages/Webinars.aspx

American Psychological Association. (2015). *Competencies for psychology practice in primary care*. Retrieved from http://www.apa.org/ed/resources/competencies-practice.pdf

Blount, F. A., & Miller, B. F. (2009). Addressing the workforce crisis in integrated primary care. *Journal of Clinical Psychology in Medical Settings, 16*(1), 113–119. https://doi.org/10.1007/s10880-008-9142-7.

Bray, J. (2004). Training primary care psychologists. *Journal of Clinical Psychology in Medical Settings, 11*(2), 101–107.

Briggs, R. D., German, M., Hershberg, R. S., Cirilli, C., Crawford, D. E., & Racine, A. D. (2016). Integrated pediatric behavioral health: Implications for training and intervention models. *Professional Psychology: Research and Practice, 47*(4), 312–319. https://doi.org/10.1037/pro0000093.

Bunik, M., Talmi, A., Stafford, B., Beaty, B., Kempe, A., Dhepyasuwan, N., & Serwint, J. R. (2013). Integrating mental health services in primary care continuity clinics: A national CORNET study. *Academic Pediatrics, 13*(6), 551–557. https://doi.org/10.1016/j.acap.2013.07.002.

Consortium for Science-Based Information on Children, Youth and Families (CSICYF). (2019, July). Retrieved from https://www.infoaboutkids.org

Colorado Housing and Finance Authority. (2018). Colorado Housing and Finance Authority. Retrieved from https://www.chfainfo.com

Dobmeyer, A. C., Rowan, A. B., Etherage, J. R., & Wilson, R. J. (2003). Training psychology interns in primary behavioral health care. *Professional Psychology: Research and Practice, 34*(6), 586–594. https://doi.org/10.1037/0735-7028.34.6.58.

Dobmeyer, A. C., Hunter, C. L., Corso, M. L., Nielsen, M. K., Corso, K. A., Polizzi, N. C., & Earles, J. E. (2016). Primary care behavioral health provider training: Systematic development and implementation in a large medical system. *Journal of Clinical Psychology in Medical Settings, 23*(3), 207–224. https://doi.org/10.1007/s10880-016-9464-9.

Dream Program. (n.d.). Dream Program. Retrieved from https://www.dreamprogram.org/

Fiscella, K., & McDaniel, S. H. (2018). The complexity, diversity, and science of primary care teams. *American Psychologist, 73*, 451–467.

Florida International University. (2018). *Miami International Child & Adolescent Mental Health Conference*. Retrieved from https://ccf.fiu.edu/training-and-education/professionals/continuing-education/micamh-conference/

Foley, K. P., Haggerty, T. S., & Harrison, N. (2015). Curriculum development: Preparing trainees to care for children and adolescents with psychiatric disorders. *The International Journal of Psychiatry in Medicine, 50*(1), 50–59. https://doi.org/10.1177/0091217415592360.

Garcia-Shelton, L., & Vogel, M. E. (2002). Primary care health psychology training: A collaborative model with family practice. *Professional Psychology: Research and Practice, 33*(6), 546–556. https://doi.org/10.1037//0735-7028.33.6.546.

Gardner, W., Murphy, M., Childs, G., Kelleher, K., Pagano, M., Jellinek, M., McInerny, T. K., Wasserman, R., Nutting, P., Chiappetta, L., & Sturner, R. (1999). The PSC-17: A brief pediatric symptom checklist with psychosocial problem subscales. A report from PROS and ASPN. *Ambulatory Child Health, 5*(3), 225–236.

Godoy, L., Long, M., Marschall, D., Hodgkinson, S., Bokor, B., Weisman, M., & Beers, L. (2017). Behavioral health integration in health care setting: Lessons learned from a pediatric hospital primary care system. *Journal of Clinical Psychology in Medical Settings, 24*, 245–258. https://doi.org/10.1007/s10880-017-9509-8.

Hall, J., Cohen, D. J., Davis, M., Gunn, R., Blount, A., Pollack, D. A., et al. (2015). Preparing the workforce for behavioral health and primary care integration. *Journal of the American Board of Family Medicine, 28*, S41–S51.

Hoffses, K., Ramirez, L., Berdan, L., Tunick, R., Honaker, S., Meadows, T., Shaffer, L., Robins, P., Sturm, L., & Stancin, T. (2016). Topical review: Building competency: Professional skills for pediatric psychologists in integrated primary care settings. *Journal of Pediatric Psychology, 41*(10), 1144–1160. https://doi.org/10.1093/jpepsy/jsw066.

Hoffses, K., Riley, A., Menousek, K., Schellinger, K., Grennan, A., Cammarata, C., & Steadman, J. (2017). Professional practices, training, and funding mechanisms: A survey of pediatric primary care psychologists. *Clinical Practice in Pediatric Psychology, 5*(1), 39–49. https://doi.org/10.1037/cpp0000173.

Hunter, C. L., & Goodie, J. L. (2010). Operational and clinical components for integrated-collaborative behavioral healthcare in the patient-centered medical home. *Families, Systems, & Health, 28*(4), 308–321. https://doi.org/10.1037/a0021761.

Kawamura, A., Mylopoulos, M., Orsino, A., Jimenez, E., & McNaughton, N. (2016). Promoting the development of adaptive expertise: Exploring a simulation model for sharing a diagnosis of autism with parents. *Academic Medicine, 91*(11), 1576–1581. https://doi.org/10.1097/ACM.0000000000001246.

Landoll, R. R., Nielsen, M. K., Waggoner, K. K., & Najera, E. (2019). Innovations in primary care behavioral health: A pilot study across the US Air Force. *Translational Behavioral Medicine, 9*(2), 266–273. https://doi.org/10.1093/tbm/iby046.

Maryland BHIPP. (2018). Maryland BHIPP. Retrieved from http://www.mdbhipp.org

McDaniel, S. H., Belar, C. D., Schroeder, C., Hargrove, D. S., & Freeman, E. L. (2002). A training curriculum for professional psychologists in primary care. *Professional Psychology: Research and Practice, 33*(1), 65–72. https://doi.org/10.1037/0735-7028.33.1.65.

MetroHealth Medical Center Psychology Internship Training Faculty. (n.d.). *Resident handbook 2018-2019*. Retrieved October 5, 2018, from https://www.metrohealth.org/upload/docs/gme/programs/psychology/2018psychologyinternshiphandbook.pdf

Montefiore: The University Hospital for Albert Einstein College of Medicine. (2018). *2018 Pediatric Behavioral Health Integrated Program (BHIP)*. Retrieved from https://www.acesconnection.com/file-SendAction/fcType/0/fcOid/473487835084039909/filePointer/473487835084039937/fodoid/473487835084039934/2018%20Training%20Institute%20Save%20the%20Date.pdf

National Association of Pediatric Nurse Practitioners. (n.d.). *Conferences*. Retrieved from https://www.napnap.org/national-conference

Njroge, W. F., Williamson, A. A., Mautone, J. A., Robins, P. M., & Benton, T. D. (2017). Competencies and training guidelines for behavioral health providers in pediatric primary care. *Child and Adolescent Psychiatric Clinics of North America, 26*(4), 717–731. https://doi.org/10.1016/j.chc.2017.06.002.

Palermo, T. M., Janicke, D. M., McQuaid, E. L., Mullins, L. L., Robins, P. M., & Wu, Y. P. (2014). Recommendations for training in pediatric psychology: Defining core competencies across training levels. *Journal of Pediatric Psychology, 39*(9), 965–984. https://doi.org/10.1093/jpepsy/jsu015.

Pisani, A. R., & Siegel, D. M. (2011). Educating residents in behavioral health care and collaboration: Integrated clinical training of pediatric residents and psychology fellows. *Academic Medicine, 86*(2), 166–173. https://doi.org/10.1097/ACM.0b013e318204fd94.

Ragunanthan, B., Frosch, E. J., & Solomon, B. S. (2017). On-site mental health professionals and pediatric residents in continuity clinic. *Clinical Pediatrics, 56*(13), 1219–1226. https://doi.org/10.1177/0009922816681136.

Reeves, S., Fletcher, S., Barr, H., Birch, I., Boet, S., Davies, N., McFayden, A., Rivera, J., & Kitto, S. (2016). A BEME systematic review of the effects of interprofessional education: BEME Guide No. 39. *Medical Teacher, 38*(7), 656–668. https://doi.org/10.3109/0142159X.2016.1173663.

Rozensky, R. H., & Janicke, D. M. (2012). Commentary: Healthcare reform and psychology's workforce:

Preparing for the future of pediatric psychology. *Journal of Pediatric Psychology, 37*(4), 359–368. https://doi.org/10.1093/jpepsy/jsr111.

Society of Clinical Child and Adolescent Psychology. (2018). *SCCAP Sponsored Conferences*. Retrieved from https://sccap53.org/sccap-sponsored-conferences/

Society of Pediatric Psychology. (2016). *2019 SPPAC*. Retrieved from https://www.societyofpediatricpsychology.org/node/726

Spirito, A., Brown, R. T., D'Angelo, E., Delamater, A., Rodrigue, J., & Siegel, L. (2003). Society of pediatric psychology task force report: Recommendations for the training of pediatric psychologists. *Journal of Pediatric Psychology, 28*(2), 85–98. https://doi.org/10.1093/jpepsy/28.2.85.

Stancin, T. (2016). Commentary: Integrated pediatric primary care: Moving from why to how. *Journal of Pediatric Psychology, 41*(10), 1161–1164. https://doi.org/10.1093/jpepsy/jsw074.

Stancin, T. (2018, May 6). *Preparing pediatricians and psychologists to work in teams: The MetroHealth Model*. In Pediatric Academic Societies Meeting. Toronto.

Stancin, T., & Perrin, E. C. (2014). Psychologists and pediatricians opportunities for collaboration in primary care. *American Psychologist, 69*(4), 332–343. https://doi.org/10.1037/a0036046.

Talmi, A., Muther, E. F., Margolis, K., Buchholz, M., Asherin, R., & Bunik, M. (2016). The scope of behavioral health integration in a pediatric primary care setting. *Journal of Pediatric Psychology, 41*(10), 1120–1132. https://doi.org/10.1093/jpepsy/jsw065.

The Regents of the University of Michigan. (2018). *Integrated health pediatric track*. Retrieved from https://ssw.umich.edu/offices/continuing-education/certificate-courses/integrated-behavioral-health-and-primary-care/pediatric-track

The University of Kansas. (n.d.). *National Conference in Clinical Child and Adolescent Psychology*. Retrieved from https://ccpp.ku.edu/2018-national-conference-clinical-child-and-adolescent-psychology

Thomas, P. A., Kern, D. E., Hughes, M. T., & Chen, B. Y. (2015). *Curriculum development for medical education: A six-step approach*. Baltimore: Johns Hopkins University Press.

United States Air Force, Air Force Medical Operations. (2014). *Primary Care Behavioral Health Services: Behavioral Health Optimization Program (BHOP) Practice Manual*.

Virginia Commonwealth University Health CME. (2017). *40th Annual Pediatric Primary Care Conference*. Retrieved from https://vcu.cloud-cme.com/aph.aspx?EID=6342&P=5

Vogel, M. E., Kanzler, K., Aikens, J., & Goodie, J. L. (2017). Integration of behavioral health and primary care: Current knowledge and future directions. *Journal of Behavioral Medicine, 40*, 69–84. https://doi.org/10.1007/s10865-016-9798-7.

Washington Chapter of the American Academy of Pediatrics. (2018). *Washington Chapter of the American Academy of Pediatrics*. Retrieved from https://wcaap.org

Zuckerman, B., Parker, S., Kaplan-Sanoff, M., Augustyn, M., & Barth, M. C. (2004). Healthy Steps: A case study of innovation in pediatric practice. *Pediatrics, 114*(3), 820–826. https://doi.org/10.1542/peds.2003-0999-L.

Financial Issues

Allen R. Miller

Introduction

For decades, rising costs in healthcare have resulted in concern from all segments of society. Multiple sources have declared that healthcare costs are unsustainable (Wilensky 2016) Corporate entities who purchase healthcare benefits for their employees and dependents have seen healthcare costs eat away at their bottom lines (Humer and Henry 2018). Total healthcare benefit costs that are made up of premiums, deductibles, and co-payments for Americans increased 33% from 2006 to 2016 (Claxton et al. 2018). Costs of healthcare in the USA have risen as a share of gross domestic product (GDP) from 5.0% in 1960 to 17.4% in 2013 (Catlin and Cowan 2015). Additionally, Medicare costs per capita are projected to grow at an annual rate of 4.6% over the next 10 years (Cubanski and Neuman 2018). Not surprisingly, healthcare cost growth has resulted in government agencies, legislators, and private enterprise calling for reductions in healthcare spending. Simultaneously, Americans want access to the latest healthcare improvements resulting from biotechnological advances, new medications, and other developments from research. The pressure to bring new products and services to the healthcare market and making them available to all Americans in a timely, cost-effective process has created tremendous stress within the healthcare industry and frustration among payers of healthcare products and services. This stress and frustration have led to increased calls for more innovation and cost reductions in the industry, which creates a perpetual cycle of searching for innovation and cost increases that, of course, leads to more stress and higher costs.

Efforts to manage costs and care for patients have resulted in pressure for primary care clinics to not only provide easy access to healthcare but also manage the care—and associated costs—for patients with chronic pain and other chronic health conditions. In this chapter, "primary care" will be used to refer to pediatric primary care practices as well as family medicine and internal medicine practices that treat children and adolescents. In the past and presently, primary care doctors quickly become overwhelmed by the increased numbers of patients they have had to manage and the complexity of the problems experienced by patients with chronic health conditions.

To manage complications in their patients, primary care doctors rely heavily on being able to refer complicated patients to medical specialists. As long as there are readily available special-

A. R. Miller (✉)
Beck Institute for Cognitive Behavior Therapy, Bala Cynwyd, PA, USA
e-mail: amiller@beckinstitute.org

ists—and the patients have some form of health insurance—our system works pretty well. When medical specialists are not available, patients do not have insurance, or patients have complicated presentations, our system gets bogged down quickly. One response to healthcare shortages has led medical schools to produce more doctors. Additionally, more support is given to primary care doctors in the form of more nurses, medical case managers, and health coaches. One unfortunate result from adding additional support is higher costs. Also, there are still unresolved issues regarding access to behavioral health professionals.

In consideration of problems experienced in the delivery of healthcare, the Institute for Healthcare Improvement undertook a review of healthcare services and outcomes, which led to its framework for the Triple Aim for healthcare systems (Berwick et al. 2008). The Triple Aim provides an approach to improve the delivery of healthcare by: improving the patient experience, improving the health of populations, and reducing the costs of healthcare. The ideas put forth in the Triple Aim were transformational for health systems who, prior to that time were, arguably, more interested in their own experience and comfort, and defensive about patient demands or expectations. At the same time that the Triple Aim concept was being developed, government funded projects focused on integrating behavioral health with primary care practices.

At least in part, the success of government-funded initiatives to integrate behavioral health and primary care was responsible for the inclusion of integration as a purpose and a goal in the Patient Protection and Affordable Care Act (ACA) of 2010 (Blount et al. 2007). The ACA contains support and incentives to states and healthcare providers to integrate primary care and behavioral healthcare. The National Committee for Quality Assurance (NCQA 2018) offers accreditation standards for health plans and providers of care to help improve the quality of services they provide to health plan members. Today, NCQA provides standards for Distinction in Behavioral Health Integration to facilitate system efforts to provide comprehensive care for patients who experience behavioral health and physical problems. The Joint Commission (TJC 2018) provides certification standards for Patient Centered Medical Homes (PCMH) that integrate behavioral health services with the goal of improving the overall level of care to primary care patients with behavioral health issues.

A number of factors put behavioral health at ground zero for recognizing problems in our healthcare system and for looking for potential solutions. Issues like chronic pain and other medical problems frequently carry with them comorbid conditions of depression and anxiety. On the flip side, conditions of depression and anxiety frequently lead to physical complaints. It would be expected that primary care practices refer their patients to mental health professionals for depression and anxiety, much like they would for any medical condition requiring the expertise of a specialist. Behavioral health, as a specialty, is wrought with all kinds of complications though. Along with the stigma that still exists about mental health problems, there are far fewer mental health professionals available than there are patients seeking their services.

Additionally, due to stigma, costs, transportation issues, and related factors, primary care has become the default mental healthcare provider in America. Patients typically find their primary care providers to be geographically closer to their homes, to have appointments times that are more readily available, to have lower costs, and to provide easier access to medications. Although these conditions are true, or because they are true, it is maddening for doctors and patients that primary care doctors do not have the time or expertise to manage either the stand-alone behavioral problems or those that accompany medical conditions in the primary care setting. In the case of behavioral health issues, the solution of having primary care manage the treatment has led to an even more overwhelmed system.

One issue not immediately recognized by the medical community, let alone the payers, is that many of the behavioral health problems presented in primary care settings are not, and cannot, be "fixed" with medications. Throughout this book, the authors provide heavy support for the use of cognitive behavioral therapy (CBT) for addressing the stand-alone psychological problems and comorbid psychological conditions that accompany medical conditions presented in primary care settings. What is not specifically addressed in the CBT treatment research are the resolving problems of access related to convenience, cost, and stigma. Having evidence-based treatments will be of little value if we do not have the means to make them available to all those in need. The next section will focus on how to make CBT more widely accessible for the public.

Delivery Model

Undoubtedly, CBT can be delivered in different settings including traditional behavioral health outpatient offices as well as in hospitals, medical specialty offices, and in primary care settings. Nonetheless, the organizational structure of how CBT therapists fit into the medical settings will differ from setting to setting. Historically, the most common setting for providing CBT has been in a traditional behavioral health outpatient office. CBT has been delivered in inpatient psychiatric and medical settings and more recently in primary care settings. However, services have not always been CBT oriented. In some cases, behavioral health services are limited to screening services, case management services, or on a single issue like depression. Some behavioral health services are based on a single treatment technique like Motivational Interviewing. Of course, services such as screenings, and individual techniques provide value of their own. The very nature of primary care is to deal with a multitude of problems in an efficient and effective manner. It is also important to recognize though that behavioral health services fit uniquely into different practice settings.

There are a number of advantages when CBT is provided in a primary care setting. By administering CBT, patients benefit by seeing a therapist close to home, in a setting that does not carry the mental health stigma, and depending on the financial model, will be less costly than going to behavioral health specialists' offices. Degrees of integration include a consultation model, co-location, and full integration (Please see Chap. 2 this volume).

A consultation model of integration involves an agreement between a primary care practice and a behavioral health provider such that the therapist gives priority to referrals made by the primary care practice. Priority status may be fulfilled by giving the patient first choice for the next available appointment or setting aside time slots to accommodate urgent patient needs. In today's world, consultations may also be conducted via secure telemedicine video sessions. By providing priority consultation times, patients benefit by being seen sooner than they otherwise would be seen. Physicians benefit because they quickly have a mental health specialist involved in the patients' treatment teams, and therapists benefit because they will receive a steady flow of patient referrals.

Co-location of CBT services provides patients and primary care staff additional advantages over a consultation model. Co-location of services typically means that CBT is provided in the same building as the primary care practice but in a different suite. However, this could also mean providing CBT in the same office suite as the primary care practice but, scheduling, billing, and documentation are done in separate information systems. It is the equivalent of offering private practice services at the same physical location as a primary care practice. The benefits to patients include the location of services in addition to the potential reduction of stigma by being in the same building as primary care. Furthermore, closer proximity promotes better communication and consultation between physicians and therapists. Within a co-location model, therapists maintain their own independence with the freedom to conduct their practice in a way that is to their liking.

Full integration of CBT services into primary care offers advantages to patients and physicians, but there are definite trade-offs for therapists who chose this model. Full integration of a CBT therapist into primary care practices means that therapists become full-fledged members of primary care treatment teams. With full integration, therapists may be employed by the practice, or by a larger health system. In addition, therapists function as members of a primary care team that is led by primary care physicians. Fully integrated practice also means that therapists are included in primary care scheduling systems, billing is completed by the primary care practice, and documentation is charted in the same medical record system. Therapists may offer appointments that are shorter in duration (e.g., 20-min sessions) or they may be available for a "warm hand-off" or "on-the-fly" consultation. For example, while meeting with patients, physicians may recognize that their patients have problems that are beyond their scope of practice and amount of time they have available. In such instances, physicians may ask therapists to join the session and after making an introduction, physicians leave therapists to conduct their session with patients. The encounter may be as short as meeting one another long enough to schedule a different meeting time (i.e., warm hand-off). At other times, therapists may spend 20 min assessing the patient's needs and providing brief interventions (i.e., on the fly consultation). In crisis situations, however, therapists may need to facilitate an admission for treatment to a higher level of care (e.g., inpatient unit). Working in a fully integrated setting changes therapists' responsibilities, their level of autonomy, and the ways in which they deliver CBT. Questions about which CBT services may be provided, and the number of sessions that will be given in primary care settings may be determined by the strategic financial model adopted by an organization. Decisions about financial models will be affected by the different forms of payments that may be available from local payers.

Payment Methods

To understand strategic financial decisions, we first must discuss options for compensation for services provided in integrated care settings. In the behavioral health arena, services may be paid as fee-for-service, as negotiated fees for being a participating member through managed care companies, case rates, and various kinds of risk arrangements including incentive payments for achieving positive outcomes.

Fee-for-service is the most straightforward and common means of being paid for services. In this arrangement, therapists provide a service (e.g., CBT session) and patients pay the stated fee. Occasionally, patients will request a receipt to submit to their insurance companies so that they can be reimbursed for paying the upfront costs of a service provided by an out-of-network provider. Therapists may charge whatever fees they believe the market will bear. What the market will bear suggests what amount patients are willing to pay for their services.

Participating member rates are established by and sometimes negotiated with third party payers. Special rates are set for those providers who are considered in-network by the payers. In this scenario, therapists apply to payers to be considered as in-network providers. In-network providers work with payers to provide services to their members. Members pay a premium to payers to receive healthcare benefits. Therapists enter into payer networks for various reasons including increased referrals from the payers, the desire to work with certain patient populations that the therapist may not otherwise have access to, and their innate belief of the importance to increase access to services. The trade-off for joining a payer network is that in exchange for the referrals you receive from the payer, you will provide your services for a reduced (negotiated) fee. Negotiated fees are often set by the payer. Thus, therapists must decide whether or not to accept or reject the set fees and the referrals that go with it. In some instances, the fees offered by payers may be negotiable and therapists may be able to obtain an agreement for the payer to give them a higher rate than what was originally offered. Higher rates are sometimes paid to therapists who provide special services not otherwise available in their network, and also to therapists who work with difficult-to-treat problems.

Case rates are more often offered for treatment provided by organizations that include program services and higher levels of care. Higher levels of care include intensive outpatient programs, partial hospital or day programs, and inpatient hospital treatment. Sometimes case rates may be available to therapists who provide a special protocol or time-limited group treatment in an outpatient setting for specific difficult-to-treat patient populations. For case-rate situations, therapists or programs are paid a set amount of money to provide needed care to patients who have a particular condition and need specialized services. Given the fixed rate agreement, if patients require more treatment than the therapist originally anticipated, the therapist is bound to the original case rate.

Case rates are a first step into risk agreements. Risk refers to a situation where there are unknowns about a patient or patient population for whom providers agree to treat for a set amount of money. Providers may accept a set fee for a particular case or for covering a population of people. The unknowns about the population determine the level of risk the providers take by entering into an agreement. If it is a healthy population of people, there may be small treatment needs and the providers may not have to provide much treatment for their payments. On the other hand, a relatively ill population may require high levels of care and in such cases, providers take the risk that they will be able to provide all the needed care for the amount of money they are being paid. If they provide more treatment than what the set payment covers, the provider loses out on any additional payments.

Risk arrangements, as already implicated, may take various forms. The risk is that providers will have to provide more services than for what they are being paid. In risk arrangements, payers agree, in advance, to pay a set amount of money to providers and in return, providers agree to provide all treatment necessary to meet the needs of individual patients or for populations of people. Risk agreements may be entered into to cover the provision of services for patients solely in an outpatient setting or, only in an inpatient setting or, in both outpatient and inpatient sites. Additionally, risk arrangements can be made to include all healthcare costs and not solely behavioral healthcare. They may include behavioral health and medical care for large populations of people. For example, a population may refer to all the people within a certain geographic region who have healthcare coverage with a certain payer (e.g., Medicare). Broad risk agreements are made by large health systems that have the resources to provide comprehensive medical and psychological care to a wide range of people. In fact, when entering a risk arrangement, it may be advantageous to serve as large a group as possible. As previously mentioned, within a population of people, a portion of members will be more healthy and some will have health challenges. For a risk arrangement to benefit both providers and payers, they need healthy people as well as less healthy people to be included in their risk population. Providers will be paid the same to take care of healthy people as they will be paid for less healthy members of the population. Providers count on having a balance of healthy and unhealthy individuals because they know that people with illnesses will likely be high utilizers of healthcare resources, whereas healthy counterparts do not. In the end, providers try to manage the needs of less healthy people without overspending the amount paid to them. The risk arrangement just described is a form of capitation (i.e., the payment amount is "capped" regardless of the amount of services provided).

Shared risk is a concept whereby both payers and providers accept risk in providing care for a certain population of people. In a shared risk arrangement, providers may agree to provide care for a set amount of money but when the health of the people in the pool is not fully understood, the payer will agree to protect the provider from losing too much money. A ceiling may be established for the maximum amount that the provider can lose, and the payer is the one who protects the providers' interests. Consequently, since both provider and payer are at risk, it is referred to as a shared risk model.

In a different scenario, the health of the population may be understood and the provider and payer enter into a risk arrangement but, this time, the payer may offer an incentive not just to provide care but for the provider to achieve positive outcomes. Providing comprehensive care and demonstrating positive outcomes with the population can result in an incentive or bonus payment to the provider for adhering to the Triple Aim of improving population health.

Outcome Measures

Consumer expectations, regulatory body oversight, and willingness of payers to offer payment incentives collectively create the motivation for providers to collect tracking results. In general, outcome measures provide an objective way to quantify the quality of the services provided. Recording outcomes is a natural occurrence within the CBT framework because of its already existing emphasis on a scientific approach to treatment. Specific data are not required but, commonly sought-after measures include ways of demonstrating achievement of the Triple Aim. Ways to capture attainment of the Triple Aim or parts thereof include obtaining feedback about the patient experience, measuring health, and assessing the reduction of costs.

Obtaining feedback about the patient experience includes more than having patients complete a satisfaction survey. Having patients complete a satisfaction survey is usually part of capturing the patient experience but it is, by itself, insufficient to offer that as a way of meeting the requirement. Indeed, patient experience surveys typically ask about how helpful were staff members, how easy it was to get appointments, how useful were the services, etc. Subjective reporting of patients' experiences should be accompanied by objective descriptors of operational processes. One question that can provide objective data is: Did patients get an appointment within the time period they requested? Examples of other objective data measures include: how many times does the telephone ring before it is answered by a staff person; how many callers hang up because they are tired of waiting for someone to answer the phone; how easy is it to get to the office location; how much time did their healthcare provider spend with patients. The list of possible objective measures could be endless. An important aspect of understanding patient experiences is identifying barriers to care at each provider location and demonstrating efforts to make improvements.

Demonstrating efforts to improve patient experiences gets into a different realm of providing healthcare services but one closely aligned with payment. There are various terms and procedures used in reference to performance improvement but, most are founded in the fundamental four-component continuous cycle of plan, do, study, and act (PDSA; Deming 1993). Planning means to collect baseline data for levels on performance that the organization has identified as needing improvement. Planning also involves consideration of various actions that could be taken to improve performance and designing an intervention to change the way things are done to improve patient experiences. At the end of the planning stage, improvement teams settle on a specific intervention to employ that they hope will have a positive impact on performance.

The next step "do," is to implement the plan that had been devised to improve performance. A necessary part of implementation is continuously measuring performance along the way. In the "study" stage, all the data collected from continuous measurement are reviewed to discover if the plan that was implemented was actually effective at improving performance. It is often not a situation of all-or-none improvement, so measures of how much performance was affected are important.

During the study stage, knowledge gained from studying the new data is used to determine whether or not the level of improvement is sufficient. If the target has been met, it must be determined what steps need to be taken to maintain it. If the target has not been met, additional actions must be taken to improve results. During the act stage, changes are implemented to maintain gains or meet new targets.

Health systems in concert with CBT therapists are encouraged to conduct performance improvement studies. Dissemination and implementation efforts by CBT therapists should employ the general PDSA cycle. Performance improvement methodology is a solid option for evaluating whether or not CBT procedures are effective with patient populations for which it has been adapted. Measurement of the impact is one requirement for winning support from health systems to integrate CBT into their settings.

Population health, the second of the Triple Aims, requires measurement of and tracking patients' symptoms and quality of life. Symptoms and health status may be captured by technology that records physiologic functions, self-report of thoughts, feelings, and behaviors, and subjective units of distress (SUDS) scales (1–100). Cognitive and behavioral measurements are regularly completed when applying evidence-based procedures. In today's healthcare environment, CBT practitioners are asked to measure whether CBT interventions are worthwhile at improving the health of large groups or populations of people. Standardized self-report scales for children and adolescents in the private domain are readily available (Beidas et al. 2015). In naturalistic settings, the rigors of randomized, controlled studies are not feasible or necessary to demonstrate effectiveness of treatments. Baseline measures before treatment, at intervals throughout treatment, at the completion of treatment, and at follow-up are sufficient to establish the effectiveness of treatment in natural settings.

One of the biggest challenges is to demonstrate that CBT delivered to patients off-sets the overall costs of healthcare, the third Triple Aim. There is some research that supports the claim that delivery of behavioral health services reduces the overall costs of healthcare (Chiles et al. 2006). Even when other health systems and researchers demonstrate that integrated behavioral health in medical settings have reduced overall medical costs, leaders in new health systems often ask a slightly different but very important question: If we do it (integration), will our costs be offset as well? This places behavioral health and CBT practitioners in somewhat of a bind. CBT practitioners cannot prove that CBT will work "here" until given a chance to demonstrate effectiveness. CBT therapists will need to create a sound argument regarding the risk the system takes by not prioritizing integrated care models.

In sum, capitated payments and various risk arrangements can be highly dependent on the outcome measures that providers, including CBT therapists, report to payers. Providing high-quality services to a population of people can make a difference in how much CBT therapists and/or the health systems that employ them will be paid in risk arrangements and can determine bonus payments when results exceed expectations.

Strategic Decisions

Strategic decisions are decided based upon many different issues. Depending on whether therapists are working in private practice or employed by a large health system or a government entity, the reasons for doing what one does may be quite different. At the beginning of this chapter, we discussed about the problems with healthcare in American society. Some problems mentioned have to do with the costs of providing CBT in a larger healthcare system. In a fee-for-service model (i.e., a situation where CBT services are delivered and fees are paid for the services), an insurer could think of this as adding to the cost of healthcare. In one scenario, payment for medical services is made and additional fees are paid for CBT services. Third-party payers may incur increased costs for CBT treatments without a clear benefit. On the other hand, when CBT treatments improve patients' abilities to better manage their lives despite having chronic medical conditions, payers may consider patients' improved functioning and less use of medical services to be worthwhile. In this second scenario, insurers may place value in CBT services that reduce overall healthcare costs.

It is true that everyone wants what is best for their wallets. So, what is best for the wallets of CBT clinicians? It depends. The largest amount of money in the shortest amount of time can be collected by having patients pay a fee out of their own pockets for CBT sessions when they take place. However, making money is not the only reason that many want to provide therapy. Professionals have other needs to be met and so for many, it is not just about making money but it also involves professional relationships, a desire to provide help to as many people as possible, and of being able to demonstrate the value of services they provide.

If CBT therapists were to treat themselves as patients, they might ask themselves to conduct a cost–benefit analysis. Accordingly, they might ask: what are the positive and negative aspects of working in a fee-for-service model versus a risk-tolerant environment? At one extreme are solo providers, working at the fee-for-service end of the spectrum. For them, the advantages are that they set their own prices, collect cash at each session, make all of their own decisions about when, where, how, and with whom to work. At the other end of that spectrum, therapists work for an organization, where they have job security with a set salary and benefits. Employees of systems may get to work on teams with dedicated providers who work long hours to provide for the needs of their communities. On the negative side, solo providers must work to establish a reputation that will generate referrals and have to manage all their own affairs or hire someone and supervise their activities. There may be ebbs and flows in referrals and income, and there may be an inability to contract on a large scale. The downside of entering into risk agreements is that individually, clinicians have little authority to make policy or procedural decisions. They have to put the team first, which may limit independence in consideration of the organization's needs.

To summarize, therapists certainly have an interest in making money, but other factors like autonomy, security, teamwork, and commitments to their communities play significant roles in deciding the setting in which they chose to work. Although there are many factors that are important for decision making, it is still important to understand the financial side of treatment.

Business Arrangements with Medical Settings

There are many challenges associated with billing mental health services in a medical setting. For example, therapists can only bill for services if various regulatory requirements are met. Regulatory requirements can vary by jurisdiction but some of the issues that can come under scrutiny include: Are patients given a mental health diagnosis that is accepted by payer? Is there complete documentation to support the interventions used to treat diagnosed problems? Are all procedures and documentation HIPAA compliant? What are the financial arrangements between primary care practices and therapists who are billing fee for services? Is it permissible for two different professionals (physician and therapist) to submit charges for the same patient from the same physical location on the same day? These questions and many others need to be answered in discussions about the larger issue of the relationship between medical practices and CBT therapists. Business relationships can be completely separate business entities. On the other hand, physicians and therapists may be employed by the one large healthcare system and all business functions blend together. CBT therapists who work in solo practices may want to do some work in medical settings. Medical providers may very much want therapists to work in their offices but, will also want to negotiate favorable financial arrangements for themselves.

How Financial Models Affect the Delivery of CBT

Many providers and payers are interested in CBT and it would be nice to think that the efficacy of CBT would be singularly responsible for decisions about integrating it into medical settings. Likely, it is not as simple as it is being automatically accepted because it is an example of good science. To some, what is just as important as the efficacy of CBT for behavioral health issues, is the potential to reduce costs. Despite the earlier statement that providing any behavioral health service can be considered an extra cost, larger systems now recognize that good CBT can be helpful for population management.

CBT therapists who work in fee-for-service settings are not going to be greatly affected by changes in payment models. A fee-for-service framework can be implemented in a private practice setting, outpatient office of a large organization, or a community mental health clinic. These settings often considered traditional behavioral health settings. In traditional settings, CBT therapists typically have an intake process in which they gather as much background information as they may need to treat individuals coming to their practice. Additionally, CBT therapists conceptualize cases using cognitive conceptualizations and/or by conducting a behavioral analysis of the presenting problems. Usually, there is at least the beginning of a conceptualization started at the onset of treatment but, conceptualizations may change over time as more information about patients' backgrounds and their response to treatment becomes available. Also, during the intake process, therapists make a provisional diagnosis and explore goals for treatment. Based upon their conceptualizations, therapists collaboratively develop treatment plans. Treatment plans contain strategically derived CBT interventions. Strategies for intervention may change over time as patients' needs change.

A qualification to the previous statement "CBT therapists may not be affected" is in order. When the need for services far exceeds the workforce's ability to meet the needs, therapists in community-oriented systems may be required to continually add new patients to their schedules. By continually adding appointments for new people, there will not be the ability to see existing cases as often as needed and everyone's care may suffer. For therapists, this scenario can be quite stressful.

Applying CBT in risk-bearing primary care settings may be even more complex. When warm hand-offs are made from primary care physicians, the process, expectations, and overall application of CBT change. Instead of having time to collect background information, develop a conceptualization and establish well thought out treatment plans, embedded clinicians must "hit the ground running." This means that in medical settings, it is important to quickly focus on the problem. It will still be necessary to exhibit understanding and good interpersonal skills, and to be collaborative in their interactions. That said, it is also incumbent on CBT therapists in fast-paced settings to quickly formulate exactly what is going on, and implement, with patients' permission, evidenced-based interventions. After intervening, feedback is requested and collaboratively, an action plan is developed for patients so that they may continue working on their problems after the session is finished. An entire session, may only last 20–30 min. This is not the way CBT clinicians were trained in the past. So, adaptations of traditional ways of doing things need to be made when practicing in risk-bearing medical settings.

Barriers to Integration

Integration of CBT into pediatric medical settings offers opportunities and at the same time, there remain challenges to accomplish these goals. Barriers to integration are not few or small. In addition to financial matters, challenges include personal preferences of therapists, attitudes of medical staff, uninformed or ill-informed decision makers, and, of course, the ever-present stigma to mental health treatment. Some of the barriers have eased over time but one should not be of the opinion that integration will be easy in a new practice or health system.

First among barriers is the simple fact that there are not enough behavioral health providers to meet the needs. Additionally, not every behavioral health provider is trained in CBT or wants to be trained in CBT, and not all clinicians want to work in medical settings. When you consider the already short supply of behavioral health professionals and whittle down the numbers to those who can provide CBT intervention, the number of available clinicians is substantially reduced. Paradoxically, the limited number of CBT therapists, instead of having increased value, can actually be a deterrent to health systems and insurers to consider integrating them into their operations. When large systems buy into an idea, they want to be assured that there is sufficient supply of the product or personnel to adopt on a scale that is large enough to serve their entire system. If there is an insufficient supply, the idea may be rejected from the onset. Too few clinicians may send large systems in search for alternative ways of meeting behavioral health needs.

There are a number of alternative means for meeting behavioral health needs. Systems and insurers may cross-train other staff members to provide someone for their patients to talk to. This may be based on their belief that the patients just need someone to talk to. For the same reason, health systems may employ less-trained behavioral health staff members to integrate into medical settings. Systems can provide online alternatives to in-person services as a way to provide quick, easy access to anything that is behavioral. If a system does decide to integrate behavioral health clinicians into medical offices, they do not have to give preference for CBT providers.

In regard to integrating behavioral health into any medical setting, there is an initial investment that must be made by a large system. Even if it is believed that by integrating CBT into a pediatric office will off-set the cost of medical treatments, those savings will not be realized immediately. A system must invest in hiring or contracting with a large number of providers to make it financially worthwhile. To back-step just a moment, if CBT clinicians are going to be a good investment, they will have to reduce costs for systems that are in a risk arrangement. If the system has solely fee-for-service contracts, the system will actually lose money if CBT is effective and patients use fewer health services. This may be a disincentive for health systems to consider integration.

Attitudes and stigma still play an important role in determining integration decisions. Some medical providers do not believe that there is a value or purpose to have behavioral health providers in their practices. They hold the belief "it is better to keep them separate." At a deeper and more disturbing level, some medical providers and members of society still believe that behavioral problems are a matter of choice and those experiencing problems just need to "pull themselves up by the bootstraps and they will be better."

Not to be minimized is the friction that will occur between medical professionals and behavioral health providers over money. Even in an ideal setting where medical personnel are enthusiastic about having behavioral health providers in their office, there will be the pertinent question about how much therapists should be compensated for their services. In large, not-for-profit systems, there may be no conflict among individuals as to where the costs will be charged and where the revenue will be credited but, for sure, there will be strong opinions about how much of the costs are charged to the medical side budget versus the behavioral health budget and who gets to claim the revenues. Ultimately, it will probably be the finance department who decides the budget issue but in an unspoken manner, where costs and revenues are credited will reflect the value that is placed on each type of service.

In a private medical setting, opinions and costs are much more personal. If the medical practice has at-risk contracts, behavioral health clinicians will be paid out of the amount of money allocated for providing all the care to a population of people. That means CBT therapists are paid from what would otherwise be profits from medical services. Of course, if CBT therapists can demonstrate that the patients they have seen utilize fewer "other" services, they will actually be saving the practice money and will be considered to have "earned" their payment.

How therapists get paid can also be an issue for patients in integrated settings. If patients have to make a co-payment or meet a deductible, they may be resistant, and their medical doctors may be less enthusiastic about having therapists in their offices.

The Triple Aim and utilizing the PDSA methodology may be unappealing to therapists. The Triple Aim and PDSA ideas are not taught in graduate schools and are not included in core competencies of CBT. Pursuing the ideals and using the methods requires thinking about different things and developing new ways of measuring as well as reporting results. As cognitive behavioral therapists, we care about receiving feedback and we typically solicit it from individuals we treat. We may use feedback from individuals or groups to improve the therapeutic relationship or to change our practices, but our results have not historically affected how much we are paid. When considering the patient experience segment of the Triple Aim, we also are concerned about how easy it is to make appointments, how long is the wait for an appointment, how patients are treated in our facilities, and whether or not patients will recommend us to their friends. Using performance improvement methodology, we need to identify what to capture, and how we can get the information. To obtain these data, we have to work with teams of people to determine what will give us the information we need and who and how it will be collected.

When we take on measuring population health, we go beyond documenting changes in symptoms of a mental health diagnosis. Depending on the focus of a particular project, we may need to capture changes in A1c levels in diabetes management or the number of suicides in a population of people. These very important figures are not things we typically have thought about when applying CBT. An assumption is that CBT therapists want everyone to have access to their therapy. Nevertheless, we rarely have been involved in efforts to reduce the costs of healthcare by designing systems for the purpose of providing easy access to everyone.

Working in an integrated setting requires multidisciplinary collaboration. When striving toward the Triple Aim and using PDSA methodology, teams of people that include medical staff, administrators, support staff, financial managers, and information system experts collaborate to determine the who, what, when, where, how, and why of every aspect of an integration initiative. Participating in such teams may be of little interest to some CBT therapists. Lack of interest in the work and learning whether or not you will be compensated for participating in teams may be huge barriers for some therapists, and they may affect the degree to which CBT will be integrated into pediatric medical settings.

Conclusion

In this chapter, we covered many of the business and financial aspects of working in a pediatric medical setting. There are advantages and disadvantages, trade-offs, and pay-offs for working in different settings. One thing that is clear is that moving CBT into medical settings requires the average clinician to expand their thinking about traditional CBT frameworks. Implicit to working within medical settings is the need to attend to larger issues than the treatment of individuals. Systemic matters regarding the patient experience, the health of populations, and reducing costs for patients are an integral part of the integration process.

Besides patient experiences and quality of care, financial considerations will always be in the backdrop because it is a measure of value that affects the practice of CBT therapists. There is no one right financial model but CBT therapists will be well advised to know various possible financial arrangements before entering negotiations with medical organizations about integration.

References

Beidas, R., Stewart, R. E., Walsh, L., Lucas, S., Downey, M. M., Jackson, K., et al. (2015). Free, brief, and validated: Standardized instruments for low resource mental health settings. *Cognitive and Behavioral Practice, 22*(1), 5–19. https://doi.org/10.1016/jcbpra.2014.02.002.

Berwick, D., Nolan, T., & Whittington, J. (2008). The Triple Aim: Care, health, and cost. *Health Affairs, 27*(3), 759–769. https://doi.org/10.1377/hlthaff.27.3.759. Health reform Revisited.

Blount, A., Schoenbaum, M., Kathol, R., Rollman, B. L., Thomas, M., O'Donohue, W., et al. (2007). The economics of behavioral health services in medical settings: A summary of the evidence. *Professional Psychology: Research and Practice, 38*(3), 290–297. https://doi.org/10.1037/0735-7028.38.3.290.

Catlin, A. C., & Cowan, C. (2015). *History of health spending in the United States, 1960-2013*. Retrieved from https://www.cms.gov/Research-Statistics-Data-and-Systems/Statistics-Trends-and-Reports/NationalHealthExpendData/Downloads/HistoricalNHEPaper.pdf

Chiles, J. A., Lambert, M. A., & Hatch, A. (2006). The impact of psychological interventions on medical cost offset: A meta-analytic review. *Clinical Psychology: Science and Practice, 6*(2), 204–220. https://doi.org/10.1093/clipsy.6.2.204.

Claxton, G., Levitt, L., Rae, M., & Sawyer, B. (2018). *Briefs*. Health Spending, Peterson-Kaiser Health System Tracker. Retrieved from https://www.healthsystemtracker.org/brief/increases-in-cost-sharing-payments-have-far-outpaced-wage-growth

Cubanski, J., & Neuman, T. (2018). *The facts on Medicare spending and financing. Issue Brief.* Henry J. Kaiser Family Foundation. Retrieved from https://www.kff.org/medicare/issue-brief/the-facts-on-medicare-spending-and-financing/

Deming, W. E. (1993). *The new economics: For industry, government, education.* Cambridge: MIT Press.

Humer, C., & Henry, D. (2018). *Amazon, Berkshire, JP Morgan partner to cut U.S. Health care costs.* Retrieved from https://www.reuters.com/article/us-amazon-healthcare/amazon-berkshire-jpmorgan-partner-to-cut-healthcare-costs-idUSKBN1FJ1NF

National Committee on Quality Assurance. (2018). Retrieved from http://www.ncqa.org/programs/recognition/practices/patient-centered-medical-home-pcmh/distinctions/behavioral-health-integration

Patient Protection and Affordable Care Act, 42 U.S.C. § 18001. (2010).

The Joint Commission. (2018). Retrieved from https://www.jointcommission.org/standards_information/bhc_requirements.aspx

Wilensky, G. (2016). *Medicare and Medicaid are unsustainable without quick action. The Opinion Pages. The New York Times.* New York. Retrieved from https://www.nytimes.com/roomfordebate/2015/07/30/the-next-50-years-for-medicare-and medicaid/medicare-and-medicaid-are-unsustainable-without-quick-action

28. Conclusion: What Have We Learned and Where Do We Go from Here?

Jennifer K. Paternostro and Robert D. Friedberg

A goal is not always meant to be reached, it often serves as something to aim at.
Bruce Lee

When we set out to edit this handbook, our goals were to alert readers to the current state of the science supporting CBT interventions with young patients diagnosed with common medical conditions and offer portable recommendations for clinical practice. We sought to collaborate with clinician-scientists who are at the top of their game and invite readers into their offices or consulting rooms to get a sense of the way they meet the challenges of providing accountable, affordable, and accessible integrated pediatric behavioral health care. So, now we reflect on our aim. What have we learned and where to go from here? In the following pages, we consider common themes shared by the individual chapters and challenges that lie ahead for CBT with children diagnosed with medical conditions.

J. K. Paternostro (✉)
Division of Developmental and Behavioral Pediatrics, Stead Family Department of Pediatrics, University of Iowa Stead Family Children's Hospital,
Iowa City, IA, USA
e-mail: jennifer-paternostro@uiowa.edu

R. D. Friedberg
Child Emphasis Area, Palo Alto University, Palo Alto, CA, USA

Common Themes

The physically and emotionally demanding nature of chronic medical conditions understandably places pediatric patients at higher risk for a number of mental health conditions. Extensive medical interventions, prolonged hospitalizations, changes in daily routines, and complex self-management requirements faced by patients with medical conditions are undoubtedly difficult when coupled with emotional distress. Delivering CBT to pediatric patients diagnosed with medical condition demands a broad lens. Integrated pediatric behavioral health care comes in a variety of flavors, including coordinated, collaborative, co-located, and fully integrated options. The diversity of care models allows for health systems to explore which model best fits the needs, values, and resources of particular clinics.

Parrish and Van Eck (Chap. 12, this volume) argued for the importance of early identification of psychological conditions and intervention in pediatric primary care settings. Psychologists located in primary care settings may help reduce stigma, optimize parent buy-in, and triage patients for more intensive intervention. By integrating pediatric psychologists into primary care offices, barriers that once prevented families from receiving psychological services are alleviated. Furthermore, CBT approaches are uniquely qualified for brief and short-term intervention. The use of objective behavioral targets, differential attention, incentives and reward structures, as well as ample psychoeducation regarding the child's condition can make an enormous difference in the lives of these families who present with mild behavioral concerns or general parenting issues.

Reliance on the Biopsychosocial Model

Chapter authors in this handbook repeatedly referred to the biopsychosocial model (Engel 1977) in their work. Indeed, the biopsychosocial model represents a paradigm shift that opened the door to integrated pediatric behavioral health care (Williams and Zahta 2017). The biopsychosocial model is inherently systemic and proposes a causally interactive model between organismic, interpersonal, psychological, and environmental factors (Alvarez et al. 2012; Melchert 2013). Accordingly, it is completely congenial with the cognitive behavioral model. Moreover, the biopsychosocial model is commonly seen as facilitating personalized and compassionate patient care by clinicians and academics alike.

Our Patients Are Diverse and Their Complaints Are Complicated

The demographic landscape is rapidly shifting in the United States and requires serious self-reflection among health-care industry professionals. Clinicians must be ready to competently care for young patients who present with diverse identities. Valenzuela, Tatum, and Lui (Chap. 3, this volume) highlighted the knowledge and skills necessary for the workforce to properly respond to various population needs. Further, Tabuenca and Basile (Chap. 25, this volume) alerted readers to various principles, processes, and practices useful in treating transgender and gender expansive youth. They explicated the many challenges transgender and gender expansive youth encounter when seeking appropriate care. Gender affirmative models of intervention have proved promising in decreasing mental health symptoms within this population. CBT models for this population are farthest along, but the existing literature base is insufficient in identifying well-established interventions.

Marginalized populations traditionally suffer from various health disparities (Arora et al. 2017; Valuenza et al. Chap. 3, this volume). Delivering accountable, affordable, and accessible pediatric behavioral health care to these vulnerable patients is a historical challenge. Valenzuela and her colleagues argue that the discrepancy in health outcomes shows no signs of self-correction and requires focused remedies. Thus, we agree the time for practice and policy changes has come. Integrated pediatric behavioral health-care services offer promise for ameliorating access, improving outcomes, decreasing stigma, and reducing costs (Reiter et al. 2018).

Further, in addition to contextual vicissitudes, pediatric patients present with varied concerns ranging from transient conditions to life-threatening illnesses. Levels of acuity and chronicity differ. Nonetheless, there are shared features. Anxiety and depression frequently walk around with most medical conditions described in this handbook. Emotional dysregulation is a transdiagnostic pathway (Essau et al. 2017) and the common target for the multitudinous CBT procedures in this book. Accordingly, Parrish, Fajer, and Papadakis (Chap. 5, this volume) discuss emotional regulation and the relevance to pediatric behavioral health care. Pain is another transdiagnostic complaint, and clinicians must respond appropriately to its dynamic nature (Chaps. 13, 14, 17, and 20, this volume). Further, disrupted sleep is a common characteristic of a myriad of physical and mental health disorders in children and adolescents. Sleep difficulties can occur independently, in direct link with, or are exacerbated by multiple disorders. Fehr, Chambers, and Ramasami (Chap. 18, this volume) assert that CBT clinicians are in an ideal position to intervene and break the negative cycle of disrupted sleep. Cognitive and behavioral interventions are widely recognized as effective in reducing sleep problems in youth.

Therefore, a unifying theory such as the biopsychological model and a comprehensive as well as flexible therapeutic approach like CBT spectrum procedures are helpful.

Change Is Hard

Changing young patients' thoughts, feelings, and behaviors is often an incredibly daunting task. Patient and family buy-in is especially important in integrated pediatric behavioral health-care settings. Moreover, this is particularly relevant since as CBT clinicians, we are in the *change business!* Motivational interviewing (MI), as described by Jeter, Gillaspy, and Leffingwell (Chap. 6), is well-suited to tackle these challenges and fits nicely within the CBT spectrum approaches. Sparking treatment engagement and igniting motivation is pivotal for patients diagnosed with co-occurring medical conditions and emotional distress. MI delicately balances both acceptance and change in order to resolve ambivalence. Therapeutic momentum is optimized by competent application of MI.

Medical noncompliance and nonadherence is more often the rule than the exception in integrated settings. Behavioral health consultants are frequently called upon to "fix" this problem and "get the patient on track" to return to health. In fact, in many settings, behavioral health consultants' ability to minimize patients' nonadherence is a measure of their worth to the team. In Chap. 25, Lemanek and Yardley provided readers with guidelines on reducing nonadherence. Collaboratively crafting individually tailored treatment plan attenuates nonadherence. Competently applying motivational interviewing and facilitating treatment adherence are essential skills for CBT-oriented clinicians working in integrated pediatric behavioral health settings.

Right Sizing the Interventions Is Essential

Koocher and Hoffman (Chap. 4, this volume) emphasize the importance of clinical accountability, professional competence, and striving to do the best we can for patients. CBT dominates the pediatric literature as a well-established psychosocial intervention for the treatment for pediatric patients with acute and chronic medical conditions. As is expected in a text entitled, *Handbook of CBT Approaches for Pediatric Medical Conditions*, CBT is repeatedly referred to as the treatment of choice. Throughout this handbook, the foundational elements of CBT are adapted to reflect the unique challenges that face pediatric patients, while fundamental CBT and DBT principles and practices are explicated (Chaps. 7 and 9, this volume), and necessary adaptations to the needs of patients diagnosed with various medical conditions are recommended (Chaps. 8 and 10, this volume).

"Flexibility within fidelity" is an axiom coined by CBT pioneer Philip Kendall and his colleagues (Kendall and Beidas 2007; Kendall et al. 2008). Simply, clinical practices that adhere to the principle of flexibility within fidelity make evidence-based CBT relevant to each individual patient. Interventions are rooted in operant, classical, social learning, and information processing paradigms as well as grounded in traditional procedural rudiments. Nevertheless, flexible techniques are responsive to contextual nuances. Variations in social emotional functioning, developmental capacities, family dynamics, real-life stressors, and cultural vicissitudes are addressed in chapters discussing musculoskeletal pain (Fussner and Lynch-Jordan), functional abdominal pain (Baber and Rodriguez), enuresis (Christophersen and Kapalu), encopresis (Kapalu and Christophersen), headache (Kaczynski), sleep difficulties (Fehr, Chambers, and Rasmaami), epilepsy (Fehr, Doss, Hughes-Scalise and Littles), cancer (Salley and Catarozoli), diabetes (Carpenter and Cammarata), asthma (Clawson, Ruppe, Nwanko, and Blair), and obesity (Bejarno, Marker, and Cushing). Work with family members is fully integrated with individually focused procedures. Indeed, a common theme throughout each chapter dealing with distinct diagnoses is to practice flexibly while faithfully sticking to CBT tenets.

Modular CBT represents a transdiagnostic approach to multiple conditions and circumstances.

As previously mentioned (Chap. 7, this volume), mCBT clusters proven procedures into conceptual categories rather than offering a particular protocol for singular diagnostic conditions (Chorpita and Daleiden 2009; Chorpita et al. 2015). This approach may potentially solve the multiple manual problem that exists within child psychotherapy (Weisz 2004). Further, mCBT is increasingly employed in integrated pediatric behavioral health-care settings (Wissow et al. 2008).

Weisberg (2018) cogently argued that most evidence-based practice used in traditional behavioral health settings requires 8–44 sessions lasting the traditional 50 min. However, in integrated pediatric behavioral health settings, sessions are typically 20–30 min long and the course of treatment spans 1–6 sessions. Strosdahl and Robinson (2018) reminded readers that many therapeutic benefits occur early in the treatment process, and shorter treatment regimens attenuate drop-out rates as well as increasing engagement. A modular approach may facilitate this necessary "right-sizing."

Moving on Down the Road: Challenges Ahead

In the rock classic *Thunder Road*, Bruce Springsteen (1975) wrote, "the door is open, but the ride ain't free." In order to fulfill the promise of delivering CBT to pediatric patients with co-occurring medical conditions, practitioners will have to figuratively pay a toll in order to get their ticket punched for traveling the new road. Graduate and postgraduate training institutions will need to make a paradigm shift in order to outfit students with proper skills. Nonspecialist baccalaureate workers must be prepared to deliver low-intensity interventions. Interdisciplinary partnerships and collaborations are imperatives. Constructing new therapeutic models to meet evolving demands and clinical research evaluating these intervention packages are indispensable. Finally, understanding the business side of the profession is vital in creating a sustainable integrated practice.

Clinical Model Development

Integrated pediatric behavioral health care in general and CBT for pediatric medical conditions is a particularly new frontier. We need more clinical models. Ideally, the chapters in this handbook serve a launching pad for clinical model development. Embedding interventions in a stepped care context is likely a future requirement (Friedberg 2017; Strosdahl and Robinson 2018). Stepped care is very congenial with the population healthcare model, which is common in IPBHC settings. Greater access to more services is a potential benefit from stepped care paradigms. Further, lower intensity interventions (relaxation/meditation groups, parental education groups, web-based and other technologically assisted programs, etc.) create the opportunities for bachelor's degree level educated para-professionals to care for patients. In this way, the nonspecialist workforce can flex up to meet increased demand (Becker-Haimes and Beidas 2018).

Delivering CBT to pediatric patients with medical complexities requires expanding one's idea of the traditional CBT framework. Fortunately, the CBT model is robust and flexible, so application to pediatric settings is relatively natural. However, more specific model building is necessary. Creating interventions that could fit within 20-min sessions and competently delivered by multiple providers from different disciplines would be welcome additions to the field.

Research

Strosdahl and Robinson (2018) emphasized, "Clinical psychology must address the theoretical and methodological challenges associated with designing, testing, and disseminating empirical supported interventions that are a good fit for integrated settings generally and health-care settings specifically (p. 1)." CBT with pediatric patients diagnosed with comorbid psychological distress undeniably requires ongoing empirical tests revealing clinical outcomes. Randomized clinical trials, meta-analyses, dismantling studies evaluating potential mediators and moderators as well as controlled case studies are important. However, as Rozbruch et al. (2017) contended, effect sizes are never enough. Various cost-studies including cost-effectiveness, cost-benefit, cost-utility, and cost-offset projects are also key.

Workforce Development

As Landoll, Elmore, Weiss, and Garza noted (Chap. 26, this volume), there are limited guidelines for training students in integrated behavioral health care. Graduate programs, internships settings, and postdoctoral training sites will need to do some heavy lifting to properly shape the workforce. However, changes must occur. Serrano et al. (2018) noted that less than half of doctoral programs and internship sites provide training in integrated care practices. Fortunately, efforts to develop large-scale, well-established training programs are on the rise.

Becker-Haimes and Beidas (2018) recommended "Graduate education (both didactic and experiential components) must not only teach trainees foundational competencies in current EBP models, but also equip clinicians with the knowledge and skills to interpret, integrate, adapt, and assess the effect of the evolving research base within their own clinical practices over time (p. 3)." The new workforce will need to make several transitions. Clinician caseloads and productivity metrics will likely shift from 5–7 patients daily to 10–14 patients (Reiter et al. 2018). Consequently, practitioners and patients will work in 15- to 20-min sessions (Asarnow et al. 2015). Moreover, Koocher and Hoffman (Chap. 4, this volume) declared that in order to successfully participate in integrated care models, clinicians should feel comfortable with basic understanding of medical conditions and their associated treatments.

Becker et al. (2014) noted that only 7% of individuals who own an undergraduate degree in psychology are employed in a behavioral health setting. This largely untapped pool of bachelor degree prepared individuals could be leveraged to scale-up low-intensity CBT interventions and meet increased patient demand (Becker et al. 2014; Brown et al. 2015). Indeed, Kazdin and Blasé (2011) referred to this as a process of task-shifting.

Behavioral health clinicians working in integrated pediatric settings will need to increase their fluency with health-care financing, pay-for-performance models, capitation, risk-cost sharing plans, return on investment principles, and documenting value-added benefits. They are well-advised to familiarize themselves with entrepreneurial skills (O'Donohue et al. 2015). Kirch and Ast (2017) urged leaders in integrated behavioral health settings to harvest potential in their staff and encourage debate during staff meetings. Leadership skills are added essentials for the emerging workforce (Friedberg et al. 2018a, b).

Better Partnerships

Pediatric psychologists must learn to effectively communicate with a wide variety of medical providers in order to provide collaborative care. Multiple chapters in this handbook urged behavioral health clinicians to build and sustain better partnerships with other health-care professionals. Jummani and Shatkin (Chap. 11, this volume) provided clinicians with a go-to resource of common pharmacological interventions for those presenting with moderate-to-severe psychopathology. Their chapter should be used as a resource for clinicians when treating pediatric patients and collaborating with medical providers.

Payment: We Need Dollars and Sense

Clinical economics is rooted in the fundamental notion that quality and financial cost of health care are not independent (Eisenberg 1989). It is well-recognized that the US health-care system is one of the world's most expensive, yet not one of the most accountable (Asarnow et al. 2015). Historically, financial and management concerns are left unaddressed in clinicians' professional development and these issues are often outsourced to other disciplines. Ultimately, this practice may be disempowering. We believe behavioral health practitioners need a seat at the management table and like Lin Manuel Miranda (2015) wrote, they need to be in the room where it happens.

Fortunately, financial and management concerns are gaining an increased amount of attention (Friedberg 2015a, b; Miller et al. 2017; Rozensky 2011, 2014). In Chap. 27 (this volume), Miller delved into the business and financial aspects of working in a pediatric medical setting. Ensuring adequate reimbursement of behavioral health services as well as demonstrating the value psychology brings to integrated care models is critical for sustainable practice. Further, a special issue of *Clinical Practice in Pediatric Psychology* explicitly focused on building an economic base for pediatric psychology services (McGrady 2018). The articles focus on various salient factors, including cost-savings, reimbursement challenges, productivity metrics, service sustainability, and demonstrating value.

Concluding Remarks

Thaler and Sunstein (2008) warned, "never underestimate the power of inertia (p. 8)." We began this handbook with a quote by Da Vinci espousing the virtue of action and thought. It is entirely appropriate to close it with a similar sentiment by contemporary thinkers such as Thaler and Sunstein. The numbers of children requiring behavioral health care will always exceed the supply of clinicians who are properly trained and equipped to help them. Nonetheless, behavioral health-care providers must take action to deliver accountable, affordable, and accessible care in an ethical fashion. The rise of integrated pediatric behavioral health-care services is encouraging. However, we must hurry to train the emerging workforce in best practices before this window of opportunity narrows. The status quo is not an option.

Inertia is a powerful force and behavioral health-care professionals must work diligently to combat its influence. The health-care environment is dynamic and fast-moving. We hope the material in the book catalyzes readers' energies toward better practice, training, theory building, and empirical investigations.

References

Alvarez, A. S., Pagani, M., & Meucci, P. (2012). The clinical application of the biopsychosocial model in mental health: A research critique. *American Journal of Physical Medicine and Rehabilitation, 91*(Suppl. 1), S173–S180.

Arora, P. G., Godoy, L., & Hodgkinson, S. (2017). Serving the underserved: Cultural considerations in behavioral health integration in pediatric primary care. *Professional Psychology: Research and Practice, 48*, 139–148.

Asarnow, J. R., Hoagwood, K. E., Stancin, T., Lochman, J. E., Hughes, J. L., Miranda, J. M., et al. (2015). Psychological science and innovative strategies for informing health care redesign: A policy brief. *Journal of Clinical Child and Adolescent Psychology, 44*, 923–933.

Becker, K. D., Chorpita, B. F., & Daleiden, E. L. (2014). Coordinating people and knowledge: Efficiency in the context of the Patient Protection and Affordable Care Act. *Clinical Psychology: Science and Practice, 21*, 106–112.

Becker-Haimes, E. M., & Beidas, R. S. (2018). Playing dissemination and implementation limbo – How long can we go? A commentary on Strosahl and Robinson. *Clinical Psychology: Science and Practice, 25*(3), e12255.

Brown, T. E., Redding, M. E. J., & Chorpita, B. F. (2015). The uncertain steps on the certain path to progress: Some guesses about the future of cognitive and behavioral therapies. *The Behavior Therapist, 38*, 144–150.

Chorpita, B. F., & Daleiden, E. L. (2009). Mapping evidence-based treatments for children and adolescents: Applications of the distillation and matching model to 615 treatment from 322 randomized trials. *Journal of Consulting and Clinical Psychology, 77*, 566–577.

Chorpita, B. F., Park, A., Tsai, K., Korathu-Larson, P., Higa-McMillan, C. K., Nakamura, B. J., et al. (2015). Balancing effectiveness with responsiveness: Therapist satisfaction across different treatment designs in the Child STEPS randomized effectiveness trials. *Journal of Consulting and Clinical Psychology, 83*, 709–718.

Eisenberg, J. M. (1989). Clinical economics: A guide to the economic analysis of clinical practices. *The Journal of the American Medical Association, 262*(20), 2879–2886.

Engel, G. (1977). The need for a new medical model: A challenge for biomedicine. *Science, 196*, 129–136.

Essau, C., Leblanc, S., & Ollendick, T. H. (Eds.). (2017). *Emotional regulation and psychopathology in children and adolescents*. Oxford: Oxford University Press.

Friedberg, R. D. (2015a). Are professional psychology training programs willing the future to economic illiterates?: A clarion call for pedagogical action. *Journal of Mental Health, 25*, 395–402.

Friedberg, R. D. (2015b). When treatment as usual gives you lemons, count on evidence based practices. *Child and Family Behavior Therapy, 37*, 335–348.

Friedberg, R. D. (2017). Care for a change: Tiered CBT for youth. *Journal of Rational-Emotive & Cognitive-Behavioral Therapy, 35*, 296–313.

Friedberg, R. D., Bearman, S. K., Miller, A., Mason, E., & Walkup, J. (2018a). 21st century skills for cognitive-behavioral clinicians interested in leading behavioral health care staffs: The importance of TEAM. *The Behavior Therapist, 41*, 294–297.

Friedberg, R. D., Nakamura, B. J., Winkelspect, C., Tebben, E., Miller, A., & Beidas, R. S. (2018b). Disruptive innovations to facilitate better dissemination and delivery of evidence-based practices: Leaping over the tar pit. *Evidence-Based Practice in Child and Adolescent Mental Health, 3*, 57–69.

Kazdin, A. E., & Blasé, S. L. (2011). Rebooting psychotherapy research and practice to reduce the burden of mental illness. *Perspectives on Psychological Science, 6*, 21–37.

Kendall, P. C., & Beidas, R. S. (2007). Smoothing the trail for dissemination of evidence-based practices for youth: Flexibility within fidelity. *Professional Psychology: Research and Practice, 38*, 13–20.

Kendall, P. C., Gosch, E., Furr, J., & Sood, E. (2008). Flexibility within fidelity. *Journal of the American Academy of Child and Adolescent Psychiatry, 47*, 987–993.

Kirch, D. G., & Ast, C. E. (2017). Health care transformation: The role of academic health centers and their psychologists. *Journal of Clinical Psychology in Medical Settings, 24*, 86–91.

McGrady, M. E. (2018). Introduction to the CPPP special issue: Building the economic evidence based for pediatric psychology services. *Clinical Practice in Pediatric Psychology, 6*, 101–106.

Melchert, T. P. (2013). Beyond theoretical orientations: The emergence of a unified scientific framework in professional psychology. *Professional Psychology: Research and Practice, 44*, 11–19.

Miller, B. F., Ross, K. M., Davis, M. M., Melek, S. P., Kathol, R., & Gordon, P. (2017). Payment reform in the patient-centered medical home: Enabling and sustaining integrated behavioral health care. *American Psychologist, 72*, 55–68.

Miranda, L. M. (2015). *The room where it happens*. New York: Broadway Music (ASCAP).

O'Donohue, W., Snipes, C., Howard, C., & Medjuck, J. (2015). The entrepreneurial professor: An oxymoron or a necessary? *The Behavior Therapist, 38*, 14–18.

Reiter, J. T., Dobmeyer, A. C., & Hunter, C. L. (2018). The primary care behavioral health (PCBH) model: An overview and operational definition. *Journal of Clinical Psychology in Medical Settings, 25*, 109–126.

Rozbruch, E. V., Mosley, C., Ghosh, S., & Friedberg, R. D. (2017). Innovative behavioral health services for children: Ready-to-use economic and business knowledge for professional psychology. In A. M. Columbus (Ed.), *Advances in psychology research* (Vol. 122, pp. 139–159). New York: Nova Publishing.

Rozensky, R. H. (2011). The institution of institutional practice of psychology: Healthcare reform and psychology's future workforce. *American Psychologist, 66*, 797–808.

Rozensky, R. H. (2014). Implications of the Affordable Care Act for education and training in professional psychology. *Training and Education in Professional Psychology, 8*, 83–94.

Serrano, N., Cordes, C., Cubic, B., & Daub, S. (2018). The state and future of primary care behavioral health model of service delivery workforce. *Journal of Clinical Psychology in Medical Settings, 25*, 157–168.

Springsteen, B. (1975). *Thunder road*. New York: Columbia Records.

Strosdahl, K. D., & Robinson, P. J. (2018). Adapting empirically supported treatment in the era of integrated care: A roadmap for success. *Clinical Psychology: Science and Practice, 25*(3), e12246.

Thaler, R. H., & Sunstein, C. R. (2008). *Nudge: Improving decisions about health, wealth, and happiness*. New York: Penguin.

Weisberg, R. B. (2018). Empirically supported treatments for this population, by the population: Commentary on Strosahl and Robinson. *Clinical Psychology: Science and Practice, 25*(3), e12256.

Weisz, J. R. (2004). *Psychotherapy for children and adolescents: Evidence-based treatment and examples*. Cambridge: Cambridge University Press.

Williams, S. E., & Zahta, N. E. (2017). *Treating somatic symptoms in children and adolescents*. New York: Guilford.

Wissow, L. S., Anthony, B., Brown, J., DosReis, S., Gadomski, A., Ginsburg, G., et al. (2008). A common factors approach to improving the mental health capacity of Primary Pediatric Care. *Administration and Policy in Mental Health and Mental Health Services Research, 35*, 305–318.

Index

A
Absorptive undergarments, 229
Acceptance, 71
   hopelessness/apathy/lack, 336
Acceptance and Commitment Therapy (ACT), 3, 336
Acculturative and traumatic stress, 29
Acetaminophen and nonsteroidal anti-inflammatory drugs, 268
Active coping, 192
Active distraction, 60
Activity pacing, 193, 194
Acute and chronic medical interventions, 151
Acute lymphocytic leukemia (ALL), 6, 323
Acute pain medications, 268
Adaptation of EBTs
   American Psychological Association, 23
   bottom-up and top-down approaches, 25
   clinical practice, 23, 25
   cultural adaptation, 23, 24
   culturally competent, 24
   culturally tailored, 24
   domains, 25
   frameworks, 25
   justifiable, 24
   local adaptation, 24
   meta-analyses, 24
   racial/ethnic minority, 25
   recommendations, 24
   risk and resilience factors, 25
   top-down/bottom-up approaches, 25
   unique risk and resilience factors, 24
ADDRESSING framework, 26
Adherence, 329–334, 336, 341
   bioassays, 410
   definition, 408
   electronic monitoring, 410
   factors, 408, 409
   HBM, 409
   health status indicators, 411
   measures, 410
   provider, 411
   quality-of-life measures, 411
   refill records, 410
   self-management, 408
   subjective reports, 411
   TPB, 409
   transtheoretical model, 409
Adjunctive nutritional goals, 244
Adolescence/young adulthood, 302, 303
Adolescents, 44
Adverse Childhood Experiences Study (ACES) questionnaire, 422
Affirmations, 72
Affirmative Cognitive Behavioral Therapy (AFFIRM), 394
Affordable Care Act (ACA), 11
African-American community, 27
African-American populations, 2
African-American Youth and Families in USA, 27–29
Alpha-1-antagonists, 153
Alpha-2-agonists, 152, 154
American Academy of Child and Adolescent Psychiatry (AACAP), 16
American Academy of Family Physicians (AAFP), 173
American Academy of Pediatrics (AAP), 173
American College of Physicians (ACP), 173
American Osteopathic Association (AOA), 173
Analgesics, 268
Antecedent-focused processes, 54
Antecedent-focused treatment targets and interventions
   attentional deployment techniques, 60
   parental differential attention, 62
   prevention
      increasing self-efficacy, 58
      meeting basic needs, 57–58
   situation modification
      negative emotional reactions, 59
      not global reassurances, 60
      pain management, 59
      primary control, 59
      problem-focused coping, 59
      provide and ask for choices, 59, 60
      soothing truth telling, 60
   situation selection, 58, 59
Anticipated adversity management, 401, 402
Antidepressant black box warning, 154, 155

Antiepileptic mood stabilizers, 154, 156
Anxiety, 41, 51, 156–158
   in childhood
      asthma-related experiences, 349
      asthma-specific assessments, 353, 354
      asthma-specific content, 362
      biological factors, 350
      case conceptualization, 349
      case formulation, 362
      comprehensive assessments, 362
      psychological factors, 350–352
      psychological functioning assessments, 354–356
      social and environmental factors, 352, 353
      vicious cycle, 350
   and depression, 14, 15, 446
Anxiety-enhancing parent behaviors, 54
Anxiety spectrum, 2, 89, 90
Anxious symptoms, 96
Anytime bathroom pass, 254
Assessment of encopresis
   interdisciplinary evaluation, 241
   medical assessment, 241, 242
   psychological/behavioral, 242
Asthma, 6, 76, 77
   action plans, 347
   affective interventions, 360, 361 (*see also* Anxiety in childhood)
   behavioral interventions, 356, 358, 359
   CBT, 356
   chronic respiratory disease, 345
   cognitive interventions, 359, 360
   control, 346
   exacerbations, 346
   factors associated with childhood, 346
   hispanic and non-hispanic, 345
   long-term controller medications, 347
   lung function measures, 346
   mental health providers, 347
   non-pharmacological interventions, 347
   psychosocial functioning, 348, 349
   quick-relief medications, 347
   severity, 346
   symptoms, 345
   systems interventions, 361, 362
   treatment nonadherence, 347, 348
Asthma Control Questionnaire, 346
Asthma Control Test, 346
Asthma-specific assessments, 353, 354
Attentional deployment techniques
   concentration, 60, 61
   distraction, 60, 61
   mindfulness, 60–62
   rumination, 60
Attention deficit disorder, 267
Attention deficit/hyperactivity disorder (ADHD), 14, 173, 179, 180, 242, 243
Autonomic nervous system (ANS), 202
Autonomy-supportive, 71

B

Basic behavioral tasks, 93, 96
Bedtime routines, 286
Bed-wetting alarm, 222, 228
Behavioral activation (BA), 93
Behavioral assessment, DE, 228
Behavioral Assessment System for Children (BASC), 221, 242
Behavioral family systems therapy for diabetes (BFST-D), 6, 333
Behavioral health
   IPBHC (*see* Integrated pediatric behavioral healthcare (IPBHC))
Behavioral health consultants (BHC), 12, 13
Behavioral Health Integration Program (BHIP), 421
Behavioral health management, 4
Behavioral insomnia of childhood (BIC)
   factors, 281
   limit setting, 282, 283
   sleep-onset associations, 281, 282
Behavioral intervention/modification, 320–322
   NE, 221
   encopresis, 246
      behavioral targets, 246
      causal factors/components, 246
      child's developmental level, 246
      education, 248
      failure of reward systems, 247
      goals, 246
      mild consequences, 247
      operant conditioning procedures, 246
      parent training, 248
      reinforcement, 247
      reluctant/nervous children, 248
      reward system, 247
      self-efficacy, 249
      self-esteem, 249
      soiling, 249
      toileting skills, 247
      toilet sits, 248
      treatment steps, 248
   NE, 221
Behavioral learning processes, 56
Behavioral rehearsal, 322
Behavioral reward systems, 6, 333, 334
Behavioral sleep medicine
   children and adolescents, 279
   circadian rhythms, 279
   cognitive abilities, 279
   nervous system, 279
   preschool-aged children, 279
   school-age children, 279
   sleep difficulties, 280
   synaptic plasticity and brain development, 279
Behavioral therapy, 14
Behavioral treatment, DE, 228
Behavior changes, 69–72, 77, 79–82
Behaviorism, 123, 124
Behavior logs, 91

Index

Bell-and-pad/urine-alarm training, 4, 221–223
Beneficence/non-maleficence, 42, 44
Beta-antagonists (blockers), 153
Biofeedback, 273
Biofeedback-assisted relaxation training, 209, 210
Biopsychosocial assessment, 316, 317
Biopsychosocial conceptualization, IDDM, 332, 333
Biopsychosocial model, 446
    adherence, 330
    blood glucose values, 330
    comorbid mental health conditions, 331
    DD, 331
    EF, 331
    glycemic control, 330
    HbA1c laboratory test, 330
    parenting and family conflict/support, 330, 331
    physiological stress response activation, 330
    puberty, 330
    variables, 330
Biosocial theory
    biological vulnerability, 121
    description, 121
    invalidating environment, 122
    transaction, 122
Bipolar disorder, 174
Blood glucose (BG), 337
Body mass index (BMI), 6
Brain–gut axis, 4, 203
Bristol Stool Scale, 241, 244
Burn injuries, 50
Business arrangements with medical settings, 440

C

Cancer diagnosis, adolescence, 151
Capitation rates, 17
Case management strategies, 128
CBT with youth
    anxious symptoms, 96
    basic behavioral tasks, 96
    clinical trials, 87
    cognitive restructuring, 96, 97
    E/E, 97
    mCBT (*see* Modular CBT (mCBT))
    meta-analyses, 87
    psychoeducation, 96
    target monitoring, 96
    theoretical foundations and empirical status
        anxiety spectrum, 89, 90
        Coping Cat program, 88
        CSH, 87
        depression, 89
        developmental, emotional and behavioral problems, 88
        disruptive behavior disorders, 88, 89
        hot cognitive content, 88
        internalizing and externalizing disorders, 88
        learning theory, 87
        mCBT, 88
        self-efficacy, 87
        training/behavior management models, 87
Central sensitization, 186
Change talk, 70, 71, 73
Chemotherapy, 61
Child Behavior Checklist (CBCL), 221, 242
Child factors, 54
Childhood Asthma Control Test, 346
Childhood cancer, 5
Child psychotherapist, 42
Children, 41–47
Children's games show, 52
Children's Hospital of Philadelphia, 421
Chinese immigrants, 30
Chronic headache disorders
    children and adolescents, 261
    family functioning, 265, 266
    functional disability, 264
    migraines (*see* Migraines)
    minor disruptions, 261
    mood, 264, 265
    NDPH, 263–264
    office complaining, 261
    pediatric (*see* Pediatric chronic headache disorders)
    peer relationships, 266
    post-concussive headache, 262, 264
    prevalence, 262
    psychosocial interventions, 261
    school, 265
    sleep, 265
    sports and other extracurricular activities, 265
    TTH, 262, 263
Chronic health conditions, 50, 51
Chronic idiopathic constipation, 240
Chronic medical conditions, 3
Chronic medical illness (CMI)
    DBT (*see* DBT-CMI)
    definition, 137
    individual feeling, 138
    NCDs, 138
    negatively reinforcing, 139
    negative reinforcement cycle of avoidance, 139
    non-adherence, 138–139
    self-management, 138
    youth living, 138–139
Chronic pain
    widespread musculoskeletal pain (*see* Widespread musculoskeletal pain)
Chronic TTH, 262, 263
Chronotherapy, 287
Circadian rhythm, 279
Client-centered counseling strategies, 69
Client-centered therapy, 46
Clinical model development, 448
Cognitive approach, 109–112
Cognitive-behavioral play intervention (CBPI), 290, 291
Cognitive-behavioral psychotherapies, 22

Cognitive behavioral therapy (CBT)
   case study, 308–310 (*see also* Epilepsy)
   chronic pain, 4
   clinical research, 44
   components, 4
   conceptualization, 332
   definition, 41
   diagnosed with medical conditions, 7
   disruptive behavior disorders, 2
   effectiveness, 44
   encopresis (*see* Encopresis)
   and emotion regulation
      affective experiences, 55
      antecedent (*see* Antecedent-focused treatment targets and interventions)
      antecedent-focused processes, 54
      assessment/functional analysis, 55–56
      child-focused and parent-implemented approaches, 54
      emotional awareness, 56, 57
      emotional understanding, 57
      include parents, 55
      one's emotional responses, 54
      response processes (*see* Response processes)
      target areas/techniques, 55
      third-wave CBT treatments, 54
   enuresis (*see* Enuresis)
   episodes of non-responsiveness, 295, 296
   ethical issues, 41, 42
   exposure-based CBT, 45
   FAPDs, 202
   framework, 3
   functional gastrointestinal symptoms, 202
   implementation, 4
   interventions, 3
   medical nonadherence, 7
   models of integrated care, 176
   musculoskeletal pain (*see* Widespread musculoskeletal pain)
   parent-training program, 43
   pediatric medical conditions, 3
   pediatric medical settings, 41, 42
   PNES (*see* Psychogenic non-epileptic seizures (PNES))
   psychological treatment, headache
      behavioral strategies, 271
      cognitive modification, 270
      comorbid symptoms, 273
      component, 272
      educating parents, 270
      family interactions, 272
      negative beliefs/fears, 270, 271
      psychoeducation, 270
      school accommodations, 273
      school stress, 271, 272
   physician prescribes, 46
   prescriptive referrals/parental preferences, 42
   sleep treatment, 288, 289
   specific knowledge and skills, 42
   with youth (*see* CBT with youth)
   young patients, 1
Cognitive behavioral therapy-based family work, 113, 114
Cognitive-behavioral treatments (CBT), 51
Cognitive change, 63
Cognitive restructuring, 93–97, 210, 318–320, 333, 336
Colorado Housing and Finance Authority (CHFA), 425
Communication skills training, 333
Comorbid behavioral health issues, 22
Comorbidities, 243
Comorbid mental health conditions, 331
Comorbid symptoms, 266
Compliance adherence, 301, 302
Comprehensive Behavior Rating Scales (CBRS), 221
Conceptualization and treatment planning, 27
Conceptualization, IDDM, 331–333
Concussion, 262, 264
Conduct disorder (CD), 173
Confidentiality, 45
Consortium for Science-Based Information on Children, Youth and Families (CSICYF), 425
Constipation, 5
   abnormal anal appearance, 241
   adulthood, 241
   biological causes, 242
   biology, 245
   children with, 240
   chronic idiopathic, 240
   chronicity, 240
   and constipation, 225
   definition, 240
   fecal incontinence, 250
   FGIDs, 240
   functional, 240, 241
   history, 220
   medical management, 243, 245
   medical treatment, 248
   NE, 220, 221
   and overflow incontinence/nonretentive encopresis, 254–255
   and overflow incontinence/retentive encopresis, 251–254
   POOP-C, 242
   prevalence, 241
   refractory, 257
   rule, 239
   and soiling, 244
   in youth, 241
Consultation team, 130
Contagion *vs.* medical causes *vs.* normative reaction, 28
Contemporary adjunctive therapy, 224
Content-specificity hypothesis (CSH), 87
Continuous glucose monitor (CGM), 329, 331
Continuous positive airway pressure (CPAP), 284
Conversion disorder, 305, 307, 308
Coping, 316–318, 320–322
Coping Cat and the C.A.T Project, 64
Coping Cat program, 88
Coping counter-thoughts, 93

Core strategies, 126
Cultural adaptations, 23–25, 33
Cultural domains
   working with
      African-American Youth and Families, 27–29
      immigrant youth and families, 29–30
      LGBTQ youth and families, 30–32
Cultural Formulation Interview (CFI), 26
Culture-bound syndromes, 29
Cyproheptadine, 269
Cystic fibrosis, 140

D
DBT-CMI
   adolescents, 141, 145
   anxiety and stress, 146
   assessment, 142
   automatic response of avoidance, 143
   clinical implications, 145, 146
   description, 142, 143
   end-stage renal disease, 145, 147, 148
   insulin pump, 147
   joint teen and parent sessions, 144
   medical non-adherence, 141
   negative reinforcement cycle, 142
   physicians, 144
   protocol, 142
   research, 144, 145
   self-monitoring, 143
   session, 142, 143
   skills, 144, 147
   T1D, 146, 147
   teen's diary card, 143
   teen's life with medical condition, 144
   transplant team reports, 145
   treatment, 142
DBT techniques for youth with chronic medical illness (DBT-CMI), 3
DDAVP, 224–226, 229
Delayed sleep–wake phase disorder, 283
Delivery model, 435, 436
Demystification, 245
Depression, 41, 89, 158–161
Depression and suicidal behavior, 22
Depressive disorders, 2
Depressive symptoms, 213
Desmopressin, 224
Developing discrepancy, 74
Diabetes Control and Complications Trial (DCCT), 329
Diabetes distress (DD), 6, 15
   avoidance of diabetes tasks, 332
   biopsychosocial model, diabetes management, 331
   cognitive restructuring, 336
   diabetes meaning-making, 336
   MI, 336
Diabetes management, 6
   biopsychosocial model (*see* Biopsychosocial model, diabetes management)
Diabetes meaning-making, 336

Diabetes task completion, 338
   behavioral reward systems, 333, 334
   problem-solving skills training, 334, 335
Dialectical behavior therapy (DBT), 3
   acceptance and change strategies, 119
   balances acceptance strategies, 137
   behaviorism, 123, 124 (*see also* Biosocial theory)
   clinical vignette, 132
   CMI (*see* Chronic medical illness (CMI))
   dialectical worldview, 124
   empirical evidence, 131, 132
   evidence-based treatment, 119, 137
   individual psychotherapy, 125–128
   medical settings, 120
   multi-family skills group format, 120
   multi-problem adolescents, 137
   "multi-problem youth" treatment, 121
   national comorbidity studies, 119
   and non-adherence
      cystic fibrosis, 140
      dialectical dilemmas, 140, 141
      endocrinology appointments, 140, 141
      family members, 140
      family unit, 140
      forcing autonomy *vs.* fostering independence, 140, 141
      middle path consensus, 140
      parental surveillance, 140
      poor judgment/decision-making, 140
      problematic/difficult, 140
      T1D, 140
      therapy-interfering behaviors, 139
      validation of emotional experiences, 139
      zoom out, 140, 142
   outpatient, 137
   school settings, 120
   treatment course, 132–134
   treatment modes and functions, 125
   treatment stages and goals, 124
Dialectical strategies, 127
Diaphragmatic breathing, 208, 269
Diary cards, 125
Diet
   behavioral interventions, 369
   health and weight status improvement, 370
   maladaptive cognitions, 374
   nutrition and, 374, 375
Dietary supplements, 268
Dihydroergotamine (DHE), 268
Disease-specific models, 26
Display rules, 52, 53
Disruptive behavior disorders, 88, 89, 174
Distraction, 60, 61
Distress, 44
Diurnal/daytime enuresis (DE)
   assessment, 229, 230
   behavioral assessment, 228
   behavioral treatment, 228
   case conceptualization, 230
   component, 227

Diurnal/daytime enuresis (DE) (cont.)
  history, 229
  incidence, 227
  medical assessment, 227, 228
  medical treatment, 228
  outcome, 230, 231
  secondary psychological problems, 227
  survey, 227
  treatment, 230
Diversity issues in PBHC
  EBTs (see Evidence-based treatments (EBTs))
  evidence-based assessment, 25–27
  minority status, 21, 22
  quality care, 32–33
"Doing" behaviors, 106
The Drinker's Check-up, 69
Dry-bed training, 223, 224
Dyadic regulation, 53

E
Eczema, 178, 179
Education/cognitive intervention
  encopresis, 244–246
Electronic medical records (EMRs), 45
Electronic record, 47
EMG biofeedback, 273
Emotional awareness, 56, 57
Emotional dysregulation, 57, 58, 61, 62, 446
Emotional regulation
  acute and chronic conditions, 49
  acute health problems, 49, 50
  and CBT (see Cognitive-behavioral therapy (CBT))
  children
    and adolescents, 64
    and families, 49
  chronic health conditions, 50, 51
  Coping Cat and the C.A.T Project, 64
  development, 52–53
  and health conditions, 51–52
  HNC program, 64
  and parents, 53–54
Emotional understanding, 57
Emotional vocabulary, 56
Emotion coaching anger, 63
Emotion management method, 52
Emotion regulation, 2
Emotion socialization, 53, 54
Encopresis, 4, 5
  assessment (see Assessment of encopresis)
  behavioral difficulties, 240
  behavioral treatment, 250
  biobehavioral/biopsychobehavioral condition, 239
  biopsychosocial treatment, 243
  case example, 255, 256
  cognitive behavioral treatment, 243
  comorbidities, 243
  constipation (see Constipation)
  diagnosis, 239
  etiology, 240

ETT, 250, 251
  maintenance of treatment gains, 251
  medical intervention, 250
  medical treatment
    adjunctive nutritional goals, 244
    bowel cleanout, 243
    bowel management program, 244
    bowel tracking log, 244, 245
    goals, 243
    maintenance medications, 243, 244
    rectal therapies, 244
  meta-analysis, 250
  overflow incontinence
    and with constipation, 251–254
    and without constipation, 254–255
  prevalence, 240
  psychological/psychosocial interventions
    behavioral (see Behavioral intervention/modification)
    education/cognitive intervention, 244–246
    goals, 244
  soiling (see Soiling)
  systematic reviews, 250
  training and supervision, 257
  treatment complicating factors, 256, 257
Endometriosis, 43
End-stage renal disease, 50, 51, 145, 147, 148
Enhanced toilet training (ETT), 250, 251
Enuresis, 4
  DE (see Diurnal/daytime enuresis (DE))
  desmopressin, 231
  inexpensive treatment, 231
  NE (see Nocturnal/nighttime enuresis (NE))
  primary, 219
  secondary, 219
  supervision, 231
  training, 231
  treatment, 231
Epilepsy, 5
  adherence, 297, 298
  adjustment, 296, 297
  adolescence/young adulthood, 302, 303
  biopsychosocial needs, population, 296
  cognitive deficits, 299
  comorbid mood and behavioral difficulties, 303
  compliance adherence, 301, 302
  defined, 296
  diagnosis, 296
  family environment, 302
  HRQOL, 296
  idiopathic, 296
  medical and psychological comorbidities, 296
  medication side effects, 301
  neuropsychological evaluation, 299
  psychosocial comorbidity, 298, 299
  sleep difficulties and daytime sleepiness, 299
  social functioning, 299
  specific variables, 300
  stress and seizures, 300
  syndromes, 296

targets of treatment, 300
treatment scenarios, 303, 304
YWE, 296
Errors, 333
Ethics
  autonomy and challenge, 43, 44
  CBT, 41, 42
  clinical competence and treatment quality, 42–43
  confidentiality, 45
  Mélange of misconduct, 45–47
  non-maleficence hazards, 45
Evidence-based assessment, 25–27
Evidence base of MI
  adherence, 76
  clinical trials, 75
  cost-effective intervention, 76
  meta-analyses, 75
  pediatric health behaviors (see Pediatric health behaviors)
Evidence-based treatments (EBTs)
  adaptation, 23–25
  BFST-D, 333
  cultural adaptations, 2
  DD, 336
  diabetes task completion, 333–335
  fear of hypoglycemia, 338
  graduated exposure, 337, 338
  injection routine chart, 337
  nonpharmacological interventions, 338
  pediatric patients and families, 22–23
Evocative, 71
Executive function (EF), 331
Exposure-based CBT, 45
Exposures and experiments (E/E), 94, 96, 97
Exposure therapies, 63
Exposure-type intervention, 44
Extensive medical interventions, 445
External anal sphincter (EAS), 251
Eye movement desensitization and reprocessing (EMDR), 46

F
Familismo, 30
Family and parent sessions, 128
Family-based intervention, 6
Family-based psychosocial treatments, 43
Family dynamics, 112, 113
Family environment, 302
Family support enhancement, 391, 393
Family systems intervention, 332
Fear of hypoglycemia, 338
Fear of Pain Questionnaire-Child Report, 190
Fecal incontinence, 4, 239–241, 250
Fecal retention, 240
Fecal soiling, 239, 240, 254
Feelings and somatic complaints, 322, 323
Feelings intensity rating system, 56
Fibromyalgia, 187, 188
"Fight or flight" response, 206

Financial issues
  ACA, 434
  behavioral health professionals, 434
  CBT integration, 441–443
  corporate entities, 433
  healthcare industry and frustration, 433
  Medicare costs per capita, 433
  outcome measures, 438, 439
  physical complaints, 434
  stand-alone behavioral problems, 434
  strategic decisions, 439, 440
  TJC 2018, 434
"Flexibility within fidelity", 447
Forcing autonomy vs. fostering independence, 140, 141
Four processes of MI, 74
Freeing Your Child from Anxiety, 96
Frequent episodic TTH, 262, 263
Functional abdominal pain disorders (FAPDs), 201
Functional constipation, 240, 241
Functional disability, 264, 265, 267, 275
Functional Disability Inventory, 190
Functional dyspepsia, 201
Functional gastrointestinal disorders (FGIDs), 4, 240
  behavioral and cognitive behavioral therapies, 202
  categories, 201
  pediatric illness (see Pediatric FAPDs)
  Rome criteria, 201
  symptoms, 201

G
Gastrocolic reflex, 248
Gastroenterology, 253
Gastrointestinal tract, 4
Gate Control Theory of Pain, 186, 191
Gender-affirmative CBT
  ABCD model, 395
  AFFIRM, 394
  clinicians, 394
  covert messages, 395
  initial sessions, 394
  research studies, 393
  support, 395
Gender-affirmative family behavior interventions, 391
Gender-affirmative lens
  child interview, 389, 390
  parent interview, 390
  referral information, 389
Gender affirmative models, 446
Gender dysphoria, 30, 386, 387
Gender expansive youth
  agency and empowerment, 399–401
  anticipated adversity management, 401, 402
  biopsychosocial, 390, 397
  case history, 395, 397
  clinicians, 385
  cognitive behavioral, 390
  diagnostic terminology, 386
  gender-affirmative models, 385
  gender dysphoria, 386, 387

Gender expansive youth (*cont.*)
  gender identity, 385
  intervention, 397, 398
  minority stress, 398, 399 (*see* Minority stress)
  professional associations, 388, 389
  TGE individuals, 385
  treatment, 385
Genetic factors, 186
GI symptom-specific anxiety, 213, 214
Graded engagement, 210, 211
Graded exposure, 211
Graduated exposure, 337, 338
Guided imagery, 60, 209

H
Headache disorders, 5
Health behaviors
  and behavior changes, 72
  pediatric (*see* Pediatric health behaviors)
The Health belief model (HBM), 409
Health disparities, 1, 21–23, 27, 29, 31–33
Health promotion, 69
Health-care, 69
  ethics, 45
  expenditures, 11
  settings, 28
  systems, 26, 27, 29, 45
The Healthy Steps program, 420
Helping the Noncompliant Child (HNC) program, 64
Hemoglobin A1c (HbA1c) laboratory test, 330
Heterosexist language, 31
Hispanic *vs.* non-Hispanic, 27
HIV report depression, 151
Home-based peritoneal dialysis, 51
Homosexuality, 30
Hot cognitions, 93
Hypothalamic-pituitary-adrenal (HPA), 202

I
Idiographic methods, 91, 92
Illness-related and iatrogenic trauma, 151
Immigrant paradox, 29
Immigrant youth and families, 2, 29–30
Immigration, 21
Incredible Years, 64
Individual psychotherapy, 125–128
Inflammatory bowel disease (IBD), 41, 89
Infrequent episodic TTH, 262, 263
Injection routine chart, 337
Insomnia, 283
Insulin-dependent diabetes
  IDDM (*see* Insulin-dependent diabetes mellitus (IDDM))
Insulin-dependent diabetes mellitus (IDDM), 6, 47
  behavioral framework, 341
  chronic illness, 341
  conceptualization, 331–333
  EBT (*see* Evidence-based treatment (EBT))
  management (*see* Diabetes management)
  psychosocial issues, 329
  T2DM, 329
  TIDM, 329
  treatment, 338–341
Integrated care, 2
  ADHD, 173, 174
  bipolar disorder, 174
  CD, 173
  characterization, 12
  definition, 12, 13
  disruptive behavior disorder, 174
  emotional and behavioral problems, 173
  mental health concerns, 174
  mental health services, 174
  models (*see* Models of integrated care)
  mood disorders, 174
  ODD, 173
  PCBH, 12, 13
  pediatric primary care visits, 174
  psychological and primary care services, 174
  psychotic symptoms, 174
  substance use disorders, 174
  suicidal behavior, 173
  value (*see* Value of IPBHC)
Integrated pediatric behavioral health-care (IPBHC), 88, 445, 446
  ACA, 11
  behavioral factors, 12
  biopsychosocial model, 12
  classification, 12
  clinics, 11
  collaborative and coordinated care options, 1
  co-located practices, 12
  coordinated care, 12
  fully integrated services, 12
  leaning initiative, 11
  mental health-care carve-out services, 11
  patient protection, 11
  in pediatric medical settings, 1
  physiological, 12
  primary and specialty (*see* Primary and specialty care)
  primary care, 12
  psychological, 12
  socio-cultural, 12
  value (*see* Value of IPBHC)
Integrative Model of Pediatric Medical Traumatic Stress, 51
Intensive medical therapy (IMT), 251
Internalizing symptoms, 60
Intervention adaptation
  CBT
    model in pediatrics, 104, 105
    protocols, 103
    limitations of, 114, 115
  cognitive approaches, 109–112
  consultation, 104
  "doing" behaviors, 106
  family dynamics, 112, 113

function of, 106, 107
medical settings, 107, 108
mental health clinician, 103
"not doing" behaviors, 106
treatment plans, 104
Invalidating environment, 122
Irritable bowel syndrome, 201

J
Jack's parents, 49

K
The Kazdin Method for Parenting the Defiant Child, 64
Kidney failure, 50
Kidney transplantation, 50, 51
Kleenex, 46

L
Learning theory, 2, 87
LGBTQ youth and families, 30–32
Local adaptation, 24

M
Maltreatment, 27
Manuals, 42
Marginalized populations, 446
Massage therapy, 188
MATCH-ADTC platform, 89
Medical adherence, 144–147
Medical assessment
 DE, 227, 228
 encopresis, 241, 242
 NE, 220
Medical compliance, 408
Medical conditions context, 106
Medical ethics, 41, 42, 44–47
Medical homes, 173
Medical nonadherence, 6, 447
Medical noncompliance, 407, 447
Medical treatment
 burns, 50
 DE, 228
 NE, 224, 225
Medication management, 14
Medication management system (MEMS), 410
Medication overuse headache (MOH), 268
Medications
 acute pain, 268
 migraines, 268
 preventive/prophylactic, 269
 symptoms of headache, 268
Mental and Behavioral Health Capacity Project (MBHCP), 13
Mental health, 70
 professionals, 46
 stigma, 12
 carve-out services, 11
Mental illness, 28
Metered dose inhaler (MDI), 410
MetroHealth system, 422, 423
Microskills, 71
Migraines
 intensity, 273
 neurobiological disorder, 263
 neurotransmitters, 263
 pain intensity, 263
 prescription medications, 263
 prevalence, 262
 prevention, 273
 rescue medications, 268
 and TTH, 263, 264, 268, 274
 viral illness, 262
MI interventions
 intervention dose, 80
 multicomponent treatment, 79
 participant characteristics, 79, 80
 pediatric health behavior change, 79
 session characteristics, 79
 standalone *vs.* complimentary intervention, 80, 81
Mind–body connection, 105
Mindfulness, 61, 62
Minority status in pediatric health, 21, 22
Minority stress
 population of children at risk, 387
 resilience, 387, 388
MiraLAX®, 253
Models of integrated care
 adaptations, 175
 adults, 175, 176
 behavioral health care, 175
 CBT, 175, 176
 community trial of Triple P, 176
 depression and anxiety, 175
 development and evaluation, 175
 individual/group-based parent-focused interventions, 176
 mental health care, 175
 meta-analysis, 175, 176
 parent-focused treatments, 176
 parent-group intervention, 176
 priorities and activities, 175
 psychological disorders, 176
 psychological treatments, 175
 psychologists, 175
 RCT, 176
 research evaluating, 176
 SAMHSA, 175
Modular CBT (mCBT), 447
 basic behavioral tasks, 93
 cognitive restructuring, 93–95
 E/E, 94, 96
 psychoeducation, 90
 target monitoring
  advantages MBC, 90–91
  clinical positioning device, 90

Modular CBT (mCBT) (*cont.*)
  idiographic methods, 91, 92
  symptom scales, 91
Monosymptomatic enuresis, 221
Montefiore Medical Center/Albert Einstein School of Medicine, 421, 422
Mood disorders, 174
Mood disruption, 5
Motivational enhancement therapy (MET), 81
Motivational interviewing (MI), 2, 27, 336, 447
  adaptations, 81, 82
  applications, 81, 82
  behavior changes (*see* Behavior changes)
  conceptualization, 70
  evidence base (*see* Evidence base of MI)
  history, 69, 70
  interventions (*see* MI interventions)
  patients talk, 70, 71
  physical activity, 69
  resistance to change, 70
  skills and strategies (*see* Skills and strategies of MI)
  style and spirit, 71
  training, 82
Multidisciplinary treatment
  activity pacing, 193, 194
  assessment, 189, 190
  caregivers, 190
  CBT, 188, 189
  clinical practice, 188
  cognitive restructuring, 194, 195
  complex condition and benefits, 188
  components, 189
  elements, 189
  healthy lifestyle habits, 195
  pain management, 188
  primary care physician, 188
  psychoeducation (*see* Psychoeducation)
  relapse prevention, 196, 197
  relaxation training, 193
  school coping
    modifications, 196
    psychologists, 196
  specialized medical providers, 188
Multi-family skills group, 129, 130
Multisite joint, 185
Multi-Systemic Therapy (MST), 88
Musculoskeletal injury, 186

N
Narcolepsy, 284, 285
National Institute of Health 2001, 280
Neurotransmitters, 263
New daily persistent headache (NDPH), 263–264, 267
Nocturnal/nighttime enuresis (NE)
  assessment, 226
    constipation role, 220, 221
    medical, 220
    psychological/behavioral, 221
  behavioral interventions, 221
  bell-and-pad/urine-alarm training, 221–223
  case conceptualization, 226
  course and prognosis, 220
  cultural issues, 220
  definition, 219
  dry-bed training, 223, 224
  history, 225, 226
  medical treatments, 224, 225
  outcome, 226, 227
  overlearning, 224
  prevalence, 219, 220
  treatment, 226
Nonadherence
  case study, 412, 413
  cognitive component, 411
  educational strategies, 411
  and medical noncompliance, 407
  prevalence, 408
Noncommunicable diseases (NCDs), 138
Non-Hispanic, 22
Non-inclusive language, 31
Non-maleficence hazards, 45
Non-medical sources, 42
Nonpharmacological interventions, 338
Nonretentive encopresis
  fecal soiling, 254
  medical assessment, 254
  psychological assessment, 255
  psychological/behavioral treatment, 255
  treatment goals, 255
  treatment guidelines, 254
  treatment plan, 255
Nonretentive fecal incontinence, 240
"Not doing" behaviors, 106
Novel Interventions in Children's Healthcare (NICH), 13

O
Obesity
  accelerometers, 373
  anxiety-specific screeners, 373
  behavioral interventions, 369
  behavior change principles, 376–378
  biological factors, 370
  biopsychosocial factors, 370
  BMI percentile, 369
  challenges, 379, 380
  chronic medical condition, 369
  comprehensive family lifestyle interventions, 373
  description, 372
  evidence-based treatments, 370
  high rates of, 369
  HRQOL, 369
  medical comorbidities, 372
  narrow-band screeners, 372
  nutrition and dietary interventions, 374, 375
  parenting strategies, 378
  physical activity and sedentary behavior, 376

psychological factors, 370, 371
psychological interventions, 373
scales and stadiometers, 372
social and environmental factors, 371, 372
social support, 377, 379
stimulus control, 373
Obsessive-compulsive disorder, 41
Obstructive sleep apnea (OSA), 284
Open-ended questions, 72
Operant conditioning, 2
Oppositional defiant disorder (ODD), 173
Orienting and commitment strategies, 126, 127
Orthopedist, 188
Overlearning, 223, 224

P
Pain-focused CBT, 188, 189
Pain gates, 191
Pain management, 59
Paradoxical contraction, 251
Parasomnias, 283
Parental differential attention, 62
Parental Opinions of Pediatric Constipation Questionnaire (POOP-C), 242
Parental socialization of emotion, 53
Parent-Child Interaction Therapy (PCIT), 3, 88
Parent-Child Interaction Training to the primary care setting (PC-PCIT), 89
Parenting strategies, 378
Parent Management Training-Oregon Model (PMTO), 88
Parker's hierarchy, 96, 97
Passive distraction, 60
Patient-Reported Outcomes Measurement Information System (PROMIS), 190
Payment methods, 436, 437
Pediatric behavior health problems
  and emotional regulation (*see* Emotional regulation)
Pediatric behavioral health care (PBHC)
  diversity issues (*see* Diversity issues in PBHC)
Pediatric bipolar disorder, 41
Pediatric burn injuries, 49
Pediatric cancer setting
  description, 317
  parents and family inclusion, 317, 318
  psychoeducation and rapport building, 318
  RCTs, 317
  treatment planning with flexibility, 318
Pediatric chronic headache disorders
  biopsychosocial formulation, 266–267
  CBT (*see* Cognitive behavioral therapy (CBT))
  complementary interventions, 273–274
  lifestyle factors, 273–274
  medications
    acute pain, 268
    migraines, 268
    preventive/prophylactic, 269
    symptoms, 268

  psychological treatment
    biofeedback, 273
    relaxation training, 269, 270
Pediatric chronic medical conditions, 141
Pediatric encopresis, 252
Pediatric epilepsy, *see* Epilepsy
Pediatric FAPDs
  CBT interventions
    biofeedback, 209, 210
    caregiver support and training, 204, 207, 208
    cognitive restructuring, 210
    diaphragmatic breathing, 208
    graded engagement, 210, 211
    graded exposure, 211
    guided imagery, 209
    PMR, 208, 209
    psychiatric comorbidities, 212
    psychoeducation, 204–207
    relaxation training, 208
    sleep problems, 211
  factors
    biological, 203
    environmental/contextual, 203
    psychological, 203
  GI symptoms, 213, 214
  psychological evaluation, 204, 205
Pediatric health
  cultural domains (*see* Cultural domains)
  minority status, 21, 22
  risk and resiliency, 27–32
Pediatric health behaviors
  accident prevention, 76
  AIDS, 76
  asthma, 76, 77
  pediatric obesity, 77, 78
  T1D, 78, 79
Pediatric medical setting
  business and financial considerations, 7
Pediatric medical stress, 49, 51, 54, 64
Pediatric obesity, 6, 77, 78
Pediatric psychology, 1, 2, 7, 296
Pediatric rheumatologist, 188
Pediatric sleep difficulties
  children and adolescents, 279
  complex cognitive abilities, 279
  effects, 280
  healthy sleep habits, 279
  initiating and maintaining, 279
  purpose of sleep, 279
  treatment (*see* Sleep treatment)
  youth sleep case example, 289–291
Pediatric sleep disturbances, 5
Per member per month (PMPM), 17
Phone coaching, 129
Physical activity, 369–373, 376–379
Physical examination, 229
Physical therapy, 188
Physician leveraging, 17
Physiological factors, 186
Physiological stress response activation, 330

Pilot training programs
    Children's Hospital of Philadelphia, 421
    clinicians, pediatric primary care, 421
    MetroHealth system, 422, 423
    Montefiore Medical Center/Albert Einstein School of Medicine, 421, 422
Pleasant activity scheduling (PAS), 93
Poor sleep, 187
Post-concussive headache, 262, 264
Post-traumatic stress disorder (PTSD), 3, 161–163
Preparing People for Change, 70
Preparing People to Change Addictive Behaviors, 69
Preventative care, 17
Preventive/prophylactic medications, 269
Primary care
    ADHD, 179, 180
    assessment and intervention strategies, 177
    and behavioral health, 173
    challenges, 177
    clinicians receive guidance, 177
    computer-based applications, 177
    eczema, 178, 179
    integrated care (*see* Integrated care)
    mobiletype, 177
    patient-centered medical homes, 173
    RCT, 177
    self-monitoring interventions, 177
    SmartCAT, 177
    and specialty care
        ADHD, 14
        adjustment and adherence, 15
        anxiety/depression, 14, 15
        parenting issues and developmental concerns, 13, 14
Primary care behavioral health (PCBH), 12, 13
Primary care physician, 188
Primary NE, 219
Problem-solving models, 93
Problem-solving skills training, 333–335, 338
Procedural distress, 338
Procedural Terminology Codes (CPT), 17
Progressive muscle relaxation (PMR), 193, 208, 209, 269
Prolonged hospitalizations, 445
PROMIS Pediatric Pain Interference, 190
Psychiatric comorbidities, 212
Psychoanalysis, 46
Psychoeducation, 90, 96
    active coping, 192
    body feels pain, 191
    body's stress response, 205–206
    CBT, 191
    Gate Control Theory of Pain, 191
    gut–brain axis, 205
    independent self-management, pain symptoms, 192
    love and support, 192
    pain gates, 191
    pain processing, 206
    pain signal, 191
    pain talk, 192
    and rapport building, 318
    reduce over-reliance, 192
    relaxation response, 191
    resuming normal routines, 193
    throughout treatment, 192
Psychogenic non-epileptic seizures (PNES), 5
    assessment, 305, 306
    biopsychosocial model, 305
    comorbidities, 306
    conversion disorder, 305
    long-term treatment, 307
    prognosis, 307
    psychological, familial, social and financial consequences, 305
    retrospective studies, 305
    somatopsychiatric risk factor profile, 305
    treatment for children, 306, 307
    treatment scenarios, 307, 308
Psychological/behavioral assessment
    encopresis, 242
    NE, 221
Psychological functioning assessments, 354–356
Psychological processes, 28
Psychological screening, 229
Psychologists, 196
Psychopharmacologic interventions
    cognitive behavioral therapy, and medication interventions, 155
    genes, environment and individual vulnerabilities, 155
    practitioners, 156
    psychiatric evaluation, 163, 164
    SSRIs, 156
    treatment, 164, 165
Psychosocial functioning, 348, 349
Psychosocial stressors, 267
Psychosocial treatment, 302
Psychotherapeutic intervention, 42
Psychotherapy, 46
Puberty, 330

Q

Quality care, 32–33
Quality of life, 370, 372, 373, 379, 380
Quantitative measures, 190

R

Race-based mistrust, 27
Racial/ethnic minority, 21–25, 32
RAIN mnemonic, 93, 94
Raising an Emotionally Intelligent Child: The Heart of Parenting, 64
Randomized controlled trial (RCT), 176, 177
Rational analysis, 93
Rational emotive therapy (RET), 46
Reattribution, 94
Reciprocal communication, 127
Rectal therapies, 244
Reflections and reflective listening, 72, 73
Relapse prevention, 196, 197

Index

Relaxation training, 193, 208, 269, 270
Rescue medications, 268
Response modulation, 63
Response processes
    cognitive change, 63
    modulation, 63
    treatment targets, 62
Resuming typical activities, 189
Retention-control training, 223
Retentive encopresis
    bowel tracking log, 253
    care coordination, 251
    gastroenterology, 253
    medical
        and behavioral factors, 252, 253
        and pharmaceutical expertise, 251
    medications, 253
    psychobiological considerations, 252
    treatment plan, 253
Retentive fecal incontinence, 240
Reward systems, 223
Rome criteria, 201
Rumination, 60

S
Salivary alpha amylase (sAA) levels, 319
SAMHSA, 175
Scaled questions/readiness rulers, 73
Scheduled awakenings, 287, 288
School settings, 120
Screen for Child Anxiety and Related Emotional Disturbances (SCARED), 96
Screening, Brief Intervention, and Referral to Treatment (SBIRT), 82
Secondary NE, 219
Second-generation antipsychotics, 153, 155
Seepage, 240
Seizure disorders, 151–152
Selective serotonin reuptake inhibitors (SSRIs), 152, 153
Self-awareness, 52
Self-consciousness emotions, 52
Self-efficacy, 87
Self-management, 138
Self-soothing, 52, 53
Serotonin-norepinephrine reuptake inhibitors (SNRIs), 152, 154
Sexual minorities, 2, 30
Sexual minority youth, 21
Shared risk concept, 437
Siblings, 267
Skill-based techniques, 93
Skilled clinician, 46
Skills and strategies of MI
    affirmations, 72
    change talk, 71, 73
    clinical example, 74–75
    developing discrepancy, 74
    four processes, 74
    microskills, 71
    open-ended questions, 72
    reflections and reflective listening, 72, 73
    rolling with resistance and developing discrepancies, 73
    scaled questions/readiness rulers, 73
    sustain talk, 71
Skills group, 129
Sleep difficulties, 446
Sleep disturbance, 5
Sleep hygiene, 285, 286
Sleep problems, 195, 211
Sleep treatment
    bedtime fading, 287
    bedtime pass, 287
    bedtime routines, 286
    BIC (*see* Behavioral insomnia of childhood (BIC))
    CBT, 288, 289
    chronotherapy, 287
    delayed sleep–wake phase disorder, 283
    estimation, 280
    extinction, 286
    factors, 281
    formal sleep assessment, 281
    image rehearsal therapy, 289
    narcolepsy, 284, 285
    OSA, 284
    parasomnias, 283
    scheduled awakenings, 287, 288
    school or work performance, 280
    sleep difficulties, 285
    sleep hygiene, 285, 286
    symptoms, 281
Sleep-onset associations, 281, 282
Sleepovers and camps, 224
SmartCAT, 177
Social learning theory, 2
Soiling
    children with and without, 249
    and constipation, 244
    demystification, 245
    fecal, 239, 240, 254
    frequency, 240, 251
    involuntary nature, 253
    parental punishment, 244
    reemergence, 251
    self-esteem, 242
    subtypes, 240
Specialty care
    and primary care (*see* Primary and specialty care)
Specific disorders
    anxiety disorders, 156–158
    depression, 158–161
    PTSD, 161–163
Standalone *vs.* complimentary intervention, 80, 81
Stigma-related stress, 31
Strength-based and affirmative approach, 31
Stress and seizures, 300
Stress reactions, 96
Stress-related symptoms, 151
Stress response, 106

Structural family therapy, 333
Style and spirit of MI, 71
Subjective units of distress (SUDS), 96
Substance Abuse and Mental Health Services Administration (SAMHSA), 174
Substance use disorders, 174
Suicidal behavior, 173
Supportive nondirective therapy (SNDT), 89
Sustain talk, 70, 71
Sympathetic statements, 61
Systemic lupus erythematosus (SLE), 152

T
Tampa Scale of Kinesiophobia, 190
Target hierarchy, 125
Target monitoring, 96
Tension-type headaches (TTH), 262–264, 268, 270, 273, 274
Theory of Motivational Interviewing, 70
Theory of planned behavior (TPB), 409
Therapeutic misconception, 44
Throughout treatment, 192
Time-consuming treatments, 51
Training issues
    competencies for practice, 419, 420
    curriculum challenges, 425, 426
    emergence of, 419
    Healthy Steps program, 420
    integration challenges, 427
    internship/postdoctoral levels, 420
    interprofessional education opportunities, 420
    pediatric adaptations, 425
    personnel challenges, 426, 427
    recommendations, 428, 429
    seminars, workshops and conferences, 423, 424
Transgender
    defined, 385
    minority stress and poor access, 387
Transtheoretical model, 70, 409
Trauma-informed diagnostic and treatment strategies, 152
Treating Tobacco Dependence, 81
Treatment for Adolescents with Depression Study (TADS), 89
Treatment nonadherence, 347, 348
Triple Aim concept, 434
Triple P-Positive Parenting Program, 88
Triptans, 268
Tuning in to Kids: Emotionally Intelligent Parenting, 65
Type 1 diabetes (T1DM), 15, 22, 78, 79, 140, 146, 147, 329, 407
Type 2 diabetes (T2DM), 329

U
Unhealthy, 70
Universal Protocol for Children (UP-C), 96
Urinary tract, 42
Urine-alarm, 225

V
Value of IPBHC
    AACAP, 16
    advantages, 15
    agreement, 16
    benefits, 15
    capitation rates, 17
    clinical efficiency, 16
    co-locating pediatric and behavioral health training programs, 16
    continuum of care, 15
    cost-savings, 17
    CPT, 17
    facilitates, 16
    global/capitated payment system, 17
    implement and sustain practices, 17
    meta-analysis, 16
    one-stop shopping, 15
    patient satisfaction and experience, 16
    payment models, 16
    physician leveraging, 17
    preventative care, 17
    workload burden, pediatricians, 16
Verbal reassurances, 60
Verbal reprimanding, 62
Veterans Affairs Health Care System, 175
Viral illness, 262
Visceral hypersensitivity, 205
Visual imagery, 270

W
Widespread musculoskeletal pain
    biopsychosocial model
        biological factors, 186, 187
        biomedical approach, 186
        gate control theory of pain, 186
        health, 186
        multidimensional processes, 186
        psychological factors, 187
        social factors, 187
    chronic and debilitating condition, 185
    multidisciplinary treatment (*see* Multidisciplinary treatment)
    multisite joint, 185
    musculoskeletal injury, 186
    primary localized pain, 185
Wind up, 187
Workforce development, 449
The World Professional Association of Transgender Health (WPATH), 388
Wound debridement, 50

Y
Young children, 282, 288
Youth Risk Behavior Surveillance (YRBS), 21
Youth sleep case example, 289–291
Youth with epilepsy (YWE), 296
Youth with medical conditions, 165